SPH

WO 445
DOD

18-6-15
HEALTH SCIENCES LIBRARY

SPH B23978

D1350791

HEALTH SCIENCES LIB
ST PETERS HOSPITAL
GUILDFORD RD, CHERTSEY
KT16 0PZ
☎01932 723213

Oxford Textbook of

Anaesthesia for the Elderly Patient

Oxford Textbooks in Anaesthesia

Oxford Textbook of Anaesthesia for the Elderly Patient
Edited by Chris Dodds, Chandra M. Kumar, and Bernadette Th. Veering

Oxford Textbook of Anaesthesia for Oral and Maxillofacial Surgery
Edited by Ian Shaw, Chandra M. Kumar, and Chris Dodds

Principles and Practice of Regional Anaesthesia, Fourth Edition
Edited by Graeme McLeod, Colin McCartney, and Tony Wildsmith

Oxford Textbook of
Anaesthesia for the Elderly Patient

Edited by

Chris Dodds

Consultant Anaesthetist
James Cook University Hospital
Middlesbrough, UK

Chandra M. Kumar

Senior Consultant in Anaesthesia
Alexandra Health Services, Khoo Teck Puat Hospital
Yishun Central, Singapore

Bernadette Th. Veering

Associate Professor
Department of Anesthesiology
Leiden University Medical Center
Leiden, The Netherlands

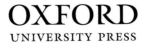

OXFORD
UNIVERSITY PRESS

OXFORD

UNIVERSITY PRESS

Great Clarendon Street, Oxford, OX2 6DP,
United Kingdom

Oxford University Press is a department of the University of Oxford.
It furthers the University's objective of excellence in research, scholarship,
and education by publishing worldwide. Oxford is a registered trade mark of
Oxford University Press in the UK and in certain other countries

© Oxford University Press 2014

The moral rights of the authors have been asserted

First Edition published in 2014

Impression: 1

All rights reserved. No part of this publication may be reproduced, stored in
a retrieval system, or transmitted, in any form or by any means, without the
prior permission in writing of Oxford University Press, or as expressly permitted
by law, by licence or under terms agreed with the appropriate reprographics
rights organization. Enquiries concerning reproduction outside the scope of the
above should be sent to the Rights Department, Oxford University Press, at the
address above

You must not circulate this work in any other form
and you must impose this same condition on any acquirer

Published in the United States of America by Oxford University Press
198 Madison Avenue, New York, NY 10016, United States of America

British Library Cataloguing in Publication Data
Data available

Library of Congress Control Number: 2013948633

ISBN 978–0–19–960499–9

Printed in China by
C&C Offset Printing Co. Ltd

Oxford University press makes no representation, express or implied, that the
drug dosages in this book are correct. Readers must therefore always check
the product information and clinical procedures with the most up-to-date
published product information and data sheets provided by the manufacturers
and the most recent codes of conduct and safety regulations. The authors and
the publishers do not accept responsibility or legal liability for any errors in the
text or for the misuse or misapplication of material in this work. Except where
otherwise stated, drug dosages and recommendations are for the non-pregnant
adult who is not breast-feeding

Links to third party websites are provided by Oxford in good faith and
for information only. Oxford disclaims any responsibility for the materials
contained in any third party website referenced in this work.

We would like to dedicate this book to those who have personally given us so much support over the years:

Chris: to my wife Ann for all her help and support

Chandra: to my wife Suchitra Kumar

Bernadette: to my special friends Caroline and Rozemarijn

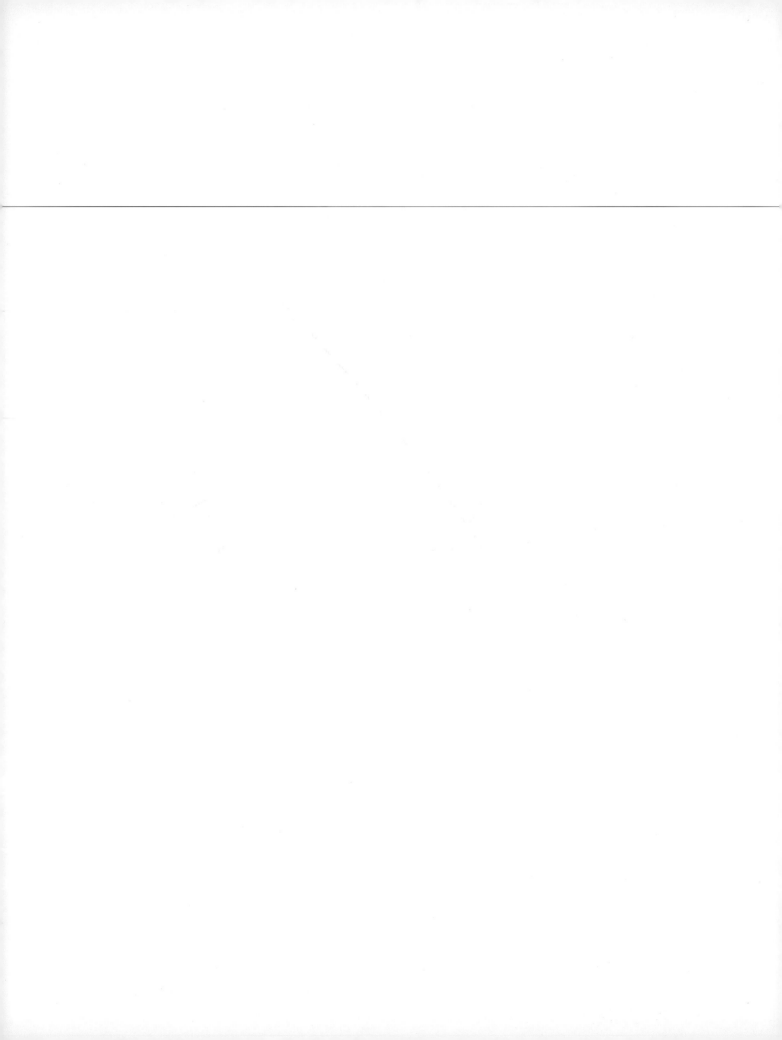

Foreword

It is a pleasure to be invited to write a foreword for this book which is comprehensive, needed, and above all else, timely.

The growth in the elderly population across the world, in both the developed and also in the developing countries, has been unprecedented over the last two decades. National bodies tasked in providing health, welfare, infrastructure, and pensions have all been caught unawares by the shift in population demographics. Nowhere, however, is the impact felt as much as by the health services that have to meet the exponential demand for greater volumes of high quality care. The problems are experienced both financially and as an uncontrollable operational delivery exercise.

At present in the UK there are nearly 15,000 people over the age of 100 years and half a million over the age of 90 years: world wide, the number of people over 65 years will exceed those aged under 5 years in two years' time—the fastest growing age group is those aged 65 and over. The chronological age at which people develop degenerative diseases is increasing and this population, when it requires anaesthesia, is presenting with more and more co-morbidities.

There is no doubt in my mind that the immediate future need of the health services is to meet the challenge of the ever-increasing elderly population with health solutions that provide high-quality care whilst simultaneously meeting the constraints of volume demand and cost-effectiveness. This book provides the way forward in anaesthesia to do just that. It is publishing at just the right time to make a maximal contribution to the problems of the immediate future. I congratulate the editors and authors and wish it every success.

Peter Hutton
Hon Professor of Anaesthesia, University of Birmingham
Consultant Anaesthetist, University of Birmingham NHS
Foundation Trust
Former President, Royal College of Anaesthetists

Preface

The balance of ages across populations throughout the world is changing. There are far more elderly people alive today than ever and they will profoundly alter the way we deliver healthcare. We will have to research, develop, and deliver appropriate anaesthesia, pain management, and intensive care to these increasingly frail and vulnerable patients. We have to recognize the fact that each elderly person is an individual whose needs vary to a far greater extent, one from another, than in other age groups. The prevention of complications and the associated loss of independence are vital in this age group and demand that we provide the highest standard of care.

The evidence base for our practice in the very old is woeful but improving and the contributors to this book have used the latest information in their chapters. There are still many unanswered questions. Our understanding of the specific problems of the elderly, and therefore our practice, must evolve year on year as new information comes to hand. Just as each elderly cohort differs from the previous one because of the variation in exposure to infection, nutritional problems, smoking, poor social services, and access to therapeutic advances, so too must our practice reflect this. It is this challenge that makes caring for an elderly patient so rewarding at an intellectual and practical level.

We hope this book will inform and enthuse those who read it to provide better care for the elderly patient and to increase the evidence base on which we inform our practice.

Contents

PART 5
Other Important Aspects

List of Abbreviations

AAA	abdominal aortic aneurysm
ABA	American Board of Anesthesiology
ABI	ankle–brachial index
ACE	angiotensin-converting enzyme
ACEI	angiotensin-converting enzyme inhibitor
ACGME	Accreditation Council for Graduate Medical Education
ADL	activities of daily living
ADP	adenosine diphosphate
AED	antiepileptic drug
AF	atrial fibrillation
AGE	advanced glycation end-product
AHA	American Heart Association
AHI	apnoea/hypopnoea index
AKI	acute kidney injury
AMT	abbreviated mental test
ANH	artificial nutrition and hydration
AQP	aquaporin
ARB	angiotensin receptor blocker
ARMDS	age-related medial degeneration and sclerosis
ART	assisted reproductive technology
AS	aortic stenosis
ASA	American Society of Anesthesiologists
ASIC	acid-sensing ion channel (receptor)
ATP	adenosine triphosphate
AVR	aortic valve surgery
BMI	body mass index
BNP	brain natriuretic peptide
CABG	coronary artery bypass grafting
CAD	coronary artery disease
CBD	case-based discussion
CBF	cerebral blood flow
CEA	carotid endarterectomy
cfPWV	carotid–femoral pulse wave velocity
CGA	comprehensive geriatric assessment
CJD	Creutzfeldt–Jakob disease
CKI	cyclin-dependent kinase inhibitor
CNS	central nervous system
COPD	chronic obstructive pulmonary disease
COX	cyclo-oxygenase
CPAP	continuous positive airway pressure
CPB	cardiopulmonary bypass
CPE	cardiopulmonary exercise

CPP	cerebral perfusion pressure
CRP	C-reactive protein
CSF	cerebrospinal fluid
CT	computed tomography
CVA	cerebrovascular attack
CYP	cytochrome P450
DBA	dobutamine stress echo
DBP	diastolic blood pressure
DLB	dementia with Lewy bodies
DLCO	diffusing capacity of the lung for carbon monoxide
DNAR	do not attempt resuscitation
DNIC	diffuse noxious inhibitory controls
ECG	Electrocardiogram
ECMO	extracorporeal membrane oxygenation
ED	emergency department
EEG	electroencephalogram
EN	enteral nutrition
eNOS	endothelium derived nitric oxide synthase
EPO	erythropoietin
ESWL	extracorporeal shock-wave lithotripsy
ET	Endothelin
EtCO$_2$	end-tidal carbon dioxide
EVAR	endovascular aneurysm repair
FEV$_1$	forced expiratory volume in 1 second
FRC	functional residual capacity
FTD	frontotemporal dementia
FVC	forced vital capacity
GABA	gamma-aminobutyric acid
GFR	glomerular filtration rate
GMC	General Medical Council
HCC	hepatocellular carcinoma
hESC	human embryonic stem cells
IABP	intra-aortic balloon pump
IASP	International Association for the Study of Pain
ICH	intracerebral haemorrhage
ICU	intensive care unit
IIS	insulin/insulin-like growth factor-like signalling
IL	Interleukin
iNOS	inducible nitric oxide synthase
IOP	intraocular pressure
LA	left atrial
LIMA	left internal mammary artery
LMA	laryngeal mask airway

LV	left ventricle	PSP	progressive supranuclear palsy
MAC	minimum alveolar concentration or mitral annular calcification	PWV	pulse wave velocity
		RAAS	renin–angiotensin–aldosterone system
MDT	multidisciplinary team	RAS	renin–angiotensin system
MEF	maximal expiratory flow	RNS	reactive nitrogen species
MEP	maximal expiratory pressure	ROS	reactive oxygen species
MET	metabolic equivalent	RSI	rapid sequence intubation
MIF	maximal inspiratory flow	RV	residual volume
MIP	maximal inspiratory pressure	SAH	subarachnoid haemorrhage
MMP	matrix metalloproteases	SBI	silent brain injury
MMSE	Mini Mental State Examination	SBP	systolic blood pressure
MR	mitral regurgitation	SDH	subdural haematoma
MRA	magnetic resonance angiography	SOAR	systolic blood pressure, oxygenation, age, and respiratory rate
MRI	magnetic resonance imaging		
MRSA	methicillin-resistant *Staphylococcus aureus*	SOD	superoxide dismutase
MS	mitral stenosis	SpO_2	haemoglobin oxygen saturation
MVR	mitral valve repair	SSI	surgical site infection
NADPH	nicotinamide adenine dinucleotide phosphate	STEMI	ST-elevation myocardial infarction
NAFLD	non-alcoholic fatty liver disease	STS	Society of Thoracic Surgeons
NF-κB	nuclear factor kappa B	SVG	saphenous vein graft
NHS	National Health Service (UK)	SVR	systemic vascular resistance
NICE	National Institute for Health and Clinical Excellence	TAP	transversus abdominis plane
		TAVI	transcatheter aortic valve implantation
NIRS	near-infrared spectroscopy	TBI	traumatic brain injury
NMDA	N-methyl-D-aspartate	TCD	transcranial Doppler
NO	nitric oxide	TGF	transforming growth factor
NP	natriuretic peptide	TIA	transient ischaemic attack
NSAID	non-steroidal anti-inflammatory drug	TLC	total lung capacity
OPCAB	off-pump coronary artery bypass	TNF	tumour necrosis factor
$PaCO_2$	partial pressure of carbon dioxide in arterial blood	TOE	transoesophageal echocardiography
PACU	post-anesthesia care unit	TOR	target of rapamycin pathway
PAD	peripheral arterial disease	TRUS	transrectal ultrasound
PaO_2	partial pressure of oxygen in the arterial blood	TTE	transthoracic echocardiography
PCNL	percutaneous nephrolithotomy	TURBT	transurethral resection of bladder tumour
PCT	procalcitonin	TURP	transurethral resection of prostate
PD	Parkinson's disease	UTI	urinary tract infection
PDD	Parkinson's disease dementia	VaD	vascular dementia
PN	parenteral nutrition	VSMC	vascular smooth muscle cell
POCD	postoperative cognitive dysfunction	WDR	wide dynamic range
POD	postoperative delirium		
POSSUM	Physiological and Operative Severity Score for Enumeration of Mortality and Morbidity		

List of Contributors

Shamsuddin Akhtar
Department of Anesthesiology,
Yale University School of Medicine,
New Haven, Connecticut

Sheila Ryan Barnett
Department of Anesthesiology,
Critical Care and Pain Medicine,
Beth Israel Deaconess Medical Center,
Boston, MA

Jaume Canet
Department of Anesthesiology,
Hospital Universitari,
Germans Trias I Pujol,
Universitat Autònoma de Barcelona,
Barcelona, Spain

Naville Chia
Department of Anesthesia,
Alexandra Health Services,
Khoo Teck Puat Hospital,
Singapore

Ipek Yalcin Christmann
Institut des Neurosciences,
Cellulaires et Intégratives UPR3212 CNRS,
Strasbourg, France

Oya Yalcin Cok
Baskent University, School of Medicine,
Department of Anaesthesiology,
Adana Research and Education Center,
Adana, Turkey

Heinrich Cornelissen
Critical Care Research Group,
Prince Charles Hospital,
Brisbane, Australia

Peter Crome
Research Department of Primary Care and Population Health,
University College London,
London, UK

Jugdeep Dhesi
Proactive care of Older People undergoing Surgery (POPS),
Department of Ageing and Health,
Guy's and St Thomas' NHS Foundation Trust,
London, UK

Chris Dodds
James Cook University Hospital,
Middlesbrough, UK

Irwin Foo
Department of Anaesthesia,
Western General Hospital,
Edinburgh, UK

John F. Fraser
Critical Care Research Group,
Prince Charles Hospital,
Brisbane, Australia;
Department of Intensive Care Medicine,
The Prince Charles Hospital, Chermside,
Queensland, Australia

Bernard Graf
Department of Anaesthesia and Intensive Care Medicine,
University Hospital of Regensburg,
Regensburg, Germany

Richard Griffiths
Department of Anaesthesia,
Peterborough and Stamford Hospitals NHS Foundation Trust,
Bretton, Peterborough,
Cambridgeshire, UK

Samuel R. Grodofsky
Department of Anesthesiology and Critical care,
Perelman School of Medicine,
University of Pennsylvania, Philadelphia, PA

Jeremy Henning
Department of Anaesthesia,
James Cook University Hospital,
Middlesbrough, UK

John Hughes
Department of Anaesthesia,
James Cook University Hospital,
Middlesbrough, UK

Uma Shridhar Iyer
Department of Anesthesia,
Alexandra Health Services,
Khoo Teck Puat Hospital, Singapore

Pragnesh Joshi
Department of Cardiac Surgery,
Sir Charles Gardiner Hospital,
Nedlands, Western Australia, Australia

Richard Keays
Director of Intensive Care,
Chelsea and Westminster Hospital
London, UK

Kwong Fah Koh
Department of Anesthesia,
Alexandra Health Services, Khoo Teck Puat Hospital,
Yishun Central, Singapore

Elke Kothmann
Department of Anaesthesia,
James Cook University Hospital,
Middlesbrough, UK

Kailash Krishnan
Clinical research fellow,
University of Nottingham, UK

Chandra M. Kumar
Department of Anesthesia,
Alexandra Health Services, Khoo Teck Puat Hospital,
Yishun Central, Singapore

Frank Lally
Institute for Science and Technology in Medicine,
Keele University,
Guy Hilton Research Centre,
Thornburrow Drive,
Hartshill,
Stoke On Trent,
Staffordshire, UK

Amjad Maniar
Department of Anesthesia,
Columbia Asia Hospitals,
Bangalore, India

Joanne McGuire
Furness General Hospital,
University Hospitals of Morecambe Bay,
Cumbria, UK

Diane Monkhouse
Department of Anaesthesia,
James Cook University Hospital,
Middlesbrough, UK

Ross J. Moy
Academic Department of Emergency Medicine,
Academic Centre, James Cook University Hospital,
Middlesbrough, UK

Stanley Muravchick
Department of Anesthesiology and Critical Care,
Hospital of the University of Pennsylvania,
Philadelphia, PA

Dave Murray
Department of Anaesthesia,
James Cook University Hospital,
Middlesbrough, UK

Onyi Onuoha
Department of Anesthesiology and Critical care,
Perelman School of Medicine,
University of Pennsylvania,
Philadelphia, PA

Anand Prakash
Medicine for the Elderly Department,
Countess of Chester Hospital, UK

James M. Prentis
Department of Perioperative and Critical Care Medicine,
Freeman Hospital,
Newcastle upon Tyne, UK

Ivan L. Rapchuk
Critical Care Research Group,
Prince Charles Hospital, Brisbane, Australia;
Department of Anaesthesia and Perfusion,
The Prince Charles Hospital, Chermside,
Queensland, Australia

Lars S. Rasmussen
Department of Anaesthesia,
Rigshospitalet,
University of Copenhagen,
Denmark

G. Alec Rooke
Department of Anesthesiology and Pain Medicine,
University of Washington,
Puget Sound Health Care System,
Seattle, Washington

Joaquin Sanchis
Department of Pneumology,
Hospital Santa Creui, Sant Pau,
Universitat Autònoma de Barcelona,
Barcelona, Spain

Edwin Seet
Department of Anesthesia,
Alexandra Health Services,
Khoo Teck Puat Hospital, Singapore

Andrew Severn
Department of Anaesthesia,
Royal Lancaster Hospital,
Lancaster, UK

Khalil Ullah Shibli
Department of Anesthesia,
Alexandra Health Services,
Khoo Teck Puat Hospital, Singapore

Sabina Shibli
Department of Anaesthesia,
Jurong Health,
Ng Teng Fong General Hospital, Singapore

Shahla Siddiqui
Department of Anesthesia,
Alexandra Health Services,
Khoo Teck Puat Hospital, Singapore

Jeffrey H. Silverstein
Department of Anesthesiology,
Icahn School of Medicine at Mount Sinai,
New York City, NY

Ashish C. Sinha
Anesthesiology and Perioperative Medicine,
Drexel University College of Medicine,
Philadelphia, PA

Chris. P. Snowden
Department of Perioperative and Critical Care Medicine,
Freeman Hospital,
Newcastle upon Tyne, UK

Sameer Somanath
University Hospital of North Durham,
Durham

Neil Soni
Respiratory and Critical Care research,
Imperial College London and Consultant in Anaesthesia and
Intensive Care,
Chelsea and Westminster Hospital,
London, UK

Aris Sophocles III
Department of Anesthesiology and Critical care,
Perelman School of Medicine,
University of Pennsylvania,
Philadelphia, PA

Barry N. Speker
Samuel Phillips Law Firm
Newcastle upon Tyne, UK

Bernadette Th. Veering
Department of Anesthesiology
Leiden University Medical Center
Leiden, The Netherlands

Ian Whitehead
Department of Anaesthesia,
James Cook University Hospital,
Middlesbrough, UK

Introduction

Chris Dodds

We face an unprecedented challenge across the world as the balance of populations tip towards ever larger proportions of older members. This trend is not likely to begin to reverse for the next 40 years and will affect every one of us both professionally and personally. This change will alter the manner in which we live as independent adults, the age at which couples start their families, and the age at which we are able to afford to stop working.

The burden of caring for dependents will increase, whether these are children, parents, or grandparents. Increasingly families require both partners to work and their ability to maintain financial stability is undermined if one of them has to restrict their hours of work to care for a previously independent family member. This comes into sharp focus when an elderly family member has a serious illness or requires surgery. Not only is there a need for immediate support to get them back to their normal level of independence but the very prolonged nature of their convalescence means that support, of a degree, may need to be provided for many months.

Complications, following all medical interventions irrespective of the procedure, are far more common in older patients, and these are likely to have the greatest impact on their independence. Some are more to be expected as predictable side effects of the necessary clinical care whereas others are unexpected serious events. We, as a profession, continue to have a duty of care to determine what may cause these complications and try whenever possible to avoid precipitating them.

Anaesthesia because of its central role in hospital medicine has the ability to influence the outcome for patients from surgery, interventional radiology, intensive care, trauma, and pain medicine amongst others. As the majority of anaesthetists will spend most of their clinical years caring for elderly patients, it is imperative to understand why they differ from younger patients, and in what ways. The increasingly unacceptable response of 'we do lots of them anyway so what is so special?' has to be replaced by an attitude of providing individually tailored care based on the latest scientific data available. This evidence base is, perhaps, the most telling insight into medical and anaesthetic research into the elderly over the years. Until very recently almost all clinical trials excluded patients over the age of 65. Exclusion criteria also included mild cognitive dysfunction and pre-existing cardiac or respiratory disease—conditions present in many elderly patients. This means that for the majority of agents used during anaesthesia, the physiological parameters which are regarded as normal and the expectations of recovery are extrapolations from data gathered on younger patients. This is simply foolhardy.

The younger, healthier, adults enrolled into trials have minimal physiological variability. It is easy to look at the data gathered and visually identify relationships even if statistical packages are used to precisely define these. The contrast to the usual elderly distribution could not be more marked. Identifying a meaningful relationship may not be visually possible at all and reliance has then to be placed on the statistical analysis. What this means is that unlike caring for a fit American Society of Anesthesiologists (ASA) grade 1 adult where the responses to induction, surgical challenges, and recovery are largely predictable, each elderly patient is an individual and their responses unpredictable and so has to be managed with a far higher level of vigilance and skill to ensure a safe outcome. The precise parameters of blood pressure, heart rate, and fluid status will vary and one patient's hypertension will be another's hypotension. Simple techniques such as spraying the larynx and vocal cords with lignocaine to ameliorate the response to laryngoscopy and intubation may cause enough lidocaine to be absorbed to cause myocardial depression and hypotension in the frail elderly patient.

Although there has been much progress since the first specialist anaesthetic society was created over 20 years ago there is still no 'normative' data published on the responses of patients over 90 years of age to routine surgery. The information that is being published at present usually refers to small studies on patients with specific problems, for instance, fractured neck of femur. Large surveys and national audits do provide an idea of scale and outcomes but their retrospective nature limits their ability to differentiate between specific anaesthetic techniques in all but the broadest manner. We are no closer to clearly understanding what causes the devastating cognitive dysfunction that occurs so commonly, affecting nearly one in four of the elderly after major surgery.

Research in the field of geriatrics is helping to provide some guidance, especially with regard to the emerging concepts about frailty as a complex entity in its own right. Genetics and stem cell biology are proving fertile fields in the quest to understand the ageing process and potential means to slow, stop, or even reverse the process. Nanotechnology and bioengineering are exploring novel solutions to help with protecting vulnerable or isolated elderly people and the almost universal access to the Internet is allowing interactive monitoring and tailored clinical advice for those with long-term medical conditions.

At a clinical and training level, awareness of the communication problems in the elderly, related to vision, hearing, and language, is improving but is still rarely taught formally across anaesthetic training schemes. Simple tests of cognition such as the abbreviated mental test (AMT) and mini-mental state evaluation (MMSE) are seldom part of routine preoperative assessment. There remains a great deal of mythology about the elderly patient's need for analgesia and what is safe and effective across nursing and medical staff.

It is for these reasons that we have embarked on creating this textbook. We have sought leading authoritative and acknowledged world experts to write the chapters in the book. There is, inevitably, a variation in both style and detail that reflects both the nature of that specialist area and also the volume of data available on that area. The sections are ordered to provide a view of the fundamental principles underlying ageing at the most basic levels, the population changes occurring and possible social consequences of those changes, the responses to drugs that change with ageing, and the potential that modern technology may hold for us. The next section covers ageing within specific organ systems, the nervous system including cognition, the cardiovascular, renal, respiratory, and hepatic systems. The third section summarizes the common areas of practice some of which are related to the surgical speciality involved. These include pre-assessment, intensive care, pain management, obesity, frailty, and palliative care as well as covering other areas such as trauma, vascular, neurosurgery, cardiovascular surgery, urological, gynaecological, and ophthalmic surgery.

Finally there are areas where the elderly demand a greater focus than currently occurs, such as training, managing infection, maintaining heat balance, and anaesthesia beyond the operating suite. There is a review of the current medicolegal system. This is primarily from a UK perspective and we assume that it reflects practice worldwide. This emphasizes the need to seek informed consent, to identify the presence of any advanced directives or legal advocates, and to assess and support competence in decision-making.

Finally we have our view of what should happen in the future as well as a possible glimpse into where practice may evolve in the not so near future.

PART 1

Basic Science

CHAPTER 1

Ageing at cellular level

Anand Prakash and Kailash Krishnan

Introduction

Ageing is a collective and progressive process. There is a gradual biological impairment of normal function due to changes at a cellular level; these changes gradually affect the various organ systems and ultimately whole body. Ageing in humans refers to a multidimensional process of physical, psychological, and social change. Ageing has been defined as the collection of changes that render human beings progressively more likely to die.[1]

The ageing process starts immediately after sexual maturity and the rate of progress of ageing is affected by intrinsic and extrinsic factors. The biological age is more important than chronological age. In the last 10 years tremendous academic interest in the processes of ageing has been generated and high-quality sophisticated research is helping our understanding of the biological basis of the ageing process and its consequences. Human premature ageing disorders provide valuable models for studying the ageing process. Some ageing processes like greying of hair have no pathological effect, whilst other ageing processes lead to changes at the cellular level and may trigger a cascade that results in damage to the cell and leads to functional impairment at tissue, organ, and system levels.

Age-related damage may alter the signalling mechanisms at cellular and molecular levels affecting genetic material, structural proteins and other vital proteins, mitochondria, cellular membranes, and ultimately result in compromise of their structures, functions, and roles. The ageing process is extremely complex and it remains incompletely understood. Cellular damage can take place due to either intrinsic or extrinsic factors. Our environment contains many toxic substances; some of them are natural and some produced by humanity. Ultraviolet radiation, ionizing nuclear radiation, industrial toxins and products, ozone, heavy metals, smoke, pollution, adulterated food or water, and infections from other organisms are all known to cause cellular damage.

Normal cellular metabolism itself generates many compounds such as free radicals, which are themselves highly damaging and there are complex pathways to limit the impact of these toxins. Ageing is associated with an impairment of these protective processes and cellular damage and dysfunction becomes more common.

The changes at cellular and molecular levels are described in the following sections. Further details that are beyond the scope of this chapter are available elsewhere.[1]

Cell senescence and cell death

Cell senescence and cellular death are two important processes that occur throughout the life of an organism. These processes help eliminate dysfunctional and damaged cells throughout life. But in later life these process may also contribute to ageing. Various factors (extrinsic and intrinsic) and mechanisms are responsible for the biological ageing at molecular and cellular levels. Cellular death is a complex process and involves apoptosis and necrosis. Many theories have been postulated for ageing. Cellular senescence is a continuous process, which includes changes in gene expression and morphology of cells. Damage to DNA, and expression of oncogenes can arrest cellular growth, alter cellular function and can make cells resistant to apoptosis.

Changes at molecular and genetic levels

Most somatic cells are programmed to divide only a limited number of times and thereafter although they do not divide they remain metabolically active. This process is termed as replicative senescence.[2] They are unable to replicate their DNA but continue to metabolize proteins and RNA. The germ line and stem cells and most cancer cells have unlimited division potential.

Why some cells undergo replicative senescence and some achieve replicative immortality and how this contributes to ageing is as yet unknown. It is likely to include some or all of the following factors: genetic mutation, metabolic changes, or intrinsic and extrinsic suppression of gene expression.

Telomere shortening and ageing

A telomere is a region of repetitive DNA sequences at the end of a chromosome, which protects the end of the chromosome from breakdown, degradation, and fusion with neighbouring chromosomes.[3] This damage can lead to a loss of genetic information and can make the genome unstable and susceptible to cell death and cancer.

Telomeres shorten progressively with each round of cell division and when they reach a critical length or are completely lost, the cell stops dividing or growing. This helps the cell avoid losing genetic information and developing genomic instability.

The enzyme telomerase reverse transcriptase maintains and stabilizes the telomere end during cell proliferation. Germ and stem cells can proliferate indefinitely as they contain large amount of the telomerase enzyme thus keeping telomere lengths stable. Somatic cells have a more limited level of telomerase enzyme which may explain why they reach senescence. Shortening of telomeres also results in impairment of immunological function.[4] Free radicals are also involved in telomeric DNA damage and shortening of telomeres.

Telomeres play a central role in both cell fate and ageing by adjusting the cellular response to stress and growth stimulation on the basis of previous cell divisions and DNA damage. Repair of critically short or 'uncapped' telomeres by telomerase or recombination is limited in most somatic cells and apoptosis or cellular senescence is triggered when too many 'uncapped' telomeres accumulate. The chance of the latter increases as the average telomere length decreases. The average telomere length is set and maintained in cells of the germ line which typically expresses high levels of telomerase. In somatic cells, the telomere length is very heterogeneous but typically declines with age, posing a barrier to tumour growth but also contributing to the loss of cells with advancing age.[5] The biotechnology industry is trying to develop therapies based on telomerase.

Codon restriction and ageing

Protein synthesis requires two steps—transcription and translation. There are three bases in the DNA code for each amino acid. The DNA code is copied to produce messenger RNA (mRNA). The order of amino acids in the polypeptide is determined by the sequence of three-letter codes in mRNA. mRNA contains genetic information. It is a copy of a portion of the DNA and carries genetic information from the gene (DNA) out of the nucleus, into the cytoplasm of the cell where it is translated to produce protein. With ageing, the process of translation gets impaired and defective proteins are created leading to various changes at cellular level impairing and compromising its function.[6,7]

Alteration in gene function with ageing

The genetic programming of cells determines the diverse functions of cells (neurons, cardiac, etc.) and the programming to produce specialized proteins (transcription). Genetic transcription is regulated by factors such as specificity factor, repressors, transcription factors, activators, and enhancers.[8] Gene expression changes when the cell reaches maturity.[9] The alteration in genetic programming may be seen at the molecular level resulting in abnormal protein production and damage.[10]

DNA is a highly complex and unstable molecule and both genomic and mitochondrial DNA is susceptible to damage and mutation. The stability of the genome depends upon the DNA repair mechanisms. This DNA repair becomes slower and less efficient in ageing cells. The longevity of an organism depends upon the efficiency of these mechanisms and its resistance to toxic factors.

Cells' ability to respond and adapt appropriately to external and internal stimuli and signals depends on intrinsic signalling pathways. Many of the molecules involved in these pathways are proteins and these are adversely affected by the mechanisms described earlier.

Mitochondria are the primary site for oxygen consumption in the cell and therefore the site for production of the majority of free radicals. Mitochondrial structure and functions decline with age due to reduced mitochondrial protein synthesis rate, control of mitochondrial membrane potential, coupling efficiency of ATP synthesis to oxygen synthesis, and control of ADP. A decrease in mitochondrial DNA content was also noted.[11]

Mitochondrial dysfunction is considered to be one of the major causative factors in the ageing process; ischaemia/reperfusion injury,

septic shock, and neurodegenerative disorders like Parkinson's disease, Alzheimer's disease, and Huntington's disease, increased free radical generation, enhanced mitochondrial inducible nitric oxide (NO) synthase activity, enhanced NO production, decreased respiratory complex activity, impaired electron transport system, and opening of mitochondrial permeability transition pores all have been suggested as factors responsible for impaired mitochondrial function.[12]

Insulin signalling pathways

A major breakthrough in ageing research in recent years has been the identification of the evolutionarily conserved role of the insulin/insulin-like growth factor-like signalling (IIS) pathway in modulating lifespan, and lowered IIS has emerged as an important means of extending lifespan. The IIS pathway has diverse functions in multicellular organisms, and mutations in it can affect growth, development, metabolic homoeostasis, fecundity, and stress resistance, as well as lifespan.[13]

Target of rapamycin pathway

The target of rapamycin pathway (TOR) is necessary for developmental growth, but upon completion of development it causes ageing and age-related diseases. Decreased TOR activity has been found to slow ageing. This signalling pathway regulates cell growth, cell proliferation, cell motility, cell survival, protein production, and transcription.[14–16]

Free radicals

A free radical is an atom or group of atoms that has at least one unpaired electron in its outermost cells and is therefore unstable and highly reactive. The free radicals containing oxygen are called reactive oxygen species (ROS) and those containing nitrogen are called reactive nitrogen species (RNS).

Ageing may be related to the deleterious side effects of free radicals produced during the course of cell metabolism. Oxidative stress and nitrosative stress are directly related to ageing. The level of free radicals in cells increases with age. The antioxidants are protective and an enhanced level increases the longevity. There is supportive evidence that the overexpression and enhancement of antioxidants extends the lifespan.[17]

Free radicals damage proteins, lipids, and nucleic acids. The amount of oxidatively damaged and modified protein increases in cells and mitochondria with age resulting in a decline in intracellular ATP level and impaired apoptosis. These produce multiple age-related disorders and diseases.[18]

The increase in oxidative modified proteins has been demonstrated with age. There is a rapid increase in levels of protein carbonyl content, protein hydrophobicity, oxidized methionine, cross-linked and glycated proteins, and also less active enzymes which are more susceptible to damage by heat and proteolysis.[19]

Protein oxidation can involve cleavage of the polypeptide chain, modification of amino acid side chains, or conversion of the protein to derivatives that are highly sensitive to proteolytic degradation. Unlike most other types of modification (except cysteine oxidation), oxidation of methionine residues to methionine sulphoxide is reversible; thus, cyclic oxidation and reduction of methionine residues leads to consumption of ROS and thereby increases the resistance of proteins to oxidation. The age-related accumulation of oxidized proteins may reflect age-related increases in rates of ROS generation, decreases in antioxidant activities, or losses in the capacity to degrade oxidized proteins.[20]

Lipids are major component of living organisms and are particularly vulnerable to damage by free radicals. There appears to be an age-associated increase in the steady state concentration of lipid peroxidation products.[21]

Protein carbonyls, 8-oxo-2'-deoxyguanosine, acrolein or 4-HNE (4-hydroxy-2 nonenal) are established biomarkers of protein, DNA, and lipid oxidation. The intracellular level of protein carbonyl has become one of the most widely accepted measurements of oxidative stress-dependent cellular damage.

Organisms contain many endogenous enzymes which act as antioxidants (such as superoxide dismutase (SOD), catalase, and glucose-6-phosphate dehydrogenase) and these enzymes counteract the deleterious effect of oxidants and act as scavengers. Aerobic organisms that use the cytochrome system have both the SOD and catalase enzymes and overexpression of these in animals are known to increase lifespan.[22–26]

A concept of nitrosative stress has emerged recently from the understanding that the interaction between oxidants and nitrosant may produce products that are more toxic and damaging than either reactant alone. The peroxynitrite molecule is a product of reaction between superoxide (ROS) and nitric oxide (RNS). This is proinflammatory and affects the nuclear factor kappa B (NF-kB) signalling process and results in age-related disorders. Nitrosylation can directly inhibit critical protein function and promote deleterious oxidative modifications. NO has been widely implicated in nitrosative stress at cellular level and is linked to cellular growth inhibition and apoptosis.[27–29]

More recently, the role of reactive nitrogen species, such as NO and its by-products—nitrate (NO_3^-), nitrite (NO_2^-), peroxynitrite ($ONOO^-$), and 3-nitrotyrosine—have been shown to have a direct role in cellular signalling, vasodilatation, and the immune response. NO is produced within cells by NO synthesis. Presently, there are three distinct isoforms of NO synthase: neuronal (nNOS or NOS-1), inducible (iNOS or NOS-2), and endothelial (eNOS or NOS-3), and several subtypes. While NO is a relatively unreactive radical, it is able to form other, more reactive, intermediates, which could have an effect on protein function and on the function of the entire organism. These reactive intermediates can trigger nitrosative damage on biomolecules, which in turn may lead to age-related diseases due to structural alteration of proteins, inhibition of enzymatic activity, and interferences of the regulatory function.[30,31] The nitrosative stress acts on several signalling pathways affecting transcription factors such as NF-kB or activator protein 1 (AP-1), and thereby influence gene expression.

Calcium homeostasis and ageing

Homeostasis of intracellular free calcium and normal signalling is vital for cellular activity and function. The transport and passage of calcium into a cell and cytoplasm is a strictly regulated process. The cellular mechanism of calcium homeostasis plays an important role in the ageing process and neurodegeneration. Altered Ca^{2+} homeostasis can account for a number of changes associated with ageing.

Ageing affects the voltage-operated calcium channels and calcium-dependent glutamate operated channels. It also affects the intracellular buffering mechanisms of calcium. Impaired calcium homeostasis alters the function of intracellular organelles such as endoplasmic reticulum (which is an important calcium store) and mitochondria.[32]

Apoptosis and necrosis

Apoptosis is a complex process characterized by genetically programmed cell death in a controlled manner. Apoptosis is an active cascade by which cell die and apoptotic bodies are removed without triggering an inflammatory process. All cells are capable of producing the intracellular mechanism necessary for apoptosis.[33–35] In contrast, necrosis is an uncontrolled passive mode of cell death due to extrinsic or intrinsic factors causing significant damage at molecular and structural levels that leads to irreversible swelling of the cell and its organelles and eventually cell lysis and death. Necrosis is associated with an acute inflammatory response.

Apoptosis eliminates damaged and dysfunctional germ cells during embryogenesis. In complex organisms, apoptosis is not only essential during embryogenesis it is also necessary for maintaining tissue homeostasis in adults and eliminating dysfunctional, damaged, and potentially cancerous cells throughout life. Failure of apoptosis can lead to an increase in incidence of cancers while excessive apoptosis can produce disorders related to degeneration.[36,37]

There are two main apoptotic pathways: the extrinsic or death receptor pathway and the intrinsic or mitochondrial pathway. They are interlinked and each pathway can influence the other. There is an additional pathway that involves T-cell mediated cytotoxicity and perforin/granzyme-dependent killing of the cell.[38]

Apoptosis can be divided into three phases: induction phase, effector phase, and degradation phase. The induction phase is initiated by physiological signals such as ROS, RNS, tumour necrosis factor (TNF), ceramide overactivation of calcium pathways, and B-cell lymphoma (Bcl)-2 family proteins.

In the effector phase, the cells become committed to die by the action of the death domain activator on the cell surface, nuclear activators such as p53, the endoplasmic reticular pathways, and activation of the mitochondrial-induced pathways.

The degradation phase involves both nuclear and cytoplasmic events. In the cytoplasm, a complex cascade of protein cleaving enzymes called *caspases* (cysteine proteases) becomes activated. In the nucleus, the nuclear envelope breaks down; endonucleases are activated, causing DNA fragmentation; and the chromatin condenses. Finally, the cell is fragmented into apoptotic bodies and phagocytosed by surrounding cells or macrophages.[39–41]

Researchers believe that mitochondria play extremely important roles in apoptosis and cell death. Mitochondria undergo major structural and functional changes and release apoptosis-inducing factors and cytochrome c that activates endonucleases and caspases. This results in the activation of various pathways and cascades.

Insufficient or excessive apoptosis due to extrinsic and or intrinsic factors can lead to disorders such as dementia, cancer, autoimmune disorders, neurodegenerative conditions, and others, which are more prevalent in the older person. Necrosis may also increase during ageing due to age-related defects at cellular and molecular levels resulting in inappropriate apoptosis.

Conclusion

The cellular and molecular mechanisms of ageing are believed to be due to the consequences of wear and tear as well as programmed changes at the level of gene expression. Damage and structural changes in vital proteins and DNA by various mechanisms compromises their function. This leads to physiological, pathological, and functional impairment in all systems of the human body.

The rate of deleterious changes depends upon various intrinsic and extrinsic factors, some are predictable and some are not. Some of us live longer and remain healthier and functionally active in comparison to others. Socioeconomic factors are very important in predicting quality ageing. Longevity does vary across species with some, such as the tortoise and sea turtles, living longer than humans, and this may be due to environmental selection.

Disease and disorders are more common in older people. Neurological ageing leads to different types of dementias. Changes in cardiac myocytes result in heart failure and many other cardiac disorders. Cancers are far more common. Changes in skeletal muscles and sarcopenia produce functional impairment and limitation of activity. The list gets longer and longer. These complex changes at molecular and cellular levels are far from being understood. Various theories and models of ageing remain controversial and the quest for an understanding of the biological process of ageing continues.

References

1. Medawar PB. *An unsolved problem of biology.* London: H.K. Lewis & Co., 1952.
2. Campisi J. Senescent cells, tumour suppression, and organismal aging: good citizens, bad neighbors. *Cell.* 2005;120(4):513–522.
3. Telomeres.net website. <http://www.telomeres.net>
4. Eisenberg DTA. An evolutionary review of human telomere biology: the thrifty telomere hypothesis and notes on potential adaptive paternal effect. *Am J Hum Biol.* 2011;23(2):149–167.
5. Aubert G, Lansdorp PM. Telomeres and aging. *Physiol Rev.* 2008;88(2):557–579.
6. Strehler B, Hirsch G, Gusseck D, Johnson R, Bick M. Codon-restriction theory of aging and development. *J Theoret Biol.* 1971;33(3):429–474.
7. Yates FE. *Theories of aging. In Birren JE (ed) Encyclopaedia of gerontology,* Volume 2 (pp. 544–545). San Diego, CA: Academic Press, 1996.
8. Austin S, Dixon R. The prokaryotic enhancer binding protein NTRC has an ATPase activity which is phosphorylation and DNA dependent. *EMBO J.* 1992;11(6):2219–2228.
9. Helfand SL, Blake KJ, Rogina B, Stracks MD, Centurion A, Naprta B. Temporal patterns of gene expression in the antenna of the adult Drosophila melanogaster. *Genetics.* 1995;140(2):549–555.
10. Cutler RG. The dysdifferentiation hypothesis of mammalian aging and longevity. In Gicobini E, Filogamo G, Giacobini G, Vernadakis V (eds) *The aging brain: cellular and molecular mechanisms of aging in the nervous system* (pp. 1–19). New York: Raven, 1982.
11. Greco M, Villani G, Mazzucchelli F, Bresolin N, Papa S, Attardi G. Marked aging-related decline in efficiency of oxidative phosphorylation in human skin fibroblasts. *FASEB J.* 2003;17(12):1706–1708.
12. Srinivasan V, Spence DW, Pandi-Perumal SR, Brown GM, Cardinali DP. Melatonin in mitochondrial dysfunction and related disorders. *Int J Alzheimers Dis.* 2011;2011:326320.
13. Broughton S, Partridge L. Insulin/IGF-like signalling, the central nervous system and aging. *Biochem J.* 2009;418(1):1–12.
14. Blagosklonny MV, Hall MN. Growth and aging: a common molecular mechanism. *Aging.* 2009;1(4):357–362.
15. Hay N, Sonenberg N. Upstream and downstream of mTOR. *Genes Dev.* 2004;18(16):1926–1945. doi:10.1101/gad.1212704.
16. Beevers C, Li F, Liu L, Huang S. Curcumin inhibits the mammalian target of rapamycin-mediated signaling pathways in cancer cells. *Int J Cancer.* 2006;119(4):757–764.
17. Ljubunicic P, Gochman E, Reznik AZ. Nitrosative stress in aging – its importance and biological implication in NF- kB signalling, In Bondy S, Maiese K (eds) *Aging and age related disorders* (pp. 27–54). Oxidative Stress in Applied Basic Research and Clinical Practice. New York: Springer, 2010.
18. Miyoshi N, Oubrahim H, Chock PB, Stadtman ER. Age-dependent cell death; the roles of ATP in hydrogen peroxide-induced apoptosis and necrosis. *Proc Natl Acad Sci USA.* 2006;103:1727–1731.
19. Stadtman ER. Protein oxidation in aging and age-related diseases. *Ann N Y Acad Sci.* 2001;928:22–38.
20. Stadtman ER. Protein oxidation and aging. *Free Radic Res.* 2006;40(12):1250–1258.
21. Praticò D. Lipid peroxidation and the aging process. *Sci Aging Knowl Environ.* 2002;50:re5.
22. McCord JM, Fridovich I. Superoxide dismutase: an enzymic function for erythrocuprein (Hemocuprein). *J Biol Chem.* 1969;244:6049–6055.
23. Keele BB Jr, McCord JM, Fridovich I. Superoxide dismutase from Escherichia coli B: a new manganese-containing enzyme. *J Biol Chem.* 1970;245:6176–6181.
24. McCord JM, Keele BB Jr, Fridovich I. An enzyme-based theory of obligate anaerobiosis: the physiological function of superoxide dismutase. *Proc Natl Acad Sci USA.* 1971;68:1024–1027.
25. McCord JM. Free radicals and inflammation: protection of synovial fluid by superoxide dismutase. *Science.* 1974;185:529–531.
26. McCord JM, Day ED Jr. Superoxide-dependent production of hydroxyl radical catalyzed by iron-EDTA complex. *FEBS Lett.* 1978;86:139–142.
27. Stamler JS, Hausladen A. Oxidative modifications in nitrosative stress. *Nat Struct Biol.* 1998;5(4):247–249.
28. Eu JP, Liu L, Zeng M, Stamler JS. An apoptotic model for nitrosative stress. *Biochemistry* 2000;39:1040–1047.
29. Marshall HE, Merchant K, Stamler JS. Nitrosation and oxidation in the regulation of gene expression. *FASEB J.* 2000;14(13):1889–1900.
30. Drew B, Leeuwenburgh C. Aging and the role of reactive nitrogen species. *Ann N Y Acad Sci.* 2002;959:66–81.
31. Kröncke KD. Nitrosative stress and transcription. *Biol Chem.* 2003 Oct–Nov;384(10–11):1365–1377.
32. Toescu EC. *Altered calcium homeostasis in old neurons.* In Riddle DR (ed) *Brain aging: models, methods, and mechanisms* (pp. 323–352). Frontiers in Neuroscience. Boca Raton, FL: CRC Press, 2007.
33. Kerr JF, Wyllie AH, Currie AR. Apoptosis: a basic biological phenomenon with wide-ranging implications in tissue kinetics. *Br J Cancer.* 1972;26(4):239–257.
34. Ellis RE, Yuan J, Horvitz HR. Mechanisms and functions of cell death. *Ann Rev Cell Biol.* 1991;7:663–698.
35. Pollack M, Leeuwenburgh C. Apoptosis and aging role of the mitochondria. *J Gerontology A Biol Sci Med Sci.* 2001;56(11): B475–B482.
36. Aravind L, Dixit VM, Koonin EV. Apoptotic molecular machinery: vastly increased complexity in vertebrates revealed by genome comparisons. *Science.* 2001;291(5507):1279–1284.
37. Thompson CB. Apoptosis in the pathogenesis and treatment of disease *Science.* 1995:267(5203):1456–1462.
38. Igney FH, Krammer PH. Death and anti-death: tumour resistance to apoptosis. *Nat Rev Cancer.* 2002;2:277–288.
39. Pollack M, Leeuwenburgh C. Apoptosis and aging role of the mitochondria. *J Gerontol A Biol Sci Med Sci.* 2001;56(11):B475–B482.
40. Warner HR, Hodes RJ, Pocinki K. What does cell death have to do with aging? *Am Geriatric Soc.* 1997;45(9):1140–1146.
41. Warner HR. Aging and regulation of apoptosis. *Curr Top Cell Regul.* 1997;35:107–121.

CHAPTER 2

Demographic and social changes

Chris Dodds

Introduction

There is a widely held belief that the population is ageing, largely due to an increased life expectancy, and it is expected that 10 per cent of the population in developed countries will be aged over 80 by 2050.[1] It is important to differentiate between lifespan, which is the maximum predicted life expectancy of the human species at about 110–120 years, and life expectancy, which is the number of years of life an individual is likely to have at any given age. The number of people aged over 65 is now greater than those under 15 in the United Kingdom. These facts have importance to us as individuals and as providers of healthcare.

The underlying principles behind these calculations and their importance to us are based on the science of demography. This allows for a numerical prediction of population changes. What is also important is the concurrent increase in the health of the ageing population. The differences between previous generations of 40-year-olds and the current one is marked and the same is true for the over 60s. Simple calculations of life expectancy do not give an indication as to how much more resources, if any, an older population will need in terms of healthcare provision but they do give a clear view on pension planning. Some countries, Japan for instance, will see a fall in their total population but an increase in their elderly subjects while others will continue to grow but with a greater proportion of elderly.[2] We need to understand the impact this will have on such societies, their healthcare,[3] and just how important maintaining independence for these people is.

Demography

Demography is a statistical science that describes the dynamic changes within populations or subpopulations over time. (It is often misquoted in medical papers to describe the characteristics of the population being studied.) The main factors that affect populations are births, deaths, ageing, and migration. Populations may be stable with little change in the ratio of people in the various age ranges, even if the total number in that population is changing. It can be stationary if there is no change in the total numbers of the population or it can be unstable with changes in either numbers or age ratios.

Data on populations may be gathered directly by gathering 'vital statistics' or by census. The first uses data from the registration of births and deaths and is a continuous data gathering process. Census is usually performed intermittently, even if regularly, by national governments. The UK population census is currently performed every 10 years.[4] Census gathering depends on a very high level of state funding and personnel resources.

The balance for any one group in a time period will be the difference between the number of births plus the net migration into that group from outside against the number who have died and those who have emigrated over the same time. These groups may be subdivided into cohorts related to, for example, age, gender, or social status.

Understanding how populations change and the challenges these pose to healthcare providers is especially important as we strive to provide safe and effective care for elderly patients. That provision of care also depends on the social changes that occur within populations.

Models for population change

There are many different models proposed to describe the features of a population and the manner in which it changes in response to internal and external forces. These may include environmental factors such as crop failure, political factors such as warfare, medical factors with epidemics such as malaria or HIV, and economic factors such as employment opportunities. Migration may occur within a nation, for example, the long-established but still growing trend for younger workers to move to urban areas away from rural ones. It may be across national boundaries and may be motivated by political or economic pressures.

The transition model

This is a model that describes changes in a population over time. It studies how birth and death rates affect the total population of a country.

Transition models are usually described as a series of stages that have implications for many aspects of the economic well-being of that population and therefore also issues such as affordability of healthcare provision.

◆ Stage 1—the total population is low but it is balanced due to high birth rates and high death rates.

◆ Stage 2—the total population is starting to rise as death rates start to fall, but birth rates remain quite high (see Fig. 2.1).

◆ Stage 3—the total population is still rising rapidly, but the gap between birth and death rates narrows. Now the natural increase is high.

◆ Stage 4—the total population is high, but it is balanced due to a low birth rate and a low death rate (see Fig. 2.2).

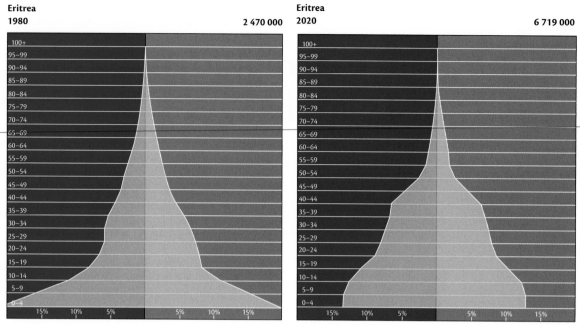

Fig. 2.1 Transition from stage 1 (1980) to stage 2 (2020) demonstrating an almost trebling of population but a falling birth rate. Reproduced with kind permission from Martin De Wulf, PopulationPyramid.net. Data from United Nations, Department of Economic and Social Affairs, Population Prospects, http://esa.un.org/wpp/

Population pyramids

One method to display these changes is through the use of population pyramids. They display males on the left and females on the right at 5-yearly intervals. They also indicate the percentage of that 5-year cohort of the total population. One of the most useful sources of these graphs is from the US Census Gateway,[5] which is frequently used by other nations as a valuable reference source for their own population projections.

Whilst the visual representation of changes in a given population over a historical period is reasonably accurate, the projection of that population into the future is less robust. The factors that influence the development of the cohorts can be assessed and attempts to quantify their effect calculated. These are often then further refined into 'life tables' and may be used to calculate risks for an individual's mortality.

An example of a historical population pyramid (Fig. 2.3) such as that for Germany after the Second World War clearly shows the reduction in both male and female cohorts aged around 19–34 years of age. The reduction in males is higher and is assumed to be due to the awful mortality within that generation at that time.

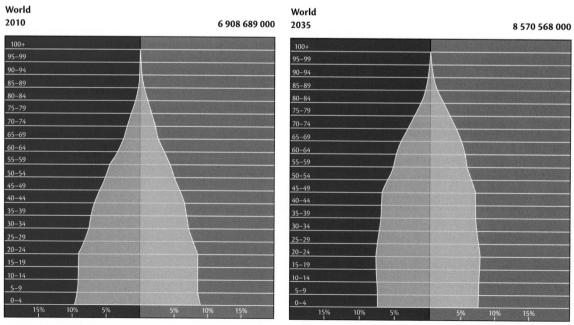

Fig. 2.2 Transition of the global population from stage 3 to stage 4 over a 20-year projection. Reproduced with kind permission from Martin De Wulf, PopulationPyramid.net. Data from United Nations, Department of Economic and Social Affairs, Population Prospects, http://esa.un.org/wpp/

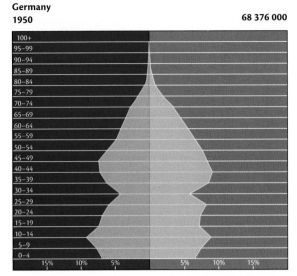

Germany
1950   **68 376 000**

Fig. 2.3 This demonstrates a reduction in numbers of young males due to casualties in the Second World War, and also a reduction in birth rate which may be due to the same cause or that may be due to the severe economic problems of that period in Germany. Reproduced with kind permission from Martin De Wulf, PopulationPyramid.net. Data from United Nations, Department of Economic and Social Affairs, Population Prospects, http://esa.un.org/wpp/

What is also clear is the strongly pyramidal shape for the elderly groups. This high mortality is likely to be related to malnutrition, limited healthcare facilities, and the minimal impact of the newly developed antibiotics on infectious diseases. Similar, but less pronounced, effects are seen across Europe and Russia. The birth rate is also low and below 'replacement level' (see 'Replacement ratio' section). This may be due to the lack of suitable males or may be a reflection of the extreme economic hardship of that time.

Changes in the German population describing the progress to date include a brief period of an increased birth rate and a lessening of the paediatric mortality. This bulge although not to the extent often seen in the 'baby boomer' years does move up the diagram over time. What is interesting is the increase in imported workers who provided a necessary workforce and a taxation income for the government. The total population of Germany is predicted to fall over the next three decades but with an increasingly old population bias.

General processes underlying the demographic changes

Birth rate

The crude birth rate, the number of children born alive each year, provides the starting point for any population. Across the world this has been falling progressively as measures such as the availability of effective contraception, education for females, and even State mandate have their effects. The ratio of boys to girls born has historically been close to equality although some states and religious groups have tried to bias the ratio in favour of more male births. Once born the next hurdle for a population relates to infant and child mortality. In the highly and moderately developed countries these have both been falling for decades, but they are still very high in the poorly developed countries.

Replacement ratio

The stability and survival of a population over time depends on enough female children surviving to childbearing age and producing the next generation of children. The exact number of children a female has to deliver to maintain the population is about 2.3 live births/female. This ratio has not been met across the majority of Europe for many years. The replacement ratio will fall slightly as infant and child mortality improves but will need to rise if there is loss of young, productive members of the population through warfare, epidemics, or natural disasters.

Fertility

In many developed countries the decision to have children is being made when the mother is in her 30s rather than late teens and early 20s as in previous generations. Whilst this frequently leads to a more financially robust family the inevitable decline in fertility related to ageing limits the numbers of births and may lead to medical interventions such as *in vitro* fertilization (IVF) to achieve one live birth. One benefit could be seen as the children born of these older parents will be working, and paying taxes, into the late old age of their parents. This may offset some of the financial risks facing many sovereign states in the future.

Death rates

We are all born to die, but life expectancy has progressively increased over the last century. European life expectancy in 1900 was approximately 40 years of age and when Germany created the concept of retirement only 1 per cent of men reached the age of 65, and the same proportion of women survived to 60 years of age. The provision of a state pension for such a small number was balanced by an inverse dependency ratio (see 'Dependency ratio' section) of almost 20:1, compared to the 4:3 expected in the coming decades as life expectancy for both males and females reaches more than 85 years of age. These figures are derived from the normal life expectancy data; others which use the concept of a productive life expectancy are more favourable.

Increased life expectancy delays the inevitable, and stretches out the population process of dying. This is seen as a fall in the elderly death rate whilst the process of extending life continues but as the population ages towards the predicted 'physiological' maximum this process will stop and the death rate will appear to rise again.

The fall in death rates across most of the globe is largely due to social and environmental changes, such as good sanitation and potable water. However, medical innovations such as antibiotics, vaccination, and screening programmes have all improved life expectancy. The impact of genetic, stem cell, and nanotechnological advances is yet to be seen; however, the predictably high cost of these therapies is likely to limit their impact on whole populations.

Dependency ratio

The dependency ratio is the number of dependent people in a population against the productive number, those in paid employment. The dependent group consist of the two ends of the age distribution: children and the elderly. The child dependency ratio is the number of children of pre-employment age, usually considered to be 0–14 years, and those in employment aged 15–65.

The elderly is similar, being those over 65 against those in employment. The total dependency ratio is simply the sum of pre-employment and retired totals over the employed number. Increasing the retirement age reduces the ratio whereas extending the period of education has the opposite effect. The higher the ratio the more precarious the state funding of care becomes. In the 1950s across the world there were 12 people working for every potential age-dependent person, this is expected to fall to 4 or lower for most of the developed world by 2050.[6]

This is compounded in the sense that the child dependency ratio described a group with the potential to become productive whereas the elderly ratio can only become more dependent as their care costs rise with advancing age. When there is a degree of equity between the numbers of children and the elderly the balance of dependency is more sustainable than when the elderly outnumber the children. This is precisely what has happened in many developed countries over the last decade (see Fig. 2.4).

The duration of education is extending and in the moderate and highly developed countries it is rarely completed by 14 years of age. Many countries have at least 50 per cent of their young adults in full-time higher education and this may also include a second degree. The costs of providing that education are met in a mixture of ways including state funding, but losing 7 or more years of paid employment is another burden on the remaining workers.

Finally, the actual lifetime productivity of an individual is always less than 100 per cent. It is usually about 70–80 per cent of their total employed lifetime. This is because of time lost from holidays and such life events as serious illness, trauma, childbearing, and caring for elderly relatives.

Migration

Geographical movements of either individuals or larger groups also affect the balance of a population. The reasons for this movement may be environmental, political, or economic. As the ability to travel, often across great distances, is a marker of independence the remaining members of that population become imbalanced towards dependency.

Environmental reasons for migration usually lead to movement of whole family groups or even communities. The less robust the local economy and social infrastructure the more likely it is that a natural event such as flooding or drought can turn into a disaster where famine follows crop failure. Major changes in the landscape will also lead to migration. Volcanic eruptions or inundation of coastal areas following earthquakes may alter previously habitable land into ones where crop cultivation or other forms of agriculture are impossible. Such events usually mark a permanent change in the geographical distribution of a population.

Political activity such as a change in regime or doctrine may dispossess individuals who flee to other countries where they are less likely to be persecuted. Initially these migrants will be affluent and able to mobilize their assets and transfer them to the 'host' country. Later migrants will be independent but much less able to take more than a few belongings with them. This leaves the state with their assets, which in the short term is an advantage, but the loss of workers may be less easily managed in the longer term.

A more devastating political force is open warfare and invasion. This combines migration with the intent to displace another population with an increased death rate in productive members of both populations. Until recently this was effectively a reduction in the male population but as more females enter active military service this may change. As the most commonly utilized cohorts in warfare are males in their late teens and early adulthood they are less likely to have contributed to maintaining the birth rate. The development of long-distance warfare with highly sophisticated remote devices such as drone aircraft does reduce the immediate attrition of infantry but increases the civilian risk.

Economic migration is where people move from a less affluent country or region to one where employment brings higher rewards. This may be controlled by state regulation, either by differentiating potential migrants who will fill skills shortage areas of work, or by limiting the absolute numbers to be admitted. Whether the immediate family of the migrant are also granted entry varies as well. Many economic migrants send a significant proportion of their earnings back home. This process has been used by many of the more developed nations to increase the number of independent workers when their own country's replacement ratio performance has fallen too low.

Impact of demographic changes

As the balance between dependent and working life changes, and in many countries individuals spend years being dependent than actually working (14 years + 30 years (retirement at 65 die at 95) vs 43 (80 per cent of 51)) the cost of delivering comprehensive, state-funded pensions becomes unsustainable and healthcare a challenge. Even where shared healthcare, between individuals and the state, exists, imbalances will become greater and health poverty may become normal for the elderly.

Social changes

The main influences on how an ageing population will lead to changes in the social fabric of a country include the demographic pattern in that country, its existing social structure, and the structure of individual family units.[7]

There are certain assumptions that have been made in other reviews; all or none of them may be true in the fullness of time. One of these is that the fundamental financial stability of a sovereign nation will not change significantly over the foreseeable future if warfare is excluded. Clearly this is no longer true.

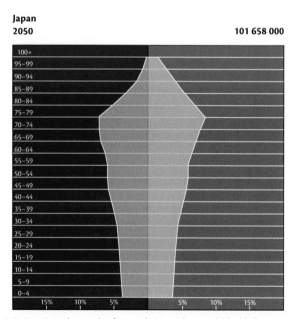

Fig. 2.4 A projected example of a population with a very high elderly bias and minimal birth rate. Note the limited number of the population of working age. Reproduced with kind permission from Martin De Wulf, PopulationPyramid.net. Data from United Nations, Department of Economic and Social Affairs, Population Prospects, http://esa.un.org/wpp/

Retirement

In many parts of the world retirement has not changed and is dependent on other family members being able to support their basic needs. Usually this includes living in the family home and is for a limited number of people as the majority die before they were far beyond active work. In many developed countries, after the start of the last century, a state-funded pension was provided. It was not until 1908 that the United Kingdom passed the 'Old-Age Pensions Act',[8] which for the first time gave a non-contributory pension to those over 70. It was set low to encourage workers to make their own arrangements for their future. To be eligible also meant passing both a means test and a 'character test' and only those of good character were eligible. Others excluded were those in receipt of poor relief, 'lunatics' in asylums, persons sentenced to prison for 10 years after their release, persons convicted of drunkenness (at the discretion of the court), and any person who was guilty of 'habitual failure to work' according to one's ability.[9] A total of nearly 600 000 pensions were awarded in a population of approximately 38 million. There are now approximately 10 million people aged over 65, all of whom are eligible for the state pension, within a population of 62 million.[10] This represents a 16-fold increase in state funding from a population that hasn't even doubled. The more the population ages the more difficult the delivery of this level of funding becomes. It is highly likely that poverty in retirement will face many elders, even in the more developed countries.

Within the demographic changes the concept of using 'productive' age rather than chronological age allows for a more accurate prediction of the actual impact that an ageing population has.[11] Productive age is usually defined as the number of years a person will survive after they become unproductive (unfit to work). This arbitrary number varies from 10 to 15 years. An example would be where a male 65-year-old has a life expectancy of 20 years. Currently this would give 20 years of retirement, whereas if a 15-year productive year calculation were used he would retire at the age of 70. This has at least two effects, firstly, the cost of providing a state pension will move more into balance because individuals will be contributing to a pension scheme for longer and the payments out to them would be for a shorter time. The implementation of laws that allow the raising of the pension age is occurring across many countries to achieve just these aims. Secondly, by identifying a smaller proportion of the population that is dependent, and no longer related to a blanket chronological age, it should be possible for states to target their financial and social support more effectively.[12]

Social effects of migration

The polarization of mobile and younger workers into cities for employment and lifestyle opportunities on one hand and the exodus of retired people into more scenic and tranquil rural retreats on the other hand exist in many countries. This leads to a progressively older and more fragile population living some distance from immediate medical and social care and a need for universal access to integrated medical records.[13,14] In some instances this can pose a serious risk to life;[15] for example, in parts of rural northern Sweden where the average age is now over 80.

This leads to the social isolation of elderly people and often means that their nearest relative capable of providing care and support is several hours' travel away. Indeed in some cases their family is not in the same country.[16] If there is a need to increase support because of an illness or injury the patient will have to be moved away from their home to their families. This may not be suitable, for example, if they live in apartments or houses with several floors and no lift. Access to opticians, chiropodists, or even pharmacies may be limited as may be access to social functions. Progressive mobility limitations and poor rural public transport further their isolation.[17] It is this generation that has been largely unmoved by the advances in computing and the Internet and are suspicious of Internet shopping and banking.[18,19] They have very limited usage of social network sites although Facebook and Skype are being occasionally used.

Healthcare

The challenge for all nations to provide adequate healthcare for their populations has always been immense. The approach towards state provision of healthcare varies across the world. There are many nations who aim to provide a basic level of care to all social groups that is independent of an individual's means. A few provide no state-supported care and leave such provision to either individuals, their families, or paid insurance schemes. Even in those states that do provide a degree of support in many cases little or no provision has been made for the increased longevity, the cost of managing long-term medical conditions, and the loss of state funding because of retirement. This is exacerbated by the speed of change in the availability of medical treatments, which shows no sign of slowing down. The cost of delivering these advances in an equitable way across a nation is daunting.[20]

The changes in the populations outlined here will have greater impact because of the fragmentation of family units that occurred throughout the latter half of the last century. There are far more elderly living alone than before and many have little close family support. The current generation of 50–60-year-olds are much more active users of the Internet and online services including healthcare. The provision of direct access for advice, possible diagnosis, and support from telephone[21] and Internet sites is easily accessible. Search engines such as Google, Yahoo, and others provide almost instantaneous information on the entire range of medical conditions and links to support groups. As this group age and become the most senior generation, in 20–30 years' time, they will still be connected to their families through the Internet and able to shop online without having to maintain a great degree of mobility. What will not change is the increasing need they will have for direct nursing and personal care as their health starts to decline.

These isolated communities will become dependent, to a far greater extent than at present, on secondary care being delivered to them as an extension of the current prehospital care models in place, although largely for trauma at present. Advanced technology (see Chapter 4) will assist, to a degree[22] in identifying the vulnerable elderly and helping them receive the assistance they need. This may simply be a call to check that they are not in trouble up to mobilizing emergency responders to visit them.

Social isolation will also occur within large urban areas[23,24] where the elderly live alone in apartments, but have no contact with their immediate neighbours. The problems of isolation[25] faced by these people may be even worse than that in isolated communities. They are often 'housebound' but are able to manage independently.

Both these groups are at a very high risk of being unable to return home if they are injured or suffer a serious medical or surgical emergency.[26] Their families increasingly have to take up the financial and caregiving role with very limited support from the state.

Conclusion

The challenge facing us is of an ageing population that is more isolated than previous generations. The data from around the world confirms that this will be a major problem to all countries for at least the next 40 years. The impact will affect people of all ages, those entering employment who will need to work for longer before retirement to pay for their pensions, those already working who may have to provide full-time care for their more elderly relatives, and the elderly themselves who may also have to care for their spouses despite being frail themselves.[27,28]

The elderly are more likely to be living independently, but are also more likely to need at least a period of direct personal support after major illnesses and may be unable to return to their home at all. The untoward consequences of medical interventions, including anaesthesia, pain therapy, and intensive care, have to be identified and all possible means of preventing them developed. That this is a very poorly researched area makes the task that much harder.

References

1. US Census Bureau. *Northern European population estimates 2050.* <http://www.census.gov/population/international/data/idb/region.php>.
2. Yashiro N. Aging of the population in Japan and its implications to the other Asian countries. *J Asian Econ.* 1997;8(2):245–261.
3. Bengtsson T, Scott K. Population aging and the future of the welfare state: the example of Sweden. *Popul Dev Rev.* 2011;37(Suppl 1):158–170.
4. Office for National Statistics UK Government. <http://www.ons.gov.uk/ons/index.html>.
5. United States Census Bureaux data. <http://www.census.gov/population/international/data>.
6. UN Population Division. *World population prospects: the 2008 revision* (2009). <http://www.un.org/esa/population/unpop.htm>.
7. Peng X. China's demographic history and future challenges. *Science.* 2011;333(6042):581–587.
8. *Old Age Pensions Act 1908.* UK Houses of Parliament.
9. Macnicol J. *The Politics of Retirement in Britain, 1908–1948* (pp. 157–158). Cambridge: Cambridge University Press, 1998

10. Office for National Statistics. *2011 census: population estimates for England and Wales.* <http://www.ons.gov.uk/ons/interactive/vp2-2011-census-comparator/index.html> (accessed 14 January 2013).
11. Rethinking age and aging. *Popul Bull.* 2008;63(4):1–16. <http://www.prb.org/pdf08/63.4aging.pdf>.
12. Miller T. Increasing longevity and Medicare expenditures. *Demography.* 2001;38(2):215–226.
13. Chen TL, Chung YF, Lin FY. Deployment of secure mobile agents for medical information systems. *J Med Syst.* 2012;36(4):2493–2503.
14. Devlin RA, Sarma S, Zhang Q. The role of supplemental coverage in a universal health insurance system: some Canadian evidence. *Health Policy.* 2011;100(1):81–90.
15. Diaz JJ, Jr, Norris P, Gunter O, Collier B, Riordan W, Morris JA, Jr. Triaging to a regional acute care surgery center: distance is critical. *J Trauma.* 2011;70(1):116–119.
16. Dhar VE. Transnational caregiving: part 1, caring for family relations across nations. *Care Manag J.* 2011;12(2):60–71.
17. Safaei J. A ride to care—a non-emergency medical transportation service in rural British Columbia. *Rural Remote Health.* 2011;11:1637.
18. Choi N. Relationship between health service use and health information technology use among older adults: analysis of the US National Health Interview Survey. *J Med Internet Res.* 2011;13(2):e33.
19. Eek M, Wressle E. Everyday technology and 86-year-old individuals in Sweden. *Disabil Rehabil Assist Technol.* 2011;6(2):123–129.
20. van der Aa NG, Kommer GJ, van Montfoort JE, Versteegh JF. Demographic projections of future pharmaceutical consumption in the Netherlands. *Water Sci Technol.* 2011;63(4):825–831.
21. Dickens AP, Richards SH, Hawton A, *et al.* An evaluation of the effectiveness of a community mentoring service for socially isolated older people: a controlled trial. *BMC Public Health.* 2011;11:218.
22. Frisardi V, Imbimbo BP. Gerontechnology for demented patients: smart homes for smart aging. *J Alzheimer's Dis.* 2011;23(1):143–146.
23. Cress ME, Orini S, Kinsler L. Living environment and mobility of older adults. *Gerontology.* 2011;57(3):287–294.
24. Iecovich E, Jacobs JM, Stessman J. Loneliness, social networks, and mortality: 18 years of follow-up. *Int J Aging Hum Dev.* 2011;72(3):243–263.
25. Ramic E, Pranjic N, Batic-Mujanovic O, Karic E, Alibasic E, Alic A. The effect of loneliness on malnutrition in elderly population. *Medicinski arhiv.* 2011;65(2):92–95.
26. Carter MW, Porell FW. The effect of sentinel injury on Medicare expenditures over time. *J Am Geriatr Soc.* 2011;59(3):406–416.
27. Noel-Miller CM. Partner caregiving in older cohabiting couples. *J Gerontol B Psychol Sci Soc Sci.* 2011;66(3):341–353.
28. Guberman N, Lavoie JP, Blein L, Olazabal I. Baby boom caregivers: care in the age of individualization. *Gerontologist.* 2012;52(2):210–218.

CHAPTER 3

Drug mechanisms in the elderly

Ipek Yalcin Christmann and Oya Yalcin Cok

Introduction

Over the past few decades, the anaesthetic management of elderly patients has been a new and significant field for research and clinical practice. Nearly all of the main issues in the perioperative management of elderly patients are the consequences of age-related physiological alterations. These physiological changes have a remarkable impact on both the pharmacokinetics and pharmacodynamics of anaesthetics resulting in significant responses in the elderly patients. Unfortunately, elderly patients have been rarely included in studies on drug mechanisms and effects.[1] Specific information on individual drugs has been limited in the elderly population. However, a thorough knowledge of 'ageing' pharmacology of anaesthetics may help anaesthetists provide safe anaesthetic management and avoid adverse events in elderly patients.

Age-related changes in the pharmacology of drugs

Ageing interferes with every aspect of the 'drug–body' interaction.[2] Drug metabolism, sensitivity, clinical and adverse effects, and drug interactions are all altered variously and specifically for each drug in individuals of advanced age.

Pharmacokinetics in the elderly

Pharmacokinetics describes the relationship between dose and concentration of a drug versus time. Briefly, it refers to what the body does to the drug, in other words, to 'the fate' of drug in the body. Pharmacokinetics of anaesthetics is largely altered by age-related physiological changes in the organ systems. Distribution, biotransformation (metabolism), and elimination are the most affected steps of pharmacokinetics of anaesthetic drugs in the elderly.

Distribution

The changes in body composition associated with age such as decreased lean body mass, increased body fat, and decreased total body water may interfere with the anaesthetic drug distribution in the central and peripheral compartments.[3–5] Since most drugs used in anaesthesia are lipid-soluble, the increased distribution volume due to increased body fat by age reduces the plasma concentration of lipophilic drugs and prolongs their elimination half-life.[6] Indeed, the increase in adipose tissue acts as a depot for these agents. Decreased muscle mass and body water reduces the distribution volume for water-soluble drugs leading to higher plasma concentrations in the elderly.

Changes in the respiratory system by age become more important especially for the uptake and distribution of volatile agents in the elderly. Loss of recoil forces and altered surfactant production increase the number of early collapsed small airways and change the distribution volume of gases in the lungs with advanced age. This results in increased ventilation in the apices and increased perfusion of bases leading to a ventilation–perfusion imbalance.[7] Other age-related changes in the respiratory system include an increase in anatomic dead space and a reduction of the diffusing capacity of the lung which may lead to a reduction in volatile agent transport and a decrease in inspired anaesthetic concentration. Cerebral weight and blood flow are also reduced in the elderly, which in turn may decrease the distribution rate of anaesthetic drugs to the central nervous system.

Changes in plasma binding proteins with age also affect the distribution of anaesthetic agents in elderly patients. The effects of altered protein binding depend on the concentration of unbound drugs and the type of protein, albumin or α_1-acid-glycoprotein. Most anaesthetics are acidic and bind to serum albumin. The concentration of albumin decreases in elderly patients resulting in an increase in unbound amount of anaesthetics such as benzodiazepines, barbiturates, and opioids.[8–10] Some chronic disease such as cardiac and renal failure can also decrease albumin levels. Decreased protein binding increases the available amount of drug for interaction with target receptors and necessitates the reduction of the dose administered.[11] Basic drugs bind to α_1-acid-glycoprotein and the level of this protein remains unaffected or increases with age.[11] If the level of α_1-acid-glycoprotein increases, this leads to a decrease in unbound level of agents and requires the use of higher doses in elderly patients.

Biotransformation (metabolism)

Biotransformation of anaesthetic drugs largely depends on enzyme reactions that occur in the liver. These reactions are classified as phase I functionalization (by oxidation or hydrolysis) and phase II biosynthetic conjugation reactions. Phase I reactions introduce functional groups to the parent compound (oxidations, reductions, and hydrolytic reactions). The cytochrome P450 enzyme system of phase I reactions is the main system responsible for the metabolism of many anaesthetics, such as inhaled agents.[12] Phase I reactions generally result in the loss of pharmacological activity. Phase II conjugation reactions lead to the formation of covalent links between a functional group on the parent compound or phase I metabolite and glucuronic acid, sulphate, glutathione, amino acids, or acetate. Phase II reactions make compounds more water-soluble and increase the excretion into urine or bile.

A decline in liver mass occurs with advanced age as well as a corresponding decrease in hepatic blood flow and intrinsic hepatic capacity in the elderly.[13] These changes reduce the rate of biotransformation and clearance of most intravenous anaesthetics.[14,15] Decreased biotransformation and clearance prolong the duration of action of anaesthetics and decrease maintenance dose requirements. Diseases related to liver insufficiency, such as cirrhosis worsen these physiological changes. In the elderly, cytochrome P450-mediated phase I reactions are more likely to be impaired than phase II metabolism influencing the pharmacokinetics of many anaesthetic drugs.

Elimination

Physiological renal changes in the elderly may interfere with the elimination of some anaesthetics which are mainly dependent on renal excretion. Renal excretion is decreased in about two-thirds of elderly subjects by a decline in glomerular filtration rate as a result of renal parenchyma loss.[16] Comorbid factors such as hypertension and coronary artery disease may also account for a decline in kidney function. Furthermore, renal blood flow decreases by approximately 10 per cent each decade. The decrease in renal clearance will obviously increase concentrations and delay the offset of action of those anaesthetics that depend on renal excretion. Reduced elimination causes drug accumulation which may lead to toxicity.

Pharmacodynamics in the elderly

Pharmacodynamics describes the relationship between the concentration and the effect of a drug versus time. Pharmacodynamics refers to how the drug affects the body and may also be altered due to age-related structural and functional changes in the target organ system.

The central and peripheral nervous systems are the actual effect-sites for many anaesthetic drugs. The changes that occur with age may affect the neuronal composition of the central nervous system, the receptors, or the signal transduction system. Consequently, age-related changes in the nervous system have an important impact on anaesthetic management. In elderly patients, brain weight is reduced by around 20 per cent, in which neuronal loss and changes in dendritic networks are observed.[17] Anaesthesia may also provoke some alterations especially in specific cognitive domains where ageing-related neuronal changes occur.[18] Spinal neuronal loss, demyelinization, and a slower peripheral conduction velocity may affect the response to anaesthetic agents when administered to the spinal cord or peripheral nerves. Furthermore, the autonomic nervous system is altered with age resulting in poor compensation of cardiovascular and nervous system effects of anaesthetics. Skeletal muscle innervation also decreases along with the loss of motor units.[1]

Ageing affects the number and function of receptors and synthesis of neurotransmitters in the central nervous system.[1] The number of gamma-aminobutyric acid (GABA) neurons and $GABA_A$ receptors decrease leading to a compensatory upregulation of inhibitory function in the elderly.[19,20] These alterations may be responsible for the high sensitivity of elderly patients to anaesthetics. On the other hand, the number of opioid receptors as well as their affinity changes in aged animals. Mu opioid receptor density and kappa opioid binding affinity decrease while delta opioid receptor affinity remains unaffected by age.[21–24] Ageing reduces N-methyl-D-aspartate (NMDA) receptor complex binding sites in the basal ganglia of ageing human brain.[25] A decline in muscarinic and nicotinic receptors has also been shown in aged humans.[26] The decreases in nicotinic receptors may contribute to the cognitive impairments observed in the elderly.[27,28]

Response to drugs in the elderly may also be modified due to changes in homeostatic mechanisms such as postural control, orthostatic circulatory responses, thermoregulation, visceral muscle function, neuroendocrine stability, and cognitive function. Perioperative stress may lead to excessive response to drug effects due to inadequate compensation mechanisms with decreased functional reserve.[1]

Pharmacokinetic and pharmacodynamic modelling in the elderly

Recent studies suggest that age is a significant co-variable that should be considered in the pharmacokinetic and pharmacodynamic modelling of any drug.[29,30] An integrated pharmacokinetic and pharmacodynamic approach may provide the appropriate selection of the right drug with the optimal dosage in elderly patients. A multi-compartment model is frequently used to explain the pharmacokinetic relationship between dose and plasma concentration. According to this method, the body is divided into three virtual compartments: the central compartment (V1) where the drug is administered, the small peripheral compartment (V2) with fast redistribution, and the large peripheral compartment (V3) with slow redistribution. In the elderly, V1 and V2 are expected to be smaller because of decreased total body water and decreased lean body mass respectively, and V3 to be larger because of increased body fat. The critical pharmacokinetic parameters in the elderly are the volume of these compartments, redistribution rate constant, metabolic rate constant, and clearance which may largely be affected by age-related physiological alterations.

When anaesthetics are considered, Emax and EC50 or MAC are the parameters of interest for the pharmacodynamic studies of these drugs. Emax is the maximum response achieved by an agonist and also refers to 'drug efficacy'. EC50 is the drug concentration at which 50 per cent of Emax is achieved and also refers to 'drug potency' for intravenous anaesthetic drugs. MAC, minimum alveolar concentration, is the analogous terminology to EC50 for inhalational anaesthetic agents. These clinically important parameters are also subject to alterations initiated by advancing age.

Age-related changes in the pharmacology of specific anaesthetics

The impact of advanced age on anaesthetic management should be considered with the continuously increasing number of elderly patients who require surgery and, as a result, anaesthesia. When anaesthetics are considered, many drugs available in many different combinations via many administration routes should be reviewed in relation with the physiological and pathophysiological status of an elderly patient. Old age alters the basic pharmacology of anaesthetic drugs. Furthermore it affects target-organ responses and exaggerates the side effects by minimizing physiological compensation mechanisms for surgical stress. The challenge is the optimization of anaesthetic drug dosing in consideration with possible interactions with aged body metabolism and altered physiology. In the following sections, age-related alterations in the pharmacology of specific anaesthetics will be discussed.

Inhaled anaesthetics

Age affects the pharmacodynamics of all inhaled anaesthetic agents. The MAC (Minimum alveolar concentration) of volatile anaesthetics decreases with age.[31] A meta-analysis by Mapleson[32] revealed that semi-logarithmic plots of MAC against age (age ≥ 1 year) for all inhalational agents were linear and parallel and the formulated alteration of MAC by age (MAC_{age}) is as follows:

$$MAC_{age} = MAC_{40} \times 10^{-0.00269(age - 40)}$$

MAC_{age}, MAC for a given age; MAC_{40}, MAC at 40 years.[32]

This formula applies to current volatile anaesthetics (Table 3.1). A decrease by 5–6 per cent in MAC and also similarly in MAC-awake, for each decade of ageing results in a potency increase by approximately 6 per cent for each decade.[31,33] This increase in potency may also be related to modifications in target receptors and neurotransmitters which provides the effects of inhaled anaesthetics in the central nervous system.

Some of the physiological respiratory changes with age, such as a small reduction in minute ventilation and a small increase in functional residual capacity, have minimal effects on the pharmacokinetics of volatile anaesthetics. Normally, alveolar anaesthetic concentration increases in an inverse proportion to the solubility of the anaesthetic when administered.[34] However, an increased ventilation–perfusion mismatch and a decreased cerebral blood flow with advanced age will probably reduce the induction speed by reducing arterial inspired concentration of the volatile anaesthetic and the perfusion of the target organ when less lipid-soluble agents are considered. This effect may be modulated by a decrease in cardiac output when more lipid-soluble volatile anaesthetics such as halothane and enflurane are used since the increased alveolar concentration due to decreased cardiac output facilitates achieving a sufficient inspired arterial concentration of these agents for clinical effects. This difference related to lipid solubility may ensure more titrability and less adverse effects due to a rapid induction in favour of less lipid-soluble volatile agents in the elderly population. A higher distribution volume and lower hepatic function in the elderly may also prolong recovery after induction and maintenance with volatile agents.[34] Ageing significantly decreases the required concentration of inhaled anaesthetics to suppress cerebral electrical activity in order to achieve a desired depth of anaesthesia. Decrease in MAC for a particular bispectral index value in the elderly has been compatible with the decrease in MAC and MAC_{awake} by age.[35] Regarding all inhaled anaesthetics, dose reduction due to increased sensitivity should always be considered in elderly patients.

Halothane

Halothane is an example of a more lipid-soluble inhalation anaesthetic and theoretically provides a rapid induction with more risk of adverse events in comparison to less lipid-soluble agents in the elderly.[36] Decreased hepatic function due to age decreases its metabolism. Halothane co-administered with nitrous oxide also impairs peripheral blood flow in the elderly.[37]

Enflurane

Enflurane exhibits similar age-related alterations to halothane in pharmacodynamics and pharmacokinetics. Furthermore, a physiological closed-circuit anaesthesia model of enflurane proved that blood gas solubility coefficients of enflurane decreased by 0.6 for each decade after 60 year, recalibrating with age-related solubility coefficients improved model predictions to align to the real pharmacology of enflurane in elderly patients.[38,39]

Isoflurane

Isoflurane has less lipid solubility providing easier titration for induction. End-tidal and arterial partial pressures of isoflurane are comparable in the elderly to those of younger patients.[40] Isoflurane with nitrous oxide also impairs peripheral blood flow in the elderly whereas it has no impact on younger patients.[37] Fig. 3.1 summarizes age-related MAC changes and corresponding end-expired isoflurane concentration when using oxygen 100 per cent, nitrous oxide 50 and 67 per cent in oxygen.

Table 3.1 Age-related MAC values for halothane, enflurane, isoflurane, sevoflurane, and desflurane

Age	$10^{-0.00269(age - 40)}$	MAC_{age}[a]				
		Halothane	Enflurane	Isoflurane	Sevoflurane	Desflurane
40	1.00	0.75[b]	1.63[b]	1.17[b]	1.80[b]	6.6[b]
50	0.94	0.70	1.53	1.10	1.69	6.20
60	0.88	0.66	1.43	1.03	1.58	5.81
70	0.83	0.62	1.35	0.97	1.49	5.48
80	0.78	0.59	1.27	0.91	1.40	5.15
90	0.73	0.55	1.19	0.85	1.31	4.82
100	0.69	0.52	1.12	0.81	1.24	4.55

[a] MAC_{age} is calculated according to the formula; $MAC_{age} = MAC_{40} \times 10^{-0.00269(age - 40)}$ where MAC_{age} represents MAC for a given age and MAC_{40} represents MAC at 40years.[32]

[b] MAC_{40} values are obtained from the article by Nickalls and Mapleson.[33]

Data from Mapleson WW (1996) Effect of age on MAC in humans: a meta-analysis. Br J Anaesth, 76(2), 179–85, and Nickalls RWD, Mapleson WW (2003) Age-related iso–MAC charts for isoflurane, sevoflurane and desflurane in man. *Br J Anaesth*, 91(2), 170–4.

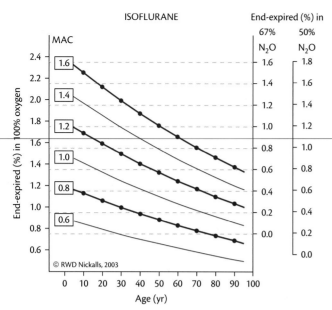

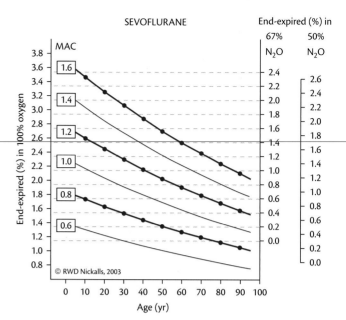

Fig. 3.1 Age-related MAC changes and corresponding end-expired isoflurane concentration when using oxygen 100 per cent, nitrous oxide 50 and 67 per cent in oxygen. Reproduced from Nickalls RWD and Mapleson WW, 'Age-related iso-MAC charts for isoflurane, sevoflurane and desflurane in man', *British Journal of Anaesthesia*, 2003, 91, 2, pp. 170–174, by permission of Oxford University Press and The Board of Management and Trustees of the British Journal of Anaesthesia.

Fig. 3.2 Age-related MAC changes and corresponding end-expired sevoflurane concentration when using oxygen 100 per cent, nitrous oxide 50 and 67 per cent in oxygen. Reproduced from Nickalls RWD and Mapleson WW, 'Age-related iso-MAC charts for isoflurane, sevoflurane and desflurane in man', *British Journal of Anaesthesia*, 2003, 91, 2, pp. 170–174, by permission of Oxford University Press and The Board of Management and Trustees of the British Journal of Anaesthesia.

Sevoflurane

Sevoflurane with a lower solubility has the advantage of a more controlled induction. End-tidal brain equilibration is prolonged in the elderly, resulting in the late onset of effect on bispectral index changes.[41,42] Fig. 3.2 summarizes age-related MAC changes and corresponding end-expired sevoflurane concentration when using oxygen 100 per cent, nitrous oxide 50 and 67 per cent in oxygen.

Desflurane

Despite its molecular structural similarity to isoflurane, desflurane has unique physical properties that provide it with the advantage of very low blood-gas solubility resulting in a very rapid induction and emergence that is also seen in the elderly population.[43] Desflurane has been reported to provide faster recovery than sevoflurane at equivalent MAC values adjusted for the elderly however, recovery of cognitive functions was comparable with both anaesthetics.[44] Fig. 3.3 summarizes age-related MAC changes and corresponding end-expired desflurane concentration when using oxygen 100 per cent, nitrous oxide 50 and 67 per cent in oxygen.

Nitrous oxide

An alteration in MAC of nitrous oxide is parallel to other inhaled anaesthetics in the elderly. A decline in MAC by 6 per cent for each decade also applies to nitrous oxide.[32] However, the metabolism of this agent has no impact on altered pharmacokinetics in the elderly since it is not metabolized in humans.

Xenon

Xenon is an inert gas which has anaesthetic properties under normobaric conditions. It is reported to have advantages of fast emergence from anaesthesia, cardiovascular and haemodynamic stability, and no metabolism in the body.[45] Interestingly, MAC of xenon has been reported to be higher in men than women.[45] A reduction of approximately 4 per cent in MAC for each decade should be considered in the elderly.[33]

Non-volatile anaesthetics

Barbiturates

Thiopentone

The pharmacokinetic alterations due to advanced age are the main factor in dose reduction requirements during thiopentone administration in the elderly. The reduced volume of distribution with age

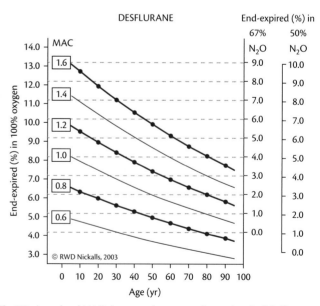

Fig. 3.3 Age-related MAC changes and corresponding end-expired desflurane concentration when using oxygen 100 per cent, nitrous oxide 50 and 67 per cent in oxygen. Reproduced from Nickalls RWD and Mapleson WW, 'Age-related iso-MAC charts for isoflurane, sevoflurane and desflurane in man', *British Journal of Anaesthesia*, 2003, 91, 2, pp. 170–174, by permission of Oxford University Press and The Board of Management and Trustees of the British Journal of Anaesthesia.

causes higher concentrations of thiopentone, since redistribution terminates the effect of a single bolus dose of the drug instead of hepatic metabolism.[46] However, metabolism by hepatic enzymes and plasma protein binding significantly affects elimination following repeated bolus doses or continuous infusion of thiopentone.[46] A 20 per cent reduction in the infusion rate is recommended to avoid a prolonged recovery.[47] The pharmacodynamics of thiopentone does not seem to change with advanced age.[47] Thiopentone provides a faster onset and better haemodynamic stability in comparison to propofol in the elderly.[48]

Methohexitone

The pharmacodynamics of methohexitone remains unchanged with ageing. However, reduced hepatic blood flow with age will decrease its elimination leading to a prolonged recovery in the elderly.[46]

Propofol

A dose reduction for propofol has been recommended in the elderly. This is due to the reduced size of the rapidly equilibrating peripheral compartment and decreased intercompartmental clearance. However, it is interesting to note that central compartment clearance and metabolism of propofol is not delayed with age. These changes increase initial blood concentration of propofol by 20 per cent in elderly patients.[49,50] Because of the interactions between pharmacokinetic and pharmacodynamic alterations for propofol with advanced age, one should anticipate an increased potency and a rapid rise and decrease in blood concentrations when administering propofol in the elderly. This may be interpreted as elderly patients requiring smaller drug doses to achieve and maintain the same level of propofol drug effect in comparison to younger patients. Due to decreased clearance and the increased intrinsic sensitivity of the drug in elderly patients, a reduction of approximately 40–50 per cent of a standard dose of propofol would be reasonable to obtain the same effects as in young patients.[50] Furthermore, female elderly patients require a 10 per cent larger dose of propofol than male patients to achieve the same blood propofol concentration.[51] The context-sensitive half-time of propofol is also affected by age and duration of infusion. A prolonged duration of propofol infusion in the elderly may result in an excessively longer context-sensitive half-time than young patients. Ageing also prolongs recovery of psychomotor functions following propofol administration.[52,53] Since ageing is a very important determinant of dose adjustments in propofol, target controlled infusion devices should provide a model using age as a covariate to administer appropriate doses for target controlled infusions of propofol in the elderly.

Etomidate

Etomidate provides haemodynamic stability. Etomidate induction doses should be halved in the elderly, since the initial volume of distribution and clearance are both decreased with age. However, sensitivity and maximal frequency slowing of the electroencephalogram (EEG) remain unchanged with advanced age.[54] Etomidate may be a safe alternative for procedural sedation in the elderly providing similar conditions and complications as in the general adult population.[55]

Benzodiazepines

Ageing impairs both pharmacokinetics and pharmacodynamics of benzodiazepines. Patients with advanced age are more sensitive to the pharmacological effects of benzodiazepines requiring significant dose adjustments.

Diazepam

Age does not influence absolute bioavailability of diazepam via various administration routes.[56] Additionally, possible enzyme induction, reduced hepatic perfusion, and clearance in the elderly may lead to accumulation of the more potent hydroxylation end-product of diazepam, desmethyldiazepam, resulting in prolonged clinical effects.[10,57]

Midazolam

Midazolam requirements are reduced by 25–75 per cent in the elderly, since both pharmacodynamics and pharmacokinetics of midazolam are altered by advanced age. EC50 for loss of response to verbal comment in elderly patients is reduced to approximately one-third of the amount required in younger patients, indicating higher sensitivity to midazolam by advanced age.[58] Decreased enzyme activity, hepatic perfusion, and an approximately 30 per cent reduction in the clearance of midazolam lead to a decrease in the formation of less potent hydroxylation end-products of midazolam prolonging offset time and clinical effects in the elderly.[59] This reflects an increased context-sensitive half-time of midazolam by twofold with advanced age. However, pharmacokinetic changes are not sufficient to explain the decreased dose requirement with midazolam. The lower doses needed in elderly patients are mainly due to pharmacodynamic changes.[60–63]

Lorazepam

Ageing decreases the volume of distribution and the total clearance of lorazepam in the elderly patients in comparison to the younger population.[64] However, the prolonged duration of clinical effects of lorazepam depends on its higher receptor affinity in the central nervous system in the elderly.[46] The results are compatible with previous evidence of increased 'sensitivity' to benzodiazepines in the elderly and suggest that a lower starting dose of lorazepam would be appropriate for older recipients.[65]

Benzodiazepine receptor antagonist
Flumazenil

Absorption, disposition, and bioavailability of flumazenil in the elderly are similar to younger patients.[66]

Ketamine

Available data about pharmacokinetics and pharmacodynamics of ketamine specific to the elderly population is limited. The reduction in the hepatic extraction ratio and microsomal enzymes may decrease the clearance and prolong clinical effects in the elderly. Structural changes in N-methyl-D-aspartate (NMDA) type glutamate receptors and increased central nervous system sensitivity may require administration of lower doses in older patients.[3]

Opioids

Managing opioid drugs in the elderly requires a thorough understanding of their unique mechanisms of action and side effect profiles. Each opioid via the various administration routes causes exaggerated physiological responses in the elderly population.[67] Although the available data about pharmacokinetics and pharmacodynamics of opioids in advanced age are limited, pharmacodynamic alterations in advanced age are more responsible for increased sensitivity to opioids than pharmacokinetic alterations in the elderly. Ageing affects opioid pharmacokinetics via altered distribution volumes and decreased liver and renal blood flows.[68] Pharmacodynamics is affected by changes in neurotransmitter synthesis and receptor site modifications with age.[69] Dose reduction is a general recommendation when elderly patients are considered.

Morphine

Dose reduction for morphine is required in the elderly since the clearance is decreased by 50 per cent with advanced age causing prolonged clinical effects and increased side effects.[70] The half-life of morphine is prolonged by approximately 50 per cent in comparison to younger adults.[71] Furthermore, clearance of morphine-6-glucuronide, an active metabolite of morphine, is dependent on renal excretion and slows down due to age-related physiological changes in the renal system. Also increased sensitivity to morphine in the elderly is responsible for increased ventilatory complications.[72] Another issue is the significant immunosuppressant effect of morphine via μ-opioid receptors which may impair the already decreased responsiveness of the immune system of elderly patients.[71]

Fentanyl

The pharmacokinetics of fentanyl in the elderly remains unchanged. Also, the blood effect-site equilibration of fentanyl does not alter by age and fentanyl has no active metabolite to accumulate in the aged body.[3] However, alterations in the pharmacodynamics of the drug with advanced age are responsible for the increased sensitivity and potency in the elderly. Dose requirements are halved in the elderly in comparison to younger patients to achieve similar clinical effects. In addition, fentanyl has immunosuppressive properties that are augmented in the elderly.[71]

Alfentanil

Age does not significantly affect the pharmacokinetics of alfentanil, but pharmacodynamics is altered in the elderly.[73] A decrease of 50 per cent in the dose administered to elderly patients is recommended in comparison to younger patients in accordance with a 50 per cent decrease in the ED50 and the increased potency of the drug by age.[73,74]

Sufentanil

Data on the pharmacodynamics and pharmacokinetics of sufentanil suggest that a very small decrease in the volume of the central compartment along with unaffected distribution and clearance may necessitate a dose adjustment for the initial few minutes in the elderly.[75–77] The difference in dose requirement between young and elderly patients has a pharmacodynamic basis. Sufentanil is roughly twice as potent in elderly patients as it is in younger patients, due to an increased brain sensitivity to opioids.[75,77]

Remifentanil

The pharmacokinetics and pharmacodynamics of remifentanil, the ultra-short-acting opioid, are affected by advancing age.[78] The central compartment and metabolic clearance is reduced by approximately 30 per cent, EC50 is decreased by 50 per cent with advanced age, and the time to reach the peak effect-site concentration is prolonged. The onset of the clinical effect of the drug is slower and the recovery is more variable in the aged population. Consequently, a bolus dose of remifentanil should be reduced by 50 per cent of the dose used in a young patient and maintenance infusion should be adjusted accordingly to achieve similar clinical effects.[78] If an adjusted dosing regimen is not used for advanced age, a more rapid

EEG activity suppression, more profound respiratory and haemodynamic depression, and a delayed recovery should be expected in the elderly.[79]

Tramadol

Tramadol is a centrally acting synthetic analgesic effective by binding to the μ-opioid receptor and by inhibiting noradrenaline and serotonin re-uptake. The half-life of tramadol is longer after the age of 75 in comparison to younger adults.[80] Dose reduction and increased duration between repeated doses has been recommended. Tramadol provides the advantage of less respiratory depression in analgesic doses. However, its use is a risk factor for postoperative delirium in the elderly.[81]

Meperidine (pethidine)

Metabolic clearance and terminal elimination half-time of this drug remain unchanged by age; however, the increased free fraction due to decreased protein binding may cause more profound clinical effects in the elderly. Another issue is accumulation of its active metabolite, normeperidine, resulting in serious central nervous system toxicity due to decreased renal function in the elderly.[82]

Neuromuscular blocking agents

The elderly population is more sensitive to the effects of neuromuscular blocking agents due to age-related alterations mainly in pharmacokinetics. Reduced distribution volume and clearance by age result in an increase in blood drug concentrations. When hydrolysis by plasma cholinesterase is responsible for the elimination of muscle relaxants such as succinylcholine and mivacurium, an age-related decrease in this enzyme level causes a longer duration of action.[83] For aminosteroid-type non-depolarizing neuromuscular agents whose elimination is dependent on hepatic and renal function and blood flow, age-related reductions in these parameters prolong the duration of action and delay the recovery in elderly patients. Age is not a covariate causing longer duration of action for muscle relaxants, such as atracurium and cisatracurium whose clearance occurs by Hofmann degradation. Decreased muscle blood flow and altered number of acetylcholine receptors due to reduced physical activity in the elderly may also delay the onset of action. Longer dosing intervals, fewer repeat doses, preference of short-acting neuromuscular agents and neuromuscular monitoring may help tailor the use of these agents in the elderly.

Depolarizing neuromuscular blocking agents

Succinylcholine

The level of plasma cholinesterase is decreased in the elderly.[83] Frail elderly patients have more impaired plasma cholinesterase levels than fit older patients.[84] Thus less hydrolysis of succinylcholine resulting in longer duration of action should be expected when it is administered to elderly patients.

Non-depolarizing neuromuscular blocking agents

Aminosteroids

Steroid-type non-depolarizing neuromuscular blocking agents are dependent on organ-based elimination and longer duration of action with these agents is expected in the elderly. Furthermore, they appear to have greater variability of duration of action in the elderly when administered during inhalation anaesthesia.[85]

Pancuronium

Although a decrease in clearance of pancuronium is expected due to the decrease in renal function with age, the results of the studies are controversial.[86] However, pancuronium is far from being the best choice since a higher incidence of residual neuromuscular block and pulmonary complications is reported with this agent in the elderly.[87]

Vecuronium

Due to decreased distribution volume and plasma clearance by age, the dose of vecuronium required to provide a stable level of blockade should be reduced by about 30 per cent in the elderly in comparison to younger population.[86] Also recovery time is expected to be 30 per cent longer in geriatric patients.[88] The main mechanism in the prolonged effect of vecuronium is decreased elimination due to decreased hepatic and renal blood flow.[89]

Rocuronium

Onset time of rocuronium is similar to that in younger patients but the duration of action is prolonged due to pharmacokinetic alterations such as decreased distribution volume and plasma clearance when rocuronium is administered. Also, decreased renal function and decreased cardiac output contribute to these effects in the elderly.[90,91]

Benzylisoquinolones

Atracurium

The pharmacodynamics and pharmacokinetics of atracurium are unchanged with age.[92] The dose and dose intervals of atracurium need not be adjusted in the elderly. Atracurium has less variability of duration of action in the elderly when used with inhaled anaesthetics when compared to an aminosteroid-type neuromuscular agent.[85,93]

Cisatracurium

Pharmacokinetic properties of cisatracurium are similar to those of atracurium except for a delayed onset of action observed with this drug in the elderly. The delayed onset is due to slower biophase equilibration.[94,95] However variability in the offset of action of cisatracurium is less in the elderly in comparison to an aminosteroid-type neuromuscular agent.[96]

Mivacurium

Clearance of mivacurium is reduced due to decreased plasma cholinesterase activity with advanced age.[97] Duration of action is prolonged by 20–30 per cent and the infusion requirement is decreased accordingly.[98]

Neuromuscular blocking agent antagonists

Reversal of residual neuromuscular blockade is an important issue in clinical practice of anaesthesia, since elderly patients are more vulnerable to complications associated with the delay in the recovery of ventilation and voluntary movements.

Anticholinesterase drugs

Age affects the pharmacology of anticholinesterase drugs used in anaesthesia practice. Neostigmine and pyridostigmine antagonize the neuromuscular blocking effect by longer-lasting carbamylation of esterase sites whereas edrophonium binds to cholinesterase active sites transiently. The most widely used anticholinesterase for antagonism of neuromuscular blockade is neostigmine. The initial volume of distribution of neostigmine is larger in the elderly than younger subjects. The duration of action of neostigmine is also prolonged.[99] Altered pharmacokinetics of pyridostigmine mainly depends on a decreased plasma clearance due to decreased renal function with ageing rather than distribution volume or elimination half-life. Pyridostigmine has a prolonged duration of action in the elderly.[100] However, the duration of action of edrophonium remains unchanged with ageing.[101,102] Neostigmine and pyridostigmine with a more prolonged duration of action in comparison to edrophonium should be preferred for elderly patients since neuromuscular blocking agents already have a prolonged duration of action with advanced age.[99]

Sugammadex

Sugammadex is a modified g-cyclodextrin selectively binding the aminosteroidal relaxant agents. The subsequently formed complex is subject to the pharmacokinetics and pharmacodynamics of sugammadex which are both altered with age. Sugammadex may bind to rocuronium and vecuronium, and to a lesser degree pancuronium.[103,104] Recovery from rocuronium-induced neuromuscular blockade is significantly longer in older than younger patients.[105] The late onset of action may be the result of reduced cardiac output and muscle blood flow in the elderly.[105] The muscle relaxant sugammadex complex is primarily excreted by the kidneys resulting in a delayed clearance and an increased effective half-life due to reduced renal function in the elderly. Clearance is halved and effective half life of sugammadex is nearly doubled in patients older than 75 years.[106] However, data about dose adjustment to improve late onset or delayed clearance is not available.

Local anaesthetics

Ageing affects the pharmacokinetics of local anaesthetics. Local absorption of local anaesthetics limits the action of drugs where therapeutic effects occur. Age-related physiological changes in the injection site may include demyelination, impairment in connective tissue or anatomical deterioration in spinal structures such as reduction in cerebrospinal fluid changes, or impaired epidural resistance and compliance. All these alterations may initiate influencing 'the fate' of local anaesthetics at the initial effect-site in the elderly. Absorption from the site of delivery to systemic circulation slows down with advanced age.[3] After local and systemic absorption, local anaesthetics tend to accumulate in highly perfused organs under normal physiological circumstances. Lung tissue rapidly extracts local anaesthetics and lowers blood concentration of these drugs and normally skeletal muscle acts as a reservoir for local anaesthetics after administration. However, all of these steps of distribution may be impaired due to decreased organ perfusion with advanced age. Equally, biotransformation of the local anaesthetic whether dependent on hydrolysis by pseudocholinesterases or enzymatic degradation in the liver is subject to physiological changes with age. Decreased enzyme levels and decreased hepatic blood flow by advanced age affect the degree of metabolism of these agents. These alterations in pharmacokinetics in the elderly may result in higher blood concentrations and longer half-lives of the drugs. However, the relationship between age and pharmacodynamics of local anaesthetics is not very clear. Altered sensitivity to local anaesthetics may be expected due to structural and functional changes in both the central and peripheral nervous systems and response to local anaesthetics may be more intense in the elderly. Consequently, duration and intensity of blockade increases with ageing, thus lower doses of local anaesthetics are required for the initial effect and maintenance infusions to avoid increased risk of adverse effects.[3]

Lidocaine

Lidocaine is the least lipophilic agent in common use and a larger fraction of this drug is absorbed into systemic circulation during the fast initial absorption phase.[107] Excessive elimination by hepatic first-pass metabolism may be reduced due to decreased cardiac output and decreased hepatic blood flow compartment while ageing. Accumulation of lidocaine in the central compartment increases serum concentration of lidocaine increasing the risk of toxicity.[108] The half-life of lidocaine in the elderly is increased by approximately 70 per cent in comparison to the half-life in the young population when administered intravenously.

Bupivacaine

When bupivacaine is administered to the epidural and subarachnoid space, the absorption occurs first a rapid initial phase followed by a slower phase. Advanced age does not affect the systemic absorption of bupivacaine after epidural administration and consequently peak plasma concentrations and the corresponding peak times of remain unchanged.[109] But a slower onset and a more profound motor blockade is observed after epidural blockade in the elderly. However, the systemic absorption of the drug after subarachnoid administration is reported to be faster with advanced age without a clinical effect on duration of action during subarachnoid anaesthesia. The total plasma clearance of bupivacaine decreases with age due to age-related decrease in serum protein binding and biotransformation by hepatic enzyme activity. The bolus and maintenance infusion doses should be reduced without causing an impaired drug effect since increased plasma concentrations and increased potency of bupivacaine is observed during subarachnoid and epidural anaesthesia in the elderly.[49] Furthermore, this kind of increased sensitivity may be due to intrinsic neuronal sensitivity and may lead to an increased risk of adverse events.

Levobupivacaine

Levobupivacaine is the pure S(−) enantiomer of racemic bupivacaine and has similar properties, clinical effects, and pharmacokinetics to racemic bupivacaine. Additionally, early absorption kinetics and equilibration rate constant of levobupivacaine are altered by ageing after epidural administration.[107,110]

Ropivacaine

The pharmacokinetics of ropivacaine is altered in the elderly since the clearance and elimination half-times are significantly decreased, by approximately twofold.[107] Decreased hepatic blood flow or decreased enzyme activity with age may be responsible for the decreased clearance since ropivacaine is mainly metabolized in the liver. Onset time and time to peak in elderly patients and adult patients are similar.[111] Additionally, age affects the pharmacodynamics of this drug. EC50 in the elderly population is significantly

less than in younger patients. Increased sensitivity to sensory and motor blocking effects of ropivacaine in the elderly should be counter-balanced by the use of smaller bolus doses and decreased continuous infusion rate in clinical practice.[79] This may also avoid accumulation of the drug by advanced age.[112]

Analgesic adjuncts in the perioperative period

Current anaesthetic practice uses many agents with analgesic properties to improve analgesia in the perioperative management. However, data about age-related alterations in the pharmacology and clinical effects of these drugs is very limited and these drugs require additional care when used in the anaesthetic management of elderly patients.[1]

Paracetamol (acetaminophen), a centrally-acting prostaglandin inhibitor, has decreased clearance in the elderly; however, its intravenous formulation is very suitable for use during the perioperative period in the elderly with unaltered clinical effects with ageing when significant renal impairment and frailty are not encountered.[56,113–115] Non-selective non-steroidal anti-inflammatory drugs (NSAIDs) such as ketorolac trigger more gastric and renal complications in patients over the age of 60 in comparison to younger adults. Dose reduction and longer dose intervals (up to 50 per cent) are recommended for the use of non-selective NSAIDs in the elderly.[116–118] Selective NSAIDs require similar caution when used in the elderly. Another issue about NSAIDs has been their possible adverse interactions with many commonly used drugs in the elderly, such as warfarin and diuretics.[3,119] Clonidine has similar effect on plasma noradrenaline and blood pressure in both older and younger patients.[120] Dexmedetomidine, a selective alpha 2-adrenoceptor agonist, had been introduced for sedation of critically ill patients but conflicting data is available about its use in the elderly.[121–124] Gabapentin is highly affected by reduced renal function in aged individuals and requires significant dose adjustments.[125,126]

Drug interactions

The amount of anaesthetic required in the elderly also depends on the presence of other anaesthetics. The clinical studies on drug utilization where multiple anaesthetics are used together show that maximum drug dosing for anaesthetic drugs have been used between 30–45 years of age and a decrease of approximately 30–50 per cent has been practised until the age of 80.[127] These findings are compatible with literature describing a decreased requirement of each individual anaesthetic with advanced age. While the pharmacology of many anaesthetics is influenced by advanced age, they also interact with each other's distribution volume, enzymatic biotransformation, receptor sites, and excretion as well as haemodynamic and neurological effects. Thus, there is a higher risk of increased adverse drug reaction with advanced age and multidrug administration.

Another concern in the elderly about drug actions is the use of multiple previously prescribed drugs. For example, the induction of liver microsomal enzymes, by, e.g. phenytoin, isoniazid, phenobarbital, alcohol or halothane, increases the metabolism of anaesthetics. The metabolism is highest with halothane (15–40 per cent of drug), followed by enflurane (2.4 per cent), sevoflurane

Table 3.2 Summary of basic pharmacological effects of ageing on anaesthetic drugs and recommended adjustments in dosing during anaesthetic management

Agents	Pharmacokinetics	Pharmacodynamics	Clinical effects	Recommendation
Volatile agents	↑ distribution volume ↓ distribution rate ↓ hepatic function Changes in respiratory system	↓ receptor numbers ↓ neurotransmitters	↓ MAC Increased alveolar concentration Late onset of effect Late recovery	Decrease MAC and end-tidal inspired concentration by 6% for each decade
Non-volatile agents				
Barbiturates	↓ distribution volume ↓ elimination ↓ clearance	Not altered	Increased blood concentration Prolonged recovery	Decrease bolus dose by 50% Reduce infusion rate by 20%
Propofol	↓ intercompartmental clearance	↓ EC50 ↑ brain sensitivity	Increased blood concentration Prolonged recovery	Decrease bolus and infusion doses by 40–50%
Etomidate	↓ distribution volume ↓ clearance	Not altered	Increased blood concentration	Decrease bolus dose by 50%
Benzodiazepines	↓ clearance ↓ hepatic function ↓ distribution volume	↓ EC50 ↑ brain sensitivity ↑ receptor affinity	Increased pharmacological effects Prolonged clinical effects Prolonged offset time	Administer lower induction doses by 25–75%
Ketamine	↓ clearance	Changes in NMDA receptor structure ↓ spinal cord neuron numbers ↑ brain sensitivity	Prolonged clinical effects	Dose reduction
Opioids	Not altered *except* ↓ clearance for *morphine* and *remifentanil* ↓ protein binding for *meperidine*	Changes in receptor number and affinity ↓ EC50 ↑ brain sensitivity	Slower onset of the clinical effects Profound physiological responses Prolonged recovery	Decrease bolus and infusion doses by 50%
Neuromuscular blocking agents (NMBAs)				
Depolarizing NMBA	↓ plasma cholinesterase	↓ acetylcholine receptors	Prolonged action	Reduce infusion rate Longer dose intervals Neuromuscular monitoring
Non-depolarizing NMBA				
Aminosteroids	↓ distribution volume ↓ clearance ↓ elimination	↓ acetylcholine receptors	Prolonged action Prolonged recovery time	Decrease dose by 30% Neuromuscular monitoring
Benzylisoquinolones	Not altered *except mivacurium* ↓ clearance ↓ plasma cholinesterase	Not altered	Delayed onset with *mivacurium*	Adjust the dose and dose intervals
NMBA antagonists				
Anticholinesterase	↓ clearance ↓ elimination rate		Prolonged action (*except with edrophonium*)	
Sugammadex	↓ clearance ↓ distribution volume ↓ elimination rate		Prolonged recovery Late onset	
Local anaesthetics	↓ clearance ↓ absorption from site of delivery ↓ metabolism ↓ elimination	↓ EC50 ↑ sensitivity to sensory and motor blocking effects	↑ serum concentration ↑ toxicity	Reduce bolus and maintenance doses Decrease continuous infusion

(2–5 per cent), isoflurane (0.17–0.2 per cent), and desflurane (0.02 per cent).[128–130] Comorbidities of elderly patients and their required medications enhance the risk of undesired interactions between drugs and lead to unexpected problems associated with anaesthetics during the perioperative period.

Conclusion

Pharmacokinetic and pharmacodynamic changes usually result in decreased metabolism and clearance and an increased sensitivity to anaesthetics in the elderly (Table 3.2). Therefore, the anaesthetic effect is often prolonged and decreased doses are adequate to achieve the clinical effect. Furthermore, age-related physiological alterations make the elderly more vulnerable to adverse drug effects. Use of short-acting anaesthetics with lower doses, slower titration, and longer intervals should be advocated to avoid the increased risk of prolonged anaesthetic action and adverse events.

References

1. Cook DJ, Rooke GA. Priorities in perioperative geriatrics. *Anesth Analg.* 2003;96(6):1823–1836.
2. Cherry KE, Morton MR. Drug sensitivity in older adults: the role of physiologic and pharmacokinetic factors. *Int J Aging Hum Dev.* 1989;28(3):159–174.
3. Coldrey JC, Upton RN, Macintyre PE. Advances in analgesia in the older patient. *Best Pract Res Clin Anaesthesiol.* 2011;25(3):367–378.
4. Vestal RE. Aging and pharmacology. *Cancer.* 1997;80(7):1302–1310.
5. Shafer SL. The pharmacology of anesthetic drugs in elderly patients. *Anesthesiol Clin North America.* 2000;18(1):1–29, v.
6. Turnheim K. Drug dosage in the elderly. Is it rational? *Drugs Aging.* 1998;13(5):357–379.
7. Lu CC, Tsai CS, Hu OYP, Chen RM, Chen TL, Ho ST. Pharmacokinetics of isoflurane in human blood. *Pharmacology.* 2008;81(4):344–349.
8. Pacifici GM, Viani A, Taddeucci-Brunelli G, Rizzo G, Carrai M, Schulz HU. Effects of development, aging, and renal and hepatic insufficiency as well as hemodialysis on the plasma concentrations of albumin and alpha 1-acid glycoprotein: implications for binding of drugs. *Ther Drug Monit.* 1986;8(3):259–263.
9. Davis D, Grossman SH, Kitchell BB, Shand DG, Routledge PA. The effects of age and smoking on the plasma protein binding of lignocaine and diazepam. *Br J Clin Pharmacol.* 1985;19(2):261–265.
10. Macklon AF, Barton M, James O, Rawlins MD. The effect of age on the pharmacokinetics of diazepam. *Clin Sci (Lond).* 1980;59(6):479–483.
11. Veering BT, Burm AG, Souverijn JH, Serree JM, Spierdijk J. The effect of age on serum concentrations of albumin and alpha 1-acid glycoprotein. *Br J Clin Pharmacol.* 1990;29(2):201–206.
12. Kharasch ED, Thummel KE. Identification of cytochrome P450 2E1 as the predominant enzyme catalyzing human liver microsomal defluorination of sevoflurane, isoflurane, and methoxyflurane. *Anesthesiology.* 1993;79(4):795–807.
13. Tonner PH, Kampen J, Scholz J. Pathophysiological changes in the elderly. *Best Pract Res Clin Anaesthesiol.* 2003;17(2):163–177.
14. Holazo AA, Winkler MB, Patel IH. Effects of age, gender and oral contraceptives on intramuscular midazolam pharmacokinetics. *J Clin Pharmacol.* 1988;28(11):1040–1045.
15. Gelman S, Reves JG, Harris D. Circulatory responses to midazolam anesthesia: emphasis on canine splanchnic circulation. *Anesth Analg.* 1983;62(2):135–139.
16. Danziger RS, Tobin JD, Becker LC, Lakatta EE, Fleg JL. The age-associated decline in glomerular filtration in healthy normotensive volunteers. Lack of relationship to cardiovascular performance. *J Am Geriatr Soc.* 1990;38(10):1127–1132.
17. Peters A. Structural changes that occur during normal aging of primate cerebral hemispheres. *Neurosci Biobehav Rev.* 2002;26(7):733–741.
18. Ancelin ML, de Roquefeuil G, Ledésert B, Bonnel F, Cheminal JC, Ritchie K. Exposure to anaesthetic agents, cognitive functioning and depressive symptomatology in the elderly. *Br J Psychiatry.* 2001;178:360–366.
19. Caspary DM, Holder TM, Hughes LF, Milbrandt JC, McKernan RM, Naritoku DK. Age-related changes in GABA(A) receptor subunit composition and function in rat auditory system. *Neuroscience.* 1999;93(1):307–312.
20. Milbrandt JC, Albin RL, Turgeon SM, Caspary DM. GABAA receptor binding in the aging rat inferior colliculus. *Neuroscience.* 1996;73(2):449–458.
21. Ueno E, Liu DD, Ho IK, Hoskins B. Opiate receptor characteristics in brains from young, mature and aged mice. *Neurobiol Aging.* 1988;9(3):279–283.
22. Hiller JM, Fan LQ, Simon EJ. Age-related changes in kappa opioid receptors in the guinea-pig brain: a quantitative autoradiographic study. *Neuroscience.* 1992;50(3):663–673.
23. Hoskins DL, Gordon TL, Crisp T. The effects of aging on mu and delta opioid receptors in the spinal cord of Fischer-344 rats. *Brain Res.* 1998;791(1–2):299–302.
24. Hess GD, Joseph JA, Roth GS. Effect of age on sensitivity to pain and brain opiate receptors. *Neurobiol Aging.* 1981;2(1):49–55.
25. Villares JC, Stavale JN. Age-related changes in the N-methyl-D-aspartate receptor binding sites within the human basal ganglia. *Exp Neurol.* 2001;171(2):391–404.
26. Marutle A, Warpman U, Bogdanovic N, Nordberg A. Regional distribution of subtypes of nicotinic receptors in human brain and effect of aging studied by (+/-)-[3H]epibatidine. *Brain Res.* 1998;801(1–2):143–149.
27. Vuyk J. Pharmacodynamics in the elderly. *Best Pract Res Clin Anaesthesiol.* 2003;17(2):207–218.
28. Tohgi H, Utsugisawa K, Yoshimura M, Nagane Y, Mihara M. Age-related changes in nicotinic acetylcholine receptor subunits alpha4 and beta2 messenger RNA expression in postmortem human frontal cortex and hippocampus. *Neurosci Lett.* 1998; 245(3):139–142.
29. Heeremans EH, Proost JH, Eleveld DJ, Absalom AR, Struys MMRF. Population pharmacokinetics and pharmacodynamics in anesthesia, intensive care and pain medicine. *Curr Opin Anaesthesiol.* 2010;23(4):479–484.
30. Derendorf H, Lesko LJ, Chaikin P, *et al.* Pharmacokinetic/pharmaco dynamicmodeling in drug research and development. *J Clin Pharmacol.* 2000;40(12 Pt 2):1399–1418.
31. Eger EI. Age, minimum alveolar anesthetic concentration, and minimum alveolar anesthetic concentration-awake. *Anesth Analg.* 2001;93(4):947–953.
32. Mapleson WW. Effect of age on MAC in humans: a meta-analysis. *Br J Anaesth.* 1996;76(2):179–185.
33. Nickalls RWD, Mapleson WW. Age-related iso-MAC charts for isoflurane, sevoflurane and desflurane in man. *Br J Anaesth.* 2003;91(2):170–174.
34. Strum DP, Eger EI, Unadkat JD, Johnson BH, Carpenter RL. Age affects the pharmacokinetics of inhaled anesthetics in humans. *Anesth Analg.* 1991;73(3):310–318.
35. Matsuura T, Oda Y, Tanaka K, Mori T, Nishikawa K, Asada A. Advance of age decreases the minimum alveolar concentrations of isoflurane and sevoflurane for maintaining bispectral index below 50. *Br J Anaesth.* 2009;102(3):331–335.
36. Hall JE, Oldham TA, Stewart JI, Harmer M. Comparison between halothane and sevoflurane for adult vital capacity induction. *Br J Anaesth.* 1997;79(3):285–288.
37. Dwyer R, Howe J. Peripheral blood flow in the elderly during inhalational anaesthesia. *Acta Anaesthesiol Scand.* 1995;39(7):939–944.
38. Takeshima R, Dohi S. Comparison of arterial baroreflex function in humans anesthetized with enflurane or isoflurane. *Anesth Analg.* 1989;69(3):284–290.

39. Vermeulen PM, Kalkman CJ, Dirksen R, Knape JTA, Moons KGM, Borm GF. Predictive performance of a physiological model for enflurane closed-circuit anaesthesia: effects of continuous cardiac output measurements and age-related solubility data. *Br J Anaesth.* 2002;88(1):38–45.

40. Dwyer RC, Fee JP, Howard PJ, Clarke RS. Arterial washin of halothane and isoflurane in young and elderly adult patients. *Br J Anaesth.* 1991;66(5):572–579.

41. Cortínez LI, Trocóniz IF, Fuentes R, *et al.* The influence of age on the dynamic relationship between end-tidal sevoflurane concentrations and bispectral index. *Anesth Analg.* 2008;107(5):1566–1572.

42. Fragen RJ, Dunn KL. The minimum alveolar concentration (MAC) of sevoflurane with and without nitrous oxide in elderly versus young adults. *J Clin Anesth.* 1996;8(5):352–356.

43. Bennett JA, Lingaraju N, Horrow JC, McElrath T, Keykhah MM. Elderly patients recover more rapidly from desflurane than from isoflurane anesthesia. *J Clin Anesth.* 1992;4(5):378–381.

44. Chen X, Zhao M, White PF, *et al.* The recovery of cognitive function after general anesthesia in elderly patients: a comparison of desflurane and sevoflurane. *Anesth Analg.* 2001;93(6):1489–1494.

45. Goto T, Nakata Y, Morita S. The minimum alveolar concentration of xenon in the elderly is sex-dependent. *Anesthesiology.* 2002;97(5):1129–1132.

46. Sadean MR, Glass PSA. Pharmacokinetics in the elderly. *Best Pract Res Clin Anaesthesiol.* 2003;17(2):191–205.

47. Stanski DR, Maitre PO. Population pharmacokinetics and pharmacodynamics of thiopental: the effect of age revisited. *Anesthesiology.* 1990;72(3):412–422.

48. Sørensen MK, Dolven TL, Rasmussen LS. Onset time and haemodynamic response after thiopental vs. propofol in the elderly: a randomized trial. *Acta Anaesthesiol Scand.* 2011;55(4):429–434.

49. Schnider TW, Minto CF, Bruckert H, Mandema JW. Population pharmacodynamic modeling and covariate detection for central neural blockade. *Anesthesiology.* 1996;85(3):502–512.

50. Schnider TW, Minto CF, Shafer SL, *et al.* The influence of age on propofol pharmacodynamics. *Anesthesiology.* 1999;90(6):1502–1516.

51. Vuyk J, Oostwouder CJ, Vletter AA, Burm AG, Bovill JG. Gender differences in the pharmacokinetics of propofol in elderly patients during and after continuous infusion. *Br J Anaesth.* 2001;86(2):183–188.

52. Keïta H, Peytavin G, Giraud O, *et al.* Aging prolongs recovery of psychomotor functions at emergence from propofol-alfentanil anaesthesia. *Can J Anaesth.* 1998;45(12):1211–1214.

53. Fredman B, Noga J, Zohar E, Yaretzky A, Jedeikin R. Influence of thiopental and propofol on postoperative cognitive recovery in the elderly patient undergoing general anesthesia. *J Clin Anesth.* 1999;11(8):635–640.

54. Arden JR, Holley FO, Stanski DR. Increased sensitivity to etomidate in the elderly: initial distribution versus altered brain response. *Anesthesiology.* 1986;65(1):19–27.

55. Cicero M, Graneto J. Etomidate for procedural sedation in the elderly: a retrospective comparison between age groups. *Am J Emerg Med.* 2011;29(9):1111–1116.

56. Divoll M, Greenblatt DJ, Ochs HR, Shader RI. Absolute bioavailability of oral and intramuscular diazepam: effects of age and sex. *Anesth Analg.* 1983;62(1):1–8.

57. Ochs HR, Greenblatt DJ, Divoll M, Abernethy DR, Feyerabend H, Dengler HJ. Diazepam kinetics in relation to age and sex. *Pharmacology.* 1981;23(1):24–30.

58. Jacobs JR, Reves JG, Marty J, White WD, Bai SA, Smith LR. Aging increases pharmacodynamic sensitivity to the hypnotic effects of midazolam. *Anesth Analg.* 1995;80(1):143–148.

59. Fujisawa T, Takuma S, Koseki H, Kimura K, Fukushima K. Recovery of intentional dynamic balance function after intravenous sedation with midazolam in young and elderly subjects. *Eur J Anaesthesiol.* 2006;23(5):422–425.

60. Bell GD, Spickett GP, Reeve PA, Morden A, Logan RF. Intravenous midazolam for upper gastrointestinal endoscopy: a study of 800 consecutive cases relating dose to age and sex of patient. *Br J Clin Pharmacol.* 1987;23(2):241–243.

61. Kanto J, Aaltonen L, Himberg JJ, Hovi-Viander M. Midazolam as an intravenous induction agent in the elderly: a clinical and pharmacokinetic study. *Anesth Analg.* 1986;65(1):15–20.

62. Platten HP, Schweizer E, Dilger K, Mikus G, Klotz U. Pharmacokinetics and the pharmacodynamic action of midazolam in young and elderly patients undergoing tooth extraction. *Clin Pharmacol Ther.* 1998;63(5):552–560.

63. Sun GC, Hsu MC, Chia YY, Chen PY, Shaw FZ. Effects of age and gender on intravenous midazolam premedication: a randomized double-blind study. *Br J Anaesth.* 2008;101(5):632–639.

64. Greenblatt DJ, Allen MD, Locniskar A, Harmatz JS, Shader RI. Lorazepam kinetics in the elderly. *Clin Pharmacol Ther.* 1979;26(1):103–113.

65. Barr J, Zomorodi K, Bertaccini EJ, Shafer SL, Geller E. A double-blind, randomized comparison of i.v. lorazepam versus midazolam for sedation of ICU patients via a pharmacologic model. *Anesthesiology.* 2001;95(2):286–298.

66. Roncari G, Timm U, Zell M, Zumbrunnen R, Weber W. Flumazenil kinetics in the elderly. *Eur J Clin Pharmacol.* 1993;45(6):585–587.

67. Aubrun F, Marmion F. The elderly patient and postoperative pain treatment. *Best Pract Res Clin Anaesthesiol.* 2007;21(1):109–127.

68. Kaiko RF, Wallenstein SL, Rogers A, Grabinski P, Houde RW. Relative analgesic potency of intramuscular heroin and morphine in cancer patients with postoperative pain and chronic pain due to cancer. *NIDA Res Monogr.* 1981;34:213–219.

69. Wilder-Smith OHG. Opioid use in the elderly. *Eur J Pain.* 2005;9(2):137–140.

70. Owen JA, Sitar DS, Berger L, Brownell L, Duke PC, Mitenko PA. Age-related morphine kinetics. *Clin Pharmacol Ther.* 1983;34(3):364–368.

71. Pergolizzi J, Böger RH, Budd K, *et al.* Opioids and the management of chronic severe pain in the elderly: consensus statement of an International Expert Panel with focus on the six clinically most often used World Health Organization step III opioids (buprenorphine, fentanyl, hydromorphone, methadone, morphine, oxycodone). *Pain Pract.* 2008;8(4):287–313.

72. Arunasalam K, Davenport HT, Painter S, Jones JG. Ventilatory response to morphine in young and old subjects. *Anaesthesia.* 1983;38(6):529–533.

73. Björkman S, Wada DR, Stanski DR. Application of physiologic models to predict the influence of changes in body composition and blood flows on the pharmacokinetics of fentanyl and alfentanil in patients. *Anesthesiology.* 1998;88(3):657–667.

74. Lemmens HJ, Burm AG, Hennis PJ, Gladines MP, Bovill JG. Influence of age on the pharmacokinetics of alfentanil. Gender dependence. *Clin Pharmacokinet.* 1990;19(5):416–422.

75. Helmers JH, van Leeuwen L, Zuurmond WW. Sufentanil pharmacokinetics in young adult and elderly surgical patients. *Eur J Anaesthesiol.* 1994;11(3):181–185.

76. Hofbauer R, Tesinsky P, Hammerschmidt V, *et al.* No reduction in the sufentanil requirement of elderly patients undergoing ventilatory support in the medical intensive care unit. *Eur J Anaesthesiol.* 1999;16(10):702–707.

77. Zhao Y, Zhang LP, Wu XM, *et al.* Clinical evaluation of target controlled infusion system for sufentanil administration. *Chin Med J (Engl).* 2009;122(20):2503–2508.

78. Minto CF, Schnider TW, Egan TD, *et al.* Influence of age and gender on the pharmacokinetics and pharmacodynamics of remifentanil. I. Model development. *Anesthesiology.* 1997;86(1):10–23.

79. KruijtSpanjer MR, Bakker NA, Absalom AR. Pharmacology in the elderly and newer anaesthesia drugs. *Best Pract Res Clin Anaesthesiol.* 2011;25(3):355–365.

80. Scott LJ, Perry CM. Tramadol: a review of its use in perioperative pain. *Drugs.* 2000;60(1):139–176.

81. Brouquet A, Cudennec T, Benoist S, *et al.* Impaired mobility, ASA status and administration of tramadol are risk factors for postoperative delirium in patients aged 75 years or more after major abdominal surgery. *Ann Surg.* 2010;251(4):759–765.

82. Fosnight SM, Holder CM, Allen KR, Hazelett S. A strategy to decrease the use of risky drugs in the elderly. *Cleve Clin J Med.* 2004;71(7):561–568.

83. Chan L. Blood cholinesterase levels in the elderly and newborn. *Malays J Pathol.* 1995;17(2):87–89.

84. Hubbard RE, O'Mahony MS, Calver BL, Woodhouse KW. Plasma esterases and inflammation in ageing and frailty. *Eur J Clin Pharmacol.* 2008;64(9):895–900.

85. Arain SR, Kern S, Ficke DJ, Ebert TJ. Variability of duration of action of neuromuscular-blocking drugs in elderly patients. *Acta Anaesthesiol Scand.* 2005;49(3):312–315.

86. Rupp SM, Castagnoli KP, Fisher DM, Miller RD. Pancuronium and vecuronium pharmacokinetics and pharmacodynamics in younger and elderly adults. *Anesthesiology.* 1987;67(1):45–49.

87. Berg H, Roed J, Viby-Mogensen J, *et al.* Residual neuromuscular block is a risk factor for postoperative pulmonary complications. A prospective, randomised, and blinded study of postoperative pulmonary complications after atracurium, vecuronium and pancuronium. *Acta Anaesthesiol Scand.* 1997;41(9):1095–1103.

88. McCarthy G, Elliott P, Mirakhur RK, Cooper R, Sharpe TD, Clarke RS. Onset and duration of action of vecuronium in the elderly: comparison with adults. *Acta Anaesthesiol Scand.* 1992;36(4):383–386.

89. Lien CA, Matteo RS, Ornstein E, Schwartz AE, Diaz J. Distribution, elimination, and action of vecuronium in the elderly. *Anesth Analg.* 1991;73(1):39–42.

90. Matteo RS, Ornstein E, Schwartz AE, Ostapkovich N, Stone JG. Pharmacokinetics and pharmacodynamics of rocuronium (Org 9426) in elderly surgical patients. *Anesth Analg.* 1993;77(6):1193–1197.

91. Bevan DR, Fiset P, Balendran P, Law-Min JC, Ratcliffe A, Donati F. Pharmacodynamic behaviour of rocuronium in the elderly. *Can J Anaesth.* 1993;40(2):127–132.

92. Parker CJ, Hunter JM, Snowdon SL. Effect of age, gender and anaesthetic technique on the pharmacodynamics of atracurium. *Br J Anaesth.* 1993;70(1):38–41.

93. Slavov V, Khalil M, Merle JC, Agostini MM, Ruggier R, Duvaldestin P. Comparison of duration of neuromuscular blocking effect of atracurium and vecuronium in young and elderly patients. *Br J Anaesth.* 1995;74(6):709–711.

94. Sorooshian SS, Stafford MA, Eastwood NB, Boyd AH, Hull CJ, Wright PM. Pharmacokinetics and pharmacodynamics of cisatracurium in young and elderly adult patients. *Anesthesiology.* 1996;84(5):1083–1091.

95. Ornstein E, Lien CA, Matteo RS, Ostapkovich ND, Diaz J, Wolf KB. Pharmacodynamics and pharmacokinetics of cisatracurium in geriatric surgical patients. *Anesthesiology.* 1996;84(3):520–525.

96. Pühringer FK, Heier T, Dodgson M, *et al.* Double-blind comparison of the variability in spontaneous recovery of cisatracurium- and vecuronium-induced neuromuscular block in adult and elderly patients. *Acta Anaesthesiol Scand.* 2002;46(4):364–371.

97. Goudsouzian N, Chakravorti S, Denman W, Schwartz A, Yang HS, Cook DR. Prolonged mivacurium infusion in young and elderly adults. *Can J Anaesth.* 1997;44(9):955–962.

98. Jones RM. Mivacurium in special patient groups. *Acta Anaesthesiol Scand Suppl.* 1995;106:47–54.

99. Young WL, Matteo RS, Ornstein E. Duration of action of neostigmine and pyridostigmine in the elderly. *Anesth Analg.* 1988;67(8):775–778.

100. Stone JG, Matteo RS, Ornstein E, *et al.* Aging alters the pharmacokinetics of pyridostigmine. *Anesth Analg.* 1995;81(4):773–776.

101. Kitajima T, Ishii K, Ogata H. Edrophonium as an antagonist of vecuronium-induced neuromuscular block in the elderly. *Anaesthesia.* 1995;50(4):359–361.

102. Matteo RS, Young WL, Ornstein E, Schwartz AE, Silverberg PA, Diaz J. Pharmacokinetics and pharmacodynamics of edrophonium in elderly surgical patients. *Anesth Analg.* 1990;71(4):334–339.

103. Peeters P, Passier P, Smeets J, *et al.* Sugammadex is cleared rapidly and primarily unchanged via renal excretion. *Biopharm Drug Dispos.* 2011;32(3):159–167.

104. Welliver M, Cheek D. An update on sugammadex sodium. *AANA J.* 2009;77(3):219–228.

105. Suzuki T, Kitajima O, Ueda K, Kondo Y, Kato J, Ogawa S. Reversibility of rocuronium-induced profound neuromuscular block with sugammadex in younger and older patients. *Br J Anaesth.* 2011;106(6):823–826.

106. McDonagh DL, Benedict PE, Kovac AL, *et al.* Efficacy, safety, and pharmacokinetics of sugammadex for the reversal of rocuronium-induced neuromuscular blockade in elderly patients. *Anesthesiology.* 2011;114(2):318–329.

107. Simon MJG, Veering BT, Stienstra R, van Kleef JW, Burm AGL. Effect of age on the clinical profile and systemic absorption and disposition of levobupivacaine after epidural administration. *Br J Anaesth.* 2004;93(4):512–520.

108. Kwa A, Sprung J, Guilder MV, Jelliffe RW. A population pharmacokinetic model of epidural lidocaine in geriatric patients: effects of low-dose dopamine. *Ther Drug Monit.* 2008;30(3):379–389.

109. Veering BT, Burm AG, Vletter AA, van den Heuvel RP, Onkenhout W, Spierdijk J. The effect of age on the systemic absorption, disposition and pharmacodynamics of bupivacaine after epidural administration. *Clin Pharmacokinet.* 1992;22(1):75–84.

110. Olofsen E, Burm AGL, Simon MJG, Veering BT, van Kleef JW, Dahan A. Population pharmacokinetic-pharmacodynamicmodeling of epidural anesthesia. *Anesthesiology.* 2008;109(4):664–674.

111. Xiao J, Cai MH, Wang XR, He P. Time course of action and pharmacokinetics of ropivacaine in adult and elderly patients following combined lumbar plexus-sciatic nerve block. *Int J Clin Pharmacol Ther.* 2010;48(9):608–613.

112. Cusato M, Allegri M, Niebel T, *et al.* Flip-flop kinetics of ropivacaine during continuous epidural infusion influences its accumulation rate. *Eur J Clin Pharmacol.* 2011;67(4):399–406.

113. Miners JO, Penhall R, Robson RA, Birkett DJ. Comparison of paracetamol metabolism in young adult and elderly males. *Eur J Clin Pharmacol.* 1988;35(2):157–160.

114. Divoll M, Ameer B, Abernethy DR, Greenblatt DJ. Age does not alter acetaminophen absorption. *J Am Geriatr Soc.* 1982;30(4):240–244.

115. Liukas A, Kuusniemi K, Aantaa R, *et al.* Pharmacokinetics of intravenous paracetamol in elderly patients. *Clin Pharmacokinet.* 2011;50(2):121–129.

116. Egbert AM. Postoperative pain management in the frail elderly. *Clin Geriatr Med.* 1996;12(3):583–599.

117. Peura DA. Prevention of nonsteroidal anti-inflammatory drug-associated gastrointestinal symptoms and ulcer complications. *Am J Med.* 2004;117(Suppl 5A):63S–71S.

118. Forrest JB, Camu F, Greer IA, *et al.* Ketorolac, diclofenac, and ketoprofen are equally safe for pain relief after major surgery. *Br J Anaesth.* 2002;88(2):227–233.

119. Barkin RL, Beckerman M, Blum SL, Clark FM, Koh EK, Wu DS. Should nonsteroidal anti-inflammatory drugs (NSAIDs) be prescribed to the older adult? *Drugs Aging.* 2010;27(10):775–789.

120. Klein CE, Gerber JG, Nies AS. Lack of an effect of age on the response to clonidine. *Clin Pharmacol Ther.* 1990;47(1):61–67.

121. Candiotti KA, Bergese SD, Bokesch PM, *et al.* Monitored anesthesia care with dexmedetomidine: a prospective, randomized, double-blind, multicenter trial. *Anesth Analg.* 2010;110(1):47–56.

122. Kunisawa T, Hanada S, Kurosawa A, Suzuki A, Takahata O, Iwasaki H. Dexmedetomidine was safely used for sedation during spinal anesthesia in a very elderly patient. *J Anesth.* 2010;24(6):938–941.

123. Lee SK. Clinical use of dexmedetomidine in monitored anesthesia care. *Korean J Anesthesiol.* 2011;61(6):451–452.

124. Gerlach AT, Murphy CV. Dexmedetomidine-associated bradycardia progressing to pulseless electrical activity: case report and review of the literature. *Pharmacotherapy*. 2009;29(12):1492–1492.

125. Schmader KE, Baron R, Haanpää ML, *et al*. Treatment considerations for elderly and frail patients with neuropathic pain. *Mayo Clin Proc*. 2010;85(3 Suppl):S26–S32.

126. McGeeneyBE. Pharmacological management of neuropathic pain in older adults: an update on peripherally and centrally acting agents. *J Pain Symptom Manage*. 2009;38(2 Suppl):S15–S27.

127. Martin G, Glass PSA, Breslin DS, *et al*. A study of anesthetic drug utilization in different age groups. *J Clin Anesth*. 2003;15(3):194–200.

128. Hatch DJ. New inhalation agents in paediatric anaesthesia. *Br J Anaesth*. 1999;83(1):42–49.

129. Walker JR. What is new with inhaled anesthetics: part 2. *J Perianesth Nurs*. 1996;11(6):404–409.

130. Pihlainen K, Ojanperä I. Analytical toxicology of fluorinated inhalation anaesthetics. *Forensic Sci Int*. 1998;97(2–3):117–133.

CHAPTER 4

Technology in an ageing society

Stanley Muravchick

Introduction

Lifespan is a species-specific biological parameter that quantifies maximum attainable age under optimal environmental conditions. For humans, it has remained constant at about 115 years for at least the past 20 centuries. Life expectancy, in contrast, is an empirical statistical estimate of typical longevity under prevailing or predicted circumstances. In fact, recent advances in medical science and basic healthcare have increased life expectancy dramatically in industrialized nations, increasing the relative 'agedness' of those societies. Currently about 500 million persons 65 years of age or older live on Earth, and the social service and healthcare systems that serve them are experiencing increasingly severe financial stress as demographic forces increase both the quantity and the intensity of services required.[1] The societal costs of age-related disability and dependence, as great as they seem, may even be underestimated: in addition to the direct healthcare costs incurred by the elderly, the lost wages and pension income incurred by an adult in the United States who must leave the workforce to care for an aged parent often exceeds a quarter of a million dollars.[2]

One pragmatic approach to managing this huge financial burden is to limit or reduce the societal costs of ageing using applied technology (gerotechnology), an approach that may also have an additional salutary socioeconomic effect as a stimulus for both scientific innovation and consumer spending. The goals of biotechnology as applied to ageing or 'gerotechnology' are several: promotion and maintenance of wellness to enable healthy older adults to enjoy 'successful ageing', a term that implies a promise of an increased portion of human lifespan during which adults remain productive and independent; early diagnosis, effective management, and perhaps even cure of age-related disease; and last, and perhaps the most ambitious, the development of technological tools capable of mitigating or even eliminating the molecular and cellular deterioration that we now know characterizes the ageing process itself.

Although there is great logical appeal to this approach, it would be naïve to believe that there are no serious obstacles to the adoption and advancement of gerotechnology, particularly with regard to establishing the primacy of 'grey' as opposed to 'green' technology agendas in contemporary society. The costs will be great and the industries and special interests that profit from the status quo are well entrenched and politically active.[3] In addition, whenever there are significant developments in basic and in applied research, concepts of intellectual property rights, regulatory issues, and appropriate legislation all need time to evolve if they are to support a social and political climate that fosters discovery and innovation with regard to human ageing. And, for the older citizens who will be the beneficiaries of society's support for gerotechnology, public perception and awareness must be continually enhanced by education in order to minimize the concerns and fears inevitably associated with large-scale adoption of biotechnology.[4] Nevertheless, the goal of the discussion to follow is to demonstrate that innovative therapies for the treatment and prevention of age-related diseases and intriguing strategies aimed at the postponement of physiological ageing are not only possible but are indeed under active development.[5]

Technological support for physiological ageing

The phenomenon of human ageing

Ageing is a universal and progressive physiological phenomenon characterized clinically by degenerative changes in both the structure and the functional capacity of organs and tissues. More specifically relevant to even 'successful' ageing, human senescence is invariably characterized by decreased muscle strength and postural balance, subtle but progressive auditory and visual sensory deficits, impairment of autonomic homeostasis, and a generalized decline in overall aerobic functional reserve.[6] These changes are believed to reflect the consequences of life-long oxidative metabolism, with subsequent damage to cellular and molecular structure produced by the by-products of metabolism that eventually manifests itself as decrements in function and functional reserve. Within mitochondria, the ubiquitous process of oxidative phosphorylation that generates the energy essential to sustain life inevitably also generates free radical species, and perhaps other toxins, that degrade membranes, proteins, and nucleic acid structures, of which a small proportion fail to undergo endogenous repair and remain damaged. This insidious process of slowly accumulating cellular and subcellular debris ultimately produces the functional degeneration over time that we know as 'normal ageing'.

For many older adults, progressive decline in cardiopulmonary aerobic capacity limits mobility and the normal daily activities and eventually makes independent living difficult or simply impractical. Nevertheless, many older adults, especially the nearly 80 million American 'baby-boomers', don't wish to have their age-related physical needs emphasized or advertised. They generally avoid buying or using products clearly aimed at the elderly customer. Hearing aids and cochlear implants, large-number telephones and display magnifiers, walkers, canes, and motorized scooters are widely accepted only when completely unavoidable. In other areas, the aggressive incorporation of gerotechnology in the form of prosthetic joints to replace those ravaged by degenerative arthritis, or ocular lens implants for those suffering from cataracts, or cardiac pacemakers and implantable defibrillators is more easily accepted because they are perceived as medical necessity.

Gerotechnology in society

Gerotechnology may also encompass items generally considered to be luxury or convenience devices, although upon closer consideration it is clear that the primary benefit for the end-user remains compensation for age-related limitations of physical or cognitive ability. Examples are particularly evident in the latest wave of automotive technology that includes automated intelligent park assist systems, radar-based cruise control, collision avoidance systems and driver attention monitoring, infrared night vision, and even pedestrian recognition systems. Though not explicitly marketed for the purpose of assisting the older adult, these systems facilitate mobility and independence in older drivers because they compensate for the mild but progressive visual impairment and increased reaction times that are inevitable with ageing. The availability of these technologies is also primarily a selling point within the luxury car segment[7,8] and it is the older, financially-established adults who comprise the largest component of the socioeconomic segment who can afford to buy these vehicles.

Older adults also appear to be willing to use their discretionary income to pay for cosmetic surgical procedures and to purchase and use dietary supplements, over-the-counter remedies, and cosmetic pharmaceuticals ('cosmeceuticals') that promise to make them look younger and feel more vital. This is reflected in the aggressive marketing of everything from 'silver' vitamin supplements, hair colouring, dietary fibre supplements and stool softeners, pharmaceuticals that treat depression and erectile dysfunction, and anti-ageing skin treatments. Many of these products, particularly those relating to skin care, are surprisingly 'high tech' in nature. *Nanomedicine* is a therapeutic strategy to apply the use of engineered or artificial nanostructures to biological systems. Modern pharmacology, in particular, has made substantial use of *nanotechnology*, the realm of materials science that refers to the design and application of physical and chemical structures that are about 1 nanometre (10^{-9} metres) in size and utilizes the unique chemical, biological, mechanical, and electrical phenomena that occur within that tiny physical realm. Nanotechnology-based preparations are already in use in both patch delivery and timed drug release applications for skin care. In fact, cosmetic industries rank high among the nanotechnology patent holders. In the United States the L'Oreal Company is an industry leader in nanomedicine patents and designates more than $600 million of its annual research budget for use in nanomedical research.[9]

Telehealth and communication technology

The quality and timeliness of healthcare for the elderly have always been compromised, to some degree, by the inability to easily access individual health records or get expert support for clinical decision-making at the site and at the moment that medical intervention is needed. One effort to overcome this limitation in the United States was a multiagency federal initiative, the High Performance Computing and Communications Program (HPCC) funded by the High Performance Computing Act of 1991. The National Library of Medicine was the first component of the National Institutes of Health to participate in HPCC[10] and it initiated a request for proposals in a wide range of communication and healthcare areas. These included standardization of medical terminology, creation and maintenance of public access medical information databases, and development of intelligent agent Internet search capability using Knowledge-Based Object Technology, or 'knowbots', software algorithms operating autonomously to seek specific information on a network or on websites.[11] Knowbots are 'mobile agents' that, in effect, travel from one website to the next using artificial intelligence in the form of knowledge-based search rules and then send a focused report of their findings back to the user's web server.

This and other dramatic, and often unpredictable, developments in information and communication technology over the past two decades have generated a bewildering list of similar-sounding terms for concepts relating to the use of these technologies for various aspects of eldercare. Terms such as *telemedicine, telecare, teleconsultation, telehomecare,*[12] even *telegeriatrics* have been created and popularized at various times, but rarely are they clearly defined. Perhaps these various concepts should be grouped under the larger umbrella of *medical informatics*, a conceptual entity better understood and widely accepted as representing the intersection between information technology and clinical decision-making.[13] Another related, somewhat broader concept is *telehealth*, defined by the United States Department of Health and Human Services[14] as 'the use of electronic information and telecommunications technologies to support long-distance clinical healthcare, patient and professional health-related education, public health and health administration'. Strategies used to achieve these goals include videoconferencing, store-and-forward imaging, Internet searches, and streaming audio and video, among others, and knowbots may soon have application in collecting important healthcare information for the patient or in collating data on a specific patient for his healthcare providers. To execute these strategies, telehealth utilizes technologies such as broadband terrestrial digital communication, electronic databases, wireless sensors and transmission systems, and a myriad of specialized software applications that are designed to accomplish specific clinical and societal goals.

Although conceptually appealing in general terms, there is not yet enough experience or outcome to endorse unequivocally the social and economic benefits of the concept of telehealth.[15] It may be more useful to consider the possible specific roles and potential uses of telehealth technology focusing upon goals that relate to healthcare and quality of life for older adults. From that perspective, telehealth has clearly been effective in a variety of clinical settings in geriatric medicine. It has the potential to greatly improve access to, and interaction with, specialists in geriatric medicine, particularly for those in assisted living facilities, frail elderly living at home with limited mobility, and older adults in rural or remote areas.[16,17] Of particular appeal is the ability to monitor elderly adults in their normal, day-to-day environment in order to manage known medical conditions and to identify impending health risks. For example, it is now feasible to easily upload electrocardiographic data from a home unit to a web-based management application that can automatically apply an algorithm for interpretation to identify impending myocardial infarction.[18] Some systems use wearable motion sensors[19] to assess walking speed and posture as well as individual gait-sensors that, with context-aware algorithms, can predict fall risks.[20] In effect, software applications can interpret sensor-derived data and identify even subtle signs of functional decline or illness in older adults and then alert healthcare providers to these changes.[21] Other inventive technology applications include automated electronic pill dispensing systems with audible reminders and a transaction log, or daily computer-generated puzzles for the mental exercise that may help to maintain cognitive function. However, as promising as the 'smart elderhome' appears with regard to reducing the need for institutionalization of patients with early cognitive impairment and even mild dementia, the impact of this strategy on long-term outcome remains to be demonstrated.[22]

Older adults, especially the affluent, appear ready to pay for these services if they provide the peace of mind associated with easy access to general health information and near-immediate contact with healthcare specialists and providers. In some new retirement, assisted-living, or nursing home complexes, video cameras and sensor networks are pre-installed and can provide intensive medical surveillance with personalized nurse intervention as needed using the Internet to transmit data from an electronic stethoscope, otoscope, dentalscope, or other device.[23] Technical requirements for acceptable wireless monitoring systems such as battery life, comfort and wearability, and data transmission range have been easily resolved by technical innovation. However, more formidable obstacles to the broader incorporation of these technologies into telehealth systems include psychological and ethical considerations such as privacy and autonomy concerns,[24] administrative issues such as licensure, liability, and uncertain reimbursement for the costs of technology,[23] as well as social and political hesitation to undertake the process of integration and storage of huge amounts of acquired monitoring data within existing healthcare system databases. In addition, many healthcare providers challenge the hypothesis that more information necessarily improves healthcare. They may also be reluctant to embrace telehealth initiatives because of concerns, perhaps justified, that it will decrease the direct physical involvement of caregivers, reducing the frequency of human interactions in institutionalized elders.[25]

Also implicit in any truly effective remote healthcare monitoring system is the need for an electronic medical record (EMR) also known as an electronic health record (EHR), a document that can be shared among several locations. Real-world experience confirms that effective telehealth requires a complex network of communication and information-exchange linkages between primary care providers and established medical institutions.[12] In Singapore, for example, their effective Tele Geriatric system requires that, for each patient event requiring consultation, a healthcare provider at the remote site must forward the patient's medical record electronically to the hospital system of the consultant geriatrician.[26] Yet in Norway, an intensive survey of regional experiences to establish which telehealth services should be implemented on a nationwide scale concluded that, based on a cost/benefit analysis, geriatrics did not deserve a priority designation.[27] Nevertheless, many of the current business models for this segment of the consumer population focus on developing communication and information system strategies, albeit primarily those that promise to facilitate social connectivity, autonomy, and the wellness essential for successful ageing.

Cardio fitness wrist watches, scales that assess body fat content as well as weight, and mobile phone applications that calculate and track dietary caloric input and expenditure take advantage of the huge business of making and selling consumer electronics designed to motivate healthy behaviour in older adults by presenting 'just-in-time' information to the user at points of decision-making and behaviour.[28]

Other initiatives that represent an indirect but important aspect of gerotechnology include the development of computer-based simulation and interactive virtual reality for medical education, as seen in the creation of an Internet-based virtual nursing college.[29] This requires the development and application of numerous complex information and communication technologies, including knowbots for information management, teleconferencing for multi-site collaboration in teaching and clinical research, remotely-accessible multimedia instructional materials, and virtual classrooms and clinics with simulated patients. Overextended medical school faculty members have found telehealth to be an effective and well-accepted technique for teaching students the skills needed to perform a history and physical examination of elderly residents in an independent living facility.[30] Weekly videoconferencing of geriatric medicine grand rounds at the University of Alberta in Canada to numerous urban and rural regional medical centres has also been shown to effectively promote continuing education in geriatric medicine both for physicians and allied health professionals.[31] Also mentioned as being of interest is the use of the Internet for 'grid computing' to support medical applications, although it is not currently clear how public collaboration to harness the unused processing cycles of a huge number of computers would actually contribute clinically to a geriatric-related telehealth environment.

Biotechnology and ageing research

Genomics, proteomics, and other -omic technologies

The extent to which lifespan is highly species-specific is strong suggestive evidence that ageing in some way reflects an evolutionary, genetically based process. One current concept maintains that the Darwinian process of natural selection favours those physical and genetic traits that promote successful species reproduction rather than those that maximize post-reproductive survival of the organism. Therefore, genetic evolution may incidentally regulate mammalian ageing by allowing the progressive post-reproductive deterioration of physiological function that generates the human ageing phenotype.[32] The Human Genome Project[33] and the ascendance of molecular biology have begun to reveal the intricacies of cellular function and the genetic basis of human biology at a level of detail far greater than was thought possible even a few decades ago. Technological advances that continue to provide faster and cheaper DNA sequencing are now, in large part, driving biological and medical research.[34] In fact, genomics and proteomics are areas of clinical investigation and technological invention that may come to dominate twenty-first century biological science and medicine.[35]

Genomics is the systematic study of complex genetic information as contained in an organism's genome, the entire inheritable complement of individual genes within chromosomal structures. If there is a genetic basis for the human ageing phenotype, the use of genomics and molecular biology to explore fully sequenced genomes will allow researchers to study the evolution of ageing in great detail. One strategy proposed to establish whether ageing reflects a relatively simple genetic mechanism[36] or a complex, multifactorial, and multigenic process[37] is comparative genomics: comparing the human genome to that of other organisms in order to understand which regions of the various genomes explain the marked differences in rates of ageing among mammalian and non-mammalian species.[38,39] The concept has been widely popularized[40] but productive application will require the use of systems biology, 'reverse engineering algorithms', and other complex computer methodologies, and it remains far from fully explored or accepted.[41] Given the huge volume of experimental genomics data produced by the newest high-throughput genetic technologies, more widespread application of systems biology may be required to incorporate information from different sources into a useful predictive ageing model.[35,37] Nevertheless, achieving the ultimate goal of identifying the specific gene loci that make humans age at a different rate than other mammals would have profound biomedical implications with regard to understanding, as well as manipulating, human lifespan.[42]

Proteomics is the study of the genetic expression of all proteins encoded in the genome (the proteome) and their physiological as well as their pathophysiological actions within cells and subcellular organelles. This discipline includes not only the detection and measurement of proteins within biological systems but also measurement of their transcription from the DNA genome by means of various messenger RNA (mRNA) systems, using techniques of *transcriptomics*.[43] Understanding the entire complex process of protein expression is essential to any proteomics endeavour related to ageing, and high-throughput proteomics using microarray technologies can examine thousands of proteins and their interactions. Protein microarrays have been used for proteome-wide analysis of protein activities and interactions in yeast, but the obvious next step is to move protein chip technology from the proteome of a simple organism to that of humans in order to explore the molecular mechanisms of human ageing and age-related disease.

The ongoing search for protein biomarkers of ageing, predictors of longevity, and early manifestations of age-related disease has been creative if somewhat unfocused and lacking in a unifying hypothesis.[44] Although the ultimate goal would be to identify an easily obtained serum profile consistently associated with longevity and 'healthy ageing', clinical proteomics is not yet at the level of reliability needed to establish generic 'biomarkers of ageing'.[45] In addition, individual molecules may not be adequate markers for processes as complex and insidious as ageing or age-related disease, although comparing large panels of a defined subset of protein molecules to establish protein patterns and changes during normal and pathological ageing might identify valuable parameters. Advances in protein profiling methods that greatly increase the detection sensitivity and accurate quantification of proteins present in very low concentrations may also be essential for individualized and predictive healthcare interventions in older adults.

Nevertheless, proteomic analysis of human oral secretions has demonstrated differences in the expression of eight proteins in men and seven in women that appear to reflect normal ageing.[46] In Japanese subjects greater than 100 years of age, proteomic analysis has shown that 18 proteins, most associated with oxidative functions, are present in plasma at levels significantly different than in young adults.[47] However, the techniques have some inherent limitations as tools that can be used to study and alter the course of ageing. These include the difficulty in separating the effects of ageing from age-related disease, tremendous intrinsic biological variability and individual diversity reflecting lifelong exposure to hundreds of environmental hazards, analytical and statistical problems associated with simultaneous determination of many different gene transcripts, and even uncertainty about the functional significance of observed changes in mRNA concentrations.[48] However, proteomic strategies continue to enhance our knowledge of the role and complexity of mitochondrial proteins and can offer an approach to testing the efficacy of antioxidants or dietary restriction in order to assess claims that they can provide older adults with an anti-ageing effect.[49]

A better understanding of post-translational protein modifications such as oxidation, glycation, and aggregation synthesis is also of particular relevance both to ageing and to age-related diseases. A recent study of human skin ageing using proteomics, rather than pure genomics, has revealed 30 proteins putatively associated with normal ageing, including several previously unrecognized, post-translationally regulated polypeptides.[50] The modification of proteins into reactive carbonyl compounds by methylglyoxal, for example, significantly increases free radicals in the form of superoxide that produce oxidative damage in renal mitochondria.[51] The phenomenon of protein aggregation in biological systems is also more ubiquitous than was previously believed. Recent evidence supports the hypothesis that generalized insolubility of proteins and protein aggregation is an inherent part of ageing itself.[52] The accumulation of oxidized proteins is now believed to be a characteristic common to the tissues of aged mammals.[53]

Combining transcriptomics and proteomics in animal models has also facilitated identification of the protein targets of trace elements. Combining *nutrigenomics* with human longevity studies may help to identify the mechanisms through which trace elements regulate the metabolic and physiological pathways altered during physiological ageing.[54] Ageing may also be consistently associated with reduced responsiveness of receptor systems to external stimuli, for example, the age-related decreased phosphorylation rate of signal transduction molecules. Cellular receptors are often multi-protein complexes that require interaction between the membrane-bound and intracellular proteins that comprise signalling complexes. Even subtle disruption of these interactions have dramatic effects on cellular and tissue function and could explain the loss of neurotransmitter responsiveness that is a general characteristic of the senescent nervous system.

Epigenetics

The role of epigenetics in ageing and age-related diseases has recently become an essential area of biotechnological development. *Epigenetics* encompasses the disciplines of both genetics and molecular biology and refers to the study of molecular and phenotypic characteristics of cells that reflect not only the underlying DNA sequence of the genome, but also the expression of that genome subject to chemical alteration and chromatin remodelling.[55] Epigenetic mechanisms such as DNA methylation dynamically modulate expression of genetic information and therefore profoundly influence cellular and tissue function throughout the body. Epigenetic processes are, in effect, molecular engines that power the continuing interactions between the genome and the environment. The resultant DNA plasticity and variability in gene expression explains much of the extreme phenotypic differences characteristic of human ageing humans that occurs despite the minimal variability of the human genome itself. Ageing can be considered as a process of lifelong genetic and epigenetic interactions at all biological levels, yet this area of clinical and basic biological research has been badly neglected in major studies of ageing.[56] When studied on a larger scale, epigenetics becomes *epigenomics*.[57] Epigenomic profiling employs genome-scale analysis with microarray-based techniques to identify cell-heritable, non-sequence-based genetic changes as well as genetic variability. This may include comparing DNA methylation levels across many DNA samples in order to identify 'target' loci consistently characterized by DNA methylation or hypomethylation.[58]

Technology and age-related disease

Epigenetic technology is now being used to explore the relationship between age-related diseases and an individual's genetic background and the environment.[59] Assuming that specific age-related epigenetic changes are functionally represented in the ageing phenotype, it can then be determined whether they are due to largely genetic, environmental, or random events and if there is evidence that they can be transmitted from one generation to the next.[60] Recent studies suggest epigenetics plays an important role in age-related pathology, especially in autoimmune and inflammatory disorders,[61] malignancy,[62] and neurodegenerative disease and stroke.[63] Proteomics has recently been used successfully to identify serum protein biomarkers which can be used to discriminate between aggressive and indolent prostatic cancers and may also identify those patients at risk of recurrence.[64] These findings complement the important advances in imaging technology being used to improve early detection of this age-related neoplastic disorder.[65]

Recent application of mass spectrometry-based proteomics has also improved our understanding of the numerous molecular pathophysiological changes that occur with major muscle diseases.[66] In contrast, proteomics has yet to be clinically reliable with regard to the diagnosis of osteoarthritis.[67] However, proteomic identification of retinal proteins under oxidative stress is giving new insights into signalling mechanisms of retinal degeneration at the molecular level.[68] The technology of proteomics has also demonstrated that peripheral concentration of apolipoprotein-E (APOE) protein and the *APOE* genotype are both associated with early pathological changes in brain regions known to be vulnerable to Alzheimer's disease even before the onset of clinical evidence of the disease. Proteomics in combination with *in vivo* brain amyloid imaging may therefore permit risk prediction for this devastating neurodegenerative disorder.[69]

Oxidative stress and the degradation or modification of protein and nucleic acids are clearly associated not only with human ageing but also with the pathogenesis of many age-related chronic disease states, especially cardiovascular and autoimmune diseases. Most importantly, proteomics may be a powerful way to establish the relevance of protein oxidation to neurodegenerative diseases including Alzheimer's and Parkinson's diseases. It is also well known that aggregation of oligomeric amyloid peptides are an important causative element in the pathogenesis of Alzheimer's disease. Peptides and proteins pre-aggregated *in vivo* in patients with Alzheimer's disease have been shown to be more resistant to the anti-aggregation effects of magnetite nanoparticles than those of age-matched controls.[70] Proteomics and nanotechnology may offer the promise of effective and focused pharmacological treatment of neurodegenerative disorders.[71] In fact, recent Canadian guidelines for the development of anti-dementia therapies urge development of nanotechnology strategies that directly target the underlying pathogenesis of these diseases, specifically through the development of protein anti-aggregants.[72]

Gene therapy is already in use in combination with nanotechnology to treat age-related macular degeneration, a difficult and debilitating phenomenon in older adults. A molecular polyionic micelle with a core containing DNA with a size of the order of 10 nanometres accumulates within choroidal neovascularization lesions and subsequently provides a photosensitizing action that permits photodynamic therapy for lesion ablation. The effect is highly specific, and subconjunctival injection of the complex followed by laser irradiation produces transgenic expression of photosensitivity only at the laser-irradiated site.[73] Other technologies that will impact the lives of middle-aged and older adults include *pharmacogenetics*, the analysis of an individual's genetic profile to predict the responsiveness and adverse effects of specific drugs or on a larger scale, *pharmacogenomics*[74] to search for consistent age-related genetic variability in drug metabolism or responsiveness. In the past, pharmacogenomic studies of the elderly were rarely performed or considered with regard to establishing drug safety and dosage, but now there are studies underway that include assessment of the polymorphism of varying genetic expression of cytochrome P450[75] a key component of many metabolic pathways, as well as investigations of the extent to which protein mutations create conformational changes that lead to a high rate of amyloid accumulation in peripheral and central nervous system tissues.[76] These approaches may soon facilitate prescription of individualized or 'designer' chemotherapy regimens and targeted nutritional supplements that meet the specific needs of an individual, adjusting, for example, for insulin resistance or chronic inflammation.

Technology of reproduction, prolongevity, and immortality

Sexual health and assisted reproduction

Historically, sexual activity has been seen as the prerogative of young adults, but ageing populations have emerged as a primary market for the various biotechnologies and pharmaceuticals that promise to enhance sexual function. In fact, there appears to be a new cultural consensus that an active sex life is an important aspect of successful ageing. Sexual function itself is often seen as an important indicator of overall health status, so-called 'virility surveillance', where age-related decline in sexual function is assumed to be indicative of compromised wellness.[77] Implicit in the term sexual function is reproduction. One aspect of ageing not often considered is the role of assisted reproductive technologies (ARTs) such as cloning. ARTs have generational consequences that are similar to the social and economic impact of lifespan extension or 'prolongevity' technologies.[78] Most would agree that prolongevity using anti-ageing technology is socially and ethically acceptable, perhaps because it also achieves the beneficent amelioration of age-related disability and disease.[79] The use of human embryonic stem cells (hESC) and cloning technologies is seen by some simply as another form of technologically-assisted prolongevity, yet is far more controversial and emotional.

If it is to be technologically assisted, human reproduction, previously determined largely by physical fitness, passion, instinct, and economic factors, may therefore need considerable regulatory governance. In the United States biotechnology research involving hESC and cloning has been funded exclusively by the private sector, effectively removing it from governmental oversight. In addition, as a complex but relatively immature field there has not been much time for clinicians and researchers to discuss and establish criteria for safety, ethical practices, or even success. Of some concern is the fact that ART may generate unintentional germ-line genetic modifications that create defective 'humanoids' or that ART will be used not solely for reproduction or life extension but rather to alter and 'correct' existing genetic information either within germ cells or somatic cells. In fact, the same biotechnologies needed for assisted reproduction can create opportunities to enhance human traits, and some feel this is inherently problematic because it alters unique individual human identity.[80] There is a similar lack of bioethical discussion on regulation of hESC in Japan with regard to prolongevity applications and some difficulty accessing resources by scientists despite relative political indifference to the topic. This appears to reflect the societal context rather than simply a focus upon religious taboos against abortion or the sanctity of embryonic life as is the case in the United States. Public policy emphasis in Japan is on resolving infertility problems in young couples in order to counteract the progressive decline in fertility rates that are driving a demographic shift towards an ever more elderly, and more dependent, Japanese society.[81]

Prolongevity and immortality

Although every nutritionally balanced diet includes some antioxidant properties, the addition of dietary antioxidant supplements to counteract ageing is an attractively simple concept. Many common antioxidants such as lycopene, coenzyme Q10, vitamin C, and vitamin E are pharmacologically active but their bioavailability through dietary supplementation depends on several factors. The major drawbacks of conventional dosage forms are poor biopharmaceutical characteristics, specifically, inadequate solubility or permeability, instability during storage, or a first-pass effect and other forms of degradation within the gastrointestinal tract.

Nanopharmacology can be used to develop novel drug delivery systems (NDDSs) that can significantly improve the effectiveness of these antioxidants when they are administered orally. NDSS technologies include the design of coupling agents, liposomes, microparticles, nanoparticles, and gel-based systems[82] although the optimal NDSS technique for any specific antioxidants is largely governed by its physicochemical and pharmacokinetic characteristics.

Using nanotechnology to remove accumulated age-related cellular and subcellular damage might also sever the link between metabolism and pathology that currently defines our understanding of physiological ageing. DNA methylation, an important process in the regulation of gene expression, is also one of the biomarkers of age-related genetic damage. Molecular nanotechnology may make possible, for the first time, the precise and purposeful re-arrangement of the genome, atom by atom. Nanobot repair of DNA that has been damaged by oxidative metabolism on a cell-by-cell basis throughout the body is not yet a reality but exists as a plausible concept.[83] Nanobots could function both as intracellular medical sensors and therapeutic devices, facilitating correction as well as detection of structural deterioration due to sustained exposure of the cellular micro-architecture to the agents of oxidative stress. Nanotechnology using cerium oxide nanoparticles as free radical scavengers[84] is already a proven approach for effectively reducing oxidative damage in biological systems. Either with current or foreseeable biotechnology, indefinite postponement of ageing[85]—'engineered negligible senescence'—may actually be possible.[86]

Cloning and tissue engineering

Biotechnological therapies involving stem cells, recombinant DNA, and therapeutic cloning are promising but complex technologies that are expected to play major roles in making successful ageing a realistic routine expectation. Generating new, undamaged cells and tissues in the bodies of older adults is an appealing strategy for achieving prolongevity and, perhaps, the ultimate antidote to ageing. Human embryonic stem cells are a more obvious reservoir of regenerative cell mechanisms than are stem cells collected from adults, but the controversial political, religious, and ethical considerations described earlier in the 'Sexual health and assisted reproduction' section with regard to ART have encouraged researchers in regenerative medicine to examine more closely the relatively primitive cells residing in the bone marrow, blood, brain, liver, muscle, and skin of adults, tissues that can be harvested without sociopolitical controversy.[87] However, any advances in prolongevity achieved through regenerative medicine will require a more thorough understanding of the molecular regulation of stem cell proliferation and cell differentiation than that which currently exists.

What is currently understood is that fully differentiated human cells have a finite capacity for mitotic division and then enter a state of viable cell cycle arrest termed senescence, a condition ultimately determined by erosion of telomeres[88] the genetic elements that stabilize the ends of chromosomes.[89] Oxidative damage, a major characteristic of ageing tissues, is also an important factor in shortening telomeres.[90] The association between cellular senescence and telomere shortening has been well established *in vitro* and evidence is now accumulating to support the concept that telomere shortening is also associated with cellular senescence *in vivo*.[91] Manipulation of the genetic expression of telomerase, the enzyme that repairs damaged or shortened telomeres and stabilizes the genetic information needed for continuing accurate cell replication, may therefore extend a cell's capacity for successive mitotic cycles.

There has been a vast increase in telomerase research over the past several years, mostly with a goal of inhibiting the activity of this enzyme as a therapeutic modality to treat malignancy.[92] In fact, many human cancer cells demonstrate both unlimited mitosis and high telomerase activity. However, facilitating telomerase activity in a controlled or modifiable way may also be a way to initiate the regrowth of tissues and organs to counter the degenerative effects of ageing. Finally, for most cells, terminal differentiation and replicative senescence are permanent postmitotic conditions. Although these states appear to be attained and maintained differently, they may share a common proliferation-restricting mechanism. In fact, many non-proliferating cells can be mitotically reactivated by the suppression of cyclin-dependent kinase inhibitors (CKIs). Suppression of CKIs has been shown to be sufficient to trigger DNA synthesis and mitosis in differentiated skeletal muscle cells, quiescent human fibroblasts, and senescent human embryo kidney cells. Manipulation of the expression of CKIs may therefore become an important tool in a biotechnological approach to the control of cell proliferation.[93]

Ethical issues

Developments in biotechnical and medical innovation and geriatric clinical intervention have profoundly impacted expectations regarding the quality as well as the quantity of life in the later adult years. These developments have greatly raised expectations regarding the possibilities for maintaining wellness, they have changed the mechanics of medical decision-making, and therefore they have greatly increased the pressures associated with family responsibility for healthcare and living arrangements in ways unforeseen a few decades ago. In what has been called the 'biomedicalization of old age'[94] technology has forced reconsideration of what constitutes 'routine' medical care and what is encompassed by the term 'heroic measures'. As the range of therapeutic options gets broader, the choices get more difficult because the differences in risk and benefit are more subtle. Even if technology makes it possible to intervene and alter the physiological process of ageing, should it? If we could live a little longer using advanced biotechnology, should we? Which has primacy, the duration of life itself or the quality of life in later years? Who determines quality of life, the elderly individual or the caregivers?

What was accepted as 'successful ageing' a few years ago now may be seen as underutilization of medical, technological, and other societal resources. The social and cultural ramifications of these changes and their ethical implications remain as an evolving and unresolved matter, but all are associated to some degree with our primal fears of mortality and isolation. These same fears appear to drive some to consider and explore the extreme applications of technology even when that technology is immature and uncertain. Cryogenics, the freezing of the deceased for the purpose of future revival, for example, may be a strategy for extreme life extension that represents the emotionally driven application of biotechnology as a response to universal concerns regarding ageing and mortality.[95]

Conclusion

It has been only a decade since the first formal textbook dedicated to this topic was published.[96] Yet the gerotechnology available today has already improved our ability to offer older adults improved disease management and a significantly compressed period of physical and mental senescence. Rather than serving as a period of debility, dependency, and decreasing health, for many people the later years of life are becoming a period of continued productivity, independence, and good health. Many older adults now have 'rehirement' rather than 'retirement' as an option, and large corporations are pooling their management and marketing expertise to form groups such as the Global Coalition on Aging to assist government agencies in establishing telehealth policies and anticipating societal trends[3] Advances in telecommunication, wireless technology and personal computing, and lifestyle choices incorporating balanced diet, exercise, stress management, and nutritional supplementation have obviously been important contributors to this phenomenon. However, biotechnological therapies involving stem cells, proteomics, therapeutic cloning, and gene-based therapies are also beginning to play major roles in promoting successful ageing. Clearly we are only at the threshold of biotechnology and nanotechnology with regard to the application of genetic reconstruction and other forms of rejuvenation therapy in geriatric medicine.[97] Yet there is little doubt that the relentless advance of biotechnology and nanotechnology therapies in the decades ahead also promises, for the first time in history, increased human lifespan and, perhaps, physical immortality.[98]

References

1. Standard and Poor's. *Global Aging 2010: an irreversible truth.* <http://www2.standardandpoors.com/spf/pdf/media/global_aging_100710.pdf> (accessed 14 August 2011).
2. Greene K. Toll of caring for elderly increases. *WSJ.* 14 June 2011.
3. Singer N. The fountain of old age. *NY Times.* 6 February 2011.
4. Chang SK. Biotechnology—updates and new developments. *Biomed Environ Sci.* 2001;14(1–2):32–39.
5. Malavolta M, Mocchegiani E, Bertoni-Freddari C. New trends in biomedical aging research. *Gerontology.* 2004;50(6):420–424.
6. Muravchick S. *Geroanesthesia: principles for management of the elderly patient.* St. Louis, MO: Mosby, 1997.
7. Lexus USA. *New vehicle highlights and safety features.* <http://www.lexus.com/models/LS/features/safety.html> (accessed 25 June 2011).
8. Mercedes-Benz USA. *Advanced technologies in new vehicles.* <http://www.mbusa.com/mercedes/innovation/advanced_technologies/overview> (accessed 14 August 2011).
9. Kaur IP, Agrawal R. Nanotechnology: a new paradigm in cosmeceuticals. *Recent Pat Drug Deliv Formul.* 2007;1(2):171–182.
10. Lindberg DA. Global information infrastructure. *Int J Biomed Comput.* 1994;34(1-4):13–19.
11. Ferrante FE. Evolving telemedicine/ehealth technology. *Telemed J E-Health.* 2005;11(3):370–383.
12. Lamothe L, Fortin JP, Labbe F, Gagnon MP, Messikh D. Impacts of telehomecare on patients, providers, and organizations. *Telemed J E-Health.* 2006;12(3):363–369.
13. Nagendran S, Moores D, Spooner R, Triscott J. Is telemedicine a subset of medical informatics? *J Telemed Telecare.* 2000;6(Suppl 2):S50–S51.
14. United States Department of Health and Human Services, Health Resources and Services Administration, Rural Health. *Telehealth.* <http://www.hrsa.gov/ruralhealth/about/telehealth/> (accessed 14 August 2011).
15. Jennett PA, Affleck Hall L, Hailey D, *et al.* The socio-economic impact of telehealth: a systematic review. *J Telemed Telecare.* 2003;9(6):311–320.
16. Brignell M, Wootton R, Gray L. The application of telemedicine to geriatric medicine. *Age Ageing.* 2007;36(4):369–374.
17. Woo J. Development of elderly care services in Hong Kong: challenges and creative solutions. *Clin Med.* 2007;7(6):548–550.
18. D'Angelo LT, Tarita E, Zywietz TK, Lueth TC. A system for intelligent home care ECG upload and priorisation. *Conf Proc IEEE Eng Med Biol Soc.* 2010;2010:2188–2191.
19. Karunanithi M. Monitoring technology for the elderly patient. *Expert Rev Med Devic.* 2007;4(2):267–277.
20. Kang HG, Mahoney DF, Hoenig H, Hirth VA, *et al.* Center for Integration of Medicine and Innovative Technology Working Group on Advanced Approaches to Physiologic Monitoring for the Aged. In situ monitoring of health in older adults: technologies and issues. *J Am Geriatr Soc.* 2010;58(8):1579–1586.
21. Rantz MJ, Skubic M, Miller SJ. Using sensor technology to augment traditional healthcare. *Conf Proc IEEE Eng Med Biol Soc.* 2009;2009:6159–6162.
22. Frisardi V, Imbimbo BP. Gerontechnology for demented patients: smart homes for smart aging. *J Alzheimers Dis.* 2011;23(1):143–146.

23. Daly JM, Jogerst G, Park JY, Kang YD, Bae T. A nursing home telehealth system: keeping residents connected. *J Gerontol Nurs.* 2005;31(8):46–51.

24. Courtney KL. Privacy and senior willingness to adopt smart home information technology in residential care facilities. *Method Inform Med.* 2008;47(1):76–81.

25. Thompson HJ, Thielke SM. How do health care providers perceive technologies for monitoring older adults? *Conf Proc IEEE Eng Med Biol Soc.* 2009;2009:4315–4318.

26. Pallawala PM, Lun KC. EMR-based TeleGeriatric system. *Stud Health Technol Inform.* 2001;84(Pt 1):849–853.

27. Norum J, Pedersen S, Stormer J, *et al.* Prioritisation of telemedicine services for large scale implementation in Norway. *J Telemed Telecare.* 2007;13(4):185–192.

28. Intille SS. A new research challenge: persuasive technology to motivate healthy aging. *IEEE Trans Inf Technol Biomed.* 2004;8(3):235–237.

29. Yensen JA, Woolery LK. A demonstration of the virtual nursing college. *Stud Health Technol Inform.* 1995;8(Pt2):1716–1716.

30. Loera JA, Kuo YF, Rahr RR. Telehealth distance mentoring of students. *Telemed J E-Health.* 2007;13(1):45–50.

31. Sclater K, Alagiakrishnan K, Sclater A. An investigation of videoconferenced geriatric medicine grand rounds in Alberta. *J Telemed Telecare.* 2004;10(2):104–107.

32. de Magalhaes JP, Church GM. Genomes optimize reproduction: aging as a consequence of the developmental program. *Physiology.* 2005;20:252–259.

33. United States Department of Energy, Office of Science. *Genomics.* <http://genomics.energy.gov/> (accessed 14 August 2011).

34. de Magalhaes JP, Finch CE, Janssens G. Next-generation sequencing in aging research: emerging applications, problems, pitfalls and possible solutions. *Ageing Res Rev.* 2010;9(3):315–323.

35. Hood L. Systems biology: integrating technology, biology, and computation. *Mech Ageing Dev.* 2003;124(1):9–16.

36. de Magalhaes JP. Is mammalian aging genetically controlled? *Biogerontology.* 2003;4(2):119–120.

37. Cevenini E, Bellavista E, Tieri P. Systems biology and longevity: an emerging approach to identify innovative anti-aging targets and strategies. *Curr Pharm Design.* 2010;16(7):802–813.

38. Ureta-Vidal A, Ettwiller L, Birney E. Comparative genomics: genome-wide analysis in metazoan eukaryotes. *Nat Rev Genet.* 2003;4(4):251–262.

39. Austad SN. Comparative biology of aging. *J Gerontol A Biol.* 2009;64(2):199–201.

40. Human Ageing Genomic Resources. <http://genomics.senescence.info/science.html>.

41. de Magalhaes JP, Toussaint O. How bioinformatics can help reverse engineer human aging. *Ageing Res Rev.* 2004;3(2):125–141.

42. Austad SN. Methusaleh's zoo: how nature provides us with clues for extending human health span. *J Comp Pathol.* 2010;142(Suppl 1):S10–S21.

43. Silvestri E, Lombardi A, de Lange P. Studies of complex biological systems with applications to molecular medicine: the need to integrate transcriptomic and proteomic approaches. *J Biomed Biotechnol.* 2011;2011:810242.

44. Schiffer E, Mischak H, Zimmerli LU. Proteomics in gerontology: current applications and future aspects—a mini-review. *Gerontology.* 2009;55(2):123–137.

45. Byerley LO, Leamy L, Tam SW, Chou CW, Ravussin E. Louisiana Healthy Aging Study. Development of a serum profile for healthy aging. *Age.* 2010;32(4):497–507.

46. Fleissig Y, Reichenberg E, Redlich M, *et al.* Comparative proteomic analysis of human oral fluids according to gender and age. *Oral Dis.* 2010;16(8):831–838.

47. Miura Y, Sato Y, Arai Y, *et al.* Proteomic analysis of plasma proteins in Japanese semisuper centenarians. *Exp Gerontol.* 2011;46(1):81–85.

48. Welle S. Gene transcript profiling in aging research. *Exp Gerontol.* 2002;37(4): 583–590.

49. Ruiz-Romero C, Blanco FJ. Mitochondrial proteomics and its application in biomedical research. *Mol Biosyst.* 2009;5(10):1130–1142.

50. Laimer M, Kocher T, Chiocchetti A, *et al.* Proteomic profiling reveals a catalogue of new candidate proteins for human skin aging. *Exp Dermatol.* 2010;19(10):912–918.

51. Rosca MG, Mustata TG, Kinter MT, *et al.* Glycation of mitochondrial proteins from diabetic rat kidney is associated with excess superoxide formation. *Am J Physiol—Renal.* 2005;289(2):F420–F430.

52. David DC, Ollikainen N, Trinidad JC, Cary MP, Burlingame AL, Kenyon C. Widespread protein aggregation as an inherent part of aging in C. elegans. *PLoS Biol.* 2010;8(8):e1000450.

53. Toda T, Nakamura M, Morisawa H, Hirota M, Nishigaki R, Yoshimi Y. Proteomic approaches to oxidative protein modifications implicated in the mechanism of aging. *Geriatr Gerontol Int.* 2010;10(Suppl 1):S25–S31.

54. Meplan C. Trace elements and ageing, a genomic perspective using selenium as an example. *J Trace Elem Med Bio.* 2011;25(Suppl 1):S11–S16.

55. Gravina S, Vijg J. Epigenetic factors in aging and longevity. *Pflug Arch.* 2010;459(2):247–258.

56. Stanziano DC, Whitehurst M, Graham P, Roos BA. A review of selected longitudinal studies on aging: past findings and future directions. *J Am Geriatr Soc.* 2010;58(Suppl 2):S292–S297.

57. Fazzari MJ, Greally JM. Introduction to epigenomics and epigenome-wide analysis. *Method Mol Cell Biol.* 2010;620:243–265.

58. Feinberg AP. Genome-scale approaches to the epigenetics of common human disease. *Virchows Arch.* 2010;456(1):13–21.

59. Rodriguez-Rodero S, Fernandez-Morera JL, Fernandez AF, Menendez-Torre E, Fraga MF. Epigenetic regulation of aging. *Discovery Med.* 2010;10(52):225–233.

60. Calvanese V, Lara E, Kahn A, Fraga MF. The role of epigenetics in aging and age-related diseases. *Ageing Res Rev.* 2009;8(4):268–276.

61. Grolleau-Julius A, Ray D, Yung RL. The role of epigenetics in aging and autoimmunity. *Clin Rev Allergy Immunol.* 2010;39(1):42–50.

62. Fernandez-Morera JL, Calvanese V, Rodriguez-Rodero S, Menendez-Torre E, Fraga MF. Epigenetic regulation of the immune system in health and disease. *Tissue Antigens.* 2010;76(6):431–439.

63. Qureshi IA, Mehler MF. Emerging role of epigenetics in stroke: part 1: DNA methylation and chromatin modifications. *Arch Neurol.* 2010;67(11):1316–1322.

64. Al-Ruwaili JA, Larkin SE, Zeidan BA, *et al.* Discovery of serum protein biomarkers for prostate cancer progression by proteomic analysis. *Cancer Genom Proteom.* 2010;7(2):93–103.

65. Fitzsimons NJ, Sun L, Moul JW. Medical technologies for the diagnosis of prostate cancer. *Exp Rev Med Devic.* 2007;4(2):227–239.

66. Ohlendieck K. Proteomics of skeletal muscle differentiation, neuromuscular disorders and fiber aging. *Expert Rev Proteomics.* 2010;7(2):283–296.

67. Ruiz-Romero C, Blanco FJ. Proteomics role in the search for improved diagnosis, prognosis and treatment of osteoarthritis. *Osteoarthr Cartilage.* 2010;18(4):500–509.

68. Lee H, Arnouk H, Sripathi S, *et al.* Prohibitin as an oxidative stress biomarker in the eye. *Int J Biol Macromol.* 2010;47(5):685–690.

69. Thambisetty M, Tripaldi R, Riddoch-Contreras J, *et al.* Proteome-based plasma markers of brain amyloid- deposition in non-demented older individuals. *J Alzheimers Dis.* 2010;22(4):1099–1109.

70. Gazova Z, Antosova A, Kristofikova Z, *et al.* Attenuated antiaggregation effects of magnetite nanoparticles in cerebrospinal fluid of people with Alzheimer's disease. *Mol Biosyst.* 2010;6(11):2200–2205.

71. Singh N, Cohen CA, Rzigalinski BA. Treatment of neurodegenerative disorders with radical nanomedicine. *Ann N Y Acad Sci.* 2007;1122:219–230.

72. Feldman HH, Gauthier S, Chertkow H, Conn DK, Freedman M, Chris M. Progress in clinical neurosciences: Canadian guidelines for the development of antidementia therapies: a conceptual summary. *Can J Neurol Sci.* 2006;33(1):6–26.

73. Tamaki Y. Prospects for nanomedicine in treating age-related macular degeneration. *Nanomedicine (Lond).* 2009;4(3):341–352.

74. Mahlknecht U, Voelter-Mahlknecht S. Pharmacogenomics: questions and concerns. *Curr Med Res Opin.* 2005;21(7):1041–1047.

75. Seripa D, Pilotto A, Panza F, Matera MG, Pilotto A. Pharmacogenetics of cytochrome P450 (CYP) in the elderly. *Ageing Res Rev.* 2010;9(4):457–474.

76. Lanni C, Racchi M, Uberti D, *et al.* Pharmacogenetics and pharmagenomics, trends in normal and pathological aging studies: focus on p53. *Curr Pharm Design.* 2008;4(26):2665–2671.

77. Marshall BL. Science, medicine and virility surveillance: 'sexy seniors' in the pharmaceutical imagination. *Sociol Health Ill.* 2010;32(2):211–224.

78. Schatten GP. Safeguarding ART. *Nat Cell Biol.* 2002;4(Suppl):s19–s22.

79. Post SG. Establishing an appropriate ethical framework: the moral conversation around the goal of prolongevity. *J Gerontol A Biol.* 2004;59(6):B534–B539.

80. DeGrazia D. Enhancement technologies and human identity. *J Med Philos.* 2005;30(3):261–283.

81. Sleeboom-Faulkner M. Contested embryonic culture in Japan—public discussion, and human embryonic stem cell research in an aging welfare society. *Med Anthropol.* 2010;29(1):44–70.

82. Ratnam DV, Ankola DD, Bhardwaj V, Sahana DK, Kumar MN. Role of antioxidants in prophylaxis and therapy: a pharmaceutical perspective. *J Control Release.* 2006;113(3):189–207.

83. Bushko RG. Fight for chromallocyte. *Stud Health Technol Inform.* 2009;149:322–331.

84. Rzigalinski BA. Nanoparticles and cell longevity. *Technol Cancer Res Treat.* 2005;4(6):651–659.

85. Wiley C. Nanotechnology and molecular homeostasis. *J Am Geriatr Soc.* 2005;53(Suppl 9):S295–S298.

86. de Grey AD, Ames BN, Andersen JK, *et al.* Time to talk SENS: critiquing the immutability of human aging. *Ann N Y Acad Sci.* 2002;959:452–462.

87. Szilvassy SJ. The biology of hematopoietic stem cells. *Arch Med Res.* 2003;34(6):446–460.

88. Kipling D. Telomeres, replicative senescence and human ageing. *Maturitas.* 2001;38(1):25–37.

89. Hamet P, Tremblay J. Genes of aging. *Metabolism.* 2003;52(10 Suppl 2):5–9.

90. Goyns MH. Genes, telomeres and mammalian ageing. *Mech Ageing Devel.* 2002;123(7):791–799.

91. Ahmed A, Tollefsbol T. Telomeres and telomerase: basic science implications for aging. *J Am Geriatr Soc.* 2001;49(8):1105–1109.

92. White LK, Wright WE, Shay JW (2001). Telomerase inhibitors. *Trends Biotechnol.* 2001;19(3):114–120.

93. Pajalunga D, Mazzola A, Salzano AM, Biferi MG, De Luca G, Crescenzi M. Critical requirement for cell cycle inhibitors in sustaining nonproliferative states. *J Cell Biol.* 2007;76(6):807–818.

94. Kaufman SR, Shim JK, Russ AJ. Revisiting the biomedicalization of aging: clinical trends and ethical challenges. *Gerontologist.* 2004;44(6):731–738.

95. Romain T. Extreme life extension: investing in cryonics for the long, long term. *Med Anthropol.* 2010;29(2):194–215.

96. Harrington TL, Harrington MK. *Gerontechnology; Why and How.* Maastricht, The Netherlands: Shaker Publishing, 2000.

97. Grossman T. Latest advances in antiaging medicine. *Keio J Med.* 2005;54(2):85–94.

98. Kurzweil R, Grossman T. Fantastic voyage: live long enough to live forever. The science behind radical life extension questions and answers. *Stud Health Technol Inform.* 2009;149:187–194.

PART 2

Ageing at a Systems Level

CHAPTER 5

Ageing at system level: neurological ageing

Anand Prakash and Kailash Krishnan

Introduction

Neurology in the ageing is being recognized increasingly as a subspecialty and with advances in medical care and improved quality of living, there is an increasing need to understand complex neurological disease in the elderly. The focus of this chapter will be on intrinsic ageing. Extrinsic factors also play an important role in secondary ageing.[1]

Ageing is not predictable either in terms of rate or sequence which is in direct contrast to the development of the central nervous system. Almost all cross-sectional studies reveal decline in physiological processes with increasing age. The magnitude of these changes varies in individuals. For the majority, these changes occur late in life. There is a strong correlation between cumulative pathological changes in the brain and cognitive decline, though there may be clinical consequences at any age.[2] The loss of neurons is the most significant change in the 'older' nervous system.[2]

The concept of brain plasticity

Neuroplasticity refers to the structural and functional adaptability of neurons and neural networks to external stimuli. This was proposed in the late eighteenth century and remained neglected for decades until revitalized in the twentieth century.

One of the key elements to neuroplasticity functioning is 'synaptic pruning'. This refers to regulatory processes, which facilitate a productive change in neural structure by reducing the overall number of neurons or connections that may involve changing the expression of neurotransmitters leaving more efficient synaptic configurations. In lay terms this could be used to describe removal of damaged or invalid neurons whilst maintaining 'efficient' neurons. Trophic interactions with target tissues are important elements of plasticity at all stages of life.

Brain

An important feature of successful ageing is intact cognition. At a cellular level in normal ageing, neuronal loss occurs only in limited areas (differential ageing) in comparison to fetal development where it occurs in all parts.[1]

The cognitive decline related to ageing does not involve a general decline in the functioning of the memory systems. Some types of memories are spared, whereas others usually decay during normal ageing. For example, frontal lobe impairment is associated with lack of attention and loss of executive functions and working memory while cell loss in the hippocampus is associated with defects in declarative learning and memory. Interestingly behavioural, electrophysiological, and morphological evidence suggest that brain plasticity continues till the end of life.

Using magnetic resonance imaging (MRI), Bartzokis et al.[3] demonstrated that grey matter volume declines linearly until old age, with no change in cerebrospinal fluid volume.

Frontal lobes

Ageing is associated with decreased activation of frontal lobes and increased activation of other cortical regions.[3] The loss of cognitive abilities suggests that the decline of the frontal lobes is the main culprit in age-related memory decline. Positron emission tomography studies revealed that the rate of blood flow in the frontal cortex was lower in older adults. Comparison of memory in old and younger adults demonstrated less activation in the left prefrontal cortex during face recognition and retrieval of words.

The dorsolateral prefrontal cortex mediates attention, sensory information, memory and problem solving skills for the purpose of navigating our external environments. The orbitomedial prefrontal cortex coordinates connections from the subcortical regions and the amygdala to the body controlling emotional processing, fear regulation, and attachment in order to navigate our inner experience. The former develops gradually over the first two decades of life and begins to decline early in adulthood whereas the latter is well maintained into adulthood. This may explain why tasks involving working memory may deteriorate, whilst those involved in emotional regulation and social processing are retained or even show improvement as we get older.

Hippocampus

It is well known that the hippocampus is impaired by ageing and that these structural and functional alterations are regional and cell-specific. Degenerative changes include neuronal cell loss in the hilus and CA regions, reduced synaptic density, and decreased glucose utilization.

Brain-derived neurotrophic factor has been associated with hippocampal-dependent learning and memory. Polymorphism of the gene involving a single amino acid substitution in codon 66 (from valine to methionine) can lead to a decreased regulated secretion.

Remarkably, the density of granule cells in the dentate gyrus increases during adulthood and remains constant during ageing, suggesting that age-related functional decline in the dentate gyrus may not be mediated by a loss of granule cells, but rather by a decline in the birth of new granule cells.

In animal models, age-related dysfunction of glucocorticoid receptors in the hypothalamo-pituitary axis contributes to hippocampal ageing and the lack of ATP production in aged hippocampus explains the profound changes in learning and memory and the altered regulation of the stress response.

There is neuropathological correlation in hippocampal sclerosis with ageing which is different to changes seen in Alzheimer's dementia. There is an accelerated loss of neurons in the pyramidal area in Alzheimer's disease when compared to controls and at any age. Granulovacuolar degenerative changes are demonstrated in dementias of Alzheimer's, Pick's disease, and Fahr's syndrome (idiopathic calcification of the basal ganglia and cerebral cortex).

Cross-sectional MRI studies have shown that patients with Alzheimer's dementia have significantly greater entorhinal cortex and hippocampal atrophy than normal subjects.

The midbrain, cerebellum, and brainstem

Normal ageing in the cerebellum is selective and regional. Volume loss of cerebellum occurs to a lesser extent when compared to the cerebral cortex. MRI amongst healthy young to older adults reveals an age-related decline in the surface area of the midbrain, cerebellum, and no changes in the pons.[3] The maximal loss occurs in the cerebellar vermis with minimal loss in the medial hemispheres. The lateral hemispheres do not appear to decline with age, no volume changes are known to occur in the midbrain, pons, and medulla.

Purkinje cell (PC) loss predominantly in the posterior cerebellar vermis occurs due to lack of neuroglobin (a neuroprotectant protein) and loss of reciprocal interaction with target neurons. It is thought that there is a decline of cell count of approximately 2.5 per cent every decade, sometimes up to 40 per cent, but this remains controversial. The greatest loss in PC densities occur in the superior cerebellar vermis. At a cellular level, there is loss of PC volume due to lack of cytoplasmic matrix, lack of nuclear elements, decrease in the width and height of dendrites, and vacuolar degeneration.

Ageing and the peripheral nervous system

Age-related changes affect all of the sensory modalities. The sensation of touch decreases with increasing age and is also directly affected by poor circulation which is more prevalent in older people.[1]

Touch receptors are fast adapting (FA) or slowly adapting (SA). These mechanoreceptors can be subclassified into: FA I (Meissner corpuscles and hair receptors), FA II (Pacinian corpuscles), SA I (Merkel cell–neurite complexes and the touch pads), and SA II (Ruffini endings). Information is processed through various channels P, NP I, NP II, and NP III. The P channel is most sensitive for vibration sense and declines with age. In older people there is loss of large nerve fibres and Meissner's corpuscles and at cellular level changes are attributed to distal axonopathy and atrophy of the sensory neurons.[4]

Decreased sensitivity of the index finger with increasing age was reported in the early 1980s. Sensitivity threshold is lowest in the lips, finger tips, and tip of the tongue, and highest in the back of the hand and feet.

The lack of touch receptors with ageing overall decreases the input to the cerebral cortex and this may account for the lack of arousal in older patients. However, sympathetic overactivity could predispose to increased anxiety in the elderly.

Pain

Changes in pain perception with ageing are complex. The issue is complicated by the physical access to drugs, polypharmacy, and comorbidity. It is thought that the elderly exhibit a higher threshold for visceral pain.[5] A study by researchers in the National University of Ageing in Australia reported that increased age was associated with differential pain perception amongst A fibres versus C fibres.[6] Interestingly, cognitive impairment is not known to affect reporting painful stimulus.[7–9]

Balance

Two problems very commonly experienced by the elderly are dizziness and falls. Increased postural sway occurs with ageing and this could be due to loss of proprioception. Maintenance of balance control is due to coordination amongst the vestibular, visual, and the somatosensory systems. Balance maintenance whilst standing on one leg shows significant changes with ageing.

Degenerative structural changes in the vestibular system involve the epithelia, Scarpa's ganglia, otoconia, vestibular nerve, and cerebellum. In the sensory receptors, there is a 40 per cent reduction in hair cells of the semicircular canals after the age of 70 and low cell density most obvious in the saccular maculae and the cristae ampullares. It is reported that there could be nearly 60 per cent loss of hair cells in the cristae. Movement of fragmented otoconia into the posterior semicircular canals is attributed to the postural imbalances. Microscopic changes describe ciliary loss, fusion, formation of vesicles, and cell shrinkage.

Studies investigating neural cell counts, volume, and nuclear density reported a 3 per cent cell loss for every decade in life after the age of 40. Atherosclerotic changes are more obvious in the vestibular apparatus in comparison to the cochlea.

Smell

Olfactory dysfunction can occur due to mechanical obstruction to the nasal passages, sensorineural damage of the lining epithelium, or damage to the central olfactory structures and their connections.

It is now known that olfactory dysfunction occurs in about half of the population between the ages of 65 and 80 years and in nearly 75 per cent of those 80 years of age and older.[10,11]

Odour identification and perception also decline with ageing.[11,12] There is no gender predisposition to this decline. The precise mechanism of this is not clearly known but suggested mechanisms include degenerative changes occurring in the olfactory epithelium, decreased number of receptors and their activity in the olfactory bulb due to lack of mucosal blanket, and defective transport in the odoriferous molecules to the olfactory cleft.

At a central level, degenerative changes occur in the central structures of the hippocampus, amygdala, the temporal lobes, and the entorhinal cortex. Disruption of odour quality coding in the cortex mediates olfactory deficits in Alzheimer's disease.[13] In Parkinson's disease patients cortical atrophy in olfactory-related brain regions correlated specifically with olfactory dysfunction.[14]

Difficulty in identifying odours predicts subsequent development of mild cognitive impairment. Olfactory dysfunction is common in Alzheimer's disease and other neurodegenerative diseases.[14–19]

Taste

Loss of taste in the elderly could be due to intrinsic factors[20] including loss of taste buds (nearly 60 per cent), though the density does not decrease. Other factors include metabolic insufficiency, changes to epithelial vascularity, lack of blood flow, atrophy of the secretory glands, and lymphatics.[21]

Extrinsic factors that may have an influence include: smoking; local disease; bacterial and fungal colonization; systemic disease including diabetes mellitus; head trauma; neoplasms; dental and otological operations which may damage the facial or glossopharyngeal nerve; and polypharmacy including antihypertensive, antineoplastic, antilipidaemic, and antirheumatic agents.

Hearing

Ageing with loss of high-frequency sounds of a Galton whistle was probably observed in the early nineteenth century.

The effects of ageing on the auditory system are bilateral and symmetrical. It is reported that 40–50 per cent of the elderly aged 75 and over have a hearing loss of 25 decibels.[22] Loss of hearing occurs earlier in men and women retain greater acuity. The cochlea is most affected by ageing.

The commonest cause of sensorineural hearing loss in the elderly is presbycusis. On a pathological basis presbycusis is broadly classified into: sensory, neural, strial, and conductive, and histological changes occur from the cochlea to the auditory cortex in the temporal lobe.

Sensory presbycusis is a slow process involving degeneration of the basal portion of the organ of Corti (loss of hair cells) and rapid decline in high-frequency thresholds, but speech discrimination remains good. The neural variety is due to loss of spiral ganglion cells, atrophy throughout the cochlea, poor speech discrimination, rapid hearing loss, and a flat audiogram.[22] Strial or metabolic presbycusis is due to atrophy of striavascularis, slowly progressive, preserved speech discrimination, and a flat audiogram. Conductive presbycusis is due to thickening of the basal membrane of the cochlea, gradually downsloping high-frequency sensory loss, and is progressive.

Vision

Vision is the last sensory system to develop and is the most complicated. Age is the leading risk factor for visual impairment, blindness, and disability.

The most common visual disability in older person is refractive errors, cataracts, glaucoma, macular degeneration, and diabetic retinopathy. Visual processing speed, light sensitivity (seeing in twilight and dark), dynamic vision (reading TV displays or digital displays), near vision, and visual search (locating a sign) become impaired with ageing. The most important functional changes are decrease in pupil size and loss of accommodation. Papillary dilatation also decreases with age. The lens, normally crystalline, thickens and turns yellow and leads to cataract. The cornea becomes thin and loses some of its transparency and curvature. The anterior chamber becomes shallow and this predisposes to glaucoma.

Colour vision diminishes with ageing and this is due to the decreased amount and spectral distribution of light. Contrast sensitivity is diminished due to drying of the eye and the small size of the pupil.

The ageing process in vitreous can make the gel more liquefied; and the vitreous can collapse and may lead to posterior vitreous detachment, retinal tears, and detachments at locations of macular holes. Sometimes calcium salts can develop in vitreous.

It is estimated that there is a loss of at least 30 per cent of the rod cells (usually 120 million) with age, though the number of cone cells remains stable. There is increased oxidative stress on the photoreceptor and ganglion cells. There is slowness and lack of blood supply to the choroid which is due to accumulation of waste and retinal pigment ischemia.

There is slowing in dark adaptation and this can be attributed to delayed rhodopsin regeneration in the retinal photoreceptors. This age-related delay in dark adaptation may also contribute to night vision problems commonly experienced by the elderly.

Ageing and the autonomic nervous system

The importance of the autonomic nervous system is much appreciated in the elderly when loss of precision in control of vital functions and deficits in effectiveness are most obvious. Systemic autonomic failure can occur as a syndrome in primary neurodegenerative disorders like Parkinson's disease, multiple systems atrophy, or secondary to complications of systemic disorders like diabetes mellitus or amyloidosis. The significant clinical effects include: orthostatic and postprandial hypotension; impaired thermoregulation; gastrointestinal problems causing dysphagia, constipation, or diarrhoea; detrusor instability; and erectile dysfunction.

Sympathetic nervous system

Much of the current knowledge about age-related changes in sympathetic nervous function is derived from studies of circulating catecholamine levels, noradrenaline kinetics and microneurographic recordings from sympathetic nerves of skeletal muscle.

There is an age-related increase in sympathetic nerve activity, males greater than females. Evidence suggests that basal plasma noradrenalin levels increase with ageing.[23] At the neurotransmitter junction, decreased sensitivity of the usual inhibitory prejunctional alpha-2 and decreased uptake of noradrenaline overrides the facilitatory effects of beta-2 adrenoreceptors. Other relevant causes include decreased local metabolism and systemic clearance.

Arterial stiffening with ageing may reduce the ability of the baroreceptors to transduce changes in pressure, diminishing the magnitude of the baroreflex. As a result, both advancing age and chronic hypertension (either or in combination) are associated with impairment of baroreflex responsiveness.[24] The elderly generally manifest a reduced responsiveness to beta adrenergic stimulation. The maximal attainable heart rate, stroke volume, ejection fraction, cardiac output, and oxygen delivery are all reduced in healthy older adults. The administration of beta adrenergic agonists elicits lesser inotropic and chronotropic responses in the elderly, while beta-blocking drugs retain their effectiveness.

As ageing impairs both the diastolic filling and the chronotropic and inotropic responsiveness of the heart, the ability of the older patient to cope with perioperative stress is predictably impaired. Increased metabolic demands, such as those imposed by sepsis or postoperative shivering, may not be met when the maximal cardiac output and tissue oxygen delivery are limited by ageing.

Parasympathetic nervous system

Not much is clearly known about the ageing in this system. Some studies have suggested that the parasympathetic system could be spared. It is also known that the sympathetic neurons modulate the synthesis of the nerve growth factor by parasympathetic neurons. Much of the decline reported related to ageing is reductions in heart rate variability in response to respiration, cough, and the Valsalva manoeuvre. Healthy ageing is associated with reductions in both baroreflex and parasympathetic modulation of heart rate, with a greater loss of the parasympathetic component.

Conclusion

Neurological disorders are more common in older people due to widespread degenerative changes in the nervous system. Cognitive decline is part of the normal and natural ageing process. Although the magnitude of these changes varies between individuals, they are affected by both extrinsic and intrinsic factors. Despite many changes the functional integrity is well maintained in older people.

References

1. Woodruff-Pak DS. *The neuropsychology of aging.* New York: Wiley-Blackwell, 1997.
2. Green MS, Kaye JA, Ball MJ. The Oregon brain aging study: neuropathology accompanying healthy aging in the oldest old. *Neurology.* 2000;54(1):105–113.
3. Bartzokis G, Beckson M, Lu PH, Nuechterlein KH, Edwards N, Mintz J. Age-related changes in frontal and temporal lobe volumes in men: a magnetic resonance imaging study. *Arch Gen Psychiatry.* 2001;58(5):461–465.
4. Lasch H, Castell DO, Castell JA. Evidence for diminished visceral pain with aging: studies using graded intraesophageal balloon distension. *Am J Physiol.* 1997;272(1 Pt 1):G1–G3.
5. Gibson SJ, Farrell M. A review of age differences in the neurophysiology of nociception and the perceptual experience of pain. *Clin J Pain.* 2004;20(4):227–239.
6. Mossey JM. Defining racial and ethnic disparities in pain management. *Clin Orthop Relat Res.* 2011;469(7):1859–1870.
7. Chakour MC, Gibson SJ, Bradbeer M, Helme RD. The effect of age on A delta- and C-fibre thermal pain perception. *Pain.* 1996;64(1):143–152.
8. Zhou Y, Petpichetchian W, Kitrungrote L. Psychometric properties of pain intensity scales comparing among postoperative adult patients, elderly patients without and with mild cognitive impairment in China. *Int J Nurs Stud.* 2011;48(4):449–457.
9. Niruban A, Biswas S, Willicombe SC, Myint PK. An audit on assessment and management of pain at the time of acute hospital admission in older people. *Int J Clin Pract.* 2010;64(10):1453–1457.
10. Winkler S, Garg AK, Mekayarajjananonth T, Bakaeen LG, Khan E. Depressed taste and smell in geriatric patients. *J Am Dent Assoc.* 1999;130(12):1759–1765.
11. Robinson AM, Conley DB, Shinners MJ, Kern RC. Apoptosis in the aging olfactory epithelium. *Laryngoscope.* 2002;112(8 Pt 1):1431–1435.
12. Kemp AH, Pierson JM, Helme RD. Quantitative electroencephalographic changes induced by odor detection and identification tasks: age related effects. *Arch Gerontol Geriatr.* 2001 ;33(1):95–107.
13. Bacon AW, Bondi MW, Salmon DP, Murphy C. Very early changes in olfactory functioning due to Alzheimer's disease and the role of apolipoprotein E in olfaction. *Ann N Y Acad Sci.* 1998;855:723–731.
14. Berendse HW, Booij J, Francot CM, *et al.* Subclinical dopaminergic dysfunction in asymptomatic Parkinson's disease patients' relatives with a decreased sense of smell. *Ann Neurol.* 2001;50(1):34–41.
15. Baloyannis SJ. Mitochondria are related to synaptic pathology in Alzheimer's disease. *Int J Alzheimers Dis.* 2011;2011:305395.
16. Braak H, Braak E. Evolution of neuronal changes in the course of Alzheimer's disease. *J Neural Transm Suppl.* 1998;53:127–140.
17. Braak H, Braak E. Development of Alzheimer-related neurofibrillary changes in the neocortex inversely recapitulates cortical myelogenesis. *Acta Neuropathol.* 1996;92(2):197–201.
18. Rapoport SI. Coupled reductions in brain oxidative phosphorylation and synaptic function can be quantified and staged in the course of Alzheimer disease. *Neurotox Res.* 2003;5(6):385–398.
19. Nava PB, Mathewson RC. Effect of age on the structure of Meissner corpuscles in murine digital pads. *Microsc Res Tech.* 1996;34(4):376–389.
20. Nordin S, Razani LJ, Markison S, Murphy C. Age-associated increases in intensity discrimination for taste. *Exp Aging Res.* 2003;29(3):371–381.
21. Jacobson A, Green E, Murphy C. Age-related functional changes in gustatory and reward processing regions: an fMRI study. *Neuroimage.* 2010;53(2):602–610.
22. Weinstein BE. *Geriatric audiology.* New York: Thieme Medical Publishers, 2000.
23. Diz DI, Arnold AC, Nautiyal M, Isa K, Shaltout HA, Tallant EA. Angiotensin peptides and central autonomic regulation. *Curr Opin Pharmacol.* 2011;11(2):131–137.
24. Kaye D, Esler M. Sympathetic neuronal regulation of the heart in aging and heart failure. *Cardiovasc Res.* 2005;66(2):256–264.

CHAPTER 6

Cardiovascular ageing

Shamsuddin Akhtar and G. Alec Rooke

Introduction

The prevalence of cardiovascular disease (hypertension, coronary artery disease, and congestive heart failure) rises exponentially with age.[1] Hypertension rises from 38 per cent of men and 38 per cent of women between ages 40–59, to 65 per cent of men and 77 per cent of women over the age of 80.[1] Similarly, coronary artery disease increases from 7 per cent of men and 7 per cent of women between ages 40–59 years, to 37 per cent of men and 23 per cent of women over the age of 80.[1] The incidence of congestive heart failure also increases exponentially.[1] Though poor cardiovascular status in the elderly is frequently attributed to the presence of concomitant cardiovascular diseases, there are many independent physiological changes that occur in the cardiovascular system with ageing that result in a lower overall cardiovascular reserve. Not only does the ageing process contribute to the development of disease, ageing appears to worsen the outcome of disease. For example, elderly patients are not only more likely to experience myocardial infarction, they are also more likely to develop heart failure as a consequence of a myocardial infarction than their younger counterparts.[2–4] Furthermore, elderly patients are also more likely to die from their myocardial infarction, develop cardiac arrest, papillary muscle rupture, acquired ventricular septal defect, and free wall rupture.[2]

This chapter addresses predominantly the physiological and pathophysiological effects of ageing on the cardiovascular system. It is difficult to clearly differentiate the ageing process from age-related diseases. In a particular patient, both processes interact to yield the specific physiological state of the system. In this chapter the age-related changes in the vascular system will be discussed first followed by changes in the heart. The general changes induced in vasculature and the heart are the same: stiffening, thickening, dilatation or enlargement, and endothelial or myocardial dysfunction. Further discussion will include the haemodynamic consequences of these changes, which involve arterial-ventricular coupling. Changes in the autonomic regulation and the neuroendocrine system, which occur with ageing, and their impact on the cardiovascular system, will then be reviewed. Finally, perioperative outcomes and general principles of cardiovascular management in the elderly will be discussed. (For respiratory diseases in the elderly, see Chapter 14.)

Vascular ageing

Vascular ageing brings together a myriad of changes that result in vascular stiffness and a predisposition to atherosclerosis. Vascular stiffness is the result of increased collagen, decreased elastin, glycosylation of proteins, free radical damage, calcification and chronic mechanical stress (also described as 'fatigue failure'). The concept of 'fatigue failure' is extrapolated from the effect of that observed in rubber tubing subjected to repetitive stretch/relaxation cycling.[5] Small vessels are affected by ageing, while altered immunological balance within the vasculature contributes to the structural and functional changes.[6–10] Endothelial dysfunction leading to vascular dysfunction is also noted with ageing. In the arteries, vascular stiffness alters the arterial waveform, most notably causing systolic accentuation, and leads to myocardial remodelling and a diminished capacity of the heart to respond to stress. Venous stiffening impairs the ability of the cardiovascular system to buffer changes in blood volume.

Atherosclerosis, in turn, contributes to the many age-related diseases such as stroke, coronary artery disease, and peripheral vascular disease. Atherosclerosis causes occlusion of the arteries. It is a heterogeneous process, in comparison to those age-related changes that happen quite uniformly throughout the conduit arteries. The severity of blood turbulence and shear stress provide a nidus for the process of atherosclerosis. Inflammation is the hallmark of atherosclerosis.[6]

Vascular stiffening

Elasticity of the vasculature primarily depends on the balance of its two major components, collagen and elastin. Elastin production essentially ceases by age 25 and collagen turnover becomes slower with ageing. With ageing, the elastic lamellae undergo thinning and fragmentation[11] with gradual transfer of mechanical forces to collagen. Collagen is 100–1000 times stiffer than elastin.[12] The possible cause of this elastin fragmentation is an alteration in transforming growth factor beta-1 (TGFβ-1) activity, metallo-proteinases activity, and chronic mechanical stress. The net result of these changes is an increase in the ratios of collagen to elastin in the vessels.[12]

The second factor that contributes to vascular stiffening is the non-enzymatic glycosylation of proteins, lipids, and nucleic acids, leading to the formation of advanced glycation end-products (AGEs). These heterogeneous groups of poorly characterized products linked together in a complicated network also contribute to the loss of vascular elasticity.[13,14] AGEs induce cross-linking of collagen, which stiffens the collagen and makes it less susceptible to normal turnover.[15] Glycation also affects elastin in the aorta, leading to similar functional consequences.[16] Accumulation of AGEs has also been linked to many age-related pathologies including oxidative stress,[16,17] progenitor cell dysfunction[18], non-vascular cell apoptosis,[19,20] and endothelial cell dysfunction.[20]

The third factor that contributes to vascular stiffening with ageing is progressive vascular calcification. This is a complicated process whereby in certain disease states, vascular smooth muscles cells, pericytes, and endothelial cells change their phenotypes to mesenchymal cells, osteoblasts, and chondrocytes.[6] All these processes can then lead to increased calcium deposition in the vasculature and cause vascular stiffness.[21]

Stiffening of the arteries is not uniform. Imaging/pulse wave measurement[22] and *in vitro*[23] studies of the aorta show that the abdominal aorta develops significant stiffness with ageing, whereas the ascending aorta lengthens and becomes dilated.[24] This may be a compensatory mechanism to maintain capacitance in the face of increased wall stiffness.

Vascular thickening

Vessels thicken with age primarily from intimal thickening and that is attributed to increases in collagen, fibronectin, proteoglycans, and migrating smooth muscle cells.[25] These changes are stimulated by TGFβ-1, angiotensin-II, and decreased levels of inhibitory cytokines and degrading enzymes.[26] Angiotensin-converting enzyme inhibitors produce beneficial effects by reducing connective tissue remodelling, smooth muscle hypertrophy and arterial stiffness.

Endothelial dysfunction

Endothelium is a biologically active organ, comprising approximately 1.5 kg.[27] It is responsible for synthesizing and releasing a wide array of molecules, which modulate arterial structure, vasoreactivity, thrombolytic and vaso-protective functions. Arterial endothelial dysfunction typically refers to changes in normal endothelial phenotype that promotes atherosclerosis and shifts the endothelium to a more vasoconstrictor, procoagulant, proliferative and proinflammatory state.[28–30]

Changes in vascular reactivity due to endothelial dysfunction have been demonstrated in functional studies in the elderly.[26,31] This is attributed to decreased production of nitric oxide (NO), which is a ubiquitous controller and modulator of many physiological processes. Endothelium-derived NO causes vasodilation and has anti-atherosclerotic properties.[31] Decreased NO production is due to reduced endothelium derived nitric oxide synthase (eNOS) and reduced eNOS expression.[32] There is some evidence to suggest that ageing also changes the expression of intracellular eNOS binding proteins.[33,34] Increased angiotensin-II decreases NO production while lower NO production decreases the ability of the vessels to dilate to mechanical stress.

Another mediator that may contribute to endothelial dysfunction is endothelin-1 (ET-1). ET-1 is 50 times more potent at vasoconstriction than noradrenaline.[34] Though the ET-1 expression is variable in different vascular beds, increased levels of ET-1 have been noted with ageing and may be responsible for the glomerulosclerosis that is observed in ageing kidneys.[35,36] ET-1-mediated vasoconstriction is augmented in older adults[37,38] and synthesis of ET-1 is greater in cultured aortic cells obtained from older when compared with younger donors.[39] There is also evidence that shows a positive association of ET-1 and oxidative stress with ageing.[37]

Increased expression of prostanoid vasoconstrictor proteins and altered cyclo-oxygenase and prostaglandin H synthase activities[40] have been shown with ageing. Vascular endothelial growth factor (VEGF) and hypoxia-induced factor (HIF) are also reduced with ageing. Endothelial dysfunction leads to an attenuated vasodilator responses in skin microvasculture[41,42] and contributes to microvascular dysfunction of the skin. The latter may predispose the elderly to impaired wound healing.[43]

Inflammation and vascular ageing

Atherosclerosis and arteriosclerosis are inflammatory processes. Increased levels of C-reactive protein and increases in erythrocyte sedimentation rate suggest an increased inflammatory propensity in the elderly.[6] Some have coined the condition as 'inflamm-aging', and the process is thought to be due to upregulation of a range of pro-inflammatory cytokines.[44,45] However, concurrent immunodeficiency has also been noted in the elderly that makes them prone to infection and immune-mediated diseases. It is not unreasonable to assume that the inflammatory milieu affects vascular ageing; however, the exact contribution of immunological balance to vascular changes in the elderly is unclear.

Small vessel pathology and ageing

Small vessel vasculature, particularly in the cerebral circulation is also affected by ageing.[46] Transcranial Doppler studies have shown evidence of increased arterial stiffness in cerebral circulation with ageing. Endothelial cells become elongated, mitochondrial content decreases, capillary number is reduced in the cerebral cortex and hippocampus, while the basement membrane thickens and becomes fibrotic.[7,8] Perivascular fibrosis, replacement of vascular smooth muscle cells by fibrohyaline material and generalized small vessel atrophy is noted with ageing. Collectively these changes lead to derangement in microcirculatory controls and predispose the elderly to ischaemic and neurological events. These small vessel changes are also closely related to the development of Alzheimer's disease, Parkinson's disease, and other neurodegenerative diseases such as cerebral autosomal dominant arteriopathy with subcortical infarcts and leucoencephalopathy.[9,10]

Vein remodelling

Like the large arteries,[5,12] veins also stiffen with increasing age.[47–49] Aged veins display subintimal fibrous thickening, fibrosis of the three media layers, a decrease in elastic tissue, increased collagen cross-linking, and hyperplasia of the smooth muscle cells.[50,51] About 70 per cent of the total blood volume is contained in the low pressure venous system.[51] The venous system is further divided into a central compartment (splanchnic) and a peripheral compartment.[51] Fluctuations in the compliance of the venous system play a very important role in the development of hypertension and compensation to hypovolaemia. An age-related decrease in venous compliance has been demonstrated, similar to that seen in the arterial system.[48] This decrease in venous compliance does not seem to be due to increased sympathetic or adrenergic influences in the elderly.[49] Other factors such as increased endothelin or myogenic factors may be responsible.[50] However, it is clear that this decrease in venous capacitance contributes to the development of hypertension in a group of patients.[52] It also impairs cardiovascular control and reduces the ability of elderly vasculature to buffer hemodynamic stresses, such as hypovolaemia.[48]

Cardiac ageing

The heart is composed of many cell types and tissues. Although cardiac myocytes contribute to the majority of the cell mass, numerically, they constitute only half of the cell population. Smooth muscle cells, endothelial cells, adipose tissue, and cardiac fibroblasts make up the other half. The heart undergoes physiological and pathophysiological ageing. The heart stiffens and potentially dilates, myocardial and endocardial dysfunction develops with ageing, and eventually some degree of systolic and diastolic dysfunction occurs. Some of the changes are due to primary modifications in the cells and tissues due to ageing, while others are in response to changes in the vasculature, for example, in response to increase stiffness of the vasculature. Yet some changes are due to pathological effects of cardiovascular disease, which are so commonly seen in the elderly.

Ventricular remodelling (stiffening and thickening)

The number of myocytes decreases with ageing. By some estimates, on average the heart has lost more than 30 per cent of its myocytes by age 80 years.[53] Greater loss of cells is noted in patients with cardiovascular disease. This is due to necrosis and apoptosis, which increase with ageing.[54] However, cardiac myocytes also hypertrophy with ageing.[53] The left ventricular wall thickens even in the absence of arterial hypertension,[55] concentric hypertrophy is noted, and the left ventricular chamber becomes more spherical.[55] The intraventricular septum also thickens which can contribute to left ventricular outflow track obstruction and further increase the afterload.[55]

Increased fibrosis is seen in older hearts.[2] The fibroblasts become more dysfunctional with ageing and show an attenuated response to growth factors (TGF-β, angiotensin-II).[56,57] Scar formation and extracellular matrix formation and healing are impaired in the elderly making them more prone to severe complications after myocardial infarction. The proportion of extracellular proteins also changes and increased expression of collagen, fibronectin, α1 and α5 integrins is noted.[26] Just as in the vasculature, collagen cross-linking increases with ageing. The resulting left ventricular hypertrophy and increased fibrosis lead to increased stiffness of the heart and potential valvular impairment and diastolic dysfunction. The reasons for these changes are complex and interrelated, and are in response to mechanical, hormonal and inflammatory stress.[58]

Excitation–contraction coupling

Functional responses in the myocardium change with ageing. Deactivation of L-type calcium channels and decreased outflow of potassium prolong cytoplasmic calcium release.[59] Reduced sarcoplasmic reticulum calcium ATPase pump activity decreases the rate of calcium re-uptake into the sarcoplasmic reticulum.[60] These phenomena lengthen the duration of contraction, and equally importantly, slow myocardial relaxation. Early diastolic filling is therefore compromised, and requires 'catch-up' in later diastole. Late diastolic filling depends on the atrial pressure and atrial contraction. In order to maintain an adequate end-diastolic volume, the atrial pressure rises, which increases backpressure in the pulmonary vasculature and can lead to cardiogenic pulmonary congestion and even pulmonary oedema when stressed by fluid overload (diastolic heart failure). Stiff ventricles further compound this problem. Elderly patients are much more prone to diastolic heart failure than their younger counterparts.[61]

In contrast to the vascular system, eNOS activity and expression are maintained in the aged heart.[62,63] However, several signal transduction pathways are impaired with ageing.[26,64,65] Anaesthetic preconditioning is reduced in the elderly due to changes in gene expression and post-translational mechanisms.[66] Myocytes become more susceptible to oxidative stress, AGE load, and the associated protein modulation by AGEs.[67]

Coronary vasomotor tone

Coronary vasomotor tone is regulated by neural control, endothelium-dependent modulation, and myogenic regulation. Though resting coronary blood flow is not significantly affected, there are some animal data to suggest that the coronary blood flow reserve is significantly reduced with ageing.[68] The adaptive reserve capacity of the endocardium is reduced compared to the epicardium and that may be responsible for the greater vulnerability of the endocardium to ischaemic episodes in the elderly.[69,70] Though vascular smooth muscle function and its neural control change with ageing,[71] myocardial oxygen demand is the principal controller of coronary blood flow even in the elderly. Hydrogen peroxide (which is a marker of cardiac metabolic activity), and local angiotensin-II production increases with ageing. Machii and colleagues have shown that ageing alters metabolic activity in cardiac myocytes, which can alter coronary vascular tone in arterioles.[68,72] However, the overall effect of ageing on coronary blood flow regulation and myocardial oxygen extraction is unknown.

Valvular changes with ageing

The thickness of the aortic and mitral valve leaflets increases with ageing. Annular dilatation is very common and 90 per cent of healthy 80-year-olds demonstrate some form of mild multivalvular regurgitation, which is typically mild, central, and present with normal appearing leaflets.[73] Specifically, the incidence of aortic regurgitation increases with age and 16 per cent of the elderly have been noted to have some form of moderate to severe aortic regurgitation.[74] The incidence of mitral annular calcification and regurgitation also increases with age. Up to 50 per cent of females and 36 per cent of males were noted to have significant mitral annular calcification.[73] It is associated with coronary events, heart failure, atrial fibrillation, endocarditis, thromboembolic strokes, and transient ischaemic attacks.[73] Similarly, the incidence of aortic stenosis increases with ageing and 80 per cent of the elderly have some degree of aortic sclerosis. This is due to increasing stiffening, scarring, and calcification of valves. The presence of significant aortic stenosis is associated with a higher incidence of new coronary events and two to three times increased risk of adverse perioperative cardiac events.[75]

Cardiac conduction system

Significant reduction in sino-atrial pacemaker cell numbers is noted with ageing. By some estimates only 10 per cent of the sino-atrial cells remain by the age 70.[76] Increased deposition of adipose tissue, amyloid, and collagen is noted, which contributes to sinus node disease. Similar changes are noted in the atrio-ventricular node and other components of the electrical system. Clinically, prolongation of the PR interval, QRS duration, and QT interval is noted. The incidence of arrhythmia, especially atrial fibrillation, sick sinus syndrome, and ventricular arrhythmias, increases significantly with ageing.[76]

Cardiac remodelling after infarction

The GISSI-2[3] and SAVE trial[4] demonstrated that older patients have a higher chance of adverse outcomes and are more likely to develop left ventricular dilatation after acute myocardial infarction than their younger counterparts. Mortality rates following acute myocardial infarction are significantly higher in older than in younger patients.[3] This discrepancy in outcomes was not due to larger infarcts. One possible explanation is that older patients have an attenuated post-infarction inflammatory response.[77] There is delayed phagocytosis of dead cardiac myocytes, and a diminished oxidative response by senescent macrophages and neutrophils.[78] Impaired scar formation in aged hearts is associated with remodelling characterized by dilatation of the ventricle and worse systolic function.[2]

Ischaemic preconditioning

Another factor contributing to poor outcomes in the elderly after infarcts could be decreased efficacy of the inherent protective mechanisms that protect against ischaemic injury (ischaemic preconditioning). Reduction in the efficacy of ischaemic preconditioning has been reported in ageing hearts in many species,[79–81] although unequivocal proof remains elusive.[82] Impaired ischaemic preconditioning may be related to increased insulin resistance, which is seen with ageing.[83–85] Anaesthetic preconditioning is decreased in the elderly.[85,86] Patients under 65 who have episodic angina prior to infarction tend to have better outcomes than those who experience their infarction with no prior history of ischaemia. In other words, chronic angina may lead to preconditioning. Overall, elderly patients have worse outcomes after an MI than younger patients, but those outcomes are not reduced by a history of angina, implying a loss of ischaemic preconditioning with age.[87] There is also some evidence that the elderly experience less pre-infarction angina and this difference may also contribute to poorer outcomes.[87]

Cardiac regeneration

Most cardiac myocytes are post-mitotic and terminally differentiated and show limited capacity for proliferation.[55] It was believed that they only respond to stress by hypertrophy. However, post-myocardial infarction studies have shown the presence of cardiac stem cells that can differentiate into myocardial cells and provide small amounts of regeneration. The potential for cardiac myocytes to regenerate is tantalizing, though the clinical significance of this finding still needs to be fully elucidated.

Neuroendocrine changes with ageing that affect the cardiovascular system

Ageing of the neuroendocrine system can have a significant effect on the cardiovascular system. Changes include the number of adrenergic receptors in the cardiac and vascular tissues, attenuation of signal transduction pathways, and changes in the balance between sympathetic and parasympathetic activity. The renin–angiotensin–aldosterone system, vasopressin, and natriuretic peptides are also affected by ageing.

Adrenergic receptors

Heart and blood vessel adrenergic receptor sensitivity to catecholamines declines with age.[88,89] A decrease in intracellular cyclic adenosine monophosphate (cAMP) production by adenylate cyclase appears to be the underlying mechanism.[90] The response to β-adrenergic receptor stimulation is reduced in the elderly.[91,92] Though the density of β-adrenergic receptors actually increase with age, coupling of the β-adrenergic receptors to the intracellullar downstream pathway is reduced.[93,94] The cardiac myocytes have β-1, β-2, and β-3 receptors. Typically, β-1 and β-2 receptors exist in an 80:20 ratio in the ventricles.[94] However, in heart failure the ratio of β-1 to β-2 receptors changes to 60:40, hence, proportionally there are more β-2 receptors in a failing heart.[94] There is some evidence that the proportions of β-3 receptors, which are implicated in the pathophysiology of heart failure and coupled to cyclic guanosine monophosphate (cGMP)/NO pathway, also increase and may depress myocardial contractile function.[95] In the elderly, isoproterenol, which has significant β-2 effects, has been shown to cause less of an increase in heart rate than in younger individuals.[92] Although this effect has not been shown consistently and to the same extent with all inotropes, it is generally considered that for the same dose of β-adrenergic agonist, chronotropic and ionotropic effects are decreased in the elderly.

Alpha-adrenergic receptors are also affected by ageing.[96–98] Decreased expression of α-1A and α-ID receptors has been noted with ageing, (which are involved in contractile function) which may be an adaptive response to cardiac hypertrophy.[99]

Baroreceptor reflex

The baroreceptor reflex, defined as the change in heart rate for a given change in blood pressure decreases with age. At least part of the explanation is the diminished response to β-receptor stimulation. However, the baroreceptor reflex encompasses many components and it is likely that the stiffening of blood vessels may contribute by reducing the stretch of the baroreceptors for a given change in blood pressure.[88,100]

Sympathetic nervous system activity

Sympathetic nervous system activity increases with age and by some estimates the sympathetic nerve activity is almost two times higher in a 65-year-old than a 25-year-old person.[100–102] This is probably due to increased catecholamine release, decreased neuronal uptake and increased sympathetic nerve activity.[103] These alterations seem to be region specific and are seen in skeletal muscle, splanchnic areas, and the heart.[104] Circulating noradrenaline concentrations increase by 1–15 per cent per decade after adulthood.[104] Similarly, the increase in noradrenaline levels during exercise is greater in elderly subjects. The decrease in catecholamine sensitivity of adrenergic receptors in the heart and blood vessels reduces the response to the increased catecholamine release.[105] In the vasculature, however, the vasoconstrictor response is at least equivalent, if not exaggerated, in comparison to younger adults.[100]

Parasympathetic nervous system activity

One way to assess autonomic outflow of the cardiovascular system is to assess the heart rate variability. Heart rate variability has two components, a high-frequency component, which is under parasympathetic control, and a low frequency component, which is under sympathetic control. Both components of heart rate variability decrease with age. Poor responsiveness to β-adrenergic receptor stimulation may explain depression in the sympathetic component, whereas low vagal output at rest is the likely mechanism behind the diminished parasympathetic, high-frequency variability.[100] The decreased heart rate response to atropine is also explained by low basal vagal tone in older adults.

Endocrine changes with ageing

The renin–angiotensin system (RAS) is central to physiological control of sodium and water homeostasis. The RAS exists not only as an endocrine system, but also as a local network in different organs, especially in the heart and brain. There, local conversion of angiotensinogen to angiotensin by regional angiotensin-converting enzyme occurs. Angiotensin-II principally mediates its effect through AT_1 and AT_2 receptors. AT_1 receptors mediate fibrosis, oxidative stress and myocardial hypertrophy among other effects. Although ageing decreases overall RAS activity via decreased levels of systemic renin–angiotensin, increased local RAS activity has been observed in the heart. In addition, both AT_1 receptors and AT_2 receptors are up regulated. These changes in the RAS system contribute to age-related changes with cardiac remodelling.[106–108] Vasopressin levels increase with age both at rest and in response to increased serum osmolality.[109,110]

Another group of hormones that are important in volume regulation are the natriuretic peptides. Atrial natriuretic peptide (ANP) is secreted primarily by the cardiac atria in response to atrial stretch, while brain natriuretic peptide (BNP) is secreted by both atrial and ventricular myocardial cells. Natriuretic peptides (NPs) are primarily counter-regulatory hormones. They antagonize the effects of a number of sympathetic hormones and the renin–angiotensin–aldosterone system.[111] Seventy per cent of all cardiac BNP is derived from the ventricles under normal conditions. In pathological conditions the proportion of BNP derived from ventricles increases significantly (up to 88 per cent).[112]

Activation of these systems is seen most frequently in congestive heart failure, although other conditions can also stimulate the release of NPs.[111,113–115] For example, increased levels of BNPs have been associated with ageing, renal insufficiency, and anaemia.[115,116] The change in peptide levels are impressive enough to warrant higher cut off levels of BNPs for diagnostic and prognostic purposes in the elderly.[116,117]

Physiological consequences of cardiovascular ageing

As the heart is closely coupled to the vascular system, it is important to note that many of the changes to the ageing heart are closely linked to progressive changes in the vascular system.[118] The vascular system serves both as a reservoir and a conductive system. It serves a critical role in buffering the effects of intermittent ejection (stroke volume). In a young person, the aorta and proximal arteries expand 10 per cent with each contraction, while the distal muscular arteries expand only 3 per cent.[119] Generalized stiffening of the arterial tree leads to increased arterial wave reflectance, increased systolic blood pressure, decreased diastolic blood pressure, and a widened pulse pressure. Some have described the vascular ageing process as four stages.[118]

Stage I

It begins with fatigue, then fracture of elastic lamellae in the proximal aorta,[120,121] which leads to aortic dilation and transfer of stresses to the stiffer collagenous fibres in the aortic wall[121] and a progressive increase in aortic systolic pressure which contributes to a widened pulse pressure. A typical increase of 20 per cent in brachial systolic pressure between 20 and 80 years of life[122,123] corresponds to a twofold increase in brachial pulse pressure and a three- to fourfold increase in aortic pulse pressure.[121]

Stage II

With progressive aortic stiffening, aortic impedance mismatch and early wave reflection develop.[121–124] At all ages, the arterial pulse wave is reflected back from the peripheral circulation by bouncing off branch points and other structures. In young adults, the reflected wave returns to the aortic root in early diastole. However, in an older individual, stiff arteries cause the wave to travel faster. Aortic impedance and pulse wave velocity increase by twofold between 20 and 80 years of life, independent of the blood pressure.[120,121,125,126] Some consider these values to be an underestimation. Magnetic resonance imaging (MRI) studies suggest as much as a tenfold increased impulse wave velocity.[127] Faster wave velocities dictate that the reflected waves will now return to the heart at, just after, or sometimes even before, the peak of ventricular ejection.[120,121,124] This leads to a secondary rise in aortic pressure, such that instead of a fall from the initial pressure peak at 100 ms,[120] there is a late systolic rise of around 30 mmHg after the original peak of ejection. This adds to the effects of increased aortic pressure at peak ejection and results in aortic pulse pressure being around three times higher (i.e. 60–70 mmHg) by 80 years of age, in comparison to the 20 mmHg, typically seen in the 20-year-old. This shift in timing of the arrival of the reflected wave from diastole into late systole leads to an increased systolic workload for the heart, alterations in ventricular–vascular coupling and 'isolated systolic hypertension' (Fig. 6.1).

A number of studies demonstrate a significant association between increased pulse wave velocity and all-cause mortality as well as adverse cardiovascular events.[128] Data from the Framingham Heart Study shows that systolic blood pressure increases by 5 mmHg per decade until the age 60 and then increases by 10 mmHg per decade, while the diastolic pressure remains the same. Widened pulse pressure is hallmark of ageing and has been seen in all ethnic groups with ageing.

Stage III

There is little change in left ventricular ejection fraction with age. However, poor buffering of cardiac pulsations by the aorta transmits more of the blood pressure increase during ejection to the peripheral arteries and microvasculature, especially organs with high blood flow, including the brain and the kidneys.[129–131] High pulsatile flow in the brain has been associated with 'white matter hyperintensities' in MRI studies.[46] Such brain lesions have been described as 'pulse wave encephalopathy'.[129,132] Similar lesions have also been seen in the kidney microvasculature and are attributed to the same phenomena.

Stage IV

The fourth stage describes the changes to the heart and occurs simultaneously with stage III. Ejecting against a higher pressure,

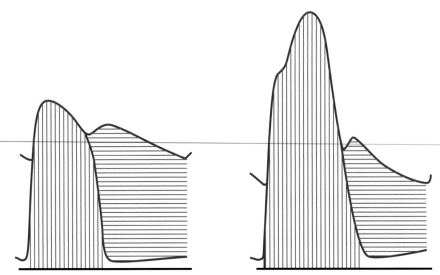

Fig. 6.1 Ascending aortic and left ventricular (LV) pressure waves shown schematically in a young subject at left and older subject with LV hypertrophy and diastolic LV dysfunction at right. In the older person, myocardial oxygen demands (vertically hatched area) are increased by the increase in LV and aortic systolic pressure and by the increased duration of systole. Myocardial oxygen supply is potentially adversely affected by a shorter duration of diastole, lower aortic pressure during diastole, and increased LV pressure during diastole caused by LV dysfunction. Reproduced from Nichols, W., 'Clinical measurement of arterial stiffness obtained from noninvasive pressure waveforms', *American Journal of Hypertension*, 18, pp. 3–10, by permission of American Journal of Hypertension, Ltd. and Oxford University Press.

especially in late systole, is sensed by cardiac myocytes, which triggers a multitude of pro-hypertrophic intracellular pathways.[133] Left ventricular mass increases by 15 per cent from age 30 to 70 years, with subsequent effects on systolic and diastolic function.[118] Diastolic dysfunction can be readily diagnosed on echocardiography.[91] Furthermore, the chronic changes make the myocardium more prone to ischaemia. There is decreased oxygen supply due to increased left ventricular diastolic pressure, decreased aortic diastolic pressure and decreased duration of diastole. Oxygen demand is increased due to myocardial hypertrophy, increased left ventricular systolic pressure, and increased duration of systole[121] (Fig. 6.2).

These changes in myocardial function are thought to explain the occasional presence of myocardial ischaemia in the elderly, even in the absence of atherosclerotic narrowing.[120,134] It also explains why tachycardia may not be well tolerated in the elderly and can easily lead to myocardial ischaemia and infarction. Ultimately, it is the presence of age-related cardiovascular changes and atherosclerotic cardiovascular disease that leads to final decompensation of the cardiovascular system in the elderly (Fig. 6.3).

Normal age-related changes in cardiovascular physiology present as decreases in peak heart rate, peak cardiac output, and peak ejection fraction.[55] Due to the overall dampening of autonomic and

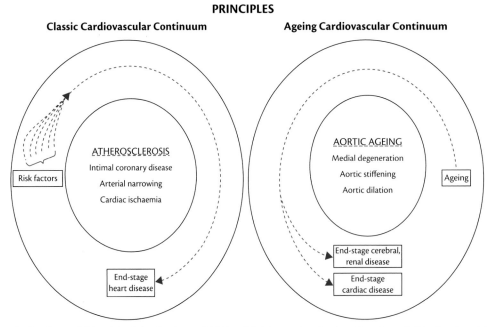

Fig. 6.2 The Cardiovascular Continuum (left) and the Aging Continuum (right), and their interaction. Reprinted from *Journal of the American College of Cardiology*, 50, 1, O'Rourke, M. and J. Hashimoto, 'Mechanical Factors in Arterial Aging: A Clinical Perspective', pp. 1–13, Copyright 2007, with permission from American College of Cardiology Foundation and Elsevier.

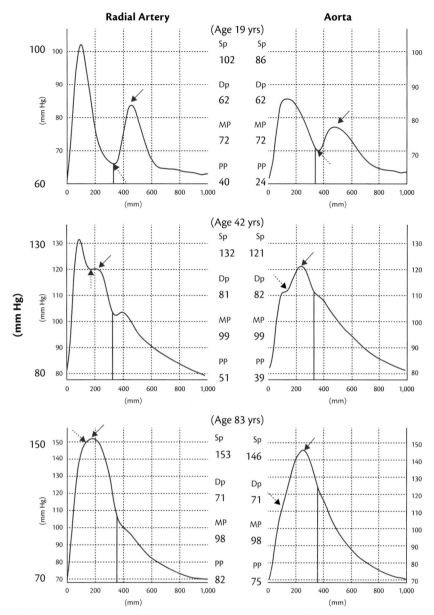

Fig. 6.3 Noninvasive recordings of radial artery pressure waves (left) and synthesized aortic pressure waves (right) in three healthy individuals to illustrate the age-related changes in wave reflection characteristics and pressure wave shapes. Solid arrows identify the peak of the reflected waves, and broken arrows indicate the beginning upstroke of the reflected waves. O'Rourke, M. F., M. E. Safar, et al., *Vascular Medicine*, 15, 6, 'The Cardiovascular Continuum extended: aging effects on the aorta and microvasculature', pp. 461–468, copyright © 2010 by Society for Vascular Medicine, reprinted by permission of SAGE.

baroreceptor activity with ageing, a decreased resting heart rate and a decreased ability to increase cardiac output with changes in heart rate is observed.[135] Compared to younger patients, increases in cardiac output in the elderly are achieved by increasing end-diastolic volume, as opposed to increasing heart rate and contractility. This results in an increased reliance on atrial filling for maintenance of cardiac output. Overall, the ability of the cardiovascular system to withstand stress is significantly decreased.[136] Aerobic capacity as evaluated by maximum body oxygen consumption decreases with ageing by 30–40 per cent per decade in healthy men and women.[137] This is due to the reductions in both maximal cardiac output and the maximal arteriovenous oxygen differences. The reduction in cardiac output is primarily due to the reduction in maximum heart rate, which is approximately 1 pulse/min/year.[91]

Structural changes in the myocardium, valves and the great vessels can be assessed by echocardiography and ultrasonography. Even the presence of calcium can be assessed in the vessels. Furthermore, systolic and diastolic function can be readily evaluated by echocardiography, which can help in early management of ischaemia and heart failure.

Outcomes after cardiac and non-cardiac surgery

Considering the burden of cardiovascular changes and limitation of cardiovascular reserve, it is not surprising that perioperative outcomes in the elderly are significantly poorer than for their younger counterparts. The operative mortality of octogenarians undergoing cardiac surgery in recent studies is reported to be in the range of 5.8–11 per cent, compared with 2.7–4.1 per cent in younger patients.[138–141] The national database also report that the operative mortality is two to five times higher in octogenarians than younger patients, a result that is similar in non-cardiac surgery.[142–144] Mortality after exploratory laparotomy can be as high as 45 per cent in the octogenarians. Though vascular procedures are known to have high risk of adverse events (5–20 per cent)[145] the risk after major orthopaedic procedures is also significant. According to one study, urgent hip fracture surgery can have a 5–7 per cent risk of adverse cardiac events while the risk after elective knee and hip arthroplasty is 1.5–3 per cent.[144]

Though the outcomes after surgery in the elderly seem acceptable when considered in terms of morbidity and in-hospital mortality, these variables alone are not adequate to reflect the overall success of the operation in the elderly. Quality of life after the operation, or functional recovery to baseline and discharge status after the operation should also be considered. In one study, after cardiac surgery only 52 per cent of the patients were discharged home with 28 per cent being discharged to an acute care facility, 12 per cent per cent to a nursing home and rest to other health facilities.[146] Though quality of life in the majority of patients who survive the operation and live independently is described as equal or better than before,[147] it is evident that a significant proportion of the elderly patients also die in the hospital, suffer significant morbidity, or may never get back to their activities of daily living after major surgery.[148]

Cardiovascular management of elderly patients

Cardiovascular management in the elderly should be governed by the fact that geriatric patients have decreased reserve to tolerate cardiovascular stress and acute haemodynamic changes. Furthermore, they are more prone to ischaemia, arrhythmias, and heart failure. Acute cardiovascular management typically involves optimization of the following components of the cardiovascular system: maintenance of optimal vascular tone, optimal fluid volume, adequate contractile function of the heart, prevention of ischaemia, and maintenance of an optimal heart rate with atrial-ventricular synchrony.

Monitoring

No study to date has clearly demonstrated a difference in outcomes with advanced monitoring techniques. Right heart catheterization, which was in vogue 10 years ago, has not been shown to improve outcomes in large randomized studies.[149,150] Intraoperative transoesophageal echocardiography may be considered in patients who develop significant and prolonged ST-changes or who demonstrate sustained severe haemodynamic disturbances.[151]

Anaesthetic management

Maintenance of the balance between myocardial oxygen demand and myocardial oxygen delivery, as well as body oxygen delivery, are probably more important than the specific anaesthetic technique or drugs selected to produce anaesthesia.[151] It is important to avoid persistent and excessive changes in heart rate and systemic blood pressure. A common recommendation is to strive to maintain the patient's heart rate and systemic blood pressure within 20 per cent of the normal awake value.[151] Nevertheless, most episodes of intraoperative myocardial ischaemia seen on the electrocardiogram

occur in the absence of haemodynamic changes.[152] Furthermore, myocardial ischaemia and dysfunction is not limited to the diseased vessels and does not correlate with the severity and distribution of coronary artery disease, suggesting that it is unlikely that non-haemodynamic myocardial ischaemia will be predictably preventable by the anaesthetist.[153] Vigilance, early detection, and treatment of myocardial dysfunction is of utmost importance.

The use of inhalational anaesthesia is associated with myocardial preconditioning and their use, especially sevoflurane, is recommended in patients with coronary artery disease.[151] Prolonged use of nitrous oxide may predispose patients to perioperative myocardial ischaemia.[149,150] A large multicentre study is currently under way to better define the harmful effects of nitrous oxide.[152,154] One of the key factors to keep in mind is that for all inhalational anaesthetics, the minimal anaesthetic concentration (MAC) decreases by approximately 6–8 per cent per decade after 40 years. Thus, MAC for an octogenarian is some 30 per cent lower than their younger counterpart.[154] Intravenous anaesthetics have a more pronounced hemodynamic effect, with smaller doses being required to achieve the same anaesthetic level. This is due to pharmacokinetic and pharmacodynamic changes in the elderly. The dose of induction agents should be decreased by 25 per cent and opioid doses may need to be reduced by 50 per cent.[155,156] Adjusting the anaesthetic dose for patient age may help reduce unnecessarily deep anaesthesia, associated hypotension and potentially reduce adverse outcomes.

Fluid therapy

Fluid therapy should not be considered routine in the elderly. It requires as much forethought as any other medication. Due to advanced atherosclerosis, stiff ventricles, diastolic dysfunction, and occult coronary artery disease, elderly patients do not tolerate hypovolaemia or hypervolaemia. Hypovolaemia leads to hypotension and organ hypoperfusion while over hydration can lead to congestive heart failure. In 1999, the United Kingdom National Confidential Inquiry into Perioperative Deaths at the extremes of age concluded that errors in fluid management (usually excess fluid) were one of the most common causes of avoidable perioperative morbidity and mortality.[157] Their report states that 'fluid management in the elderly is often poor; they should be accorded the same status as drug prescription. Multidisciplinary reviews to develop good local working practices are required'. The most recent report from 2010 re-emphasizes the same issue. It discusses it in the context of preventing acute kidney injury.[157]

Though not specifically addressed in elderly patients, goal-directed fluid therapy seems to improve outcomes. One of the primary goals of fluid therapy is to achieve adequate cardiac index/stroke volume, for a particular clinical situation, by maintaining optimal preload. In the perioperative setting, one of the biggest challenges has been to determine accurately (and easily) the fluid status of the patient. Static markers of preload (central venous pressure, pulmonary artery wedge pressure, etc.) were used for decades and are still used to guide fluid therapy. However, these markers are not very accurate.[158] Non-invasive, dynamic indices like pulse pressure variation (PPV), systolic pressure variation (SPV), and stroke volume variation (SVV) may be better predictors of volume status.[159] Though the British guidelines recommend using flow directed monitors to determine fluid status, one should keep in mind that most of these studies are small and results may not be applicable to elderly patients.

Vasopressor therapy

Elderly patients have diminished responses to commonly used adrenergic drugs. Responses to ephedrine and phenylephrine are reduced[91] and higher doses may be required to achieve the desired effect especially after induction of general anaesthesia or to overcome the sympatholytic effect of neuraxial blockade.[91] As with all drugs, inotropic agents should be titrated to effect.

Rhythm therapy

Many elderly patients suffer from supraventricular, ventricular arrhythmias or high-degree conduction blocks. They may be receiving anti-arrhythmic agents and/or have implantable devices (permanent pacemakers or cardioverter/defibrillators). Anti-muscarinic agents should be administered cautiously in patients with atrial fibrillation. These drugs may initiate a rapid ventricular rate, which may require treatment with beta-blockers, calcium channel blockers, or amiodarone.[160] Management of implantable devices should be based on recommended guidelines and institutional practices.

Conclusion

Ageing reduces the reserve of the cardiovascular system. The elderly become less responsive to catecholamine stimulation, and more dependent on their volume status, even while it becomes more difficult to maintain the correct level of volume so as to avoid decreased cardiac output or pulmonary congestion. Rhythm disturbances may make maintenance of a reasonable heart rate problematic. Other changes predispose the elderly to patient to disease and increase the risk of perioperative complications and worsened long-term mortality and quality of life. It is hoped that by keeping in mind the physiological impact of age-related cardiovascular changes and cardiovascular ailments, practitioners will be able to manage the elderly patients more effectively and reduce the risk of adverse outcome.

References

1. Roger VL, Go AS, Lloyd-Jones DM, *et al.* Heart disease and stroke statistics—2011 update: a report from the American Heart Association. *Circulation.* 2011;123(4):e18–e209.

2. Chen W, Frangogiannis NG. The role of inflammatory and fibrogenic pathways in heart failure associated with aging. *Heart Fail Rev.* 2010;15(5):415–422.

3. Maggioni AP, Maseri A, Fresco C, *et al.* Age-related increase in mortality among patients with first myocardial infarctions treated with thrombolysis. The Investigators of the Gruppo Italiano per lo Studio della Sopravvivenza nell'Infarto Miocardico (GISSI-2). *N Engl J Med.* 1993;329(20):1442–1448.

4. St John Sutton M, Pfeffer MA, Moye L, *et al.* Cardiovascular death and left ventricular remodeling two years after myocardial infarction: baseline predictors and impact of long-term use of captopril: information from the Survival and Ventricular Enlargement (SAVE) trial. *Circulation.* 1997;96(10):3294–3299.

5. Zieman SJ, Melenovsky V, Kass DA. Mechanisms, pathophysiology, and therapy of arterial stiffness. *Arterioscler Thromb Vasc Biol.* 2005;25(5):932–943.

6. Kovacic JC, Moreno P, Nabel EG, Hachinski V, Fuster V. Cellular senescence, vascular disease, and aging: part 2 of a 2-part review: clinical vascular disease in the elderly. *Circulation.* 2011;123(17):1900–1910.

7. Farkas E, Luiten PG. Cerebral microvascular pathology in aging and Alzheimer's disease. *Progress in neurobiology.* 2001;64(6):575–611.

8. Iadecola C, Park L, Capone C. Threats to the mind: aging, amyloid, and hypertension. *Stroke.* 2009;40(3 Suppl):S40–S44.

9. Thompson CS, Hakim AM. Living beyond our physiological means: small vessel disease of the brain is an expression of a systemic failure in arteriolar function: a unifying hypothesis. *Stroke.* 2009;40(5):e322–e330.

10. Kalaria RN. Linking cerebrovascular defense mechanisms in brain ageing and Alzheimer's disease. *Neurobiol Aging.* 2009;30(9):1512–1514.

11. Li Z, Froehlich J, Galis ZS, Lakatta EG. Increased expression of matrix metalloproteinase-2 in the thickened intima of aged rats. *Hypertension.* 1999;33(1):116–123.

12. Greenwald SE. Ageing of the conduit arteries. *J Pathol.* 2007;211(2):157–172.

13. Goh SY, Cooper ME. Clinical review: the role of advanced glycation end products in progression and complications of diabetes. *J Clin Endocrinol Metabo.* 2008;93(4):1143–1152.

14. Rojas A, Morales MA. Advanced glycation and endothelial functions: a link towards vascular complications in diabetes. *Life Sci.* 2004;76(7):715–730.

15. Verzijl N, DeGroot J, Thorpe SR, *et al.* Effect of collagen turnover on the accumulation of advanced glycation end products. *J Biol Chem.* 2000;275(50):39027–39031.

16. Konova E, Baydanoff S, Atanasova M, Velkova A. Age-related changes in the glycation of human aortic elastin. *Exp Gerontol.* 2004;39(2):249–254.

17. Yamagishi S, Nakamura K, Matsui T, Ueda S, Fukami K, Okuda S. Agents that block advanced glycation end product (AGE)-RAGE (receptor for AGEs)-oxidative stress system: a novel therapeutic strategy for diabetic vascular complications. *Expert Opin Investig Drugs.* 2008;17(7):983–996.

18. Scheubel RJ, Kahrstedt S, Weber H, *et al.* Depression of progenitor cell function by advanced glycation endproducts (AGEs): potential relevance for impaired angiogenesis in advanced age and diabetes. *Exp Gerontol.* 2006;41(5):540–548.

19. Mercer N, Ahmed H, Etcheverry SB, Vasta GR, Cortizo AM. Regulation of advanced glycation end product (AGE) receptors and apoptosis by AGEs in osteoblast-like cells. *Mol Cell Biochem.* 2007;306(1-2):87–94.

20. Xiang M, Yang M, Zhou C, Liu J, Li W, Qian Z. Crocetin prevents AGEs-induced vascular endothelial cell apoptosis. *Pharmacol Res.* 2006;54(4):268–274.

21. Kovacic JC, Randolph GJ. Vascular calcification: harder than it looks. *Arterioscler Thromb Vasc Biol.* 2011;31(6):1249–1250.

22. Hickson SS, Butlin M, Graves M, *et al.* The relationship of age with regional aortic stiffness and diameter. *JACC Cardiovasc Imaging.* 2010;3(12):1247–1255.

23. Haskett D, Johnson G, Zhou A, Utzinger U, Vande Geest J. Microstructural and biomechanical alterations of the human aorta as a function of age and location. *Biomech Model Mechanobiol.* 2010;9(6):725–736.

24. Rose JL, Lalande A, Bouchot O, *et al.* Influence of age and sex on aortic distensibility assessed by MRI in healthy subjects. *Magn Reson Imaging.* 2010;28(2):255–263.

25. Lakatta EG. Arterial and cardiac aging: major shareholders in cardiovascular disease enterprises: Part III: cellular and molecular clues to heart and arterial aging. *Circulation.* 2003;107(3):490–497.

26. Maruyama Y. Aging and arterial-cardiac interactions in the elderly. *Int J Cardiol.* 2012;155(1):14–19.

27. Ruschitzka FT, Noll G, Luscher TF. The endothelium in coronary artery disease. *Cardiology.* 1997;88(Suppl 3):3–19.

28. Barton M. Obesity and aging: determinants of endothelial cell dysfunction and atherosclerosis. *Pflugers Arch.* 2010;460(5):825–837.

29. Barton M. Ageing as a determinant of renal and vascular disease: role of endothelial factors. *Nephrol Dial Transplant.* 2005;20(3):485–490.

30. Barton M. Aging and biomedicine 2005: where should we go from here? *Cardiovasc Res.* 2005;66(2):187–189.

31. Smith AR, Visioli F, Frei B, Hagen TM. Age-related changes in endothelial nitric oxide synthase phosphorylation and nitric oxide dependent vasodilation: evidence for a novel mechanism involving

sphingomyelinase and ceramide-activated phosphatase 2A. *Aging Cell.* 2006;5(5):391–400.

32. Briones AM, Salaices M, Vila E. Ageing alters the production of nitric oxide and prostanoids after IL-1beta exposure in mesenteric resistance arteries. *Mech Ageing Dev.* 2005;126(6-7):710–721.

33. Yoon HJ, Cho SW, Ahn BW, Yang SY. Alterations in the activity and expression of endothelial NO synthase in aged human endothelial cells. *Mech Ageing Dev.* 2010;131(2):119–123.

34. Levin ER. Endothelins. *N Engl J Med.* 1995;333(6):356–363.

35. Goettsch W, Lattmann T, Amann K, *et al.* Increased expression of endothelin-1 and inducible nitric oxide synthase isoform II in aging arteries in vivo: implications for atherosclerosis. *Biochem Biophys Res Commun.* 2001;280(3):908–913.

36. Lattmann T, Shaw S, Munter K, Vetter W, Barton M. Anatomically distinct activation of endothelin-3 and the L-arginine/nitric oxide pathway in the kidney with advanced aging. *Biochem Biophys Res Commun.* 2005;327(1):234–241.

37. Seals DR, Jablonski KL, Donato AJ. Aging and vascular endothelial function in humans. *Clin Sci (Lond).* 2011;120(9):357–375.

38. Thijssen DH, Rongen GA, van Dijk A, Smits P, Hopman MT. Enhanced endothelin-1-mediated leg vascular tone in healthy older subjects. *J Appl Physiol.* 2007;103(3):852–857.

39. Tokunaga O, Fan J, Watanabe T, Kobayashi M, Kumazaki T, Mitsui Y. Endothelin. Immunohistologic localization in aorta and biosynthesis by cultured human aortic endothelial cells. *Lab Invest.* 1992;67(2):210–217.

40. Woodman CR, Price EM, Laughlin MH. Selected contribution: aging impairs nitric oxide and prostacyclin mediation of endothelium-dependent dilation in soleus feed arteries. *J Appl Physiol.* 2003;95(5):2164–2170.

41. Tew GA, Klonizakis M, Saxton JM. Effects of ageing and fitness on skin-microvessel vasodilator function in humans. *Eur J Appl Physiol.* 2010;109(2):173–181.

42. Gates PE, Strain WD, Shore AC. Human endothelial function and microvascular ageing. *Exp Physiol.* 2009;94(3):311–316.

43. Holowatz LA, Houghton BL, Wong BJ, *et al.* Nitric oxide and attenuated reflex cutaneous vasodilation in aged skin. *Am J Physiol Heart Circ Physiol.* 2003;284(5):H1662–H1667.

44. Franceschi C, Bonafe M, Valensin S, *et al.* Inflamm-aging. An evolutionary perspective on immunosenescence. *Ann N Y Acad Sci.* 2000;908:244–254.

45. Fagiolo U, Cossarizza A, Scala E, *et al.* Increased cytokine production in mononuclear cells of healthy elderly people. *Eur J Immunol.* 1993;23(9):2375–2378.

46. Brown WR, Thore CR. Review: cerebral microvascular pathology in ageing and neurodegeneration. *Neuropathol Appl Neurobiol.* 2011;37(1):56–74.

47. Fu Q, Iwase S, Niimi Y, *et al.* Age-related changes in vasomotor reflex control of calf venous capacitance response to lower body negative pressure in humans. *Jpn J Physiol.* 2002;52(1):69–76.

48. Olsen H, Lanne T. Reduced venous compliance in lower limbs of aging humans and its importance for capacitance function. *Am J Physiol.* 1998;275(3 Pt 2):H878–H886.

49. Young CN, Stillabower ME, DiSabatino A, Farquhar WB. Venous smooth muscle tone and responsiveness in older adults. *J Appl Physiol.* 2006;101(5):1362–1367.

50. Greaney JL, Farquhar WB. Why do veins stiffen with advancing age? *J Appl Physiol.* 2011;110(1):11–12.

51. Gelman S. Venous function and central venous pressure: a physiologic story. *Anesthesiology.* 2008;108(4):735–748.

52. Fink GD. Arthur C. Corcoran Memorial Lecture. Sympathetic activity, vascular capacitance, and long-term regulation of arterial pressure. *Hypertension.* 2009;53(2):307–312.

53. Bernhard D, Laufer G. The aging cardiomyocyte: a mini-review. *Gerontology.* 2008;54(1):24–31.

54. Anversa P, Palackal T, Sonnenblick EH, Olivetti G, Meggs LG, Capasso JM. Myocyte cell loss and myocyte cellular hyperplasia in the hypertrophied aging rat heart. *Circ Res.* 1990;67(4):871–885.

55. Karavidas A, Lazaros G, Tsiachris D, Pyrgakis V. Aging and the cardiovascular system. *Hellenic J Cardiol.* 2010;51(5):421–427.

56. Flanders KC. Smad3 as a mediator of the fibrotic response. *Int J Exp Pathol.* 2004;85(2):47–64.

57. Shivakumar K, Dostal DE, Boheler K, Baker KM, Lakatta EG. Differential response of cardiac fibroblasts from young adult and senescent rats to ANG II. *Am J Physiol Heart Circ Physiol.* 2003;284(4):H1454–H1459.

58. Cieslik KA, Taffet GE, Carlson S, Hermosillo J, Trial J, Entman ML. Immune-inflammatory dysregulation modulates the incidence of progressive fibrosis and diastolic stiffness in the aging heart. *J Mol Cell Cardiol.* 2011;50(1):248–256.

59. Josephson IR, Guia A, Stern MD, Lakatta EG. Alterations in properties of L-type Ca channels in aging rat heart. *J Mol Cell Cardiol.* 2002;34(3):297–308.

60. Lindner M, Bohle T, Beuckelmann DJ. Ca^{2+}-handling in heart failure—a review focusing on Ca^{2+} sparks. *Basic Res Cardiol.* 2002;97(Suppl 1):I79–I82.

61. Miller TR, Grossman SJ, Schectman KB, Biello DR, Ludbrook PA, Ehsani AA. Left ventricular diastolic filling and its association with age. *Am J Cardiol.* 1986;58(6):531–535.

62. Zieman SJ, Gerstenblith G, Lakatta EG, *et al.* Upregulation of the nitric oxide-cGMP pathway in aged myocardium: physiological response to l-arginine. *Circ Res.* 2001;88(1):97–102.

63. van der Loo B, Bachschmid M, Labugger R, *et al.* Expression and activity patterns of nitric oxide synthases and antioxidant enzymes reveal a substantial heterogeneity between cardiac and vascular aging in the rat. *Biogerontology.* 2005;6(5):325–334.

64. Swinnen M, Vanhoutte D, Van Almen GC, *et al.* Absence of thrombospondin-2 causes age-related dilated cardiomyopathy. *Circulation.* 2009;120(16):1585–1597.

65. Inuzuka Y, Okuda J, Kawashima T, *et al.* Suppression of phosphoinositide 3-kinase prevents cardiac aging in mice. *Circulation.* 2009;120(17):1695–1703.

66. Liu L, Zhu J, Glass PS, Brink PR, Rampil IJ, Rebecchi MJ. Age-associated changes in cardiac gene expression after preconditioning. *Anesthesiology.* 2009;111(5):1052–1064.

67. Li SY, Du M, Dolence EK, *et al.* Aging induces cardiac diastolic dysfunction, oxidative stress, accumulation of advanced glycation endproducts and protein modification. *Aging Cell.* 2005;4(2):57–64.

68. Machii H, Saitoh S, Kaneshiro T, Takeishi Y. Aging impairs myocardium-induced dilation in coronary arterioles: role of hydrogen peroxide and angiotensin. *Mech Ageing Dev.* 2010;131(11–12):710–717.

69. Hachamovitch R, Wicker P, Capasso JM, Anversa P. Alterations of coronary blood flow and reserve with aging in Fischer 344 rats. *Am J Physiol.* 1989;256(1 Pt 2):H66–H73.

70. Nunez E, Hosoya K, Susic D, Frohlich ED. Enalapril and losartan reduced cardiac mass and improved coronary hemodynamics in SHR. *Hypertension.* 1997;29(1 Pt 2):519–524.

71. Vanhoutte PM. Aging and vascular responsiveness. *J Cardiovasc Pharmacol.* 1988;12(Suppl 8):S11–S19.

72. Lang MG, Noll G, Luscher TF. Effect of aging and hypertension on contractility of resistance arteries: modulation by endothelial factors. *Am J Physiol.* 1995;269(3 Pt 2):H837–H844.

73. Aronow WS. Heart disease and aging. *Med Clin North Am.* 2006;90(5):849–862.

74. Nassimiha D, Aronow WS, Ahn C, Goldman ME. Association of coronary risk factors with progression of valvular aortic stenosis in older persons. *Am J Cardiol.* 2001;87(11):1313–1314.

75. Kertai MD, Bountioukos M, Boersma E, *et al.* Aortic stenosis: an underestimated risk factor for perioperative complications in patients undergoing noncardiac surgery. *Am J Med.* 2004;116(1):8–13.

76. Jones SA. Ageing to arrhythmias: conundrums of connections in the ageing heart. *J Pharm Pharmacol.* 2006;58(12):1571–1576.

77. Swift ME, Burns AL, Gray KL, DiPietro LA. Age-related alterations in the inflammatory response to dermal injury. *J Invest Dermatol.* 2001;117(5):1027–1035.

78. Ding A, Hwang S, Schwab R. Effect of aging on murine macrophages. Diminished response to IFN-gamma for enhanced oxidative metabolism. *J Immunol.* 1994;153(5):2146–2152.

79. Jahangir A, Sagar S, Terzic A. Aging and cardioprotection. *J Appl Physiol.* 2007;103(6):2120–2128.

80. Pepe S. Dysfunctional ischemic preconditioning mechanisms in aging. *Cardiovasc Res.* 2001;49(1):11–14.

81. Lakatta EG, Sollott SJ. The 'heartbreak' of older age. *Mol Interv.* 2002;2(7):431–446.

82. Abete P, Cacciatore F, Testa G, *et al.* Ischemic preconditioning in the aging heart: from bench to bedside. *Ageing Res Rev.* 2010;9(2):153–162.

83. Lechleitner M. Obesity and the metabolic syndrome in the elderly—a mini-review. *Gerontology.* 2008;54(5):253–259.

84. Mozaffarian D, Kamineni A, Prineas RJ, Siscovick DS. Metabolic syndrome and mortality in older adults: the Cardiovascular Health Study. *Arch Intern Med.* 2008;168(9):969–978.

85. Mio Y, Bienengraeber MW, Marinovic J, *et al.* Age-related attenuation of isoflurane preconditioning in human atrial cardiomyocytes: roles for mitochondrial respiration and sarcolemmal adenosine triphosphate-sensitive potassium channel activity. *Anesthesiology.* 2008;108(4):612–620.

86. Riess ML, Camara AK, Rhodes SS, McCormick J, Jiang MT, Stowe DF. Increasing heart size and age attenuate anesthetic preconditioning in guinea pig isolated hearts. *Anesth Analg.* 2005;101(6):1572–1576.

87. Abete P, Ferrara N, Cacciatore F, *et al.* Angina-induced protection against myocardial infarction in adult and elderly patients: a loss of preconditioning mechanism in the aging heart? *J Am Coll Cardiol.* 1997;30(4):947–954.

88. Czuriga D, Papp Z, Czuriga I, Balogh Á. Cardiac aging—a review. *Eur Surg.* 2011;43:69–77.

89. Hotta H, Uchida S. Aging of the autonomic nervous system and possible improvements in autonomic activity using somatic afferent stimulation. *Geriatr Gerontol Int.* 2010;(10 Suppl 1):S127–S136.

90. Farrell SR, Howlett SE. The age-related decrease in catecholamine sensitivity is mediated by beta(1)-adrenergic receptors linked to a decrease in adenylate cyclase activity in ventricular myocytes from male Fischer 344 rats. *Mech Ageing Dev.* 2008;129(12):735–744.

91. Rooke GA. Cardiovascular aging and anesthetic implications. *J Cardiothorac Vasc Anesth.* 2003;17(4):512–523.

92. Lakatta EG. Alterations in the cardiovascular system that occur in advanced age. *Fed Proc.* 1979;38(2):163–167.

93. Docherty JR. Cardiovascular responses in ageing: a review. *Pharmacological reviews.* 1990;42(2):103–125.

94. Brodde OE, Michel MC. Adrenergic and muscarinic receptors in the human heart. *Pharmacol Rev.* 1999;51(4):651–690.

95. Birenbaum A, Tesse A, Loyer X, *et al.* Involvement of beta 3-adrenoceptor in altered beta-adrenergic response in senescent heart: role of nitric oxide synthase 1-derived nitric oxide. *Anesthesiology.* 2008;109(6):1045–1053.

96. McCloskey DT, Turnbull L, Swigart P, O'Connell TD, Simpson PC, Baker AJ. Abnormal myocardial contraction in alpha(1A)- and alpha(1B)-adrenoceptor double-knockout mice. *J Mol Cell Cardiol.* 2003;35(10):1207–1216.

97. Turnbull L, McCloskey DT, O'Connell TD, Simpson PC, Baker AJ. Alpha 1-adrenergic receptor responses in alpha 1AB-AR knockout mouse hearts suggest the presence of alpha 1D-AR. *Am J Physiol Heart Circ Physiol.* 2003;284(4):H1104–H1109.

98. O'Connell TD, Ishizaka S, Nakamura A, *et al.* The alpha(1A/C)- and alpha(1B)-adrenergic receptors are required for physiological cardiac hypertrophy in the double-knockout mouse. *J Clin Invest.* 2003;111(11):1783–1791.

99. Cao XJ, Li YF. Alteration of messenger RNA and protein levels of cardiac alpha(1)-adrenergic receptor and angiotensin II receptor subtypes during aging in rats. *Can J Cardiol.* 2009;25(7):415–420.

100. Wichi RB, De Angelis K, Jones L, Irigoyen MC. A brief review of chronic exercise intervention to prevent autonomic nervous system changes during the aging process. *Clinics (Sao Paulo).* 2009;64(3):253–258.

101. Negrao CE, Moreira ED, Santos MC, Farah VM, Krieger EM. Vagal function impairment after exercise training. *J Appl Physiol.* 1992;72(5):1749–1753.

102. Dinenno FA, Jones PP, Seals DR, Tanaka H. Limb blood flow and vascular conductance are reduced with age in healthy humans: relation to elevations in sympathetic nerve activity and declines in oxygen demand. *Circulation.* 1999;100(2):164–170.

103. Esler MD, Turner AG, Kaye DM, *et al.* Aging effects on human sympathetic neuronal function. *Am J Physiol.* 1995;268(1 Pt 2):R278–R285.

104. Stratton JR, Levy WC, Caldwell JH, *et al.* Effects of aging on cardiovascular responses to parasympathetic withdrawal. *J Am Coll Cardiol.* 2003;41(11):2077–2083.

105. Eckberg DL, Drabinsky M, Braunwald E. Defective cardiac parasympathetic control in patients with heart disease. *N Engl J Med.* 1971;285(16):877–883.

106. Heymes C, Swynghedauw B, Chevalier B. Activation of angiotensinogen and angiotensin-converting enzyme gene expression in the left ventricle of senescent rats. *Circulation.* 1994;90(3):1328–1333.

107. Corman B, Michel JB. Renin-angiotensin system, converting-enzyme inhibition and kidney function in aging female rats. *Am J Physiol.* 1986;251(3 Pt 2):R450–R455.

108. Basso N, Cini R, Pietrelli A, Ferder L, Terragno NA, Inserra F. Protective effect of long-term angiotensin II inhibition. *Am J Physiol Heart Circ Physiol.* 2007;293(3):H1351–H1358.

109. Davis PJ, Davis FB. Water excretion in the elderly. *Endocrinol Metab Clin North Am.* 1987;16(4):867–875.

110. Weidmann P, De Myttenaere-Bursztein S, Maxwell MH, de Lima J. Effect on aging on plasma renin and aldosterone in normal man. *Kidney Int.* 1975;8(5):325–333.

111. Martinez-Rumayor A, Richards AM, Burnett JC, Januzzi JL, Jr. Biology of the natriuretic peptides. *Am J Cardiol.* 2008;101(3A):3–8.

112. Mukoyama M, Nakao K, Saito Y, *et al.* Human brain natriuretic peptide, a novel cardiac hormone. *Lancet.* 1990;335(8692):801–802.

113. Liang F, O'Rear J, Schellenberger U, *et al.* Evidence for functional heterogeneity of circulating B-type natriuretic peptide. *J Am Coll Cardiol.* 2007;49(10):1071–1078.

114. Goetze JP. Biosynthesis of cardiac natriuretic peptides. *Results Probl Cell Differ.* 2009;50:97–120.

115. Balion CM, Santaguida P, McKelvie R, *et al.* Physiological, pathological, pharmacological, biochemical and hematological factors affecting BNP and NT-proBNP. *Clin Biochem.* 2008;41(4-5):231–239.

116. Remme WJ, Swedberg K. Comprehensive guidelines for the diagnosis and treatment of chronic heart failure. Task force for the diagnosis and treatment of chronic heart failure of the European Society of Cardiology. *Eur J Heart Fail.* 2002;4(1):11–22.

117. Maisel A, Mueller C, Adams K Jr, *et al.* State of the art: using natriuretic peptide levels in clinical practice. *Eur J Heart Fail.* 2008;10(9):824–839.

118. O'Rourke MF, Safar ME, Dzau V. The Cardiovascular Continuum extended: aging effects on the aorta and microvasculature. *Vasc Med.* 2010;15(6):461–468.

119. Boutouyrie P, Laurent S, Benetos A, Girerd XJ, Hoeks AP, Safar ME. Opposing effects of ageing on distal and proximal large arteries in hypertensives. *J Hypertens. Suppl.* 1992;10(6):S87–S91.

120. Nichols WW, O'Rourke MF. *McDonal's blood flow in arteries: theoretical, experimental and clinical principles.* 5th ed. London: Hodder Arnold, 2005.

121. O'Rourke MF, Hashimoto J. Mechanical factors in arterial aging: a clinical perspective. *J Am Coll Cardiol.* 2007;50(1):1–13.

122. Franklin SS, Gustin Wt, Wong ND, *et al.* Hemodynamic patterns of age-related changes in blood pressure. The Framingham Heart Study. *Circulation.* 1997;96(1):308–315.

123. McEniery CM, Yasmin, McDonnell B, *et al.* Central pressure: variability and impact of cardiovascular risk factors: the Anglo-Cardiff Collaborative Trial II. *Hypertension.* 2008;51(6):1476–1482.

124. Borlaug BA, Melenovsky V, Redfield MM, *et al.* Impact of arterial load and loading sequence on left ventricular tissue velocities in humans. *J Am Coll Cardiol.* 2007;50(16):1570–1577.

125. Avolio AP, Chen SG, Wang RP, Zhang CL, Li MF, O'Rourke MF. Effects of aging on changing arterial compliance and left ventricular load in a northern Chinese urban community. *Circulation.* 1983;68(1):50–58.

126. Lakatta EG, Levy D. Arterial and cardiac aging: major shareholders in cardiovascular disease enterprises. Part I: aging arteries: a 'set up' for vascular disease. *Circulation.* 2003;107(1):139–146.

127. Redheuil A, Yu WC, Wu CO, *et al.* Reduced ascending aortic strain and distensibility: earliest manifestations of vascular aging in humans. *Hypertension.* 2010;55(2):319–326.

128. Vlachopoulos C, Aznaouridis K, Stefanadis C. Prediction of cardiovascular events and all-cause mortality with arterial stiffness: a systematic review and meta-analysis. *J Am Coll Cardiol.* 2010;55(13):1318–1327.

129. Bateman GA. Pulse-wave encephalopathy: a comparative study of the hydrodynamics of leukoaraiosis and normal-pressure hydrocephalus. *Neuroradiology.* 2002;44(9):740–748.

130. O'Rourke MF, Safar ME. Relationship between aortic stiffening and microvascular disease in brain and kidney: cause and logic of therapy. *Hypertension.* 2005;46(1):200–204.

131. Safar ME, Lacolley P. Disturbance of macro- and microcirculation: relations with pulse pressure and cardiac organ damage. *Am J Physiol Heart Circ Physiol.* 2007;293(1):H1–H7.

132. Henry Feugeas MC, De Marco G, Peretti, II, Godon-Hardy S, Fredy D, Claeys ES. Age-related cerebral white matter changes and pulse-wave encephalopathy: observations with three-dimensional MRI. *Magn Reson Imaging.* 2005;23(9):929–937.

133. Lakatta EG, Levy D. Arterial and cardiac aging: major shareholders in cardiovascular disease enterprises. Part II: the aging heart in health: links to heart disease. *Circulation.* 2003;107(2):346–354.

134. Panting JR, Gatehouse PD, Yang GZ, *et al.* Abnormal subendocardial perfusion in cardiac syndrome X detected by cardiovascular magnetic resonance imaging. *N Engl J Med.* 2002;346(25):1948–1953.

135. Julius S, Amery A, Whitlock LS, Conway J. Influence of age on the hemodynamic response to exercise. *Circulation.* 1967;36(2):222–230.

136. Fleg JL, O'Connor F, Gerstenblith G, *et al.* Impact of age on the cardiovascular response to dynamic upright exercise in healthy men and women. *J Appl Physiol.* 1995;78(3):890–900.

137. Pimentel AE, Gentile CL, Tanaka H, Seals DR, Gates PE. Greater rate of decline in maximal aerobic capacity with age in endurance-trained than in sedentary men. *J Appl Physiol.* 2003;94(6):2406–2413.

138. Krane M, Voss B, Hiebinger A, *et al.* Twenty years of cardiac surgery in patients aged 80 years and older: risks and benefits. *Ann Thorac Surg.* 2011;91(2):506–513.

139. Krane M, Bauernschmitt R, Hiebinger A, *et al.* Cardiac reoperation in patients aged 80 years and older. *Ann Thorac Surg.* 2009;87(5):1379–1385.

140. Tsai TP, Nessim S, Kass RM, *et al.* Morbidity and mortality after coronary artery bypass in octogenarians. *Ann Thorac Surg.* 1991;51(6):983–986.

141. Yashar JJ, Yashar AG, Torres D, Hittner K. Favorable results of coronary artery bypass and/or valve replacement in octogenarians. *Cardiovasc Surg.* 1993;1(1):68–71.

142. Collart F, Feier H, Kerbaul F, *et al.* Valvular surgery in octogenarians: operative risks factors, evaluation of Euroscore and long term results. *Eur J Cardiothorac Surg.* 2005;27(2):276–280.

143. Kolh P, Kerzmann A, Honore C, Comte L, Limet R. Aortic valve surgery in octogenarians: predictive factors for operative and long-term results. *Eur J Cardiothorac Surg.* 2007;31(4):600–606.

144. Mantilla CB, Horlocker TT, Schroeder DR, Berry DJ, Brown DL. Frequency of myocardial infarction, pulmonary embolism, deep venous thrombosis, and death following primary hip or knee arthroplasty. *Anesthesiology.* 2002;96(5):1140–1146.

145. Fleischmann KE, Beckman JA, Buller CE, *et al.* 2009 ACCF/AHA focused update on perioperative beta blockade: a report of the American college of cardiology foundation/American heart association task force on practice guidelines. *Circulation.* 2009;120(21):2123–2151.

146. Bardakci H, Cheema FH, Topkara VK, *et al.* Discharge to home rates are significantly lower for octogenarians undergoing coronary artery bypass graft surgery. *Ann Thorac Surg.* 2007;83(2):483–489.

147. Craver JM, Puskas JD, Weintraub WW, *et al.* 601 octogenarians undergoing cardiac surgery: outcome and comparison with younger age groups. *Ann Thorac Surg.* 1999;67(4):1104–1110.

148. Avery GJ, 2nd, Ley SJ, Hill JD, Hershon JJ, Dick SE. Cardiac surgery in the octogenarian: evaluation of risk, cost, and outcome. *Ann Thorac Surg.* 2001;71(2):591–596.

149. Sandham JD, Hull RD, Brant RF, *et al.* A randomized, controlled trial of the use of pulmonary-artery catheters in high-risk surgical patients. *N Engl J Med.* 2003;348(1):5–14.

150. Cowie BS. Does the pulmonary artery catheter still have a role in the perioperative period? *Anaesth Intensive Care.* 2011;39(3):345–355.

151. Fleisher LA, Beckman JA, Brown KA, *et al.* 2009 ACCF/AHA focused update on perioperative beta blockade incorporated into the ACC/AHA 2007 guidelines on perioperative cardiovascular evaluation and care for noncardiac surgery: a report of the American college of cardiology foundation/American heart association task force on practice guidelines. *Circulation.* 2009;120(21):e169–e276.

152. Galal W, Hoeks SE, Flu WJ, *et al.* Relation between preoperative and intraoperative new wall motion abnormalities in vascular surgery patients: a transesophageal echocardiographic study. *Anesthesiology.* 2010;112(3):557–566.

153. Subramaniam B, Subramaniam K. Not all perioperative myocardial infarctions can be prevented with preoperative revascularization. *Anesthesiology.* 2010;112(3):524–526.

154. Nickalls RW, Mapleson WW. Age-related iso-MAC charts for isoflurane, sevoflurane and desflurane in man. *Br J Anaesth.* 2003;91(2):170–174.

155. Kazama T, Ikeda K, Morita K, *et al.* Comparison of the effect-site k(eO)s of propofol for blood pressure and EEG bispectral index in elderly and younger patients. *Anesthesiology.* 1999;90(6):1517–1527.

156. Schnider TW, Minto CF, Shafer SL, *et al.* The influence of age on propofol pharmacodynamics. *Anesthesiology.* 1999;90(6):1502–1516.

157. Powell-Tuck J, Gosling P, Lobo D, *et al. British Consensus Guidelines on Intravenous Fluid Therapy for Adult Surgical Patients.* 2008. <http://www.ics.ac.uk/ics-homepage/guidelines-standards/>.

158. Marik PE, Baram M, Vahid B. Does central venous pressure predict fluid responsiveness? A systematic review of the literature and the tale of seven mares. *Chest.* 2008;134(1):172–178.

159. Marik PE, Cavallazzi R, Vasu T, Hirani A. Dynamic changes in arterial waveform derived variables and fluid responsiveness in mechanically ventilated patients: a systematic review of the literature. *Crit Care Med.* 2009;37(9):2642–2647.

160. Barnett SR. Polypharmacy and perioperative medications in the elderly. *Anesthesiol Clin.* 2009;27(3):377–389.

CHAPTER 7

Respiratory ageing

Jaume Canet and Joaquin Sanchis

Introduction

A recent study concluded that the life expectancy of individuals born in the industrialized world at the start of the twenty-first century will exceed 100 years, and what is more important, their quality of life will be good for the most part.[1] Yet, because of the inexorable physical deterioration that comes with time, most medical and surgical interventions will still be concentrated in the last quarter of a person's life.[2] Surgery after the age of 70 years has become increasingly common: on the one hand, persons of advanced age now account for a larger percentage of the population, and on the other, improvements in surgical and anaesthetic techniques have made them less invasive than they once were. We can foresee that these trends will continue, leaving us to cope with a growing demand in treatment for older patients, who will require diagnostic and therapeutic procedures similar to those we now perform on our youngest patients.

From the 6th week of gestation to the age of 8 years, the lung is growing exponentially in both size and complexity as the respiratory bronchioles and alveolar ducts branch out to increase by several orders of magnitude. By the end of this process of development the lung will have around 300 million alveoli, tenfold more than at birth. Lung function and capacity reaches its height at around the age of 20 years and is maintained for about 10 more years in men and 20 in women.[3] Deterioration then sets in, as some 10 per cent of capacity is lost with each decade of life, even in athletes whose level of physical activity remains vigorous.[4,5] At that rate of loss, it is estimated that a level of functional reserve that would be incompatible with life would be reached at some point between the age of 120 and 150 years. Deterioration originates mainly in the loss of the elastic properties of the lung itself and in the increase in chest wall rigidity that also comes with age. This process brings about a significant reduction in the surface available for gas exchange and, thus, a tendency to hypoxaemia.

The anaesthetist must understand such age-related changes in depth because declining lung function is exacerbated by many surgical and anaesthetic factors, including the body positions required for surgery, the mechanical factors related to muscle injury, and the residual effects of anaesthetics and analgesics.[6] Furthermore, a higher incidence of cognitive decline in the early postoperative period in older patients makes it difficult for them to cooperate with measures to prevent and treat pulmonary complications.[7] Such complications are as common as cardiovascular ones but when the respiratory system is affected the observed mortality is higher, at around 20 per cent in one recently compiled general surgical population.[8]

This chapter reviews the changes that age imposes on the physiology of the respiratory system, with emphasis on the aspects that are most relevant to the practice of anaesthesia. Readers wishing to go beyond the scope of this chapter will find several extensive reviews available in the literature.[9–14]

Structural changes

The mechanics of the respiratory system are conventionally studied by separately analysing the physical properties of the chest wall and those of the lung itself. The chest wall is composed of two elements: the bony and cartilaginous structures of the wall (the rib cage) and the muscles that move them. The compliance of the bony and cartilaginous structures diminishes with age, probably as a result of loss of elasticity as calcification develops in spinal and costal ligaments and in the cartilage that secures the ribs. The resulting rigidity makes it more difficult to mobilize these structures. In addition, partial or complete fractures of dorsal vertebrae due to age-related osteoporosis, observed in 60 per cent of women and 30 per cent of men by the age of 80 years,[15] will make kyphosis more pronounced. As a result, the thorax becomes rounder as its anteroposterior diameter increases.[16] These geometric changes, along with diminished chest wall compliance, produce a right shift of the pulmonary pressure-volume curve, inducing a slight increase in functional residual capacity (FRC).

With increased anteroposterior diameter, the dome of the diaphragm loses as much as 23–25 per cent of its height in older patients in comparison with young adults,[17,18] impairing the muscle's ability to generate force.[16] The nutritional deficiencies that are so common in the elderly also have a deleterious effect on the respiratory muscles and their ability to generate maximal inspiratory and expiratory pressures (MIP and MEP)[19] and an acceptable level of maximal voluntary ventilation.[20]

The course of respiratory muscle deterioration has been seen to keep pace with the decline of other musculoskeletal structures,[21] such that lower MIP and MEP values closely correlate with hand-grip weakening.[19] Various changes in both muscle fibres and nerve structures account for weakness in the elderly.[22,23] The area of the muscle cross-section shrinks, and there are reductions in the number of muscle fibres (particularly type II fast twitch muscles) and motor nerve fibres (with selective denervation of type II muscle fibres). Changes in neuromuscular junctions also take place, and peripheral motor neurons diminish in number.[22,23]

Malnutrition, malabsorption, and comorbidity are common findings in patients of advanced age. Studies of the impact of poor nutrition on respiratory muscle structure and function have revealed a correlation between these deficiencies and diaphragm weight and both MIP and MEP.[24] Neuromuscular disorders such as Parkinson's disease and cerebral-vascular abnormalities[25,26] and the observed increase in the frequency of heart failure[27] all have very significant effects on the strength of respiratory muscles. The relationship between strength and duration of diaphragmatic contraction—the tension/time index (TTI)—is altered such that older patients with heart failure have a higher TTI, leading to rapid onset of muscle fatigue on effort.[28] These changes can complicate ventilator weaning after an operation or lead to ventilator insufficiency.

Age-related deterioration of the pulmonary parenchyma is not attributable to the physical properties of the surfactants covering alveolar surfaces, as these fluids seem to remain unaffected by age. Nor have changes in type II pneumocytes or the number and function of Clara cells been detected. Therefore, an explanation for the declining performance of the parenchyma must be looked for in the elastic properties of lung tissues. Elastic recoil—7–9 cmH$_2$O measured at 60 per cent of total lung capacity (TLC) at its peak at around the age of 20 years—begins to decrease at a rate of 0.2 cmH$_2$O each year after that, leading to a loss of 50 per cent at around the age of 50 years.[29] The likely cause is the spatial arrangement and crosslinking of elastic fibres or perhaps the presence of pseudoelastin.[30] Alveolar ducts dilate as a result, leading to so-called senile hyperinflation, somewhat misleadingly referred to as senile emphysema. Since older non-smokers show no signs of tissue destruction or infiltration, age-related emphysema is distinguishable from the pathologic emphysema that comes with smoking.[31] Pressure-volume curves rise and shift farther to the left than the curves of 20-year-olds.[32] After the age of 60 years, some of the elastic fibres of respiratory bronchioles and alveoli will have ruptured, leading to alveolar degeneration and shrinkage, particularly around alveolar ducts, which appear dilated and more homogeneous. This finding is distinct from the irregular distribution seen in smoking-related emphysema. Morphometric studies show that distances between alveolar walls are greater after the 3rd decade of life and that the surface area where gas exchange takes place decreases progressively per unit volume. Observed loss has ranged from 75 m^2 at age 30 years to 60 m^2 at age 75 years (30), and by the age of 90 years 30 per cent of the surface available at the age of 30 years may have been lost.[31,33]

Deep within the lung, at the most distal portions of the bronchial-bronchiolar tree and infundibular zones approaching the alveoli, bronchioles are anchored to the surrounding thin alveolar walls that lend them support. Thus, the calibre of bronchioles depends on the tethering action of the alveolar wall, and loss of its elastic recoil will promote a corresponding narrowing of the bronchiole. When an area of the lung collapses, air ceases to enter the alveoli and neighbouring bronchi, but when it is primarily the bronchioles that close, air may remain trapped in the alveolar and infundibular region even in the absence of lung collapse. Air trapping in the young adult caused by closure of terminal bronchioles only occurs in interdependent regions of the lung, usually toward the end of maximal expiration.[34] This phenomenon is accentuated at advanced age, and eventually comes to affect most of the lung after the age of 70 years, when lung volume approaches residual volume (RV). Increased air trapping is largely attributable to the loss of elastic retraction[29] but is also promoted by the ageing bronchiolar wall's diminished resistance to collapse.[35] Given that long-term clearance of surface material from the small airways also decreases with age,[36] this factor may also play a part in raising the prevalence of respiratory symptoms in the elderly.

Lung function

Closing volume (CV) is defined as the difference in lung volume at the beginning of airway closure and at RV.[14] Closing capacity (CC) is the sum of CV and RV. Both CV and CC can be fairly easily estimated by administering a bolus of tracer gas[37] or measuring the single-breath concentration of a resident gas (molecular nitrogen),[38] provided RV is also known. As early as 1970, Leblanc and colleagues[39] studied CC in 80 non-smokers aged 18–82 years, demonstrating changes related to age and body posture. CC increases with age until it eventually reaches FRC and can be seen to be present throughout resting tidal breathing (CC > FRC, referred to as resting tidal closure) (Fig. 7.1). A portion of the airway will open at the beginning of inspiration, while other portions will open toward the end or remain closed throughout the cycle when the individual is at rest. This phenomenon is more evident in the decubitus position, leading to less efficient gas mixing in the lung, among other deleterious effects, and should be taken into account when protective pre-oxygenation is provided before anaesthetic induction in patients over the age of 65 years. For these older patients, breathing 100 per cent oxygen for three minutes or longer will clearly be more beneficial than taking the usual four maximal inspirations of 100 per cent oxygen, the technique used for younger patients.[42]

Lung volumes

Although TLC diminishes slightly between the ages of 20 and 70 years in absolute terms, height also decreases over the same period as intervertebral discs become thinner. Therefore, TLC hardly changes when height is also taken into account. However, vital capacity (VC) is reduced by 25 per cent between the ages of 20 and 60 years,[43] and RV increases proportionally, from 25 per cent of TLC in the young adult to 40 per cent in the 70-year-old[12] (Fig. 7.1). The changes in the elasticity of lung tissue that have been mentioned are somewhat greater than chest wall changes, explaining why the FRC/TLC relation increases slightly in older individuals.[29] Thus, at rest a person of advanced age breathes at a volume that is closer to maximal volume than it is in the young adult. This situation overloads the respiratory muscles, which must begin to contract during inspiration when part of their capacity for shortening has already been used. The energy expended in breathing by a 60-year-old is therefore about 20 per cent greater than that expended by a young adult of 20 years.[44]

Spirometry

After the maximum value of forced expiratory volume in 1 second (FEV$_1$) is reached around age 20 years in healthy women and between 25 and 27 years in men, this volume will decrease with age at a rate of 20 ml per year until the age of 40 years; after the age of 65 years loss occurs at a rate of 38 ml per year.[43] We can expect to see a 25 per cent reduction of an individual's maximum FEV$_1$ by the time a woman reaches 55 years and a man reaches 60 years.[43,45] Given that forced vital capacity (FVC) declines somewhat more rapidly than FEV$_1$, the FEV$_1$/FVC ratio rises slightly with age.[46] Deterioration in spirometric variables is more marked in men than in women and is more pronounced in smokers even before pulmonary disease becomes evident. If smokers reach the age of 90 years, their FEV$_1$ will be half what it was when they were 65 years old,

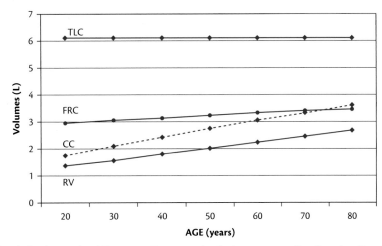

Fig. 7.1 Lung volumes for a normal male (height 1.7 m) at different ages. The conventional volumes were predicted based on Quanjer and colleagues;[40] CC values were based on Buist and colleagues.[41] CC: closing capacity; FRC: functional residual capacity; RV: residual volume; TLC: total lung capacity. Data from Quanjer PH, Tammeling GJ, Cotes JE, Pedersen OF, Peslin R, Yernault JC (1993) Lung volumes and forced ventilatory flows. Report Working Party "Standardization of Lung Function Tests". European Coal and Steel Community. *EurResp J*, Suppl. Mar(16), 5–40 and Buist AS, Ross BB (1973). Predicted values for closing volumes using a modified single breath test. *Am Rev Respir Dis*, 107(5), 744–752.

when it was already significantly lower than that of non-smokers of the same age and height.[46–48]

The prevalence of chronic obstructive pulmonary disease (COPD) has been found to be two- to threefold higher in persons over 60 years of age,[49] an alarming statistic that requires careful consideration. The 2010 update of the Global Initiative on Obstructive Lung Disease (GOLD) proposes diagnostic criteria based on post-bronchodilator spirometry: $FEV_1/FVC < 70$ per cent and $FEV_1 \leq 80$ per cent of its reference value.[50] If these cut offs were applied, approximately 35 per cent of healthy never-smokers would have COPD at age 70 years or older and in the population over the age of 80 years, about 50 per cent would have COPD.[51] Therefore, to minimize over diagnosis, the GOLD spirometric criteria must be used in conjunction with age-specific reference values, that is, values obtained from healthy populations of the same age. Nonetheless, even elderly subjects classified as healthy normals using a lower level of normal for FEV_1 but with a ratio of FEV_1/FVC <70 per cent may show a higher risk of death and of COPD-related hospitalizations.[52]

While maximal inspiratory and expiratory flow (MIF and MEF) rates decrease with age, their variability increases, making it difficult to quantify loss precisely.[53] When researchers have measured negative expiratory pressure, a technique that is less dependent on a patient's active cooperation, they have been able to demonstrate the presence of expiratory flow limitation in 32.5 per cent of elderly men and 38 per cent of elderly women who are otherwise healthy.[54] The age-related decline of MEF is attributable to the concurrent reduction in lung elastic recoil.[55] A lower MEF and a higher FRC are key determinants of mechanical limitations on exercise tolerance in the older adult.[56] In a submaximal exercise tolerance test, an elderly individual must breathe faster than a younger person. Another element that considerably curtails an older individual's possibility of increasing ventilation other than by increasing respiratory frequency is a disproportionately high end-expiratory lung volume in comparison to the young.[56] During exercise a major consequence of the loss of elastic recoil with age may be the sacrifice of optimal length of inspiratory muscles and an increased cost of breathing.[57] The mechanical limits age places on expiratory flow and inspiratory

pressure are present even in highly fit older subjects.[58] For these reasons, fatigue sets in sooner in the person of advanced age.

Finally, regarding non-specific airway responsiveness, older age has been directly related to the slope of the methacholine dose–response curve, but only in elderly individuals who are former smokers and not in current smokers or non-smokers.[59]

Maximum inspiratory pressure and maximum expiratory pressure

Respiratory muscle force is measured by recording the pressure that develops on blocking a forced maximal inspiration at FRC or RV and during a forced maximal expiration at TLC. MIP values over 80 cmH$_2$O in men or over 70 cmH$_2$O in women rule out significant muscle weakness,[60] but large studies such as those of Enright and colleagues[19] show that the MIP of a subject over the age of 75 years is well below those levels, providing evidence of reduced muscle force in even the fittest and most active older individuals. Lower MIP may be clinically important in situations that lead to respiratory muscle overload, such as pneumonia[30] or congestive heart failure.[61] Nutritional deficiency is another factor related to increased muscle dysfunction.

When assessing the functional status of an elderly patient the physician has to take into account that, beyond the deterioration of spirometric variables as a result of the functional decline of the lung, difficulties arise from age-related psychomotor and cognitive deficits, which interfere with patient cooperation and lead to worse results in about a fifth of elderly patients.[62,63]

Gas exchange

Regional imbalances in ventilation–perfusion relationships in the lung are exacerbated with age. Mismatching may be due to an excess in the number of ventilated alveoli with poor perfusion (dead space effect) or to excess perfusion from alveoli receiving reduced ventilation (shunting effect). Both types of mismatching increase the alveolar–arterial difference in oxygen tension ($P_{(A-a)}O_2$)[64] to a degree that is described by the equation proposed by Sorbini and colleagues:[65]

$$P_{(A-a)}O_2 = 14.5 - 0.057 \times age$$

where pressure is expressed in kilopascals and age in years, or

$$P_{(A-a)}O_2 = 109 - 43 \times age$$

where pressure is expressed in millimetres of mercury and age in years. Appropriately lower PaO_2 reference values must therefore be used when assessing function in patients of advanced age. Over the age of 65 years an acceptable reference range would be 10.5–11.3 kPa (80–90 mmHg),[66] so for individuals aged 82 years, a PaO_2 of 9.8 kPa (73.7 mmHg) would indicate only slightly altered gas exchange. Because of the sigmoidal shape of the oxygen–haemoglobin dissociation curve, changes in PaO_2 above 9.3 kPa (70 mmHg) are poorly detected when arterial oxygen saturation is monitored by pulse oximetry, although it is possible to detect a progressive age-related reduction in that variable when very large population samples are studied (Fig. 7.2).

$PaCO_2$, on the other hand, remains comparatively unchanged. The diffusing capacity of the lung for carbon monoxide (DLCO) also diminishes with age, however, as do the reference ranges used, as described by the equation of Guènard and Marthan:[67]

$$DLCO = 126 - 0.90 \times age$$

where DLCO is expressed as millilitres per minute per $PaCO_2$ in kilopascals ($r = 0.54$, p <0.001).

Lung perfusion

The capillary bed of the lung diminishes with age, leading to a 30 per cent rise in mean pulmonary arterial pressure as well as a rise in pulmonary vascular resistance.[68] Attenuation of the hypoxic pulmonary vasoconstriction reflex occurs as a result of the greater rigidity of pulmonary vessels, leading to changes in the ventilation–perfusion relationship in older patients.[12] These slight abnormalities become highly relevant when one-lung ventilation is required.[69]

The upper airway

The impaired cough and swallowing reflexes seen in greater frequency in persons over the age of 70 years[70] probably arise from a variety of contributing factors: increased pharyngeal and subglottic resistance in men (but not in women),[71] loss of muscle supporting the pharyngeal wall, delayed swallowing reflex, comorbidity (COPD, cerebrovascular stroke, cognitive decline, and hypothyroidism), and loss of bronchial epithelial cilia. In addition, the tracheobronchial tree becomes less able to recognize foreign bodies or substances[72] and the cough itself is less efficient in terms of volume, force, and expiratory flow. These impaired cough and swallowing mechanisms, especially in the presence of poor mouth care or in edentulous individuals, put the older patient at more risk for tracheobronchial aspiration of oral, pharyngeal, or gastric contents and, therefore, at greater risk for aspiration pneumonia.[70] In a large study of hospitalized patients with community-acquired pneumonia a fivefold rise in incidence of this diagnosis was observed as age increased from 65–69 to 90 years; associated mortality doubled over the same age range.[73] Risk rises further when the patient is placed in the decubitus position for prolonged periods and when sedatives or general anaesthetics are used.

The association of central respiratory depression with increased pharyngeal collapsibility during sleep in both sexes may be the basis for a higher incidence of sleep disordered breathing, particularly in men.[74,75] Repeated upper airway obstructive events during sleep occur in 24 per cent to 75 per cent of older adults.[76]

Central regulation

Minute ventilation in the adult of advanced age is similar to that of a young person with similar physical characteristics and in similar condition, but the older individual's tidal volume is lower

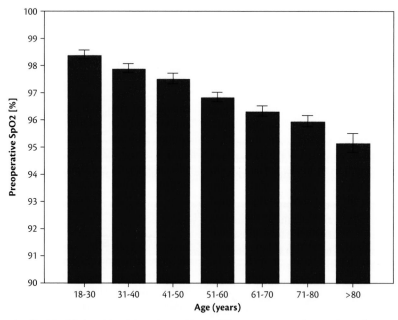

Fig. 7.2 Mean arterial oxygen saturation (SpO_2) while breathing air in supine position in different age ranges. The error bars refer to standard error. This broad surgical population included patients with healthy and diseased lungs.[8] Data from Canet J, Gallart L, Gomar C, Paluzié G, Vallès J, Castillo J, Sabaté S, Mazo V, Briones Z, Sanchis J, ARISCAT Investigators (2010) Prediction of postoperative pulmonary complications in a population-based surgical cohort. Anesthesiology, 113(6), 1338–50.

and respiratory frequency is higher.[77] The ventilatory response to hypoxia is clearly attenuated in an elderly person and the response to hypercapnia is also reduced. Central respiratory drive is usually estimated by measuring the pressure generated in the first 100 ms of an occluded breath, a measure unaffected by the compliance of the respiratory system. At advanced age, in response to hypercapnia this pressure has been seen to be about half what it would have been in youth and in response to hypoxia less than half; these findings are not explained by muscle weakness.[78] The observed decline suggests that information from chemical and mechanical receptors is processed with difficulty in the older adult and that activity along efferent neural pathways toward muscles is inadequate. Decreased perception of elastic and resistive loading during breathing has also been reported.[79,80] The summary effect is one of depressed regulation of breathing control, which leads to considerable attenuation of warning systems and adaptive processes.

Conclusion

Ageing is marked by significant changes in the respiratory system. Lung function gradually declines after the age of 30 years, and respiratory reserve is drastically reduced after the age of 80 years. Advanced age therefore increases individual risk during any medical event such as surgery. The most important physiologic changes in the thorax are decreased compliance of the chest wall, reduced elastic recoil of the lungs, and diminished respiratory muscle force. Together these developments lead to a 20 per cent reduction in the surface area available for gas exchange and a change in the ventilation–perfusion ratio. PaO_2 and ventilatory reserve are both reduced as a result. Also important are declining reflexes governing cough and swallowing and diminished sensitivity to hypoxia and, to a lesser degree, to hypercapnia.

The anaesthetist must bear all these changes in mind in order to cope with the challenges that arise in the perioperative management of the elderly patient to assure that the outcome of surgery is successful.

References

1. Christensen K, Doblhammer G, Rau R, Vaupel JW. Ageing populations: the challenges ahead. *Lancet*. 2009;374:1196–1208.
2. Sabaté S, Canet J, Gomar C, Castillo J, Villalonga A, ANESCAT Investigators. Cross-sectional survey of anaesthetic practices in Catalonia, Spain. *Ann Fr Anesth Reanim*. 2008;27(5):371–383.
3. Burrows B, Cline MG, Knudson RJ, *et al.* A descriptive analysis of the growth and decline of the FVC and FEV₁ .*Chest*. 1983;83(5):717–724.
4. McClaran SR, Babcock MA, Pegelow DF. Longitudinal effects of aging on lung function at rest and exercise in healthy active fit elderly adults. *J Appl Physiol*. 1995;78(5):1957–1968.
5. Pollock ML, Mengelkoch LJ, Graves JE. Twenty-year follow-up of aerobic power and body composition of older track athletes. *J Appl Physiol*. 1997;82(5):1508–1516.
6. Canet J, Mazo V. Postoperative pulmonary complications. *Minerva Anestesiol*. 2010;76(2):138–143.
7. Manku K, Bacchetti P, Leung JM. Prognostic significance of postoperative in-hospital complications in elderly patients. I. Long-term survival. *Anesth Analg*. 2003;96(2):583–589.
8. Canet J, Gallart L, Gomar C, *et al.* Prediction of postoperative pulmonary complications in a population-based surgical cohort. *Anesthesiology*. 2010;113(6):1338–1350.
9. Wahba WM. Influence of aging on lung function – clinical significance of changes from age twenty. *Anesth Analg*. 1983;62(8):764–776.
10. Smith TC. Respiratory effects of aging. *Semin Anesth*. 1986;5(1):14–22.
11. Janssens JP, Pache JC, Nicod LP. Physiological changes in respiratory function associated with ageing. *Eur Respir J*. 1999;13(1):197–205.
12. Zaugg M, Lucchinetti E. Respiratory function in the elderly. *Anesthesiol Clin*. 2000;18(1):48–58.
13. Sprung J, Gajic O, Warner DO. Review article: age related alterations in respiratory function—anesthetic considerations. *Can J Anesth*. 2006;53(12):1244–1257.
14. Milic-Emili J, Torchio R, D'Angelo E. Closing volume: a reappraisal (1967–2007). *Eur J Appl Physiol*. 2007;99(6):567–583.
15. Gunby MC, Morley JE. Epidemiology of bone loss with aging. *Clin Geriatr Med*. 1994;10(4):557–571.
16. Edge J, Millard F, Reid L, Simon G. The radiographic appearance of the chest in persons of advanced age. *Br J Radiol*. 1964;37(10):769–774.
17. Polkey MI, Harris ML, Hughes PD, *et al.* The contractile properties of the elderly human diaphragm. *Am J Respir Crit Care Med*. 1997;155(5):1560–1564.
18. Tolep K, Higgins N, Muza S, Criner G, Kelsen S. Comparison of diaphragm strength between healthy adult elderly and young men. *Am J Respir Crit Care Med*. 1995;152(2):677–682.
19. Enright PL, Kronmal RA, Manolio TA, Schenker MB, Hyatt RE. Respiratory muscle strength in the elderly: correlates and reference values. *Am J Respir Crit Care Med*. 1994;149(3 Pt1):430–438.
20. Arora NS, Rochester DF. Respiratory muscle strength and maximal voluntary ventilation in undernourished patients. *Am Rev Respir Dis*. 1982;126(1):5–8.
21. Bassey EJ, Harries UJ. Normal values for handgrip strength in 920 men and women aged over 65 years, and longitudinal changes over 4 years in 620 survivors. *Clin Sci*. 1993;84(3):331–337.
22. Tolep K, Kelsen S. Effect of aging on respiratory skeletal muscles. *Clin Chest Med*. 1993;14(3):363–378.
23. Brown M, Hasser E. Complexity of age-related change in skeletal muscle. *J Gerontol A Biol Sci Med Sci*. 1996;51(2):B117–B123.
24. Wilson DO, Rogers RM, Hoffman RM. Nutrition and chronic lung disease. *Am Rev Respir Dis*. 1985;132(6):1347–1365.
25. Brown L. Respiratory dysfunction in Parkinson's disease. *Clin Chest Med*. 1994;15(4):715–727.
26. Vingerhoets F, Bogousslavsky J. Respiratory dysfunction in stroke. *Clin Chest Med*. 1994;15(4):729–737.
27. Mancini D, Henson D, LaManca J, Levine S. Respiratory muscle function and dyspnoea in patients with chronic heart failure. *Circulation*. 1992;86(3):909–918.
28. Stassijns G, Lysens R, Decramer M. Peripheral and respiratory muscles in chronic heart failure. *Eur Respir J*. 1996;9(10):2161–2167.
29. Turner J, Mead J, Wohl M. Elasticity of human lungs in relation to age. *J Appl Physiol*. 1968;25(6):664–671.
30. Crapo RO. The aging lung. In Mahler DA (ed) *Pulmonary disease in the elderly patient*, Vol. 63 (pp. 1–21). New York: Marcel Dekker, 1993.
31. Verbeken E, Cauberghs M, Mertens I, Clement J, Lauweryns JM, Van de Woestijne KP. The senile lung. Comparison with normal and emphysematous lungs. 1: Structural aspects. *Chest*. 1992;101(3):793–799.
32. Verbeken E, Cauberghs M, Mertens I, Clement J, Lauweryns JM, Van de Woestijne KP (1992). The senile lung. Comparison with normal and emphysematous lungs. 2. Functional aspects. *Chest*. 1992;101(3):800–809.
33. Gillooly M, Lamb D. Airspace size in lungs of lifelong nonsmokers: effect of age and sex. *Thorax*. 1993;48(1):39–43.
34. Milic-Emili J, Henderson JA, Dolovich MB, Trop D, Kaneko KMB. Regional distribution of inspired gas in the lung. *J Appl Physiol*. 1966;21(3):749–759.
35. Holland J, Milic-Emili J, Macklem PT, Bates DV. Regional distribution of pulmonary ventilation and perfusion in elderly subjects. *J Clin Invest*. 1966;47(1):81–92.
36. Svartengren M, Falk R, Philipson K. Long-term clearance from small airways decreases with age. *Eur Respir J*. 2005;26(4):609–615.

37. Dollfuss RE, Milic-Emili J, Bates DV. Regional ventilation of the lung studied with boluses of 133 Xenon. *Respir Physiol.* 1967;2(2):234–246.

38. Anthonisen NR, Danson J, Robertson PC, Ross WR. Airway closure as a function of age. *Respir Physiol.* 1969;8(1):58–65.

39. Leblanc P, Ruff F, Milic-Emili J. Effects of age and body position on "airway closure" in man. *J Appl Physiol.* 1970;28(4):448–451.

40. Quanjer PH, Tammeling GJ, Cotes JE, Pedersen OF, Peslin R, Yernault JC. Lung volumes and forced ventilatory flows. Report Working Party 'Standardization of Lung Function Tests'. European Coal and Steel Community. *Eur Resp J Suppl.* 1993;16:5–40.

41. Buist AS, Ross BB. Predicted values for closing volumes using a modified single breath test. *Am Rev Respir Dis.* 1973;107(5):744–752.

42. Valentine SJ, Marjot R, Monk CR. Preoxygenation in the elderly: a comparison of the four-maximal-breath and three-minute techniques. *Anesth Analg.* 1990;71(5):516–519.

43. Schmidt CD, Dickman ML, Gardner RM, Brough FK. Spirometric standards for healthy elderly men and women: 532 subjects, ages 55 through 94 years. *Am Rev Respir Dis.* 1973;108(4):933–939.

44. Tzankoff SP, Norris AH. Longitudinal changes in basal metabolism in man. *J Appl Physiol.* 1978;45(4):709–717.

45. Milne JS, Williamson J. Respiratory function tests in older people. *Clin Sci.* 1972;42(3):71–81.

46. Griffith KA, Sherrill DL, Siegel EM, Manolio TA, Bonekat HW, Enright PL. Predictors of loss of lung function in the elderly: the Cardiovascular Health Study. *Am J Respir Crit Care Med.* 2001;163(1):61–68.

47. Anthonisen NR, Connett JE, Murray RP, for the Lung Health Study Research Group. Smoking and lung function of Lung Health Study Participants after 11 Years. *Am J Respir Crit Care Med.* 2002;166(5):675–679.

48. Edwards R. ABC of smoking cessation. The problem of tobacco smoking. *BMJ.* 2004;328(7433):217–219.

49. Buist AS, McBurnie MA, Vollmer WM, *et al.* International variation in the prevalence of COPD (the GOLD Study): a population-based prevalence study. *Lancet.* 2007;370(9589):741–750.

50. Global Initiative for Chronic Obstructive Lung Disease. *Update 2010.* <http://wwgoldcopd.org> (accessed 31 August 2011).

51. Hardie JA, Buist AS, Vollmer WM, Ellingsen I, Bakke PS, Morkve O. Risk of over-diagnosis of COPD in asymptomatic elderly never-smokers. *Eur Resp J.* 2002;20(5):1117–1122.

52. Manino DM, Buist AS, Vollmer WM. Chronic obstructive disease in the older adult: what defines abnormal lung function? *Thorax.* 2007;62(3):237–241.

53. Enright P, Burchette R, Peters J, Lebowitz M, McDonnell W, Abbey D. Peak flow lability: association with asthma and spirometry in an older cohort. *Chest.* 1997;112(4):895–901.

54. de Bisschop C, Marty ML, Tessier JF, Barbeger-Gateau P, Dartigues JF, Guénard H. Expiratory flow limitation and obstruction in the elderly. *Eur Respir J.* 2005;26(4):594–601.

55. Babb TG, Rodarte JR. Mechanism of reduced maximal expiratory flow with aging. *J Appl Physiol.* 2000;89(2):505–511.

56. DeLorey DS, Babb TG. Progressive mechanical ventilator constraints with aging. *Am J Respir Crit Care Med.* 1999;160(1):169–177.

57. Johnson BD, Reddan WG, Pegelow DF, Seow KC, Dempsey A. Flow limitation and regulation of functional residual capacity during exercise in a physical active aging population. *Am Rev Respir Dis.* 1991;143(5):960–967.

58. Johnson BD, Reddan WG, Seow KC, Dempsey A. Mechanical constraints on exercise hypernea in a fit aging population. *Am Rev Respir Dis.* 1991;143(5):968–977.

59. Sparrow D, O'Connor GT, Rosner B, Segal M, Weiss ST. The influence of age and level of pulmonary function in nonspecific airway responsiveness. *Am Rev Respir Dis.* 1991;143(5):978–982.

60. Polkey M, Green M, Moxham J (1995). Measurement of respiratory muscle strength. *Thorax.* 1995;50(11):1131–1135.

61. Evans S, Watson L, Hawkins M, Cowley A, Johnston I, Kinnear W. Respiratory muscle strength in chronic heart failure. *Thorax.* 1995;50(6):625–628.

62. De Filippi D, Tana F, Vanzati S, Balzarini B, Galetti G. Study of respiratory function in the elderly with different nutritional and cognitive status and functional ability assessed by plethysmographic and spirometric parameters. *Arch Gerontol Geriatr.* 2003;37(1):33–43.

63. Allen SC. Spirometry in old age. *Age Ageing.* 2003;32(1):4–5.

64. Cardús J, Burgos F, Diaz O, *et al.* Increase in pulmonary ventilation–perfusion inequality with age in healthy individuals. *Am J Respir Crit Care Med.* 1997;156(2 Pt 1):648–653.

65. Sorbini CA, Grassi V, Solinas E, Mulesan G. Arterial oxygen tension in relation to age in healthy subjects. *Respiration.* 1968;25(1):3–13.

66. Delclaux B, Orcel B, Housset B, Whitelaw WA, Derenne J. Arterial blood gases in elderly persons with chronic obstructive pulmonary disease (COPD). *Eur Respir J.* 1994;7(5):856–861.

67. Guénard H, Marthan R. Pulmonary gas exchange in elderly subjects. *Eur Respir J.* 1996;9(12):2573–2577.

68. Davidson WR Jr, Fee EC. Influence of aging on pulmonary hemodynamics in a population free of coronary artery disease. *Am J Cardiol.* 1990;65(22):1454–1458.

69. Weening CS, Pietak S, Hickey RF, *et al.* Relationship of preoperative closing volume to functional residual capacity and alveolar-arterial oxygen difference during anesthesia with controlled ventilation. *Anesthesiology.* 1974;1(1):3–7.

70. Marik PE, Kaplan D. Aspiration pneumonia and dysphagia in the elderly. *Chest.* 2003;124(1):328–336.

71. White DP, Lombard RM, Cadieux RJ, Zwillich CW. Pharyngeal resistance in normal humans: influence of gender, age and obesity. *J Appl Physiol.* 1985;58(2):365–371.

72. Pontoppidan H, Beecher HK. Progressive loss of protective reflex in the airway with the advance of age. *JAMA.* 1960;31(174):2209–2213.

73. Kaplan V, Angus DC, Griffin MF, Clermont G, Watson RS, Linde-Zwirble WT. Hospitalized community-acquired pneumonia in the elderly. *Am J Respir Crit Care.* 2002;165(6):766–772.

74. Young T, Shahar E, Nieto FJ, Redline S, *et al.* Predictors of sleep disordered breathing in community-dwelling adults: the sleep health study. *Arch Intern Med.* 2002;192(8):893–900.

75. Eikermann M, Jordan AS, Chamberlin NL. The influence of aging on pharyngeal collapsibility during sleep. *Chest.* 2007;131(6):1702–1709.

76. Ancoli-Israël S, Coy T. Are breathing disturbances in elderly equivalent to sleep apnea syndrome? *Sleep.* 1994;17(1):77–83.

77. Krumpe PE, Knudson RJ, Parsons G, Reiser K. The aging respiratory system. *Clin Geriat Med.* 1985;1(1):143–175.

78. Peterson DD, Pack AI, Silage DA, Fishman AP. Effects of aging on ventilatory and occlusion pressure responses to hypoxia and hypercapnia. *Am Rev Respir Dis .* 1981;124(4):387–391.

79. Tack M, Altose MD, Cherniack NS. Effect of aging on respiratory sensations produced by elastic loads. *J Appl Physiol.* 1981;50(4):844–850.

80. Tack M, Altose MD, Cherniack NS. Effect of aging on the perception of resistive ventilatory loads. *Am Rev Respir Dis.* 1982;126(3):463–467.

CHAPTER 8

Renal changes with ageing

Chris Dodds

Introduction

The functions of the kidneys and urinary tract are fundamental to the integrity of the biochemical balance of all cells. This balance is one of the most resilient homeostatic systems within the body and is essential for the effective functions of all other systems. Unsurprisingly, there is a close relationship between a falling glomerular filtration rate (GFR) and mortality and morbidity.[1] Although the decline in performance of the kidneys occurs as early as 20 years of age it is only in later life that this decline erodes the renal reserve to the degree that homeostasis is compromised. The precise incidence of chronic kidney failure in the elderly is uncertain because it is diagnosed on the estimated GFR (eGFR) using values derived from younger populations. Certainly fewer elderly than would be expected develop end-stage renal failure.

The endocrine functions of the kidney relating to erythropoietin and renin produced by the juxtaglomerular apparatus and calcitriol from cells in the proximal tubule are also affected by ageing.

It is important to recognize that changes in kidney function will be present in the elderly due directly to ageing even though the degree of change may vary depending on other life events such as diet, infection, or hypertension. The anatomical changes are probably due to a combination of small vessel endothelial damage that is caused by the same mechanisms as occur in the neurological and cardiovascular systems (see Chapters 5 and 6) and podocyte dysfunction, parietal epithelial injury, and mesangial cell damage as more specific renal pathology.

Changes in the ageing kidney

The anatomical changes in the kidney with age were described many years ago but in common with so much related to the elderly these descriptions were based on a limited number of subjects and no account was made of other concurrent diseases.

How much of the anatomical changes (see Fig. 8.1) and functional effects are due to age alone rather than disease states is only now starting to become clearer.[2] Changes due to ageing alone may include intracellular changes such as falls in protein production due to transcription errors or increases in 'protective' elements to ameliorate the effects of increasing reactive oxidative products. One of the changes that appear to be affected by ageing alone[3] is that linked to increases in nuclear factor kappa beta (NF-kB), predominantly in glomeruli, and affects all glomerular cell types; podocytes, parietal epithelial, endothelial and mesangial cells. Why this occurs is unclear but it is one of the few changes that appear to be purely age related.

With ageing the glomerulus enlarges, with an increase in numbers of epithelial and mesangial cells. As podocytes are limited in their ability to be replaced by cell division, although they do

hypertrophy, this leads to relative podocyte depletion in proportion to other cell types. As hypertrophy is a process that also has a finite capacity, the relative depletion is finally associated with glomerulosclerosis. This process of podocyte dysfunction is related to other factors than just ageing.

Several animal models are used to investigate the effects of ageing on the kidneys, one of which is the US National Institute on Aging model using Fischer 144 rats. Rats have some known differences from humans in that calorie restriction does lead to increased longevity and better organ preservation, which has not been conclusively demonstrated in primates. Also, rats appear not to develop hypertension or diabetes, the two commonest associated conditions in the elderly human. However, they do get glomerulosclerosis when not calorie restricted.[4]

Gene expression techniques were used in this rodent model to compare the calorie-restricted group with the free-feeding one. The results were worse for all genetic study sets in the latter group. Reductions were seen in podocyte transcription factor,[5] nephrin,[6]

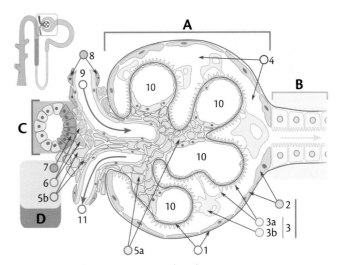

A—Renal corpuscle.
B—Proximal tubule.
C—Distal convoluted tubule.
D—Juxtaglomerular apparatus.
1. Basement membrane (basal lamina).
2. Bowman's capsule—parietal layer.
3. Bowman's capsule—visceral layer.
3a. Pedicels (foot processes from podocytes).
3b. Podocyte.
4. Bowman's space (urinary space).
5a. Mesangium—intraglomerular cell.
5b. Mesangium—extraglomerular cell.
6. Granular cells (juxtaglomerular cells).
7. Macula densa.
8. Myocytes (smooth muscle).
9. Afferent arteriole.
10. Glomerulus capillaries.
11. Efferent arteriole

Fig. 8.1 Diagram of renal corpuscle structure. Reproduced with kind permission from Michal Komorniczak, MD—medical illustrations—Poland.

and podocyte apical membrane protein tyrosine phosphatase[7] as well as other factors. This damage to the podocytes and parietal epithelium is probably linked to free radicals, as the calorie-restricted group showed far fewer examples of cell damage with ageing.

The intimal thickening of vessels within the kidney by increased collagen, smooth muscle cells, as well as fibronectin and proteoglycans, is in part due to increased levels of angiotensin-II and transforming growth factor beta-1. There is also an imbalance because of a concurrently reduction in the local levels of inhibitory cytokines and other protective enzymes.[8] The vascular endothelium in the kidney appears to be particularly susceptible to the action of endothelin-1. This highly potent vasoconstrictor is linked to oxidative stress and is increased in the elderly patient.[9,10] This is likely to be one of the major vascular factors in glomerulosclerosis. The vascular endothelial damage leading to glomerulosclerosis seems to predominately affect the more cortically placed nephrons and their associated juxtaglomerular bodies rather than those nearer the medullary zone.

Functions of the nephron

The kidneys in the healthy elderly person maintain all the necessary homeostatic functions of the body, but, as with other organ systems their ability to respond to stresses becomes increasingly limited. This limitation is in both speed and degree of response.

Glomerular filtration

Glomerulosclerosis leads to a reduction in the surface area available for filtration and a thickening of the basement membrane and these lead to a decrease in the volume of filtration. Absolute measurements of GFR using markers such as inulin are rarely performed clinically and surrogate markers are more commonly used to calculate the eGFR. These include creatinine and cystatin C.[11] Both have limitations (see Table 8.1) in the elderly.[12] Serum levels of creatinine are dependent on production largely in muscles and renal elimination. Single estimates are poor guides to renal function and creatinine clearance is a more accurate investigation. However, it is reasonably only performed when there is a high suspicion of kidney failure. Cystatin C is a small molecular-weight protein that is produced in all nucleated cells. Like creatinine it is freely filtered and not resorbed. Serum values therefore do reflect glomerular filtration. It is not believed to be affected by age and muscle mass, unlike creatinine, although it may be affected by body composition. There are several formulae that use either the serum creatinine or cystatin C to more accurately calculate GFR but with few exceptions,[13] they have been developed in patient groups that do not have a high proportion of elderly subjects. The normal decline in

Table 8.1 GRF and chronic kidney failure

Normal	>90 ml/min/1.73m^2
Stage 1	>90 ml/min/1.73m^2 plus proteinuria
Stage 2	60–90 ml/min/1.73m^2
Stage 3	30–60 ml/min/1.73m^2
Stage 4	15–30 ml/min/1.73m^2
Stage 5 (end stage)	<15 ml/min/1.73m^2

Reprinted from *American Journal of Kidney Diseases*, 39, 2, 'KDOQI Guideline on stratification and classification of CKD', pp. S46–S75, Copyright 2002, with permission from the National Kidney Foundation and Elsevier.

filtration with ageing means that many otherwise healthy subjects are defined as being in stage 2–3 kidney failure. This misdiagnosis has enormous revenue implications for heathcare as well as possible adverse effects on the individual concerned.

The fall in eGFR in the elderly is more likely to be dependent on their reduced metabolic rate for body surface area than a pathological cause. Although there is a reduction in the total number of functioning glomeruli those remaining increase their individual filtration rates.

Water balance

Hydration is the balance between water intake and output; this includes water lost through the kidney combined with the non-renal losses, which are largely through sweat and gastrointestinal losses. Although the mean water intake falls in men slightly, this is offset by reductions in the non-renal losses[14] and overall hydration is generally well maintained in healthy elderly subjects.

Water balance in the kidney is a tightly regulated process involving the ability of the kidney to respond to water loads and depletion by producing urine that varies from highly dilute to very concentrated depending on the change in plasma osmolarity. This complex process encompasses filtration through the glomerulus and then passive diffusion back through the proximal tubule with sodium, chloride, and potassium after filtration, along the high osmotic gradient maintained in the medulla through the thin descending and ascending portions of the loop of Henle, through the aldosterone-dependent systems in the distal tubule to the vasopressin regulated collecting ducts.

The movement of water, through cells in the convoluted tubules and collecting ducts, is through specific water channels; the aquaporins (AQPs) (see Fig. 8.2). AQP1 is expressed in the descending limb of the loop of Henle as well as the proximal tubule. AQP2 is the vasopressin responsive water channel and is located in the apical plasma membrane and subapical vesicles in the principal cells of the collecting duct. Once in the cells the water leaves via the AQP3 and AQP4 channels.

The hyperosmotic gradient within the medulla is dependent on sodium reabsorption and urea secretion and the counter current multiplier in the deep medulla. The maximum osmolarity in the deep medulla falls with ageing from the normal level of 1200–1400 mOsmol to approximately 800 mOsmol.

Several processes affect the osmotic gradient within the medulla with ageing.

The loss of surface cortical nephrons leaves a predominance of the shorter more juxtamedullary nephrons and that reduces overall length of the tubules. The effective shunting of the afferent to efferent renal capillaries where glomerulosclerosis has occurred and the reduction in the efferent capillary vasa recti around the nephrons reduce the counter current osmotic gradient within the medulla. This decreases the effectiveness of the loop of Henle, the ascending tubule, and collecting ducts. Equally, there are changes in the superficial medulla in sodium and urea transporters with ageing.[15]

Sodium reabsorption occurs actively, with chloride and potassium, through the sodium/potassium co-transporter NKCC2/BSC1 in the outer medulla. There is a decrease in the absolute amount of this cotransporter with ageing. In rats, the normal response to fluid restriction of an increase cotransporter is also reduced with age. Both these effects will reduce the kidneys ability to maintain the hypertonic medullary gradient.

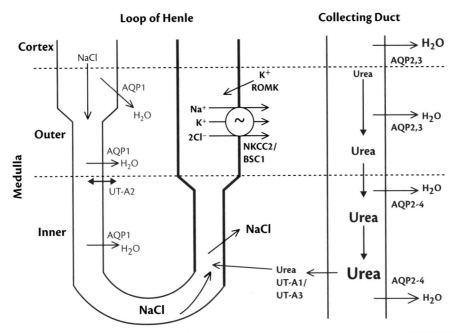

Fig. 8.2 Transport proteins involved in the urinary concentrating mechanism. In the outer medulla, active NaCl reabsorption via NKCC2/BSC1 in the thick ascending limb of the loop of Henle generates a hypertonic medullary interstitium. This concentrates NaCl in the lumen of the thin descending limb of the loop of Henle by osmotically removing water via AQP1 water channels. In the inner medulla, passive NaCl reabsorption exceeds urea secretion. Water is reabsorbed from the collecting duct, in the presence of vasopressin via AQP2 in the apical plasma membrane and AQP3 and AQP4 in the basolateral plasma membrane. Urea is concentrated in the collecting duct lumen until the fluid reaches the urea-permeable terminal inner medullary collecting duct where urea is reabsorbed into the inner medullary interstitium via the UT-A1 and UT-A3 urea transporters. Reprinted from *Seminars in Nephrology*, 29, 6, Jeff M. Sands, 'Urinary Concentration and Dilution in the Aging Kidney', pp. 579–586, Copyright 2009, with permission from Elsevier.

Urea transporters are present in the inner medullary collecting ducts and they contribute to the normal hypertonicity of the deep medulla as well as responding to vasopressin by increasing urea permeability. They, like the sodium transporters, decline in numbers with age and are also likely to contribute to the fall in medullary tonicity.

Vasopressin is released from the posterior hypothalamus in response to stimulation from osmoreceptors within the hypothalamus. This response does not appear to decline with ageing and may even by heightened. Vasopressin is active on two receptor types, V_1 (expressed in two forms, a and b) and V_2. $V_{1(a, b)}$ is expressed in the brain, vasculature, and the liver whereas the V_2 receptor is expressed in the collecting duct principal cells. The V_2 receptor is a G-protein, which generates the second messenger cyclic AMP leading to activation of the protein kinase A (cAMP/PKA) pathway. The regulation of AQP2 via the V_2 receptor occurs throughout the collecting duct and activation of V_2 receptors by vasopressin causes a movement of AQP2 channels from storage in the subapical vesicles to the apical membrane, which then increases the water uptake of the cells. Potentially, a reduction in either responsiveness or abundance of the V_2 receptors could account for the reduced urine concentrating ability seen with ageing, but no robust evidence is available at present for this.

Endocrine functions

The kidney has several important endocrine roles and these are also altered in the ageing kidney.

The renin–angiotensin–aldosterone system (RAAS) and its control of circulating volume and electrolyte balance are altered during ageing even in the absence of hypertension or other cardiovascular

Table 8.2 Effects of stimulation of the angiotensin AT_1 receptor

Renin suppression
Vasoconstriction
Water retention
Sodium retention
Reactive oxygen species (ROS) formation
Sympathetic nervous system augmentation:
• Inotropic
• Chronotropic
• Arrhythmogenic
Inflammation
Fibrosis
Cell growth and proliferation

diseases. Circulating levels of renin fall with advancing age and this is believed to mirror the degree of glomerulosclerosis with involvement of the juxtaglomerular apparatus. A similar reduction is also seen with aldosterone. Both of these falls reduce the efficiency of potassium balance and cause a tendency towards hyperkalaemia with ageing. An increase in angiotensin-II has profound effects throughout the body and also reduces bradykinin leading to a relatively unopposed vasoconstriction (see Table 8.2).

With advancing age there is an imbalance between the parasympathetic and sympathetic limbs of the autonomic system. This results in reduced baroreceptor sensitivity and heart rate variability. This is due, in part, to increases in angiotensin-II activity within the dorsal medulla. The renal action of angiotensin-II is directly on the tubular resorption of sodium and through receptors within the adrenal glands to secrete aldosterone. Aldosterone stimulates electrolyte and water resorption in the distal tubule.

There is strong evidence that blockade of the RAAS that reduces renin and aldosterone as well as angiotensin-II improves cardiovascular performance. It is also protective against new onset diabetes through their effect on insulin regulation. RAAS blockade also improves proteinuria and delays progression of chronic kidney disease especially if there is diabetes or hypertensive glomerulosclerosis. However, it does cause a rise in plasma potassium and creatinine so close monitoring is needed. There is concern that in the very elderly patient with chronic kidney disease the use of angiotensin-converting enzyme inhibitors (ACEIs) or angiotensin receptor blockers causes a further deterioration in renal function. In younger patients there is a protective effect, but one small study[16] that included patients over the age of 70 with more severe (stage 4/5 disease) demonstrated an improvement in eGFR on cessation of treatment with RAAS blockage.

Erythropoietin

Erythropoietin (EPO) is produced in the kidney and to a much lesser degree in the liver. It is present in low levels in the plasma but can rise over 1000-fold in response to oxidative stress. The production of EPO is from the peritubular epithelial cells in the renal cortex. As described earlier, the cortex is the area most vulnerable to age-related glomerulosclerosis and nephrosclerosis, and the scale of response to hypoxia is reduced in the elderly. Hypoxia reduces the oxygen-dependent hydroxylation of the hypoxia inducible transcription factor, altering the feedback regulation leading to an increased production of EPO.

EPO is essential for the production of red cells. It binds to EPO receptors on red cell progenitor cells and their precursors such as pro-erythroblasts in the bone marrow. This differentiation from multipotential progenitor cells into the erythroid cell line, through burst forming (BFU-E) and colony forming unit erythroids (CFU-E), is totally dependent on EPO for subsequent maturation. Although there are no EPO receptors on the surface of mature red cells, longevity of these cells is enhanced by circulating EPO.[17] Although EPO is essential for red cell production this is also limited by the availability of appropriate iron stores, which may be depleted in the elderly with nutritional problems.

EPO has other roles in addition to red cell function. It is protective of the renal blood vessels and mitigates against oxidative stress and atherosclerosis progression.[18] There are EPO receptors on T and B lymphocytes [19] within the brain and in small peripheral blood vessels. These affect immunological function, recovery after primary hypoxic brain damage and wound healing though influences on angiogenesis.

Replacement therapy with recombinant EPO or continuous erythropoietin receptor activator (CERA) restores red cell numbers and increases haematocrit towards normal. This normalization of haemoglobin restores the buffering function of the blood to oxidative stress and reduces left ventricular hypertrophy.[20]

Replacement therapy does have significant side effects, including hypertension and thrombosis secondary to a raised plasma viscosity. Some patients develop a resistance to the replacement therapy[21]

and very rarely may develop antibodies against EPO, leading to loss of red cell production and aplastic anaemia.[22]

Calcitriol

Calcitriol (1,25-dihydrocholecalciferol) is an active form of vitamin D and is produced by cells in the proximal convoluted tubule by hydroxylation of calcidiol (25-hydroxycholecalciferol) by 1-alpha hydroxylase. There is accumulating evidence that calcidiol is also an active hormone with low levels being associated with some cancers.[23,24] This hydroxylation process is regulated by parathyroid hormone as an important step in calcium homeostasis. The main renal action of parathyroid hormone is on phosphate excretion, which is the counter ion of calcium. Phosphate balance is also maintained by fibroblast growth factor 23 (FGF-23), which is a recently described regulator of phosphate metabolism and a counter regulator of the renal 1-alpha hydroxylase. FGF-23 is linked with the *Klotho* gene,[25] which has been itself identified as an anti-ageing gene. Involution of the nephrons in the renal cortex reduces the kidney's ability to form calcitriol,

The actions of calcitriol increase circulating levels of calcium and include directly increasing gastrointestinal uptake of dietary calcium and renal tubular resorption of calcium. It also acts indirectly on osteoclasts that release calcium from bone. These actions are mediated through the nuclear calcitriol receptors, which are also called vitamin D receptors (VDRs). Binding of calcitriol forms receptor/ligand complexes, which, acting as transcription factors, cause nuclear expression of calcium binding proteins. There are VDRs in most tissues and low calcitriol has effects on many common disorders including osteoporosis, musculoskeletal pain and weakness, malignancies of prostate, colon, and breast,[26] as well as diabetes and cardiovascular disease. For many of these diseases there is a U-shaped distribution against serum calcitriol concentrations, identifying that there is likely to be an optimal circulating level of calcitriol and values that are either too low or too high are either not beneficial or may be actively harmful.

There are several examples of the benefit of supplementing calcitriol to within the normal range. Falls in the elderly, which are one reflection of failing muscle function, are influenced by calcitriol and replacement supplementation reduced the incidence[27,28] by 20–50 per cent. Osteoporosis is one of the most commonly occurring diseases with ageing. The reduction in bone density frequently results from a reduction in serum calcium because of reduced intestinal absorption and calcitriol deficiency due to low body stores from low exposure to sunlight in temperate climates. This combination stimulates parathyroid hormone secretion and release of calcium from bone. Treatment with calcitriol alone reduces the rate of bone loss[29] and this is further improved with calcium supplementation.[30]

Conclusion

The ageing kidney becomes increasingly vulnerable to acute injury by hypotension or hypoxia. Kidneys are progressively scarred from a combination of vascular, endothelial, and glomerular changes with age. This leads to a reduction in filtration and a blunting of water and electrolyte homeostasis. The endocrine functions that govern many essential processes from prevention of hypoxia to maintaining muscle strength and bone integrity are also limited by the loss of cortical nephrons. The RAAS in particular plays a fundamental role in maintaining body fluid balance and disordered function increases the risk of hypertension, heart failure, new-onset diabetes mellitus, and further renal failure.

These facts require anaesthetists to understand the likely functional renal reserve of their elderly patients and of the limitations of current tests to define chronic kidney disease, especially measurements of the eGFR. There are implications for drug handling, fluid and electrolyte therapy, and the complex interactions of the renally active drugs used to treat many diseases common in the elderly such as ACEIs and non-steroidal anti-inflammatory drugs.

References

1. Weiner DE, Tighiouart H, Elsayed EF, *et al*. Inflammation and cardiovascular events in individuals with and without chronic kidney disease. *Kidney Int*. 2008;73:1406–1412.

2. Wiggins JE. Aging in the glomerulus. *J Gerontol A Biol Sci Med Sci*. 2012;67(12):1358–1364.

3. Wiggins JE, Patel SR, Shedden KA, *et al*. NFkappaB promotes inflammation, coagulation, and fibrosis in the aging glomerulus. *J Am Soc Nephrol*. 2010;21:587–597.

4. Yu BP, Masoro EJ, McMahan CA. Nutritional influences on aging of Fischer 344 rats: I. Physical, metabolic, and longevity characteristics. *J Gerontol*. 1985;40:657–670.

5. Ruf RG, Schultheiss M, Lichtenberger A, *et al*. Prevalence of WT1 mutations in a large cohort of patients with steroid-resistant and steroid-sensitive nephrotic syndrome. *Kidney Int*. 2004;66:564–570.

6. Patrakka J, Tryggvason K. Nephrin—a unique structural and signaling protein of the kidney filter. *Trends Mol Med*. 2007;13:396–403.

7. Thomas PE, Wharram BL, Goyal M, Wiggins JE, Holzman LB, Wiggins RC. GLEPP1, a renal glomerular epithelial cell (podocyte) membrane protein-tyrosine phosphatase. Identification, molecular cloning, and characterization in rabbit. *J Biol Chem*. 1994;269:19953–19962.

8. Maruyama Y. Aging and arterial-cardiac interactions in the elderly. *Int J Cardiol*. 2012;155(1):14–19.

9. Gottsch W, Lattmann T, Amann K, *et al*. Increased expression of endothelin-1 and inducible nitric oxide synthase isoform II in aging arteries in vivo: implications for atherosclerosis. *Biochem Biophys Res Commun*. 2001;280(3):908–913.

10. Lattmann T, Shaw S, Munter K, Vetter W, Barton M. Anatomically distinct activation of endothelin-3 and the L-arginine/nitric oxide pathway in the kidney with advanced aging. *Biochem Biophys Res Commun*. 2005;327(1):234–241.

11. Christensson A, Elmstahl S. Estimation of the age-dependent decline of glomerular filtration rate from formulas based on creatinine and cystatin C in the general elderly population. *Nephron Clin Pract*. 2011;117(1):c40–c50.

12. Bottomley MJ, Kalachik A, Mevada C, Brook MO, James T, Harden PN. Single estimated glomerular filtration rate and albuminuria measurement substantially overestimates prevalence of chronic kidney disease. *Nephron Clinical Pract*. 2011;117(4):c348–c352.

13. Schaeffner ES, Ebert N, Delanaye P, *et al*. Two novel equations to estimate kidney function in persons aged 70 years or older. *Ann Intern Med*. 2012;157(7):471–481.

14. Manz F, Johner SA, Wentz A, Boeing H, Remer T. Water balance throughout the adult life span in a German population. *Br J Nutr*. 2012;107(11):1673–1681.

15. Sands JM. Urinary concentration and dilution in the aging kidney. *Semin Nephrol*. 2009;29(6):579–586.

16. Ahmed AK, Kamath NS, El Kossi M, El Nahas AM. The impact of stopping inhibitors of the renin-angiotensin system in patients with advanced chronic kidney disease. *Nephrol Dial Transplant*. 2010;25(12):3977–3982.

17. Korell J, Vos FE, Coulter CV, Schollum JB, Walker RJ, Duffull SB. Modeling red blood cell survival data. *J Pharmacokinet Pharmacodyn*. 2011;38(6):787–801.

18. Fujiwara N, Nakamura T, Sato E, *et al*. Renovascular protective effects of erythropoietin in patients with chronic kidney disease. *Intern Med*. 2011;50(18):1929–1934.

19. Lisowska KA, Debska-Slizien A, Bryl E, Rutkowski B, Witkowski JM. Erythropoietin receptor is expressed on human peripheral blood T and B lymphocytes and monocytes and is modulated by recombinant human erythropoietin treatment. *Artif Organs*. 2010;34(8):654–662.

20. Hayashi T, Suzuki A, Shoji T, *et al*. Cardiovascular effect of normalizing the hematocrit level during erythropoietin therapy in predialysis patients with chronic renal failure. *Am J Kidney Dis*. 2000;35(2):250–256.

21. Khankin EV, Mutter WP, Tamez H, Yuan HT, Karumanchi SA, Thadhani R. Soluble erythropoietin receptor contributes to erythropoietin resistance in end-stage renal disease. *PLoS One*. 2010;5(2):e9246.

22. Shimizu H, Saitoh T, Ota F, *et al*. Pure red cell aplasia induced only by intravenous administration of recombinant human erythropoietin. *Acta Haematol*. 2011;126(2):114–118.

23. Tuohimaa P. Vitamin D and aging. *J Steroid Biochem Mol Biol*. 2009;114(1–2):78–84.

24. Tuohimaa P. Vitamin D, aging, and cancer. *Nutr Rev*. 2008;66(10 Suppl 2):S147–S152.

25. Nabeshima Y, Imura H. alpha-Klotho: a regulator that integrates calcium homeostasis. *Am J Nephrol*. 2008;28(3):455–464.

26. Holick MF. Vitamin D and sunlight: strategies for cancer prevention and other health benefits. *Clin J Am Soc Nephrol*. 2008;3(5):1548–1554.

27. Dawson-Hughes B. Serum 25-hydroxyvitamin D and muscle atrophy in the elderly. *Proc Nutr Soc*. 2012;71(1):46–49.

28. Zittermann A, Gummert JF, Borgermann J. Vitamin D deficiency and mortality. *Curr Opin Clin Nutr Metab Care*. 2009;12(6):634–639.

29. Peppone LJ, Hebl S, Purnell JQ, *et al*. The efficacy of calcitriol therapy in the management of bone loss and fractures: a qualitative review. *Osteoporos Int*. 2010;21(7):1133–1149.

30. Bischoff-Ferrari HA, Staehelin HB. Importance of vitamin D and calcium at older age. *Int J Vitam Nutr Res*. 2008;78(6):286–292.

CHAPTER 9

Ageing and hepatic function

James M. Prentis and Chris. P. Snowden

Introduction

Ageing is accompanied by marked changes in the physiology of many organ systems. Unlike many other organs, the liver has remarkable reserve and regeneration capabilities. Even so, these unique properties may be altered by advancing age and although simple hepatic function is retained, recent evidence suggests that there is an increased susceptibility to liver disease and an exaggerated effect of environmental factors in the elderly population. This chapter starts with a brief review of normal liver function at vascular (macro and micro) and cellular level. The effect of ageing on each component is then described and the effect of exposure to disease and environmental factors are reviewed.

Hepatic structure and blood supply

Anatomy

Morphologically, the liver is divided into a large right and smaller left lobe by the falciform ligament. However, a more functional division divides the liver into left and right hemi-livers along a line that passes through the gall bladder bed towards the vena cava and through the right axis of the caudate lobe. This follows the line of division of the portal venous inflow. Further subdivisions of the portal inflow divide each hemi-liver into two sectors and then each sector into two segments. Divisions in the bile duct and hepatic artery mirror the divisions of the portal inflow forming a series of portal trinities.

Fig. 9.1 demonstrates the relations of the eight segments of the liver often referred to in surgical resections. The left liver comprises segments II and III (also referred to as the left lateral segment) plus IV (which in combination with segment III forms the quadrate lobe). The right liver comprises segments V to VIII. The caudate lobe is a distinct anatomical segment (segment I) and receives blood supply from both the left and right liver draining independently into the vena cava.

The right hepatic vein drains independently into the vena cava but the middle and left hepatic veins usually join prior to draining into the vena cava. There are often a few small veins draining posteriorly, and occasionally two or three inferior right hepatic veins of moderate size.

Blood supply

Macrovascular

The liver is supported by blood flow from the hepatic artery and the portal vein. The contribution of each supply is variable but is usually 75 per cent from the portal vein and 25 per cent from the hepatic artery. Hepatic oxygenation is provided in a 50:50 ratio due to the hepatic artery containing a higher percentage of oxygenated blood.

Reduction in hepatosplanchnic blood flow may be demonstrated in globally reduced cardiac output states with redistribution towards vital organs and with more regional changes in vascular resistance of other vascular beds. Importantly, hepatic blood flow may be significantly reduced wherever central venous pressure rises above portal venous critical closing pressure (approximately 3–5 mmHg). Avoidance of an excessive rise in central venous pressure is also important in blood conservation strategies during liver surgery.

Regional hepatosplanchnic blood flow is altered by hormonal, metabolic, and neurological factors. A major influence on regional hepatic flow during operative procedures is the effect of surgical

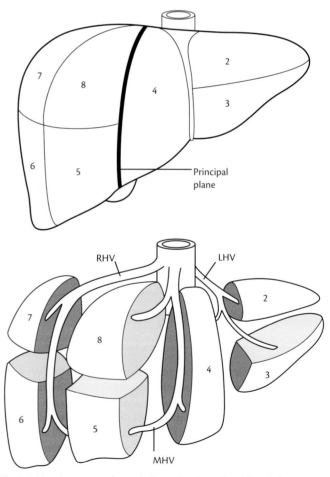

Fig. 9.1 Hepatic segments for surgical resection. Reproduced from Robert Sutcliffe et al., *Oxford Specialist Handbook of Liver and Pancreatobiliary Surgery: with Liver Transplantation*, 2009, Figure 1.1 and 1.2, page 3, with permission from Oxford University Press.

stress and regional analgesia on the autonomic nerve components of the hepatosplanchnic area. However, some degree of regional autoregulation of the hepatic blood flow occurs via the hepatic 'arterial buffer' response. Wherever portal flow is reduced, hepatic artery flow is increased to maintain liver blood flow. The mechanism of this response is incompletely understood but is related to hepatic adenosine washout.[1] Unfortunately, this blood flow compensatory arrangement is not reciprocal in that the portal vein does not have any such mechanism to increase hepatic blood flow. Therefore, whenever hepatic arterial pressure falls, there is a reciprocal decrease in liver blood flow. The buffer response is maintained in even severe cirrhosis.[2,3] Volatile agents suppress the hepatic artery buffer response to varying extents whilst pneumoperitoneum also ablates the buffer response in an experimental setting.[4] In most situations, oxygen delivery is surplus to demand and minor reductions in blood flow are inconsequential. However, in some circumstances (e.g. sepsis, reduced liver reserve including fatty liver), oxygen dependency may apply and increased demand has to be met by increased oxygen extraction.

Microvascular

The hepatic microcirculation includes all vessels with a diameter less than 300 micrometres. The hepatic artery and portal vein divide repeatedly within the liver to form their respective terminal branches (hepatic arterioles and portal venules). These both supply blood to hepatic sinusoids, which allow the mixing of oxygen-rich hepatic arterial blood with the nutrient-rich blood from the portal vein. This is the principal site for uptake, secretion, and multiple other processes between the blood and the adjacent hepatocytes.

The sinusoid epithelium is highly specialized with multiple dynamic fenestrations. These act as a selective sieve whose diameters are affected by luminal blood pressure, vasoactive substances, drugs, and toxins. In addition, they generally lack a basal lamina during health so that solutes and small particles have direct access to the perisinusoidal space (space of Disse). The fenestrations allow the free passage of chylomicron remnants between the plasma and the space of Disse. This means that they play an important role in the control mechanism for blood cholesterol levels and lipid metabolism.

Microcirculatory vascular changes are controlled by multiple hormonal influences including nitric oxide, endothelins (ETs), and carbon monoxide production, which derive predominantly from the hepatic vascular endothelial cells. It has been suggested that a critical balance between vasoconstrictor and vasodilator substances must exist to maintain a balanced flow at the microcirculatory level. All volatile agents have the potential to cause microcirculatory vasoconstriction and thereby reduce flow,[5] although this is minimal with isoflurane and desflurane.[6] Various agents have been used to promote specific hepatosplanchnic vasodilatation including dopexamine, prostacyclin, and ET-1 receptor antagonists.[7] However, none of these agents have a proven clinical role in hepatosplanchnic protection.

Cellular anatomy and function

Hepatocytes

The hepatocytes are the main cell body of the liver accounting for 70–80 per cent of the cellular mass. They have multiple functions including the synthesis of albumin, fibrinogen, multiple clotting factors, lipoproteins, ceruloplasmin, transferrin, complement, and glycoproteins. They also have important roles in carbohydrate and lipid metabolism, bile salt formation, and drug excretion.

Kupffer cells

The liver receives multiple toxic, infective, and foreign substances from portal blood. The Kupffer cells, a form of macrophage found in the sinusoid epithelium, have a crucial role in the body's immune response. They not only produce a variety of beneficial vasoactive mediators but are also capable of removing these potentially harmful substances before they enter the systemic circulation.

Stellate cells

Stellate cells are fat storing cells and also are a major storage site of retinoids including vitamin A. They are not located in the endothelium itself but they do extend throughout the space of Disse. They are thought to play a role in the local regulation of blood flow through the hepatic sinusoids and have been implicated in the aetiology of hepatic fibrosis.

Hepatic regeneration

The liver is a unique tissue that is able to regenerate itself. Regeneration occurs as a reaction to surgical or chemical injury and is a compensatory liver growth caused by division of existing hepatocytes, rather than cellular hypertrophy. Regeneration is highly regulated by various complex signal transduction pathways, which require activation by specific genes.

Hepatic structure and blood supply: age-related changes

Unlike the vast majority of other organs, the ageing process does not promote major specific changes in structure, blood supply, or basic hepatic function [8]. However, there is increasing evidence that at a microvascular level there are subtle changes that may predispose to certain pathologies and have clinical relevance in certain situations.

Blood supply

Overall liver blood supply reduces with advancing age. A reduction in liver volume goes some way to explaining this, but even when taken per unit liver volume, there remains some flow reduction. After the mid 20s, the blood supply to the liver is reduced 0.3–1.5 per cent every year.[9] The blood flow through the liver at the age of 60 years is reduced by 40–50 per cent.

Sinusoidal endothelium

Despite the evidence that the macrovascular flow diminishes with age, the sinusoidal perfusion rate, at least in animal experiments, remains stable throughout life.[10] However, it is becoming increasingly recognized that there are morphological changes in the sinusoidal endothelium and the space of Disse directly associated with the ageing process. The endothelial cells show marked thickening and a reduction in the number of fenestrations with increasing age. The diameter of endothelial fenestrations is also reduced. Sporadic deposition of collagen in the extracellular space of Disse and increased numbers of fat engorged, non-activated stellate cells are seen with advancing age.[11] In addition, there is endothelial upregulation of von Willebrand factor and intercellular adhesion molecule (ICAM)-1[12] with reduced expression of caveolin-1 (important in the control of fenestration size).[13] These changes have been termed age-related 'pseudocapillarizations' as the sinusoidal endothelium begins to resemble those seen frequently in non-fenestrated capillary beds.[14]

Cellular changes

Hepatic compliance and weight decreases with increasing age. The number of liver cells also reduces sharply after the age of 60 years. In addition to a reduction in cellular mass, there are also morphological changes. However, high interindividual variability may obscure the relevance of some age-related differences.

Hepatocytes

Despite age being associated with reduced hepatic volume, blood flow, and changes at the sinusoidal level, the impact of ageing on hepatocyte function is not clear. Histological changes occur in the hepatocytes. Their volume increases[15] as do certain cellular constituents. The cell nuclei appear larger and often become double or multinuclear.[16] The cytoplasm also accumulates more lysosomes and lipofuscin (a pigment associated with ageing),[17] whilst there is a reduction in the smooth endoplasmic reticulum,[18] the site for a number of important enzymes involved in metabolism.

Kupffer cells

A number of reports have demonstrated increased numbers of Kupffer cells associated with increasing age. Indeed, this is not unexpected due to ageing being associated with an increase in systemic markers of inflammation. However, actual phagocytic activity is reduced by approximately one-third with increasing age.[19,20] This may be one explanation for the increase in the susceptibility to infections seen in the elderly.

Stellate cells

Age also affects the stellate cell population. It is a common finding that these cells are fat engorged in the elderly population often ballooning into the lumen of the sinusoid with the potential to block or reduce blood flow.[21] The effects of these changes are unknown.

Hepatic regeneration and age

The most clinically relevant age-related change in liver physiology is the result of a marked decline in the rate of hepatic regeneration.[22] There is no change in the ability to regenerate. However, it was noted many decades ago that there is a considerable reduction in there generative response of old livers to partial hepatectomy.[23] In animal models, 99 per cent of hepatocytes regenerate after partial hepatectomy in young mice, compared to only 30 per cent in older mice.[24] These findings have stimulated much research interest in defining the aetiological mechanisms behind age-related changes in regeneration ability.

Increase in intracellular lipofuscin

Hepatocytes in the elderly have increased levels of lipofuscin.[17] This reflects the inability of the older cells to be able to eliminate cellular waste products and this accumulation impairs cellular function. However, as cells expand with ageing and the lipofuscin compartment accounts for only 1 per cent of the total volume, it seems unlikely that this is a major factor in reduced regenerative activity.

Telomere length

Telomeres are specialized nucleoprotein structures at the end of eukaryotic chromosomes which have a specific role in regeneration and replication. Telomere DNA of human somatic cells shortens during each cell division thus leading to finite cell proliferation. This evolved as a mechanism to protect cells from continuous divisions leading to multiple mutations. With age there is a reduction in telomere length and the rate of telomere shortening is significantly higher in the hepatocyte compared to other cell types.[25] The shortening of telomeric ends of chromosomes correlates with ageing and the decline in the replicative potential of the cell. There has also been a recent study showing that telomerase reactivation in an enzyme-deficient mouse reversed certain well-documented age-related deficits.[26]

Growth factors

The proliferative response of hepatocytes to growth factors is diminished in older animals. It has long been hypothesized that the ageing process impairs either the growth-regulating molecules or their receptor sites. It has been shown that liver cells from older animals did not respond to epidermal growth factor (EGF) stimulation as well as cells from younger animals.[27] Furthermore, there may also be a decline in the EGF binding capacity with age to the hepatocyte plasma membrane.[28] Growth hormone (GH) has also been implicated in the reduced regenerative capacity of the liver. Endogenous hepatocellular levels of GH and receptor sites decline with age. It has been reported that GH treatment of old rats after partial hepatectomy enhances hepatocyte proliferation compared to similar aged cohorts.[29]

Pseudocapillarization

As discussed, age-related pseudocapillarization is important in the development of age-related liver disease.[14] A recent paper has suggested that this process may also impact upon the regenerative response. Older mice treated with serotonin receptor agonist, showed enhanced liver regeneration. This response correlated with an increase in the number of endothelial cell fenestrations.[30] This data suggests that serotonin agonist enhances endothelial cell fenestration diameter, improves hepatic perfusion, and restores the hepatic regenerative capacity.

Hepatic physiology: age-related changes

Effect of age on normal hepatic functions

The liver is an organ with considerable reserve and in health the ageing process does not cause significant alteration in clinical function. Clotting processes and protein synthesis are not directly altered. However, certain functions are implicated with advancing age:

Glucose metabolism

Hepatic glucose production (HGP) plays a major role in glucose homeostasis, both in the fasting and in the postprandial states.[31] The liver is exquisitely sensitive to insulin and hepatic glucose production is completely suppressed at plasma insulin levels well below the commonly used insulin dose in patients with diabetes. There is no difference in basal glucose production or hepatic glucose suppression by insulin between young and old individuals.[32] However, with low-dose insulin infusions, glucose production is more rapidly suppressed in the elderly, perhaps due to a delayed suppression of endogenous insulin release in the older individuals. Hepatic insulin resistance does not seem to play a significant role in decreased glucose tolerance of elderly people.[32]

Enzyme and drug metabolism

The liver plays a major role in drug clearance and ageing has been reported to diminish this capacity. Initially, most interest was centred on the clearance of drugs that undergo mandatory oxidation by the microsomal cytochrome P450-dependent mono-oxygenase systems. A number of animal studies have documented significant age-related declines in the amounts, specific activities, and rates of induction of these systems.[33] However, most in vitro studies using human liver tissue have failed to detect age-related deficiencies in cytochrome P450-dependent microsomal mono-oxygenases.[34] Reduction in liver volume and blood flow in the elderly may explain the disparity between these findings. Age-related decline in liver volume and blood flow may contribute to diminished clearance of drugs that exhibit extensive first-pass kinetic profiles.

Endocytic activity

Blood clearance of a variety of waste macromolecules takes place in hepatic sinusoidal endothelial cells (SECs). Given the extensive range of substrates metabolized by the liver, age-related changes in the hepatic sinusoid and microcirculation have important systemic implications for ageing and age-related diseases. Reduced endocytosis, demonstrated in an elderly animal model, may increase systemic exposure to potential harmful waste macromolecules.[11] Loss of endothelial fenestration leads to impaired transfer of lipoproteins from blood to hepatocytes. This is further exacerbated by a reduction in bile acid synthesis and decreased bile flow which leads to reduced excretion and also a decline in low-density lipoprotein metabolism. These factors all contribute to provide a mechanism for impaired chylomicron remnant clearance, postprandial hyperlipidaemia, hypercholesterolaemia, and increased frequency of gallstone formation seen in elderly patients.

Susceptibility to environmental factors and liver disease

Mitochondrial structural integrity remains mostly unchanged with ageing. However, mitochondrial DNA may be injured through persistent endogenous free radical generation and prolonged duration of exposure in the elderly may lead to an accumulation of oxidative DNA damage. In turn, this may increase susceptibility to disease or environmental factors promulgating further oxidative injury. Since the liver is the central metabolic organ, an ageing liver is uniquely positioned to be severely susceptible to disease and environmental factors (e.g. diet, alcohol intake, and viruses) that promote oxidative damage.

Non-alcoholic fatty liver disease

Fat storage and metabolism is an important part of liver function but the abnormal retention of lipids in hepatocytes is a pathological phenomenon termed steatosis. Severe steatosis has a greater effect on the micro- than the macrovascular circulation. The lipid swollen hepatocytes and stellate cells distort the sinusoidal lumens resulting in inefficient blood flow. These factors result in impairment of tissue oxygenation and increased susceptibility to oxidative forms of liver injury.

The most common cause of steatosis in clinical practice, and an increasing burden in Western societies, is non-alcoholic fatty liver disease (NAFLD). NAFLD is a metabolic syndrome closely related to obesity, type 2 diabetes, hypertension, and dyslipidaemia. It is the result of overnutrition and physical inactivity which is an increasing problem in the developed world. It is a progressive disease leading from simple steatosis through to steatohepatitis and cirrhosis. A number of risk factors have been shown to predict this progression including obesity, diabetes, AST:ALT ratio greater than 1 and age over 45 years. Whilst only 10–25 per cent of patients actually progress to cirrhosis, the high prevalence of the disease, the ageing population and the obesity epidemic will ensure that this will become a huge burden to health services in the future.

Alcoholic liver disease

Currently, regular alcohol usage in the elderly is lower than in other age groups (70 per cent for 20–34 years compared to 30 per cent for >75 years).[35] However, this rate is increasing as is the rate of potentially harmful alcohol use.[36] Despite conventional practice suggesting alcoholic liver disease typically affects patients between the ages of 50 to 60 years, recent studies have found that 20–30 per cent of patients with alcoholic cirrhosis were elderly.[37] Psychosocial deprivation alone, caused by the increasing age of the population has the potential to increase the rate of alcohol consumption and abuse in the elderly population.

Elderly patients often have multiple associated comorbidities and have less reserve to be able to cope with the stress of illness. Elderly patients with ALD have increasing severe symptoms and complications including portal hypertension.[37] They are also at increased risk of mortality. Three-year survival in with cirrhosis patients aged under 60 years was 76 per cent, compared to 46 per cent in those aged over 60 years. Those over 70 years with cirrhosis, have a markedly reduced survival rate (25 per cent at 1 year).[38]

Alcohol excess has the potential to cause alcoholic fatty liver disease which is a reversible state. However, approximately one-third will go on to develop alcoholic steatohepatitis and 10–20 per cent will progress to end-stage cirrhosis. An important factor in the development of alcoholic steatosis is the production of reactive oxygen species and the elderly are more prone to oxidative stress, mechanisms promoting an increase in oxygen free radicals may be related to the increased severity of alcoholic liver disease seen in elderly patients. These may be produced by alcohol-induced intestinal luminal injury leading to toxin translocation into the portal circulation. This triggers the release of various interleukins, growth factors, and cytokines, predominantly from Kupffer cells. In addition, several enzymatic systems have been implicated in the increased severity of alcoholic-induced liver disease in the elderly. In animal experiments, specific inhibitors of the cytochrome P450 (CYP)-2E1 pathway can result in improvement of alcoholic liver disease. Reduction in hepatic size and blood flow combined with a reduction in the effective volume of distribution with age alters alcohol elimination and results in higher blood alcohol concentrations per unit consumed. Concomitant polypharmacy in the elderly, with drugs metabolized via the CYP pathway (especially those eliminated via the CYP2E1 pathway such as paracetamol, methotrexate and phenytoin) may compete with alcohol metabolic pathways. Chronic alcohol usage increases the oxidative capacity of this pathway leading to decreased serum drug concentrations but with a subsequent increase in potentially toxic metabolites.

Hepatitis C and age

Hepatitis C virus (HCV) is a RNA virus which it is estimated has infected 170 million people worldwide.[39] As it is mainly transmitted via the parenteral route, the seroprevalence of anti-HCV was fourfold lower for patients over 70 years compared to individuals aged 30–40 years.[40] Prolonged chronic infection can lead to fibrosis and the development of cirrhosis. The main risk factor for the development of fibrosis is the age at infection. In two studies, examining in total 5000 people, the rate of fibrosis progression was highest and disease severity was greater in those individuals aged over 50 at infection.[41,42] An increased prevalence of hepatitis C-associated cirrhosis in the elderly population is to be expected, at least in the next 20 years. However, the introduction of newer antiretrovirals and monitoring methods to distinguish those at risk of progression to cirrhosis may alleviate the massive increase in disease prevalence.

Hepatocellular carcinoma

Hepatocellular carcinoma (HCC) is the most common consequence of cirrhosis in the elderly.[43] It is clear that cirrhosis of any underlying aetiology has the potential for malignant transformation. The rate of this transformation is especially high in viral hepatitis especially hepatitis C and co-infection with hepatitis B and C.[44] The exact mechanisms for the development why HCV predisposes to HCC is not yet fully understood, although it is hypothesized that various viral protein–host cell interactions play a direct role in the malignant transformation. Older patients have been shown to be at higher risk for malignant change. In patients with HCV infection, even when stratified for degree of fibrosis, there was a 15-fold increase in the incidence of HCC.[45] Elderly patients often develop HCC before other complications of cirrhosis become apparent and HCC was the cause of death in 71 per cent of patients in one study.[46]

Age,[47] obesity,[48] and diabetes,[49] the main risk factors for NAFLD, are all risk factors for the development of HCC. Again, the exact mechanism behind the development of HCC in NAFLD like HCV infection, remains unclear. Insulin resistance is associated with inflammatory cascade initiation with increased release of cytokines such as tumour necrosis factor alpha (TNFα), interleukin 6 (IL6), and NF-kb that are likely to contribute to the carcinogenic potential of NAFLD[50]). The development of NAFLD is also associated with oxidative stress due to the changes in the microvasculature. This causes a release of reactive oxygen species which may also increase the risk of malignancy.[51] Alcohol intake further increases the risk of malignancy.

Clinical relevance to anaesthesia in the elderly

In health, there is minimal evidence that advancing age per se adversely affects normal liver function and physiology to any major extent. The direct clinical effect of the subtle age-related structural and cellular changes defined has yet to be elucidated.

Even so, reduced hepatic blood supply and cellular mass, in conjunction with a reduction in the rate of hepatic regeneration, combine to reduce functional hepatic reserve in the elderly population. Furthermore, prolonged exposure to oxidative stress through dietary and environmental factors ensures that the elderly liver is inherently susceptible to further insult (e.g. major surgery). There are several situations where reduced hepatic reserve in the elderly may be particularly important. These include liver resection, response to severe infection and in relation to liver donation in transplantation.

Liver resection

Liver resection creates a unique surgical situation where pre-existing liver reserve becomes crucially important. Increasing longevity of the population ensures that more patients surviving primary oncological resection will present for resection of secondary hepatic metastases at an older age. By definition, liver resection will reduce liver volume. The volume of liver that can be safely resected in humans is approximately 80 per cent. Under normal circumstances, the human liver initiates regeneration within 3 days and has reached its original size by 6 months,[52] although some studies have shown full restoration at 3 months. Rapid regeneration may allow complete functional recovery within 2–3 weeks after partial hepatectomy.[53] However, this assumes good function in the remaining liver. Wherever there is already limited hepatic reserve or where ischaemia–reperfusion manoeuvres are required during the resection (leading to significant oxidative stress), the functional reserve of the remaining liver will be an important component of good postoperative recovery. If there is a predicted risk of liver failure developing after a procedure then pre-emptive manoeuvres such as portal embolization of the affected segments some weeks prior to resection can stimulate regeneration in the proposed liver remnant prior to surgery, thereby enhancing postoperative liver function. An increase of 40–60 per cent in the size of the non-embolized liver can be anticipated in non-cirrhotic livers.[54] Similarly chemoembolization can be used in potentially unresectable hepatocellular carcinoma to reduce the tumour mass and increase residual function to an extent which may permit definitive resection. However, wherever the regenerative capacity is reduced, as in some elderly patients, this may not provide adequate liver reserve to cope with large resections.

Liver transplantation

Liver transplantation criteria are expanding alongside the number of patients requiring transplantation. Given the lack of suitable donors in the UK, organs of more marginal quality are being used. Long-term graft survival is related to several factors, of which donor age and the degree of steatosis are the most important. The common interrelationship between these two factors means that donation of organs from elderly donors often leads to poor outcome. Patients receiving livers with severe steatosis (>60 per cent) have a rate of post transplantation primary non-function of up to 80 per cent compared to 2.5 per cent in those with steatosis <30 per cent.[55] The likely cause, as for NAFLD, is the disruption to the microvasculature and sinusoidal flow leading to decreased tolerance of oxidative stress. As well as primary non-function, donor age is also predictive of the severity of recurrent liver HCV-related disease upon the graft.[56]

Sepsis

The incidence and mortality rate of severe sepsis increases dramatically with increasing age.[57] Although the process is initiated by an infectious process, it is the changes at a microvascular level that affects oxygenation and tissue perfusion. The liver has an important mechanism in actively modifying this process; however, it can also be directly affected as a result of hepatosplanchnic hypoperfusion. Kupffer cells release a host of inflammatory mediators that can induce tissue injury whilst the sinusoidal endothelium is also damaged, and can become plugged with fibrin clots and blood cells. This increases liver injury, coagulopathy, microvascular ischaemia, cell death, and hepatocellular failure. The ageing liver, despite having preserved function is already at risk of ischaemic injury due to the changes seen at a microvascular level namely thickening of the endothelium, alterations in sinusoidal blood flow and reduction in its regenerative capacity. These factors may explain the increased susceptibility of the elderly to sepsis and increased mortality.

Conclusion

Unlike other organs, liver function is relatively well preserved into advancing age and changes seen both on a macro- and microvascular scale are more often of pathological and physiological interest. However, more subtle changes in the liver ultrastruture and reduced rates of cellular regeneration may reduce hepatic reserve and render the ageing liver more susceptible to oxidative stress and injury. This may not only promote increased overt liver disease in the elderly, but increases the risk of liver dysfunction and failure following surgery. Increases in the ageing population that require more complex forms of surgery and critical care will ensure that existing liver reserve will become a more important consideration to patient outcome in the future. Therapies to reduce injury and preserve liver function will be of benefit to the elderly population.

References

1. Lautt WW, McQuaker JE. Maintenance of hepatic arterial blood flow during hemorrhage is mediated by adenosine. *Can J Physiol Pharmacol.* 1989;67:1023–1028.
2. Gulberg V, Haag K, Rossle M, Gerbes AL. Hepatic arterial buffer response in patients with advanced cirrhosis. *Hepatology.* 2002;35:630–634.
3. Richter S, Mucke I, Menger MD, Vollmar B. Impact of intrinsic blood flow regulation in cirrhosis: maintenance of hepatic arterial buffer response. *Am J Physiol Gastrointest Liver Physiol.* 2000;279:G454–G462.
4. Richter S, Olinger A, Hildebrandt U, Menger MD, Vollmar B. Loss of physiologic hepatic blood flow control ('hepatic arterial buffer response') during CO2-pneumoperitoneum in the rat. *Anesth Analg.* 2001;93:872–877.
5. Grundmann U, Zissis A, Bauer C, Bauer M. In vivo effects of halothane, enflurane, and isoflurane on hepatic sinusoidal microcirculation. *Acta Anaes Scand.* 1997;14(6):760–766.
6. O'Riordan J, O'Beirne HA, Young Y, Bellamy MC. Effects of desflurane and isoflurane on splanchnic microcirculation during major surgery. *Br J Anaes.* 1997;78(1):95–96.
7. Renton MC, Snowden CP. Dopexamine and its role in the protection of hepatosplanchnic and renal perfusion in high-risk surgical and critically ill patients. *Br J Anaesth.* 2005;94(4):459–467.
8. Bulter JM, Begg EJ. Free drug metabolic clearance in the elderly. *Clin Pharmacokinet.* 2008;47:297–321.
9. Wynne HA, Cope LH, Mutch E, Rawlins MD, Woodhouse KW, James OFW. The effect of age upon liver volume and apparent liver blood flow in healthy man. *Hepatology.* 1989;9:297–301.
10. Vollmar B, Pradarutti S, Richter S, Menger MD. In vivo quantification of ageing changes in the rat liver from early juvenile to senescent life. *Liver.* 2002;22:330–341.
11. Ito Y, Sorensen KK, Bethea NW, et al. Age-related changes in the hepatic circulation of mice. *Exp Gerontol.* 2007;48:789–797.
12. McLean AJ, Cogger VC, Chong GC, et al. Age related pseudocapillarization of the human liver. *J Pathol.* 2003;200:112–117.
13. Jamieson H, Hilmer SN, Cogger VC, et al. Caloric restriction reduced age related pseudocapillarization of the hepatic sinusoid. *Exp Gerontol.* 2007;42:374–378.
14. Le Couteur DG, Fraser R, Cogger VC, McLean AJ. Hepatic pseudocapillarization and atherosclerosis in ageing. *Lancet.* 2002;359:1612–1615.
15. Schmucker DL, Mooney JS, Jones AL. Stereological analysis of hepatic fine structure in the Fisher 344 rat. Influence of sublobular location and animal age. *J Cell Biol.* 1978;78:319–337.
16. Schmucker DL. Aging and the liver: an update. *J Gerontol.* 1998;53:B315–B320.
17. Schmucker DL, Sachs H. Quantifying dense bodies and lipofuscin as a function of ageing: a morphologist' perspective. *Arch Gerontol Geriatr.* 2002;34:249–261.
18. Schmucker DL, Woodhouse KW, Wang RK, et al. Effects of age and gender on in vitro properties of human liver microsomal monooxygenases. *Clin Pharmacol Ther.* 1990;48:436–443.
19. Videla LA, Tapia G, Fernandez V. Influence of ageing on Kupffer cell respiratory activity in relation to particle phagocytosis and oxidative stress parameters in the mouse liver. *Redox Rep.* 2001;6:155–159.
20. Yamano T, DeCicco LA, Rikans LE. Attenuation of cadmium-induced liver injury in senescent male Fisher 344 rats: role of Kupffer cells and inflammatory cytokines. *Toxicol Appl Pharmacol.* 2000;162:68–75.
21. Durham SK, Brouwer A, Barelds RJ, Horan MA, Knook DL. Competitive endotoxin-induced hepatic injury in young and aged rats. *J Pathol.* 1990;162:341–349.
22. Schmucker DL, Sanchez H. Liver regeneration and aging: a current perspective. *Curr Gerontol Geriatr Res.* 2011:526379.
23. Bucher NLR. The influence of age upon the incorporation of thymidine-2C14 into the DNA of regenerating rat liver. *Cancer Res.* 1964;118:225–232.
24. Stocker E, Heine WD. Regeneration of liver parenchyma under normal and pathological conditions. *Beiyr Path.* 1971;144:400–408.
25. Takubo K, Nakamura K, Izumiyama N, et al. Telomere shortening with aging in human livers. *J Gerontol.* 2000;55:B533–B536.
26. Jaskelioff M, Muller FL, Paik JH, et al. Telomerase reactivation reverses tissue degeneration in aged telomerase-deficient mice. *Nature.* 2011;469:102–107.
27. Sawada N. Hepatocytes from old rats retain responsiveness of c-myc expression to EGF in primary culture but do not enter S phase. *Exp Cell Res.* 1989;181(2):584–588.
28. Marti U. Handling of epidermal growth factor and number of epidermal growth factor receptors are changed in aged male rats. *Hepatology.* 1993;18(6):1432–1436.
29. Krupczak-Hollis K, Wang X, Dennewitz MB, Costa RH. Growth hormone stimulates proliferation of old-aged regenerating liver through forkhead box m1b. *Hepatology.* 2003;38(6):1552–1562.
30. Furrer K, Rickenbacher A, Tian Y, et al. Serotonin reverts age-related capillarization and failure of regeneration in the liver through a VEGF-dependent pathway. *Proc Natl Acad Sci USA.* 2011;108(7):2945–2950.
31. Wahren J, Ekberg K. Splanchnic regulation of glucose production. *Annu Rev Nutr.* 2007;27:329–345.
32. Scheen AJ. Diabetes mellitus in the elderly: insulin resistance and/or impaired insulin secretion? *Diabetes Metab.* 2005:31:5S27–5S34.

33. Schmucker DL, Wang RK. The effect of aging on kinetic profile of rat liver microsomal NADPH cytochrome c reductase. *Exp Gerontol.* 1984;18:313–321.

34. Schmucker DL, Woodhouse KW, Wang RK, *et al.* Effects of age and gender on in vitro properties of human liver microsomal monooxygenases. *Clin Pharmacol Therapeut.* 1990;48(4):365–374.

35. Schoenborn CA, Cohen BH. *Trends in smoking, alcohol consumption and other health practices among US adults 1977–1983* (pp. 173–177). Ulm: Fisher Verlag.

36. John W, Culberson MD. Alcohol use in the elderly: beyond the CAGE. *Geriatrics.* 2006;61:23–27.

37. James OFW. Parenchymal liver disease in the elderly. *Gut.* 1997;41:430–432.

38. Potter JR, James OFW. Clinical features and prognosis of alcoholic liver disease in the respect of advancing age. *Gerontology.* 1987;33:380–387.

39. WHO. Hepatitis C: global prevalence. *Wkly Epidemiol.* 1997;72:341–344.

40. Alter MJ. Epidemiology of hepatitis C. *Hepatology.* 1997;26(suppl 1):62S–65S.

41. Poynard T, Bedossa P, Opolon P. Natural history of liver fibrosis progression in patients with chronic hepatitis C. *Lancet.* 1997;349:825–832.

42. Roudot-Thoraval F, Bastie A, Pawlotsky JM, *et al.* Epidemiological factors affecting the severity of hepatitis C virus-related liver disease: a French study of 6,664 patients. The study group for the prevalence and epidemiology of hepatitis C virus. *Hepatology.* 1997;26:485–490.

43. Ikeda K, Saitoh S, Suzuki Y, *et al.* Disease progression and hepatocellular carcinogenesis in patients with chronic viral hepatitis: a prospective observation of 2,215 patients. *J Hepatol.* 1998;28:930–938.

44. Chiaramonte M, Stroffolini T, Vian A, *et al.* Rate of incidence of hepatocellular carcinoma in patients with compensated viral cirrhosis. *Cancer.* 1999;85:2132–2137.

45. Asahina Y, Tsuchiya K, Tamak Ni, *et al.* Effect of aging on risk for hepatocellular carcinoma in chronic hepatitis C virus infection. *Hepatology.* 2010;52:518–527.

46. Benvegnu L, Gios M, Alberti A. Natural history of compensated viral cirrhosis: a prospective study on the incidence and hierarchy of major complications. *Gut.* 2004;53:744–749.

47. Hui JM, Kench JG, Chitturi S, *et al.* Long term outcomes of cirrhosis in non-alcoholic steatohepatitis compared with hepatitis C. *Hepatology* 2003;38:420–427.

48. Caldwell SH, Crespo DM, Kang HS, Al-Osami AM. Obesity and hepatocellular carcinoma. *Gastroenterology.* 2004;127:S97–S103.

49. Adami HO, Chow WH, Nyren O, *et al.* Excess risk of primary liver cancer with diabetes mellitus. *J Natl Cancer Inst.* 1996;88:1472–1477.

50. Sakurai T, Maeda S, Chang I, Karin M. Loss of hepatic NF-kappa B activity enhances chemical hepatocarcinogenesis through sustained c-Jun N-terminal kinase 1 activation. *Proc Natl Acad Sci USA* 2006;103:10544–10551.

51. Bugianesi E. Non alcoholic steatohepatitis and cancer. *Clin Liver Dis* 2007;11:191–207.

52. Gove CD, Hughes RD. Liver regeneration in relationship to acute liver failure. *Gut.* 1991;Suppl:S92–S96.

53. Nagasue N, Yukaya H, Ogawa Y, Kohno H, Nakamura T. Human liver regeneration after major hepatic resection. A study of normal liver and livers with chronic hepatitis and cirrhosis. *Ann Surg.* 1987;206:30–39.

54. Kawasaki S, Makuuchi M, Kakazu T, *et al.* Resection for multiple metastatic liver tumors after portal embolization. *Surgery.* 1994;115:674–677.

55. Ploeg RJ, D'Alessandro AM, Knechtle SJ, *et al.* Risk factors for primary dysfunction after liver transplantation—a multi-variate analysis. *Transplantation.* 1993;55:807–813.

56. Baccarani U, Adani GL, Toniutto P, *et al.* Liver transplantation from old donors into HCV and non-HCV recipients. *Transpl Proc.* 2004;36:527–528.

57. Angus DC, Linde-Zwirble WT, Lidicker J, Clermont G, Carcillo J, Pinsky MR. Epidemiology of severe sepsis in the United States: analysis of incidence, outcome and associated costs of care. *Crit Care Med.* 2001;29:1303–1310.

CHAPTER 10

Cognitive aspects of geriatric anaesthesia

Lars S. Rasmussen and Jeffrey H. Silverstein

Introduction

Brain function may be depressed in surgical patients as a result of numerous factors, of which sedatives and general anaesthetics are only a few. A small number of patients, based primarily on anecdotal reports, may suffer profound deterioration in the perioperative period. In the community of caregivers of patients with dementia, there is a strongly held opinion that anaesthesia is directly linked to significant impairment (see, for example, the Alzheimer's Association Online community at <http://www.alz.org>).[1] There is very little known about these cases. Fairly extensive research suggests that some lesser degree of brain dysfunction is common after surgery, especially in the elderly. Immediately following major procedures with anaesthesia, recovery of basic brain function is monitored in the post-anaesthesia care unit. However, sometimes the recovery of brain function is delayed and deterioration may also occur after recovery has taken place. When a change in behaviour is present or the change is significant, deterioration may be noted by the staff, by the relatives, and by the patient. However, more subtle changes may not be noticed until the patient has returned to his home or work environment. If the impairment causes substantial disability, it is extremely important to investigate the severity of impairment and search for possible reversible factors. The crucial question is whether the postoperative level of functioning is really different from the preoperative level. It is natural to attribute any deficit to unusual events such as surgery and anaesthesia but that may not be a correct interpretation. Unfortunately, very few surgical patients' brain function is well documented as a part of the preoperative investigation so it is frequently impossible to verify that a change has in fact occurred.

The anaesthesia clinician should be able to perform simple evaluations of brain function, to diagnose or identify the most common types of perioperative brain dysfunction and to provide patients and families with relevant counselling perioperatively. The aim of this chapter is therefore to provide the clinician with a basic knowledge about perioperative cognitive disorders and a number of definitions, risk factors, and suggested aetiological factors with emphasis on the elderly surgical patient.

Consciousness

Humans experience daily cycles of wakefulness and sleep. Wakefulness is an aroused brain state in which an individual is conscious and engages in coherent cognitive and behavioural responses. Consciousness involves awareness and orientation to self and surroundings. Alterations in consciousness are considered part of most anaesthetic regimens, either in the form of sedation or general anaesthesia. Upon completion of anaesthesia two different forms of disturbance of consciousness have been observed. These alterations have been categorized as emergence delirium and inadequate emergence. As opposed to a change in cognitive function, as described in the following 'Cognition' section, the diagnosis of delirium is made by observation.

Cognition

Cognition is a higher brain function involved in processing of information. Sensory input must be interpreted and acted upon, if relevant. Cognitive function is essential to select, store, and retrieve information to allow an adequate response. Cognitive function depends on active neurons connected in a network with synapses and transmitters. It is usual to describe several different cognitive domains such as memory, executive function, etc. These domains are not entirely independent and do not map onto any well-defined brain regions.[2] The test instruments available do not clearly discriminate between specific domains. For example, memory can be profoundly impaired without significant deficits in other domains but the detection of such impairment requires testing which will also demand information processing and responding. The so-called memory tests will therefore also require a certain amount of attention and a coordinated response involving, for instance, a presentation of recalled items or words from a list. Likewise, an attention test will require that the patient is able to recall the instructions.

Ageing is associated with some loss of neurons and synapses but, more importantly, with a change in synaptic physiology and diminished integration of activation.[3] Cognitive ability declines with increasing age in numerous studies, but it can be problematic to simply compare age groups at the same time point (cross-sectional design) because this approach will not take into account that the two groups have been exposed to different environments during life, to different educational systems, and that society and language changes over time. Any detected difference must be carefully interpreted with these confounders in mind before it can be concluded that age per se is the explanation. Age-related decline can also be examined in longitudinal studies looking at within-person changes, but practice effects must then be considered.[4]

Cognitive function may be well preserved even at a very high chronological age in individuals who have an ability to compensate for age-related changes and pathology. Necropsy may reveal severe brain pathology in elderly people in whom no dementia was diagnosed[5] and there is a huge variability in the clinical consequences of brain damage in terms of cognitive function. Cognitive reserve is 'the capacity to sustain the effect of disease or injury sufficient to cause clinical dementia in an individual possessing less cognitive reserve'.[6] The conception is that cognitive reserve allows an individual to compensate for brain damage, perhaps by recruitment of other brain areas. A greater cognitive reserve is associated with a high level of education, higher socioeconomic status, and an active lifestyle.[7]

Brain function changes over time and there is an ongoing formation of new synapses, modification of synaptic transmission, of gene expression, and of neural network organization. These changes occur through life and are referred to by a common term, neuroplasticity, which not only provides adaption to changes in the environment and new challenges, but also may serve to restore function if needed. The ageing brain does, therefore, possess a remarkable ability to maintain function, but ageing is associated with a decline in the repair capacity, including neurogenesis. Even the adult brain contains neural stem cells which may give rise to neurons as well as glia, and there appear to be neural stem cells near the lateral ventricles and in the hippocampus, where they may be important for memory function. Neurogenesis declines with increasing age and this could be a key factor in age-related impairment of learning and memory,[8] although the exact regulation of neurogenesis remains to be determined. Alterations in neuroplasticity appear particularly sensitive to stress in an elderly mouse model that may have relevance to postoperative cognitive dysfunction (POCD).

Assessing cognition

Questionnaires

It is not easy to obtain reliable information about cognitive function from subjects by asking them. Many normal individuals consider themselves forgetful[9] and in demented subjects it is usual that no significant complaints are presented since only the relatives may notice the deficits. Subjective symptoms may be early signs of cognitive decline but they may also reflect expectations, self-esteem, anxiety, or depression.[10] Questionnaires are therefore difficult to use and do not produce consistency between the scores obtained and the objective results recorded in detailed neuropsychological tests.

Neuropsychological tests

There is a wide range of different neuropsychological tests that can be combined into various tests batteries and they can be modified to a greater or lesser degree by the clinicians and researchers, for instance by slight changes in the instructions. All these tests provide some information and it is important to consider that they are all useful but that they assess different aspects of cognition with different sensitivity, meaning that the chance of detecting a deficit will be related to the composition of the test battery and the characteristics of the subjects. The interpretation of the results is greatly facilitated if data from appropriate controls are available.

Screening tests

A simple and short-lasting test can be useful for screening purposes, and a more comprehensive test battery can then be applied if one suspects that there is a cognitive deficit.

Screening tests include the Mini Mental State Examination,[11] where ten different items related to orientation, memory, attention, etc. are recorded and the maximum score is 30 points. Another test is the clock-drawing test, where the patient is given a piece of paper with a pre-drawn circle and asked to add the numbers so it looks like a clock. Then the patient should add arms so that the clock indicates a certain time, for instance '10 minutes after eleven'. Such brief testing can give an idea whether the patient has severe cognitive impairment, but none of the two tests can be classified as more than rather crude screening instruments.

Neuropsychological testing in surgical patients

A more detailed examination will include the administration of a whole test battery by a specially trained examiner.[12] This will allow a much more accurate assessment with a higher sensitivity, and the recorded quantitative results are suitable for a statistical analysis and to compare with previous or subsequent tests sessions. The purpose is to obtain the best possible result for the particular subject, so the examination must take place in an undisturbed setting with consideration of the need for reading glasses and hearing aids. The examiner must be able to judge if the patient is fit for testing and well motivated. It is questionable if a reliable assessment of baseline performance can be achieved immediately prior to surgery, and it is not easy to decide when the postoperative performance can be examined. There is a risk of confounding if the patient is examined so soon that he or she is still under the influence of opioids, sedative, or even general anaesthetics. Sleep deprivation and pain are other factors than can impair performance.

The selection of the appropriate tests is a major challenge since there are so many to consider. There is a trade-off between obtaining a high probability of detecting decline, if present (sensitivity) versus the risk of chance findings if a very large test battery is administered. Large test batteries are very time-consuming and will be perceived as highly inconvenient. Furthermore, the difficulty of the tasks must be well suited to the population. No change can be detected if the tests are either too easy or too difficult, and the examiner must be sure that the subject is following the instructions. Computer-aided testing helps in standardizing the procedure and may allow testing without the need of an examiner.

Definitions of syndromes and their detection

Some types of cognitive impairment, like dementia, are well-defined conditions with published criteria in the World Health Organization (WHO) International Classification of Diseases (ICD-10) or the *Diagnostic and Statistical Manual of Mental Disorders* from the American Psychiatric Association (DSM-V). These criteria may, however, not be easy to use in the clinical setting. For other types of cognitive impairment (like POCD), there are no agreed upon criteria, and this causes substantial difficulty in summarizing research findings and elucidating the aetiology.

Dementia

Dementia is a syndrome due to disease of the brain, usually of a chronic or progressive nature, in which there is disturbance of multiple higher cortical functions, including memory, thinking, orientation, comprehension, calculation, learning capacity, language, and judgement. Consciousness is not clouded. The impairments of cognitive function are commonly accompanied, and occasionally preceded, by deterioration in emotional control, social behaviour, or motivation. This syndrome occurs in Alzheimer's disease, in cerebrovascular disease, and in other conditions primarily or secondarily affecting the brain. Based on individual cases, there has been concern that anaesthesia and surgery can exacerbate dementia. A number of retrospective studies of patients followed for Alzheimer's disease have not found a correlation between surgery, anaesthesia, and dementing illness. There are no large prospective studies that have evaluated this issue. Laboratory evidence that anaesthetic agents can have an impact on the biochemistry of neurofibrillatory tangles and hyperphosphorylated tau have led to additional speculation that anaesthetic agents are neurotoxic, leading to POCD and dementia. Recent data has added to this concern, but the issue remains speculative.[13]

Delirium (defined according to ICD-10)

An aetiologically non-specific organic cerebral syndrome characterized by concurrent disturbances of consciousness and attention, perception, thinking, memory, psychomotor behaviour, emotion, and the sleep–wake schedule. The duration is variable and the degree of severity ranges from mild to very severe.

Criteria for postoperative cognitive dysfunction

This condition is not well defined. It has been used to describe the postoperative deterioration in cognitive function, which has been reported by patients or relatives. It is usually subtle and not apparent until the patient is discharged from hospital and tries to resume normal activity. The phenomenon is difficult to verify since a preoperative examination of cognitive function is not normally available. In the context of ICD-10, it is probably most appropriate to classify it as a 'mild cognitive disorder' although this may not be without problems. Most research in this field is based on a comparison of performance in neuropsychological test results before and after surgery and anaesthesia. A deficit may be detected by consideration of changes in the individual patients in one or more tests. There is much discussion how this should be done, and also how data should be analysed and interpreted.[12]

Large and comprehensive test batteries will probably be more sensitive but it is not straight forward to decide which of the variables that should be taken into account in the statistical analysis. More important, however, is the decision regarding what a significant decline means. A statistically significant difference in a single test may be clinically unimportant, and there is a risk of chance findings when numerous variables are analysed.[14] It is therefore common to define POCD as a deterioration of a certain magnitude, for instance, a 25 per cent deterioration in a test.[15] Another commonly used definition is 'A deterioration of one standard deviation in at least two tests'.[16,17] That standard deviation is calculated from the preoperative test and is a measure of variability in the population of surgical patients prior to the procedure. It would be more relevant to obtain measures of the expected, normal variability between sessions in order to separate normal variation from important deterioration. It has been shown that the definitions given here are rather liberal and the POCD incidence will therefore be relatively large in studies using these criteria.[18,19] Other definitions have been based on data obtained by neuropsychological testing of healthy controls to assess not only expected variability between sessions, but also to correct for the practice effects that are well known to occur when subjects are exposed repeatedly to a task. The statistics are rather complicated but will allow the researcher to express a single patient's change in performance in a single number, the so-called Z-score. This indicates the number of standard deviations which that particular patient deviated from the expected. That standard deviation is a measure of variability between two sessions in healthy controls, and a Z-score exceeding 1.96 would be expected in less than 2.5 per cent of subjects with no change in performance.[12] A similar approach is used in the so-called 'Reliable Change Index'.[20,21]

Detection of cognitive deterioration after surgery

Postoperative delirium

Postoperative delirium is a common complication, especially in elderly patients. Numerous predisposing and eliciting factors have been identified (Table 10.1).[22] The incidence after major surgery is between 10 and 20 per cent but delirium is also frequent during hospitalization for medical conditions. The condition is usually fluctuating over the day and the typical duration is a couple of days. The incidence of delirium may be reduced in high-risk elderly patients if they are managed in close cooperation between surgeons, anaesthesiologists, and specialists in internal medicine, preferably in dedicated wards with specially trained nursing staff.[23,24]

Postoperative delirium is a serious complication that is associated with an inability to cooperate, and intravenous catheters, drains, etc. may be lost by accident. Compliance with medication is also problematic in a delirious patient and there is a risk of fractures and head trauma because patients may fall. Other postoperative complications are more common, including mortality, and hospitalization is prolonged. It is, however, somewhat difficult to separate risk factors for delirium from those important for other adverse outcomes.

Patients at high risk should therefore be identified preoperatively. If delirium occurs, then the clinician should carefully examine the patient to detect precipitating factors that can be corrected.

Emergence delirium is a special type where the patient fulfils the criteria immediately after surgery.

During the emergence process, it is fairly common for patient to regain gag reflexes and react physically to the presence of an endotracheal tube before reacting in a meaningful way to commands. A smaller group can be distinguished in which, even after extubation, thinking is highly confused and the patient may be partially or fully combative. This second state is referred to as emergence delirium or emergence excitation. It is common across all age group but perhaps more frequent in children. Recently, Radtke has described a state in the elderly he describes as inadequate emergence, which may be a corollary of hypoactive postoperative

Table 10.1 Risk factors and eliciting factors for postoperative delirium

Risk factors
Increasing age
Pre-existing cognitive impairment
Acute surgery
Femoral neck fracture

Eliciting factors
Medication
Withdrawal states
Fluid and electrolyte disturbance
Hypoxaemia
Pain
Sensory deprivation
Lack of sleep
Infection
High or low blood glucose

delirium.[25] Delirium is a term defined in the DSM-IV (and the soon to be released DSM 5) and can be detected by the Confusion Assessment Method (CAM)[26] (Table 10.2). In elderly patients, delirium tends to appear between days 1 and 4 following an operation and following a prolonged period of lucidity in which their behaviour is normal.

Treatment

Treatment of delirium should be focused on supportive measures to protect the patient, including a general consideration of ventilation, oxygenation, circulation, hydration, pain, medication, and restoration of a normal sleep-awake cycle. It can be necessary to give small doses (0.5–1 mg intravenously) of haloperidol to enable adequate cooperation.

Postoperative cognitive dysfunction

Cognitive impairment after surgery and anaesthesia has been described for more than 50 years but was primarily based on anecdotal reports because it was difficult to study and verify.[27]

Table 10.2 Confusion Assessment Method (CAM)

Delirium is present if 1 and 2, AND either 3a or 3b are positive
1. Acute onset and fluctuating course
Is there evidence of an acute change in mental status from baseline?
2. Inattention
3a. Disorganized thinking
Thinking disorganized or incoherent: such as rambling or irrelevant conversation, unclear or illogical flow of ideas, or unpredictable switching from subject to subject?
3b. Altered level of consciousness
A patient with a depressed level of consciousness is more easily not recognized as being delirious (hypoactive form) whereas the hyperactive type is much more obvious

Copyright © 2002, E. Wesley Ely, MD, MPH and Vanderbilt University, all rights reserved, reproduced with permission.

Cross-sectional and case–control studies have been conducted but it is not easy to obtain conclusive results and most have been unable to show an association between cognitive performance and exposure to anaesthesia. Such studies are limited by several issues. A major proportion of all elderly has been exposed to anaesthesia, but there is usually no assessment of baseline performance, and the subjects may not even recall reliably when or if they had surgery, if it was a minor or major procedure, and the interval between the test and the anaesthetic is often not well known.[28] Age at exposure is probably also very important.[29]

Prospective cohort studies with neuropsychological testing before and after surgery have most often been done in cardiac surgery patients where deterioration has been reported repeatedly. Incidences of deterioration between 30 and 80 per cent have been reported early after such surgery, and deficits have been detected in 10–60 per cent even several months postoperatively.[30–33] The duration of cardiopulmonary bypass, valve surgery, poor cardiac function, and increasing age have been identified as risk factors and it has often been assumed that brain embolization was an important aetiological underlying this brain dysfunction. It has, interestingly, been very difficult to verify this assumption and POCD does not seem to be less common after coronary artery bypass surgery without cardiopulmonary bypass. Many other interventions have been assessed in an attempt to reduce the incidence of POCD after cardiac surgery, but only a few have been effective, and the pharmacological approach in particular has shown disappointing results.[34]

Non-cardiac surgery constitutes a much larger proportion of the surgical spectrum but POCD has not been so well studied in this area. A typical question has been whether regional anaesthesia should be preferred in the elderly, and it has been suggested that regional techniques would lead to better preservation of cognitive function after surgery. To date, multiple randomized studies have not been able to document a difference. The early studies of POCD within non-cardiac surgery used different criteria and had difficulty in detecting any deterioration, especially if the methodology from the cardiac surgery studies was applied.

The use of control groups, other tests, and analyses has enabled better detection of cognitive deterioration after non-cardiac procedures (Fig. 10.1), with approximately 25 per cent of elderly patients fulfilling the criteria at 1 week and 10 per cent at 3 months after major surgery with general anaesthesia.[35] The incidence seems to be lower in middle-aged patients and after minor surgery.[36,37]

The most important risk factors for POCD after non-cardiac surgery seem to be increasing age, low level of education, and postoperative complications. The type of anaesthesia is probably less important, and no randomized studies have documented a lower incidence of POCD after regional anaesthesia beyond the 1st week.[38–40]

Few studies have compared general anaesthetics, but a few recent studies suggest that inhalational anaesthesia may be associated with less POCD than total intravenous anaesthesia.[41,42]

The clinical relevance of POCD has been questioned as one could ask whether a minor deterioration in neuropsychological test results means anything to a patient. A significant correlation between POCD and activities of daily living has been found,[35] but it also seems that POCD is associated with a higher long-term mortality, withdrawal from the labour market, and a higher need for social transfer payment.[43,44] Several aspects of quality of life seem also to be affected by POCD.[45]

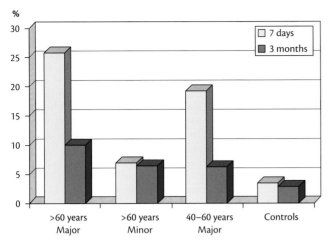

Fig. 10.1 Incidence of postoperative cognitive dysfunction in various groups of patients undergoing non-cardiac surgery. Reprinted from *The Lancet*, 351, 9106, Moller JT, Cluitmans P, Rasmussen LS et al., 'Long-term postoperative cognitive dysfunction in the elderly: ISPOCD1 study', pp. 857–861, Copyright 1998, with permission from Elsevier.

It is less clear as to whether POCD is associated with dementia. No significant association has been found in epidemiological studies of subjects who have completed neuropsychological testing on several occasions over several years during which some underwent surgery and anaesthesia.[46]

There are many pitfalls in POCD research. Generally, only patients at a high level of functioning are included and some may decline follow-up examination. The reported incidences of POCD are therefore most likely underestimated. There is a poor consistency regarding which patients fulfil POCD criteria at the postoperative test sessions. One may, for instance, assume that those with POCD at 3 months all had POCD early after surgery as well. In contrast, only a minor proportion display POCD at all postoperative sessions, meaning on one hand, that there is a good chance of recovery, but on the other hand that POCD may only be detected after long-term follow-up where numerous other factors than surgery and anaesthesia may be important.[47]

Another interesting consideration is to focus on the proportion of subjects displaying improvement after surgery, since variability alone could lead to high proportions showing improvement or deterioration. Only a small proportion of surgical patients show improvement early after surgery, but these figures are seldom presented.[47]

Several possible aetiologies have been proposed to explain why POCD occurs (Table 10.3).[48,49]

Studies using animal models and cell cultures have found an association between exposure to general anaesthetics and various forms of cell injury such as apoptosis and neuronal degeneration.[50–52] Animals exposed to these drugs also have displayed behavioural deficits with impaired learning and memory function compared with control animals.[53] Inhalational anaesthetics increase the levels and aggregation of the Alzheimer's disease-associated amyloid beta-protein and also production of inflammatory markers in mice brain tissue.[54–57] Interestingly, we have no convincing data showing that regional anaesthesia offers any long-term advantage regarding cognitive function in humans. This combined with the limited amount of evidence supporting that POCD is a problem occurring a long time after surgery should

Table 10.3 Suggested aetiology underlying postoperative cognitive dysfunction

Neurotoxicity of general anaesthetics
Hypoxaemia
Hypoperfusion
Thrombosis and embolism
Inflammation and stress
Psychological and environmental factors

lead to a cautious interpretation of the earlier mentioned findings in animal and cells models. It must, however, be kept in mind that the clinical studies have very little data on the frail elderly with preoperative cognitive impairment, and the follow-up is not complete in such studies. Therefore, patients with deficits may not have been assessed after surgery.

Arterial hypoxaemia and brain hypoperfusion can cause cerebral hypoxia and this may have serious consequences. Short episodes of modest hypoxaemia and hypotension are quite common perioperatively but they have not been shown to be significant risk factors for POCD.[35] Brain perfusion is unfortunately not easy to measure.

Brain embolism can occur in connection with numerous types of surgical procedures, either as a result of manipulation of cerebral arteries, use of cardiopulmonary bypass, or as paradoxical embolism caused by entry of, for example, air or bone marrow particles during joint surgery or procedures where the surgical field is above heart level.[17] Emboli are typically easy to detect but difficult to count and it has been very difficult to show a significant association between emboli counts and cognitive impairment.[58] POCD also occurs even if no emboli are detected so this is unlikely to be the most important explanation.

Conclusion

The elderly brain is sensitive to insults arising directly from coexisting diseases such as the vascular changes in hypertension or diabetes and more subtly from the effects of surgical procedures. The causes of the latter are becoming tantalizingly clearer although, in reality, little has changed over the last 60 years. This is despite the dramatic improvements in anaesthetic practice, monitoring, and drugs for instance, and in minimally invasive surgical techniques. Inflammation and stress are probably some of the most relevant factors to address in the elucidation of POCD pathophysiology. These mechanisms are most pronounced in connection with major procedures where POCD is most common and elderly have an altered response with difficulty in coping with long-term elevated levels of inflammatory mediators and cortisol.[59,60] A few studies have supported these mechanisms but this needs to be studied in more detail. Psychological factors and the hospital environment should also be considered as it has been done for delirium.

We may be a lot closer to an understanding of the aetiology of acute cognitive dysfunction in the ill elderly patient and that raises the hope that preventative or supportive strategies will be possible in the near future.

References

1. Alz.Org®. Alzheimer's Association. <http://www.alz.org/> (accessed 17 December 2012).

2. Zakzanis KK, Mraz R, Graham SJ. An fMRI study of the Trail Making Test. *Neuropsychologia*. 2005;43(13):1878–1886.

3. Bishop NA, Lu T, Yankner BA. Neural mechanisms of ageing and cognitive decline. *Nature*. 2010;464(7288):529–535.

4. Salthouse TA. Selective review of cognitive aging. *J Int Neuropsychol Soc*. 2010;16(5):754–760.

5. Neuropathology Group of the Medical Research Council Cognitive Function and Ageing Study (MRC CFAS). Neuropathology Group. Medical Research Council Cognitive Function and Aging Study. Pathological correlates of late-onset dementia in a multicentre, community-based population in England and Wales. *Lancet*. 2001;357(9251):169–175.

6. Whalley LJ, Deary IJ, Appleton CL, Starr JM. Cognitive reserve and the neurobiology of cognitive aging. *Ageing Res Rev*. 2004;3(4):369–382.

7. Stern Y. Cognitive reserve. *Neuropsychologia*. 2009;47(10):2015–2028.

8. Lazarov O, Mattson MP, Peterson DA, Pimplikar SW, van Praag H. When neurogenesis encounters aging and disease. *Trends Neurosci*. 2010;33(12):569–579.

9. Commissaris CJ, Ponds RW, Jolles J. Subjective forgetfulness in a normal Dutch population: possibilities for health education and other interventions. *Patient Educ Couns*. 1998;34(1):25–32.

10. Newman S, Klinger L, Venn G, Smith P, Harrison M, Treasure T. Subjective reports of cognition in relation to assessed cognitive performance following coronary artery bypass surgery. *J Psychosom Res*. 1989;33(2):227–233.

11. Folstein MF, Folstein SE, McHugh PR. Mini-Mental State: a practical method for grading the cognitive state of patients for the clinician. *J Psychiatr Res*. 1975;12(3):189–198.

12. Rasmussen LS, Larsen K, Houx P, et al. The assessment of postoperative cognitive function. *Acta Anaesthesiol Scand*. 2001;45(3):275–289.

13. Liu Y, Pan N, Ma Y, et al. Inhaled sevoflurane may promote progression of amnestic mild cognitive impairment: a prospective, randomized parallel-group study. *Am J Med Sci*. 2013;345(5):355–360.

14. Ancelin ML, de Roquefeuil G, Ledésert B, Bonnel F, Cheminal JC, Ritchie K. Exposure to anaesthetic agents, cognitive functioning and depressive symptomatology in the elderly. *Br J Psychiatr*. 2001;178:360–366.

15. Heyer EJ, Adams DC, Solomon RA, et al. Neuropsychometric changes in patients after carotid endarterectomy. *Stroke*. 1998;29(6):1110–1115.

16. Treasure T, Smith PL, Newman S, et al. Impairment of cerebral function following cardiac and other major surgery. *Eur J Cardiothorac Surg*. 1989;3(3):216–221.

17. Pugsley W, Klinger L, Paschalis C, Treasure T, Harrison M, Newman S. The impact of microemboli during cardiopulmonary bypass on neuropsychological functioning. *Stroke*. 1994;25(7):1393–1399.

18. Keizer AM, Hijman R, Kalkman CJ, Kahn RS, van Dijk D; Octopus Study Group. The incidence of cognitive decline after (not) undergoing coronary artery bypass grafting: the impact of a controlled definition. *Acta Anaesthesiol Scand*. 2005;49(9):1232–1235.

19. Mahanna EP, Blumenthal JA, White WD, *et al.* Defining neuropsychological dysfunction after coronary artery bypass grafting. *Ann Thorac Surg*. 1996;61(5):1342–1347.

20. Kneebone AC, Andrew MJ, Baker RA, Knight JL. Neuropsychologic changes after coronary artery bypass grafting: use of reliable change indices. *Ann Thorac Surg*. 1998;65:1320–1325.

21. Evered L, Scott DA, Silbert B, Maruff P. Postoperative cognitive dysfunction is independent of type of surgery and anesthetic. *Anesth Analg*. 2011;112(5):1179–1185.

22. Steiner LA. Postoperative delirium. Part 1: pathophysiology and risk factors. *Eur J Anaesthesiol*. 2011;28(9):628–636.

23. Siddiqi N, Stockdale R, Britton AM, Holmes J. Interventions for preventing delirium in hospitalised patients. *Cochrane Database Syst Rev*. 2007;18(2):CD005563.

24. Bjorkelund KB, Hommel A, Thorngren K-G, Gustafson L, Larsson S, Lundberg D. Reducing delirium in elderly patients with hip fracture: a multi-factorial intervention study. *Acta Anaesthesiol Scand*. 2010;54(6):678–688.

25. Radtke FM, Franck M, Hagemann L, Seeling M, Wernecke KD, Spies CD. Risk factors for inadequate emergence after anesthesia: emergence delirium and hypoactive emergence. *Minerva Anestesiol*. 2010;76(6):394–403.

26. Inouye SK, van Dyck CH, Alessi CA, Balkin S, Siegal AP, Horwitz RI. Clarifying confusion: the confusion assessment method. A new method for detection of delirium. *Ann Intern Med*. 1990;113(12):941–948.

27. Bedford PD. Adverse cerebral effects of anaesthesia on old people. *Lancet*. 1955;269(6884):259–263.

28. Dijkstra JB, Van Boxtel MP, Houx PJ, Jolles J. An operation under general anesthesia as a risk factor for age-related cognitive decline: results from a large cross-sectional population study. *J Am Geriatr Soc*. 1998;46(10):1258–1265.

29. Bohnen N, Warner MA, Kokmen E, Kurland LT. Early and midlife exposure to anesthesia and age of onset of Alzheimer's disease. *Int J Neurosci*. 1994;77(3–4):181–185.

30. Savageau JA, Stanton BA, Jenkins CD, Frater RWM. Neuropsychological dysfunction following elective cardiac operation. II. A six-month reassessment. *J Thorac Cardiovasc Surg*. 1982;84(4):595–600.

31. Savageau JA, Stanton BA, Jenkins CD, Klein MD. Neuropsychological dysfunction following elective cardiac operation. I. Early assessment. *J Thorac Cardiovasc Surg*. 1982;84(4):585–594.

32. Shaw PJ, Bates D, Cartlidge NEF, et al. Early intellectual dysfunction following coronary bypass surgery. *Q J Med*. 1986;58(225):59–68.

33. Shaw PJ, Bates D, Cartlidge NEF, et al. Long-term intellectual dysfunction following coronary artery bypass graft surgery: a six month follow-up study. *Q J Med*. 1987;62(239):259–268.

34. Hogue CW Jr, Palin CA, Arrowsmith JE. Cardiopulmonary bypass management and neurologic outcomes: an evidence-based appraisal of current practices. *Anesth Analg*. 2006;103(1):21–37.

35. Moller JT, Cluitmans P, Rasmussen LS, *et al.* Long-term postoperative cognitive dysfunction in the elderly: ISPOCD1 study. *Lancet*. 1998;351(9917):857–861. Erratum in: *Lancet*. 1998;351:1742.

36. Canet J, Raeder J, Rasmussen LS, *et al.* Cognitive dysfunction after minor surgery in the elderly. *Acta Anaesthesiol Scand*. 2003;47(10):1204–1210.

37. Johnson T, Monk T, Rasmussen LS, *et al.* Postoperative cognitive dysfunction in middle-aged patients. *Anesthesiology*. 2002;96(6):1351–1357.

38. Wu CL, Hsu W, Richman JM, Raja SN. Postoperative cognitive function as an outcome of regional anesthesia and analgesia. *Reg Anesth Pain Med*. 2004;29(3):257–268.

39. Rasmussen LS. Postoperative cognitive dysfunction: incidence and prevention. *Best Pract Res Clin Anaesthesiol*. 2006;20(2):315–330.

40. Bryson GL, Wyand A. Evidence-based clinical update: general anesthesia and the risk of delirium and postoperative cognitive dysfunction. *Can J Anaesth*. 2006;53(7):669–677.

41. Royse CF, Andrews DT, Newman SN, *et al.* The influence of propofol or desflurane on postoperative cognitive dysfunction in patients undergoing coronary artery bypass surgery. *Anaesthesia*. 2011;66(6):455–464.

42. Schoen J, Husemann L, Tiemeyer C, *et al.* Cognitive function after sevoflurane- vs propofol-based anaesthesia for on-pump cardiac surgery: a randomized controlled trial. *Br J Anaesth*. 2011;106(6):840–850.

43. Steinmetz J, Christensen KB, Lund T, Lohse N, Rasmussen LS; ISPOCD Group. Long-term consequences of postoperative cognitive dysfunction. *Anesthesiology*. 2009;110(3):548–555.

44. Monk TG, Weldon BC, Garvan CW, *et al.* Predictors of cognitive dysfunction after major noncardiac surgery. *Anesthesiology*. 2008;108(1):18–30.

45. Newman MF, Grocott HP, Mathew JP, *et al.* Report of the substudy assessing the impact of neurocognitive function on quality of life 5 years after cardiac surgery. *Stroke*. 2001;32(12):2874–2881.

46. Avidan MS, Searleman AC, Storandt M, *et al.* Long-term cognitive decline in older subjects was not attributable to noncardiac surgery or major illness. *Anesthesiology*. 2009;111(5):964–970.

47. Rasmussen LS, Siersma VD, ISPOCD group. Postoperative cognitive dysfunction: true deterioration versus random variation. *Acta Anaesthesiol Scand.* 2004;48(9):1137–1143.

48. Krenk L, Rasmussen LS, Kehlet H. New insights into the pathophysiology of postoperative cognitive dysfunction. *Acta Anaesthesiol Scand.* 2010;54(8):951–956.

49. Culley DJ, Xie Z, Crosby G. General anesthetic-induced neurotoxicity: an emerging problem for the young and old? *Curr Opin Anaesthesiol.* 2007;20(5):408–413.

50. Jevtovic-Todorovic V, Hartman RE, Izumi Y, et al. Early exposure to common anesthetic agents causes widespread neurodegeneration in the developing rat brain and persistent learning deficits. *J Neurosci.* 2003;23(3):876–882.

51. Jevtovic-Todorovic V, Beals J, Benshoff N, Olney JW. Prolonged exposure to inhalational anesthetic nitrous oxide kills neurons in adult rat brain. *Neuroscience.* 2003;122(3):609–616.

52. Young C, Jevtovic-Todorovic V, Qin YQ, et al. Potential of ketamine and midazolam, individually or in combination, to induce apoptotic neurodegeneration in the infant mouse brain. *Br J Pharmacol.* 2005;146(2):189–197.

53. Wiklund A, Granon S, Faure P, Sundman E, Changeux JP, Eriksson LI. Object memory in young and aged mice after sevoflurane anaesthesia. *Neuroreport.* 2009;20(16):1419–1423.

54. Xie Z, Dong Y, Maeda U, et al. The common inhalation anesthetic isoflurane induces apoptosis and increases amyloid beta protein levels. *Anesthesiology.* 2006;104(5):988–994.

55. Eckenhoff RG, Johansson JS, Wei H, et al. Inhaled anesthetic enhancement of amyloid-beta oligomerization and cytotoxicity. *Anesthesiology.* 2004;101(3):703–709.

56. Wu X, Lu Y, Dong Y, et al. The inhalation anesthetic isoflurane increases levels of proinflammatory TNF-α, IL-6, and IL-1β. *Neurobiol Aging.* 2012;33(7):1364–1378.

57. Xie Z, Culley DJ, Dong Y, et al. The common inhalation anesthetic isoflurane induces caspase activation and increases amyloid beta-protein level in vivo. *Ann Neuro.* 2008;64(6):618–627.

58. Liu YH, Wang DX, Li LH, et al. The effects of cardiopulmonary bypass on the number of cerebral microemboli and the incidence of cognitive dysfunction after coronary artery bypass graft surgery. *Anesth Analg.* 2009;109(4):1013–1022.

59. Ramlawi B, Rudolph JL, Mieno S, et al. C-reactive protein and inflammatory response associated to neurocognitive decline following cardiac surgery. *Surgery.* 2006;140(2):221–226.

60. McEwen BS, Sapolsky RM. Stress and cognitive function. *Curr Opin Neurobiol.* 1995;5(2):205–216.

CHAPTER 11

Pain mechanisms in the elderly

Khalil Ullah Shibli and Sabina Shibli

Introduction

Pain is one of the commonest symptoms in medicine. Pain may continue beyond its protective and diagnostic usefulness, either because the source of the pain is itself incurable or irreversible anatomical changes lead to continuing noxious stimulation long after the initial cause has ended. Pain control irrespective of its nature and description, is now a major concern especially with population ageing and the associated pain of the chronic degenerative conditions of the elderly. Basic scientific research into pain mechanisms is increasing and has revealed numerous novel targets for the advent of new pain therapies. Despite this increased interest causative factors are not always identified. Truly effective treatment can only be achieved if the underlying pain mechanisms following identified causes are known. This chapter will focus on mechanisms of pain in the elderly and will include definitions, types, and descriptions of pain, how the pain is initiated or caused, detected, transmitted, facilitated, inhibited, modulated, and finally perceived. The 'physiology of pain' will be discussed at peripheral, spinal (dorsal horn), and central (supraspinal) level to elucidate the mechanisms of pain. Ageing affects the characteristics and morphology of pain fibres, their ability to respond to nociceptive information processing, the expression of ion channels and receptors, neurotransmitter release, spinal modulation, and finally altered perception and reporting of pain in elderly people.

Pain and the elderly

The National Institute of Aging (NIA), in collaboration with the National Institutes of Health (NIH) pain consortium, described pain in older patients as 'a complex and serious condition which affects their physiological, psychological and social well-beings significantly' in their executive summary.[1] They opined that despite recent developments in the understanding of the molecular entities and neural pathways involved in pain sensation, very little is known about how ageing affects parts of the nervous system that detect and transmit painful stimuli and express painful experiences at a mechanistic level.[1] Apart from altered pain perception, expression, and dampened modulation, the elderly have similar biological pain mechanisms to their younger counterparts. However, the elderly are more vulnerable to the deleterious effects of persistent pain. Yezierski eloquently described the ageing process as a loss of 'buffering' capacity in which compensatory, homeostatic mechanisms are rendered ineffective thus leading to a permissive biological environment for the development of pain.[2]

The bio-psychosocial model of pain described by Loeser[3] sees the whole process with nociception as a trigger, pain as a result, suffering as a consequence, and pain behaviour as an observable and measurable element. Biological responses alone to a noxious stimulus cannot be interpreted as pain. Before going any further it is important to understand what pain is.

Description of pain

Definition

The definition of pain varies widely but one accepted definition—'pain is an unpleasant sensory and emotional experience associated with actual or potential tissue damage, or described in terms of such as damage'—is defined by the International Association for the study of pain (IASP) which also avoids tying the pain to stimulus.[4]

Types of pain

Pain may be categorized as physiological or clinical (pathophysiological) and there are several other description of pain.

Physiological pain

Physiological pain is transmitted via the same fibres and pathways as clinical pain (see later) but has a protective function, acts as a warning for potential and impending tissue damage, and is transient and predominantly localized. The human response to physiological pain is to either 'withdraw' or 'immobilize'.

Clinical pain

Clinical pain is pathological. It shares the same pathways and fibres as physiological pain, but may be associated with tissue injury, inflammation, or direct nerve damage. The hallmark of clinical or pathological pain is the feature of peripheral and central sensitization with spread to the undamaged areas. Clinical (pathophysiological) pain persists even after the cessation of stimulus[5] and can present as an acute or chronic pain.

Acute pain

Acute pain results from tissue injury and is inflammatory in nature. It is mainly adaptive and reparative and comes as a warning sign with healing prospects. It may result from an accidental tissue or bone trauma, a surgical procedure, visceral inflammation, and ischaemia. It could even be as simple as muscular pains and sprains. In acute pain (predominantly nociceptive), the nervous system is usually intact and not unduly perturbed.

Chronic pain

Chronic pain is an outcome of ongoing peripheral or central pathology, chronic inflammation with or without any obvious lesion, tissue damage, or degenerative process. It may involve both sensory and autonomic nervous system. It can be spontaneous, provoked, or persistent and may be autonomous and independent of the initiating stimulus.

Nociceptive pain (inflammatory and trauma)

Nociceptive pain refers to acute inflammatory pain as a result of normal tissue trauma in response to a noxious stimulus. A noxious stimulus is one that is damaging to normal tissues.[4] An example of nociceptive pain is physiological pain.

Neuropathic pain

Neuropathic pain is initiated or caused by a primary lesion or dysfunction in the nervous system and can be peripheral or central in origin. Peripheral neuropathic pain is initiated or caused by a primary lesion or dysfunction in the peripheral nervous system whereas central pain is initiated or caused by lesion or dysfunction in the central nervous system.[4] A hallmark feature of neuropathic pain is generally sensory hypersensitivity and probable later involvement of the autonomic nervous system.

Peripheral pain

Pain sensation from the periphery to the spinal cord is carried by small diameter thinly myelinated or unmyelinated nerve fibres termed 'nociceptors'. Nociceptors are 'neurons' preferentially sensitive to a noxious stimulus or to a stimulus which would become noxious if prolonged.[4]

Nociception is a somatosensory response of the peripheral and central nervous system to a harmful mechanical, electrical, thermal, or chemical stimulus. Peripheral nociceptors belong to the group of A-delta and C fibres with their cell bodies in the dorsal root ganglion (DRG) or trigeminal ganglion. These are present in the skin, muscles, connective tissues, blood vessels and thoracic and abdominal viscera.

There are three main types of sensory fibres in the peripheral nervous system: A-beta, A-delta, and C fibres. Each fibre has different properties allowing them to respond to and transmit different types of sensory information.

A-beta fibres are large in diameter and highly myelinated, therefore, quickest to conduct action potentials from their peripheral to central terminals. These fibres have low activation thresholds and normally respond to light touch and are responsible for conveying tactile information. Under normal conditions, rapidly conducting A-beta fibres (conduction velocities >30 m/sec) are mainly concerned with non-noxious input from specialized encapsulated receptors.[6] The large A-beta low threshold fibre activation closes the 'gate' at spinal level by activating inhibitory interneurons and inhibiting messages from small diameter fibres thus blocking ascending pain transmission.

A-delta fibres are smaller in diameter (2–5 µm), thinly myelinated, and slower-conducting than A-beta fibres and have a higher activation threshold. They respond to both thermal and mechanical stimuli. A-delta fibre conduction velocity is 5–30 m/s and their pain is described as fast, first, sharp, and pricking.

C fibres are the smallest (<2 µm) type of primary afferents and are unmyelinated with conduction velocities 0.5–2.5 m/s thus making them the slowest conducting fibres. They have the highest threshold for activation and therefore, detect selectively nociceptive or 'painful' stimuli. Most C fibres show polymodal responses. Some are exclusively chemosensitive under normal conditions and do not respond to mechanical and thermal stimuli although responsive to noxious thermal (>45°C) stimuli.

A small proportion of 'silent' or 'sleeping' nociceptors identified in the skin as well as visceral organs are unmyelinated primary afferent neurons. These may be unresponsive, even to intense stimuli.[7] However, in the presence of inflammatory mediators and chemical irritants they become responsive and discharge spontaneously to induce changes in receptive field and play a significant role in sensitization.

Under normal circumstances fine afferent C fibres' and A-delta fibres' activation by brief high-intensity stimuli induces little or no tissue damage or structural change but may cause a short-lasting transient pain which serves as a physiological warning. These events can also be considered as a physiological protective response as nociceptive system reverts back to normal once the initial and underlying injury is healed.[7] In clinical settings these may be post-operative pain, visceral inflammation, infection, and mild tissue damage. A-delta and C-afferent fibres are activated by even lower intensity stimuli and produce pain that differs in quality and is more persistent. If left untreated, it is capable of inducing longer-lasting morphological and functional changes in the peripheral and central nervous system. Chronic postsurgical pain (>2 months) is one category that can be described as 'primarily acute post-operative pain which was poorly or under treated, thus turned chronic and persistent'.

As already described, A-delta and C fibres transduce noxious stimuli into action potentials and propagate these to the dorsal horn of the spinal cord. The nociceptors (central terminals of primary afferent fibres) terminate in an orderly manner in layers of substantia gelatinosa (laminae) of the dorsal horn. The peripheral afferent fibres termination and organization will be discussed (see later) in dorsal horn mechanisms of pain.

Inflammatory pain

Kidd and Urban[6] described three functions of primary peripheral afferent neurons with respect to their role in nociception i.e. *transduction*, *conduction*, and *transmission*. Transduction is the detection of noxious or damaging stimuli while conduction is the passage of resulting sensory input from peripheral terminals to the dorsal horn of spinal cord. Transmission is the synaptic transfer of this input to neurons within specific laminae of the dorsal horn.

In peripheral inflammatory pain mechanisms, transduction or detection of painful stimuli will be examined first to illustrate the initiation of afferent barrage of noxious stimuli and its consequent effects. Conduction and transmission processes will be elaborated while describing the role of peripheral afferent nociceptors and dorsal horn mechanisms (see later).

The tissue trauma and subsequent inflammation cause changes in local blood flow, hyperaemia, an increase in vascular permeability and oedema formation along with activation and migration of immune cells from surrounding tissues and changes in the release of growth and trophic factors. As a result of tissue injury, several inflammatory mediators are released peripherally and a few are synthesized. The so called inflammatory 'soup' is either directly algogenic or may act indirectly by sensitizing peripheral afferents to even lower intensity, mechanical, non-noxious stimuli leading to increased responsiveness termed 'peripheral sensitization'. Subsequent involvement of the surrounding injury area causes primary hyperalgesia.[7,8] Primary hyperalgesia is the extreme sensitivity of the uninjured area surrounding injury to even non-noxious stimuli.

Visceral pain

Visceral afferents transmit noxious information to dorsal root ganglia where cutaneous afferents also terminate. Visceral pain fibres travel with parasympathetic and sympathetic fibres, and are therefore associated with the autonomic nervous system activity because of C fibres' mediated effects on stimulation. Increase in heart and respiratory rate, sweating, and rise in blood pressure are associated with visceral pain. Although no clear boundaries exist, visceral pain can be distinguished from cutaneous or peripherally induced somatic pain. Visceral pain is vague, deep, and 'diffuse' in nature. It has the characteristics of escalation in intensity, summation, and spread, and may turn into referred pain. Referred pain arises as a result of the convergence and co-localization of visceral and peripheral (cutaneous/dermatomal) afferents in the dorsal horn.[5] The sensation of visceral pain declines with age and elderly people exhibit a delayed response in reporting visceral pain.[9] Their primary noxious stimulus is either visceral distention or inflammation.

Key features of pain mechanisms

It is commonly believed that pain is activated in the periphery only by nociceptors in response to an adequate noxious stimulus. This may be true of nociceptive pain under normal circumstances but it is perhaps too simplistic to attribute pain hypersensitivity or spontaneous pain to this. Here, a number of different input channels can lead to the pain sensation[10] (Table 11.1). The different pain-evoked input channels represent the operation of multiple mechanisms[10] (Table 11.2). However, keeping in view the scope of this chapter, only selected inputs and their operations are discussed here.

Table 11.1 Input channels for pain

- Mechanical, thermal, or chemical stimuli
- Activation of sensitized nociceptors in the periphery by low-intensity stimuli
- Ectopic discharge in nociceptors originating at a neuroma, dorsal root ganglion, peripheral nerve, or dorsal root
- Low-threshold afferent activation in the periphery by low-intensity mechanical–thermal stimuli, in combination with central sensitization, synaptic reorganization, or disinhibition
- Ectopic discharge in low-threshold afferents originating at a neuroma, dorsal root ganglion, peripheral nerve, dorsal root (peripheral nerve injury associated with central sensitization, synaptic reorganization, or disinhibition)
- Spontaneous activity in central neurons (in the dorsal horn, thalamus, or cortex), ectopic discharge in low-threshold afferents originating at a neuroma, dorsal root ganglion, peripheral nerve, dorsal root and spontaneous activity in central neurons (in the dorsal horn, thalamus, or cortex).

Adapted from Woolf CJ, Max M B., 'Mechanism-based pain diagnosis: issues for analgesic drug development', *Anesthesiology*, 95, pp. 241–249, copyright 2011, with permission from Wolters Kluwer and the American Society of Anesthesiologists.

Table 11.2 Different input channels representing operation of multiple mechanisms

- Activation of high-threshold receptor, ion channel transducers in nociceptor peripheral terminals•Change in threshold sensitivity of receptor, ion channel transducers in nociceptor peripheral terminals (peripheral sensitization)
- Changes in ion channel expression, phosphorylation, or accumulation in primary afferents (altered sensory neuron excitability)
- Posttranslational changes in ligand- and voltage-gated ion channel kinetics in central (spinal cord and brain) neurons, changing their excitability and the strength of their synaptic inputs (central sensitization)
- Alterations in the expression of receptors–transmitters–ion channels in peripheral and central neurons (phenotype modulation)
- Modification of synaptic connections caused by cell death or sprouting (synaptic reorganization)
- Loss of local inhibition at different relay levels in the neuraxis and of descending inhibition originating in the forebrain and brainstem and terminating in the brainstem and spinal cord, caused by decreased activation of neurons, downregulation of receptors–transmitters, and cell death (disinhibition)

Adapted from Woolf CJ, Max M B., 'Mechanism-based pain diagnosis: issues for analgesic drug development', *Anesthesiology*, 95, pp. 241–249, copyright 2011, with permission from Wolters Kluwer and the American Society of Anesthesiologists.

There are two major phenomena that need to be discussed here in detail to delineate the effects of type and nature of injury on the induction of pain. Both the processes begin with either soft tissue and bone trauma alone or accompanied with a nerve injury. It is interesting to note here that the majority of accidental or surgical trauma and other injuries do not follow a pure physiological script in the development of either inflammatory (nociceptive) or nerve injury (neuropathic) pain. There is a significant overlap of events during the process of transduction, conduction and transmission depending on the magnitude of the injury (intensity of noxious stimuli), bodily responses to the insult (ageing effect and threshold), and the timely intervention of injury and pain containment (treatment). However, the inflammatory processes (acute or chronic) are considered as the beginning of the sequence of events in pain generation.

Inflammatory mediators

In the event of injury, damaged cells release their intracellular contents; these include macrophages, lymphocytes, and mast cells. Thus the afferent nerve terminals are exposed to painful inflammatory mediators, such as potassium and hydrogen ions, 5-hydroxytryptamine (5-HT), histamine, bradykinin, purines, cytokines, substance P, neurokinin A, calcitonin gene related peptide (CGRP), adenosine triphosphate (ATP), and nitric oxide. Inflammation activates the arachidonic acid pathway to produce leukotrienes and prostaglandins. Bradykinin causes activation and sensitization of primary afferent neurons and produces pain, inflammation and hyperalgesia. Cytokines may act directly on nociceptors or indirectly stimulates release of prostaglandins. Pro-inflammatory cytokines, tumour necrosis factor alpha (TNFα), interleukin (IL)-1, IL-6, and chemokine IL-8, may produce mechanical and thermal hyperalgesia.[6,8]

Prostaglandins play a major role as mediators of inflammation, fever, and pain. They are mainly sensitizing agents and sensitize the primary afferent neurons to bradykinin and other pro-inflammatory mediators. Prostaglandins can also directly activate nociceptors and reduce their activation threshold and enhance their responses to other stimuli. 5-HT released from mast cells and platelets can cause direct excitation of sensory afferent neurons during injury and ongoing stimuli. Histamine released from mast cell degranulation acts on sensory neurons and produces itch in low and pain in high concentrations.[11]

Substance P degranulates mast cells to cause histamine release and also induces the release of prostaglandin (PGE$_2$), both are the mediators of pain.[6]

Damage to a peripheral nerve during tissue injury, will also produce several biochemical, physiological, and morphological changes. Nerve damage increases production of a neurotrophic peptide—the nerve growth factor (NGF) which plays a significant role in the development of peripheral sensitization. Axonal transport of NGF to the dorsal horn plays a significant role in central sensitization.[5]

Primary (peripheral) afferent nociceptor activation

Peripheral tissue or nerve injury results in primary afferent nociceptor activation and the release of excitatory peptides, expression of receptors, and ion channels.

Expression of receptors and transduction

The process of transduction or detection of painful stimuli reveals a series of ion channel-linked receptors including heat-activated *vanilloid receptors, acid-sensing ion channel receptors* (ASICs), and *purinergic receptors.*[6]

The vanilloid receptors belong to a group of transient receptor potential (TRP) ion channels permeable to Ca^{2+} ion.[6] The vanilloid receptor-related TRP channels (TRPV) are sensitive to capsaicin, heat, acid, inflammation, and are responsive to thermal stimuli (>43°C). Vanilloid receptors are distributed in small-diameter peripheral afferent neurons and in the central nervous system.

The ASICs respond to low pH and present throughout the nervous system. ASICs are activated by heat, acid, ischaemia, and inflammation.

The purinoreceptors are ionotropic ligand-gated ion channels mediating fast synaptic transmission by extracellular ATP.[12] ATP activates sensory neurons and causes sharp transient pain.

Expression of ion channels and transduction

The nerve fibres possess voltage-gated sodium (Na$^+$) channels which are important for normal nerve conduction. The excitation of primary afferent neurons is controlled by opening and closing of the voltage-gated sodium (Na$^+$ inward current) and potassium (K$^+$ outward current) channels. The Na$^+$ channels open rapidly and transiently to allow membrane depolarization and generation of an action potential. Activation of these cationic channels is responsible for the generation of nociceptive signals. Abnormal ectopic firing is also mediated by the Na$^+$ channels which are classified as tetrodotoxin sensitive (TTX-S) and tetrodotoxin resistant (TTX-R). The larger diameter fibres express TTX-S sodium channels while the small diameter nociceptive neurons express both.[13] Prostaglandin E2, adenosine, and serotonin also enhance channel sensitivity.[14] It has been suggested that Na$^+$ channel blockers may be used to treat pain but their side effects may limit their clinical use. Selective blockade

of TTX-R has been proposed as an option for treating neuropathic and chronic pain states.[6]

The potassium (K$^+$) channels are present in the sensory neurons and stabilize the membrane potential by maintaining hyperpolarization (outward current). The downregulation of K$^+$ channels may result in a hyperexcitable state of sensory neurons.[5]

The voltage-gated calcium (Ca^{2+}) channels (VGCCs) are involved in sensory transduction and transmitter release. VGCCs cause a prolonged excitatory state by increasing intracellular Ca^{2+} in response to an action potential. VGCC activation causes release of substance P and CGRP which are potent mediators of pain.

Dorsal horn pain mechanisms

The primary afferents terminate in the dorsal horn of the spinal cord. Most nociceptive thinly myelinated A-delta fibres end in laminae I and V whereas the unmyelinated nociceptive C fibres terminate superficially in the outer laminae 1 and II, the underlying substantia gelatinosa, with a smaller number reaching the deeper lamina V as well. The large tactile A-beta fibres terminate in deeper laminae and predominantly innervate laminae III–VI. The primary role of peripheral fibres was proposed by Melzack and Wall[15] (1965) in their *'gate control theory of pain'*. According to the gate control theory, central transmission (T) cells are present in the spinal cord that transmits pain to higher centres via brainstem and thalamus to the cortex for perception. Peripheral trauma activates A-delta and C fibres and their impulses excite central transmission T cells. Central transmission cells also receive input from large A-beta mechanoreceptors and their simultaneous stimulation closes the gate on T cells, which is opened by nociceptive stimuli from A-delta and C fibres, thus causing inhibition of ascending nociception. Le Bars et al.[16] described a similar inhibitory system triggered by noxious (not innocuous) stimulation which is activated by the stimulation of A-delta and C fibres, termed diffuse noxious inhibitory controls or DNIC. Riley et al.[17] described the basic principle of DNIC as 'pain inhibition by pain' and coined the term 'conditioned pain modulation' (CPM).

Therefore the modulation of nociceptive information, i.e. the facilitation of pain and descending inhibition, takes place in the dorsal horn.

Ascending pathways

The spinothalamic tract (STT) is considered the most important pain projection pathway in the system.[18] Laminae I and V neurons provides cells of origin of STT and the majority of STT fibres cross over near their spinal levels of origin.

There are two main divisions of the spinothalamic tract (neospinothalmic and paleospinothalamic). The neospinothalamic tract is also referred to as the lateral STT and transmits distinct information regarding location, intensity, and duration of noxious stimuli. It projects to the posterior nuclei of the thalamus. The paleospinothalamic tract forms the medial portion of the pathway and projects to the medial thalamic nuclei. It is concerned with the autonomic and unpleasant emotional aspects of pain.

The spinoreticular tract produces arousal associated with pain perception and mediates motivational, affective and autonomic responses to pain.

The spinomesencephalic tract projects to the midbrain reticular formation and evokes non-discriminative painful sensation. This tract may be important in the activation of descending anti-nociception processes.

The spinocervical tract is located in the dorsolateral funiculus and its fibres ascend uncrossed to the lateral cervical nucleus, a fibre relay to the contralateral thalamus.

The dorsal columns are mainly associated with carrying non-painful sensation nevertheless some fibres are responsive to noxious stimuli. Large A-beta fibres travel in this pathway.

The nociceptive information carried by small myelinated and unmyelinated fibres is processed in the dorsal horn before its further relay to the higher centres. The dorsal horn is a seat of complex interactions where the peripheral high-threshold sensory fibres interact with the local intrinsic spinal interneurons and descending fibres from the brain. There are two main classes of neurons activated by these peripheral fibres, i.e. nociceptive specific (NS) and multi-receptive wide dynamic range (WDR) neurons. NS cells are mostly found superficially and synapse with A-delta and C fibres only. The NS or high threshold neurons are activated exclusively by noxious stimuli and fire action potentials when a painful stimulus is detected at the periphery. The multi-receptive, convergent or WDR neurons are located in the deeper laminae of the dorsal horn. These neurons respond to nociceptive as well as non-nociceptive input and their firing increases with an increase in intensity of the stimulus. WDR activity is generated by nociceptive input and transferred after processing in the dorsal horn, directly or via brainstem relay nuclei to the thalamus and onto the cortex.[19] Simultaneously, parallel outputs from the dorsal horn reach ventral horn to activate flexor motor neurons to initiate 'withdrawal flexion reflex' hence both the sensation of physiological pain and the flexion withdrawal reflex occur together.[20]

WDR neurons receive input from all three types of sensory fibres, and therefore respond to the full range of stimulation, from light touch to noxious pinch, heat, and chemicals. WDR neurons fire action potentials in a graded fashion depending on stimulus intensity, and also exhibit 'wind-up', a short-lasting form of synaptic plasticity.

Central sensitization and neuroplasticity

The increase in excitability of spinal neurons after peripheral injury is termed central sensitization. The arrival of nociceptive information from tissue or nerve injury, which is acute, continuous, and persistent, results in the release of excitatory amino acids, *glutamate* and *aspartate* from the nociceptive central terminals. Glutamate causes alpha-amino-5-hydroxy-5-methyl-4-isoxazole propionic acid (AMPA) receptor activation to initiate a baseline response in the dorsal horn to noxious and tactile stimuli akin to physiological processing of sensory information. Repetitive high-frequency C fibres stimulation activates N-methyl-D-aspartate (NMDA) receptors, which would not have been activated under normal physiological conditions. NMDA receptors are normally blocked (plugged) by magnesium (Mg^{2+}) ion to prevent depolarization and activation. Sodium influx at AMPA receptors removes the Mg^{2+} block by membrane depolarization and allows channels to open. The loss of Mg^{2+} block with eventual entry of calcium into the cell results in immediate early gene induction (IEG—c *fos* and c-*jun*),[21] activation of protein kinase C (PKC) and protein tyrosine kinases (PTKs) which phosphorylates the NMDA receptor to produce medium or long-term changes. NMDA receptor involvement induces and maintains a state of *central sensitization* and *secondary hyperalgesia*.

If this stage is not treated effectively, long-term morphological and chemical changes will occur with structural reorganization, sprouting, expansion of receptive fields, and neuronal cross talking and results in the development of memory of pain (plasticity).[10]

Dorsal horn inhibition (modulation) of pain

According to Melzack and Wall's gate control theory, the first inhibitory system exists within the peripheral afferent fibres. A-delta and C fibres relay nociceptive information to the dorsal horn and the peripheral co-stimulation or co-activation of large A-beta fibres blocks it at the spinal (transmission cells) level. The closure of the pain gate by A-beta fibres may be temporary until the stimulus becomes intense and persistent, resulting in loss of inhibition. The nociceptive information released ascends to the supraspinal level to activate descending inhibitory and modulatory systems. However, the second line of defence against nociception is the release of inhibitory neurotransmitters GABA (gamma-amino-butyric-acid) and glycine and the activation of opioid and alpha-adrenoceptors in the dorsal horn. The inhibitory neurotransmitters, GABA and glycine decrease the response of NS and WDR cells, thus influencing the output of the dorsal horn.

GABA and glycine cause tonic inhibition of nociceptive input in the dorsal horn. $GABA_A$ receptors mediate postsynaptic inhibition while $GABA_B$ presynaptically inhibits excitatory amino acids in the dorsal horn. GABA agonists work at the chloride channel to cause hyperpolarization of the membrane and have a 'calming effect' on the membrane potential. Along with several other contributors, the loss of GABA inhibitory control also contributes to the development of *allodynic* pain.

In response to peripheral injury and inflammation and as a result of stress and immune responses, opioid peptides including B-endorphin, met-enkephalin, dynorphin, and endomorphins are released at the site of the injury and into the circulation. Opioid peptides bind to the opioid receptors which are expressed in dorsal root ganglia and transported intra-axonally to the peripheral nerve terminals. In the spinal dorsal horn, opioid receptors are present at both presynaptic and postsynaptic locations. Activation of the presynaptic receptors inhibits the release of 'algogenic' excitatory neurotransmitters including substance P. The postsynaptic opioid receptors mediated activation of potassium channels causes hyperpolarization of WDR and NS neurons. However, the opioid receptor sensitivity is severely affected in neuropathic pain and therefore opioid's effective use seems to be limited in chronic persistent pain. Prolonged use of exogenous opioids may also interfere with the opioid receptor mechanism and may cause hyperalgesia, which is secondary to NMDA receptor activation.[5]

The descending inhibitory modulatory system produces analgesia by activating presynaptic alpha adrenoceptors and endogenous release of noradrenaline in the dorsal horn. The opioid and alpha adrenoceptor agonists work synergistically. Clonidine, an alpha agonist drug, produces analgesia on spinal administration. Additionally, adenosine receptors also modulate dorsal horn nociceptive processing.

Descending inhibition or modulation

The peripheral fibres organization in the dorsal horn and their ascending route to supra spinal structures were discussed earlier (see 'Ascending pathways'). The second-order neurons from the dorsal horn ascend and terminate in brainstem, thalamus, and the cortex. The main ascending nociceptive pathways are spinothalamic and spinoreticular pathways. The descending pain modulatory fibres arise from the rostral ventromedial medulla (RVM) and projects to the spinal dorsal horn. They possess both excitatory and inhibitory characteristics. The main supraspinal areas involved in anti-nociception and pain modulation are the hypothalamus, periaqueductal grey (PAG) matter (opioids), the locus coeruleus (noradrenaline), the nucleus raphe magnus (serotonin/GABA), and the nucleus reticularis paragigantocellularis lateralis (serotonin). They travel down via dorsolateral funiculus to the spinal cord. The nociceptive information relay to the earlier mentioned supraspinal regions and nuclei results in their stimulation and subsequent release of specific inhibitory neurotransmitters at various levels to modulate pain at the dorsal horn.

Cortex role in pain perception and expression

Nociception has also been defined as the detection of noxious stimuli and its subsequent transmission of encoded information to the brain and the *pain* being a *perceptual process* that arises as a result of such activity.[6] The cortical contribution in pain perception and modulation provides the basis for several non-drug therapies and treatments for managing complex pains. Those include TENS, acupuncture, behaviour modification and the motivational strategies. The higher cortical centres have controls of perceptual (somatosensory) and affective (cingulate cortex) components of pain processing, perception and expression. Noxious, painful stimulus results in activation of sensory, motor, premotor, parietal, frontal, occipital, insular, and anterior cingulate regions of the cortex.[5] The limbic system controls the motivational and behavioural responses while frontal cortex has strong perceptual controlling mechanisms. The pain perception, pain expression and the pain behaviour all rely on cortical integration. Pain as opposed to nociception, is created in the brain.[22]

Neuroanatomical, physiological, and functional changes in pain mechanisms in elderly

Gagliese and Farrell[9] described in detail the effects of ageing on neuroanatomy, variations in peripheral inflammatory mediator release and responses, perturbed central neurotransmitter release, and altered facilitatory and inhibitory modulatory functions.

The neurobiology of ageing has a considerable influence over nociception, anti-nociception, and pain under normal physiological conditions.[9] Ageing does affect pain processing with demonstrable non-uniform morphological and biochemical changes throughout the peripheral and central nervous system. The peripheral nerves of both animals and humans, notably and selectively, lose myelinated fibres with signs of spontaneous axonal damage and wallerian degeneration.

There are three models of age-related changes in pain prevalence which influences pain mechanisms at different stages in life. Anderson et al.[23] described the first model as an increase in pain with increasing age until the 6th decade with primary aetiology of mechanical and occupational origin. The second model is of degenerative disease processes which apparently occur after

normal working age or post retirement. The third model is age independent and includes chest pain, back pain, stomach aches, and headaches, which do not necessarily have mechanical component aetiology.

Later in life, it may be the alterations in neurophysiology,[24,25] dementia, lack of pain reporting, and stoicism[26] altered perception of pain or neuroanatomical changes in nociceptors which may result in the reduced reporting of pain in older people.

Chakour et al.[24] reported a reduction in A-delta fibre numbers in elderly people, which becomes apparent in later life because of its diminished contribution in pain transmission. The loss of A-delta fibres leads to recruitment of C nociceptive fibres. This, along with continued peripheral stimulation, results in the late transmission of pain sensation with a poor reaction time in elderly population. This phenomenon contributes to the development of chronic pain in the elderly.

Gagliese and Farrell[9] reviewed animal and human experimental literature on ageing effects in pain. Ageing results in diminished levels of neuropeptides, substance P, CGRP, and somatostatin in the dorsal horn along with low levels of the inhibitory neurotransmitters, 5HT, and noradrenaline which reflects an impaired peripheral and spinal descending inhibitory (modulatory) mechanism. The concentration of opioid receptors in cortex, striatum, and hypothalamus decreases with age with decreased levels of circulating B-endorphins in elderly population.

The NMDA receptor function and binding also decline with age in animal studies.[9] The reversal of centrally mediated sensitization in older adults also suggests decrements in the effectiveness of endogenous inhibitory processes. This would also be consistent with an age-related decrease in pain tolerance. Recently it has been suggested that age-related changes in pain perception are not significant, but that pain tolerance does change and declines with advancing age.[2]

The integrated homeostatic body systems that include endocrine, immune, and autonomic nervous systems are also affected by age, and when combined with changes and alterations in inflammatory responses, oxidative stress, and cell death contribute to the development of persistent pain in elderly.[2] The cellular and molecular mechanisms responsible for ageing and pain provide evidence that the induction and maintenance of chronic pain depends on the integrated function of the sympathetic and parasympathetic nervous systems along with coordinated interaction with the hypothalamic–pituitary–adrenal axis.[2] Therefore, the tissue injury or nerve damage is responsible for a perturbed autonomic nervous system which is involved in the generation of sympathetically maintained pain, complex regional pain syndromes, persistent pain, and neuralgias in elderly populations.

It has been suggested that there are deficits in endogenous pain inhibition (spinal and supraspinal) in older humans. The failure of DNIC system in elderly population shows as an increase in thermal pain ratings during noxious cold stimulation and unmasks a net facilitatory effect of noxious stimuli when compared to younger subjects.[2]

Elderly adults who are cognitively impaired may also have difficulty modulating pain stimuli simply because the cortical centres responsible for cognitive processing and activation of descending pain modulating systems are compromised in older adults resulting in the loss of descending pain-modulation.

Conclusion

Pain in the elderly remains a complex issue and full understanding requires a holistic approach towards understanding pain with ageing process. Pain in the elderly means a dynamic and intertwined relationship of an 'aged' anatomy of pain transmission, with declining physiological functions, involving physicochemical process with compromised coping mechanisms. Although in the elderly the initiation, aggravation, maintenance, excitation, and inhibition at the spinal cord level and descending modulation of pain occur in a similar way to younger people the functional, biological, and psychological responses may not be the same.

References

1. NIA, NIH. Workshop Executive Summary 2008. <http://painconsortium.nih.gov> (accessed 22 January 2013).
2. Yezierski RP. Pain and aging research: what's on the horizon? *IASP Newsletter*. 2011;July.
3. Loeser JD. Pain and suffering. *Clin J Pain*. 2000;16(2):S2–S6.
4. International Association for the Study of Pain. *IASP taxonomy*. <http://www.iasp-pain.org/Content/NavigationMenu/GeneralResource Links/PainDefinitions/default.htm>.
5. Siddall PJ, Cousins MJ. Physiology of pain. In Power I, Kam, P (eds) *Principles of physiology for the anaesthetists*, 2nd edn (pp. 381–398). London: Hodder Arnold, 2008.
6. Kidd BL, Urban LA. Mechanisms of inflammatory pain. *Br J Anaesth*. 2001;87(1):3–11.
7. Dray A. Inflammatory mediators of pain. *Br J Anaesth*. 1995;75:125–131.
8. Woolf CJ. Somatic pain-pathogenesis and prevention. *Br J Anaesth*. 1995;75:169–176.
9. Gagliese L, Farrell MJ. The neurobiology of aging, nociception, and pain: an integration of animal and human experimental evidence. In Gibson SJ, Weiner DK (eds) *Pain in older persons. Progress in pain research and management*, Vol. 35 (pp. 25–44). Seattle, WA: IASP Press, 2005.
10. Woolf CJ, Max MB. Mechanism-based pain diagnosis. *Anesthesiology*. 2001;95:241–249.
11. Simone DA, Alrejo M, LaMotte RM. Psychophysical studies of the itch sensation and itchy skin ('allokenis') produced by intracutaneous injection of histamine. *Somatosens Motor Res*. 1991;8:271–279.
12. Burnstock G, Wood JN. Purinergic receptors: their role in nociception and primary afferent neurotransmission. *Curr Opin Neurobiol*. 1996;6:526–532.
13. Gold MS, Reichling DB, Shuster MJ, Levine JD. Hyperalgesic agents increase a tetrodotoxin-resistant Na⁺ current in nociceptors. *Proc Natl Acad Sci USA* 1996; 93: 1108–1112.
14. England S, Bevan SJ, Docherty RJ. Prostaglandin E2 modulates the tetrodotoxin-resistant sodium current in neonatal rat dorsal root ganglion neurones via the cyclic AMP-protein kinase A cascade. *J Physiol*. 1996;495:429–440.
15. Melzack R, Wall PD. Pain mechanisms: a new theory. *Science*. 1965;150:971–979.
16. Le Bars D, Dickenson AH, Besson JM. Diffuse noxious inhibitory controls (DNIC). Effects on dorsal horn convergent neurones in the rat. *Pain*. 1979;6:283–304.
17. Riley JL, King CD, Wongb F, Fillingim RB, Mauderli AP. Lack of endogenous modulation and reduced decay of prolonged heat pain in older adults. *Pain*. 2010;150:153–160.
18. Abram SE. Pain pathways and mechanisms. In Abram SE, Haddox JD (eds) *Pain Clinic Manual*, 2nd edn (pp. 13–20). Philadelphia, PA: Lippincott Williams & Wilkins, 2000.
19. Willis WD, Coggeshall RE. *Sensory mechanisms of the spinal cord*. New York: Plenum Press, 1991.
20. Willer JC. Comparative study of perceived pain and nociceptive flexion reflex in man. *Pain*. 1979;3:69–80.
21. Munglani R, Hunt SP. Molecular biology of pain. *Br J Anaesth*. 1995;75:186–192.
22. Melzack R. Gate control theory: on the evolution of pain concepts. *Pain Forum*. 1996;5:128–138.
23. Anderson HI, Ejlertsson G, Leden I, Rosenberg C. Chronic pain in a geographically defined population; studies of differences in age, gender, social class, and pain localization. *Clin J Pain*. 1993;9(3):174–182.
24. Chakour MC, Gibson SJ, Bradbeer M, Helme RD. The effect of age on A delta and C- fibre thermal pain perception. *Pain*. 1996;64(1):143–152.
25. Gibson SJ, Farrell M. A review of age differences in the neurophysiology of nociception and the perceptual experience of pain. *Clin J Pain*. 2004;20(4):227–239.
26. Helme RD, Gibson SJ. Pain in older people. In Crombie IK, Croft PR, Linton SJ, Le Resche L, Von Korff M (eds) *Epidemiology of Pain* (pp. 103–112). Seattle, WA: IASP Press, 1999.

PART 3

Applied Science and Diseases of the Elderly

CHAPTER 12

Neurological disorders in the elderly

Anand Prakash and Kailash Krishnan

Introduction

With an increase in age expectancy, older persons are more vulnerable to chronic conditions including brain dysfunction with manifestations of progressive cognitive decline and behavioural disturbance. This chapter will describe in brief the important and common neurological conditions in older people.

Dementia

The commonest syndrome is dementia, characterized by impairment of at least two cognitive functions including short-term and long-term memory, language, judgement, and abstract thinking. The greatest risk factor is age but diabetes, hypertension, stroke, traumatic head injury, and a low formal level of education are also associated risk factors.

Alzheimer's dementia

Alzheimer's dementia (AD) is the commonest type of dementia and affects nearly half a million people in the UK. Nearly 400 000 people have Alzheimer's disease in England and Wales. Incidence generally begins in the seventh decade of life and is estimated to be 4.9 per 1000 person-years and doubles with every 5 years afterwards. Prevalence is estimated at 40 per cent in persons aged 85 and above. Mean time from onset of symptoms to diagnosis is between 2 and 3 years.

The known risk factors are age, smoking, female sex (African American and Hispanic descent), trisomy 21, family history of the disease, and presence of the epsilon 4 allele (especially in homozygotes) of the apolipoprotein E (APOE) gene on chromosome 19.[1,2]

Cerebral atrophy occurs especially in the temporal and parietal lobes. Loss of cholinergic neurons occurs in the nucleus basalis of Meynert and serotonergic cells of the raphe nuclei. This may correlate with lack of attention and higher-order cognitive processing. Abnormal accumulation of extracellular amyloid protein due to defective proteolytic processing of the amyloid precursor protein and intracellular microtubular-associated hyperphosphorylated tau proteins[3] are considered as hallmark events in the pathogenesis.[4] These are visualized in large numbers (in comparison to normal older people) as plaques and neurofibrillary tangles using a modified silver stain and seen predominantly in the hippocampus and the neocortex.[5,6]

Memory impairment is often the first presenting sign and is mandatory for diagnosis.[1,2] Impairment of constructional skills and naming can also be affected during the early stages. Mild dementia often involves memory and language impairment[7] whereas behavioural abnormalities including nocturnal agitation and wandering occur in moderate disease. Psychiatric manifestations of anxiety, depression, delusions, florid psychosis, and hallucinations may occur and are difficult for family and carers to manage. All intellectual faculties are impaired as the condition progresses and death is usually due to pneumonia or coexisting medical illness. Essentially, the diagnosis is clinical and aided by neuropsychological tests. The clinical criteria for diagnosis was proposed by the *Diagnostic and Statistical Manual of Mental Disorders*, fourth edition (DSM-5), National Institute of Neurological and Communicative Disorders and Stroke and the Alzheimer's Disease and Related Disorders Association (NINCDS-ADRDA) in 1984 and revised earlier this year.[1,2] Positron emission tomography and single-photon emission computed tomography (SPECT) images analyse glucose metabolism and are useful in differentiating dementia subtypes.

Frontotemporal dementia

Frontotemporal dementia (FTD) is a syndrome which includes Pick's disease, semantic dementia, and progressive non-fluent aphasia.[8] Approximately 40 per cent of patients have a family history of depression and less than 10 per cent are inherited. An autosomal dominant mode of inheritance occurs through mutations in the microtubule-associated tau protein (MAPT) or progranulin gene, both on chromosome 17.

The most important clinical characteristics are changes in personal character, social behaviour, lack of insight, early emotional blunting, and loss of speech output. Visuospatial skills, calculation, and memory are preserved in the early stages.[9] Progressive fluent aphasia, inability to comprehend word meaning, anomia, and speech devoid of content are noted.[8] Primitive signs of sucking, grasp, and pout reflexes occur early in FTD.[10]

Vascular dementia

The onset of vascular dementia (VaD) is usually within 3 months of a stroke and prevalence is from 11 to 20 per cent. Risk factors include increasing age, male sex, diabetes mellitus, hypertension, smoking, cardiac disease, a low level of formal education, and family history.[11] Interestingly the presence of APOE epsilon 4 increases the risk of VaD and pathological studies have reported overlap between AD and VaD. Small vessel disease can cause subcortical syndromes of senile leucoencephalopathy and lacunar states or affect the frontal lobes.[12,13] In Biswanger's disease there is extensive white matter ischaemic injury to the cerebral hemispheres.

Dementia with Lewy bodies

Dementia with Lewy bodies (DLB) is the second most common variety of degenerative dementia. DLB, Parkinson's disease (PD), multisystem atrophy, pure autonomic failure, rapid eye movement (REM) sleep behaviour disorder, and Hallervorden–Spatz disease may all belong to a spectrum of disorders called synucleinopathies. The hallmark of these disorders is Lewy bodies and Lewy neuritis which contain fibrillary aggregates of alpha synuclein protein. In PD such inclusions are present in the brainstem whereas in DLB they are present in the brainstem, neocortex, and limbic system. There may be concurrent AD pathology. In DLB there is a reduction in cholinergic transmission from the basal forebrain and brainstem nuclei.

Clinical manifestations include cortical and subcortical features of fluctuations in cognition but preserved memory in the early stages, recurrent visual hallucinations, features of parkinsonism, marked postural instability leading to falls, and extreme neuroleptic sensitivity. Other features may include autonomic dysfunction, REM sleep disorders, delusions, hallucinations, and depression. Neuroimaging reveals white matter changes similar to AD, but preserved temporal lobe and hippocampus.

Corticobasal degeneration

Corticobasal degeneration is a tauopathy (a class of neurodegenerative disease) mainly affecting the frontal and parietal lobes and substantia nigra. It may overlap with FTD or AD. Clinical features are unique involving cortical and subcortical structures presenting with executive dysfunction, visuospatial disturbances, difficulties in memory retrieval, and progressive non-fluent aphasia.

Parkinson's disease dementia

Cognitive impairment may be a non-motor manifestation of PD[14] and is a significant determinant of neuropsychiatric manifestations.[15,16]

Risk factors for dementia in PD are old age, duration of PD, presence of akinetic rigid profile, and depression.[17] Parkinson's disease dementia (PDD) could be considered as an extended spectrum of synucleinopathies with early manifestations of impaired executive function, attention, visuospatial, and visuoperceptive problems (such as drawing figures, identifying television personalities). These patients use verbal switching less effectively but more effective semantic clustering in comparison to Alzheimer's disease. Excessive daytime sleepiness and REM sleep disorder are common.[18]

Progressive supranuclear palsy, spinocerebellar degeneration, Wilson's disease, and striatonigral degeneration exhibit combinations of parkinsonism, ataxia, chorea, and ophthalmoplegia.[19–23] The parkinsonism dementia complex of Guam is characterized by dementia of Alzheimer's type, PD, and amyotrophic lateral sclerosis.

Prion disease

These are a group of rare, invariably fatal, neurodegenerative disorders (spongiform encephalopathies) with prolonged incubation periods affecting humans and animals. These include Creutzfeldt–Jakob disease (CJD), Kuru, fatal and sporadic familial insomnia, and Gerstmann–Straussler–Scheinker disease.

CJD is the commonest human prion disease (80 per cent). Disease acquisition may be sporadic, familial, iatrogenic, or variant. The commonest variety is sporadic. CJD is characterized by a rapidly progressive dementia associated with myoclonic jerks with variable pyramidal, extrapyramidal, and cerebellar signs. Though some overlap exists amongst the two, neuropsychiatric manifestations (depression, anxiety, apathy, depression) occur early in variant CJD.

Drug-induced dementia

Psychotropics, anticholinergics, anticonvulsants, and cardiac drugs are associated with dementia syndromes. Alcohol abuse can lead to cognition decline and neuropsychiatric symptoms. Prefrontal and frontal damage occur due to long-term alcohol abuse leading to memory loss and executive dysfunction. Other areas affected are the hypothalamus, cerebellum, and white matter. Heavy metals such as lead, arsenic, manganese, or mercury are unusual causes of dementia in the elderly. A recent study suggested that iron deposition could lead to disruption of white matter in AD and abnormal accumulation of iron, copper, and zinc lead to oxidative stress and macromolecular damage.

Chronic infections

Chronic meningitis due to bacterial (tuberculosis, Whipple's disease), parasitic (malaria, cysticercosis, toxoplasmosis), or fungal (*Histoplasma, Cryptococcus, Candida, Coccidioides, Aspergillus*) organisms can lead to dementia syndrome with cranial nerve deficits. Syphilis can cause dementia either by chronic meningitis or meningovascular syphilis. Diagnosis is by laboratory examination and examination of the cerebrospinal fluid (CSF).

Other systemic illnesses

Other systemic illnesses that could cause dementia syndromes include cardiac failure, pulmonary failure, uraemia, and hepatic encephalopathy. Dysfunction of thyroid, parathyroid, and adrenals are also known causes. Vitamin B_{12} deficiency is a rare cause of dementia. Temporal arteritis and vasculitis are unusual causes. Neoplasms both intrinsic and metastatic especially involving the frontal lobe can present with dementia. Traumatic brain injuries leading to subdural and extradural haematomas or obstructive hydrocephalus can produce dementia syndromes.

The treatment goals include management of cognitive and behaviour symptoms with the aim to improve overall functioning, education, training, support, and counselling of carers. The treatment for cognitive symptoms of dementia is limited. The drugs used in treatment at present belong to either of two categories: acetyl cholinesterase inhibitors (donepezil, galantamine, and rivastigmine) and NMDA (N-methyl D-aspartate) receptor antagonist memantine.[2]

Risk factor management especially regarding hypertension (as revealed by the European Systolic Hypertension trial) reduces white matter damage in VaD. Not much evidence exists for the use of lipid lowering therapy.

Atypical and typical neuroleptics, antidepressants, mood stabilizers, and benzodiazepines have all been used in management of behaviour symptoms.[1,2] Neuroleptics should be avoided in DLB due to extreme sensitivity. In addition to pharmacotherapy, the non-pharmacological management of patients with behavioural disturbance may include speech therapy, retraining, and rehabilitation.

Stroke

The World Health Organization definition of stroke is 'the clinical syndrome of rapid onset of focal cerebral deficit, lasting more than 24 hours or leading to death, with no apparent cause other than a vascular one'. It can be classified into two categories: ischaemia due to thrombosis or arterial embolism and haemorrhage. The incidence increases with age with the risk doubling for both men and women for each successive decade after 55. Up to age 75 men have more strokes and related deaths compared to women with a reversal afterwards. Each year in England, approximately 110 000 people have a first or recurrent stroke and a further 20 000 people have a transient ischaemic attack (TIA). TIA is a focal loss of neurological function due to temporary ischaemia lasting up to 24 hours.[24,25] Modern imaging reveals that deficits lasting more than an hour are due to irreversible cortical infarcts.[26,27]

Risk factors include age, male sex, smoking, alcohol abuse, obesity, hypertension, diabetes, hyperlipidaemia, cardiac diseases (myocardial infarction, atrial fibrillation, left ventricular hypertrophy), peripheral vascular disease, previous TIA/stroke, and family history.[13,28]

Hypertension is the leading risk factor for both ischaemic and haemorrhagic stroke with nearly two-thirds of global stroke burden due to suboptimal control.[11] Antihypertensive therapy reduces the risk of stroke by more than 30 per cent. It remains unclear as to what would be an optimal range for the over 80 age group.[29,30]

Atrial fibrillation (AF) is the commonest arrhythmia in the elderly with prevalence increasing from 0.1 per cent in those younger than 55 to 10 per cent in people older than 80. It is an independent risk factor for stroke with the relative risk increased by 5 per cent. Strokes that occur due to AF cause more neurological disability. Patients with type 2 diabetes mellitus have at least a two-fold risk in increased risk of stroke and this is further increased by smoking, hypertension, and atrial fibrillation. The CHADS$_2$[31] and CHA$_2$DS$_2$VASc scoring system is a useful tool in predicting risk factor of stroke with non-rheumatic atrial fibrillation.[32,33] Unless there is a significant contraindication, anticoagulation is the preferred treatment in the elderly in preventing stroke.

A major risk factor for the elderly due to atherosclerosis is symptoms due to a stenotic carotid lesion greater than 50 per cent. The risk of stroke in these patients is 20–30 per cent. Carotid endarterectomy (CEA) is beneficial for symptomatic patients with recent non-disabling carotid artery ischaemic events and ipsilateral 70 per cent to 99 per cent carotid artery stenosis. Carotid stenting can be considered in patients who are medically unwell for CEA, high level stenosis or risk of stenosis is high after CEA.[34,35]

Ischaemic stroke

Ischaemic stroke accounts for nearly 80 per cent of all strokes. Causes of ischaemic stroke in the elderly include atheromatous disease, lacunar infarction, cardiac embolism secondary to AF, mural thrombus in the left ventricle, bacterial endocarditis, prosthetic valve thrombosis, coronary artery bypass graft or coronary angiography, mitral or aortic valve repair, cardiac arrest, hyperviscosity states, and syphilis. The commonly used Bamford classification helps to localize stroke lesions on clinical findings and aids to identify pathology and prognosis.

Stroke 'mimics'

Stroke 'mimics' are common conditions which may present like a stroke and include metabolic disturbances including hypo- and hypernatremia, hypo- and hyperglycaemia; seizures; and other central nervous system disorders including subdural haematoma, brain abscess, primary brain tumour, migraine, previous stroke with a residual deficit, and sometimes functional disorders.

Cerebral computed tomography (CT) and magnetic resonance imaging (MRI) are indicated for localizing the vascular territory of infarcts and distinguishing from haemorrhage.[36] Some patients with transient or even persisting neurological symptoms may have a normal CT scan. Magnetic resonance angiography and spiral CT scans are used in imaging intra- and extracranial arteries. B-mode ultrasound and Doppler are used to quantify severity of disease in the internal carotid and vertebral artery.

The initial management of a patient with stroke involves stabilization of the airway and adequate oxygen therapy. Full blood count, urea, electrolytes, coagulation screen, and an electrocardiogram are considered routine. Urgent CT of head is performed to rule out haemorrhage or for signs of early ischaemic change. Blood pressure is usually monitored closely. Thrombolysis with intravenous tissue plasminogen activator has been effective in improving functional outcomes following an acute ischaemic stroke.[37] New methods of catheter-based thrombolysis and clot retrieval measures and devices are being evaluated.

Haemorrhagic stroke

These include subarachnoid (SAH) and intracerebral haemorrhage (ICH). SAH accounts for about 8 per cent of all strokes. CT scan is the test of choice in diagnosis and identifying source of haemorrhage with sensitivity of 90 per cent in the first 24 hours. If in doubt, lumbar puncture should be performed and the CSF is analysed using spectrophotometry to check for xanthochromia. Cerebral angiography is indicated to detect any underlying aneurysm and identify the size and location.

ICH occurs at least twice as commonly as SAH, with age and hypertension being the most important risk factors. Trauma, underlying coagulopathy, and amyloid angiopathy are other recognized risk factors. The typical presentation is focal neurological deficit that progresses over minutes to hours with accompanying headache, nausea, vomiting, decreased consciousness, and elevated blood pressure.[38,39] Seizures (6–7 per cent) are more common in lobar haemorrhage. It rarely occurs during sleep. CT is the imaging of choice and MRI is equally effective in detecting haemorrhage. The prognosis of ICH is worse than ischaemic stroke with 30-day mortality of 40 per cent as compared to 20 per cent.[40]

Epilepsy in the elderly

Epilepsy is the third commonest neurological diagnosis with a major psychosocial and economic burden on older people and society.[41] Seizures and epilepsy in this population are much more common than is often realized. The prevalence of epilepsy increases with age and is greatest in patients older than 75 years. The diagnosis of epilepsy in the elderly is challenging and misdiagnosis can occur in up to 30 per cent of cases.[42] There may be lack of aura, automatisms, and rarely transition from focal to generalization. Intermittent confusional episodes or light headedness, dizziness, and cramps could be clinical manifestations. Status epilepticus is more common compared to the young. The causes of late-onset epilepsy are cerebrovascular disease[43] (most common cause), neurodegenerative disorders, trauma, and brain tumours. Seizure risk increases up to 20-fold in the first year following a stroke and is more common in the haemorrhagic variety.

Seizure 'mimics'

Seizure mimics can happen during syncope, TIA, transient global amnesia, cardiac arrhythmia, drop attacks, hypoglycaemia, panic attacks, cataplexy associated with narcolepsy, migraine, and sleep disorders.

The most reliable method of diagnosis is an accurate history.[44] It is important to investigate for metabolic disturbances, side effects of drugs and withdrawal, and substance abuse. Epilepsy protocol MRI is the imaging of choice and is indicated in patients with refractory partial seizures or tumours.[45] A normal electroencephalogram (EEG) does not rule epilepsy.[42] If in doubt, a video EEG or inpatient monitoring is recommended.[45,46]

There is lack of data in terms of effective seizure control with antiepileptic drugs (AEDs) in the elderly. Factors to be taken into consideration are age-related physiological changes in the nervous system, other comorbidities, and age-related decrease in hepatic blood flow and glomerular filtration rate, drug interactions, and pharmacokinetics, compliance, and nutritional state may influence absorption or promote drug toxicity. The principles of treatment are seizure control with minimal side effects.[47] Lamotrigine and gabapentin are the drugs of choice in partial seizures. Lamotrigine, sodium valproate,[48,49] levetiracetam, and topiramate are recommended for generalized seizures (International League against Epilepsy guidelines).[47,50] Levetiracetam has been suggested for the treatment of status epilepticus in elderly people when comorbidity and respiratory insufficiency does not permit the use of benzodiazepines or phenytoin.

Parkinson's disease and parkinsonism

Parkinsonism is a broad term to describe any of two or more of akinesia, rigidity, resting tremor,[51] and postural instability. It includes PD and other neurodegenerative disorders.[52]

Idiopathic PD is a clinicopathological correlate with levodopa responsive parkinsonism, loss of dopaminergic pigmented neurons especially in the ventrolateral and ventromedial nuclei of the substantia nigra, and Lewy body inclusions. The motor manifestations tend to occur when 60 per cent or more of the dopaminergic reserve is depleted.[15,53] PD is typically an asymmetric disease and initial symptoms may include loss of dexterity on fine tasks of fingers, tremor, and generalized slowing down. Akinesia or bradykinesia is essential for diagnosis. Other features may include micrographia, mask-like face, reduced blink rate, soft and monotonous speech, drooling of saliva, and lead pipe rigidity. Resting tremor is common

in both PD and drug-induced parkinsonism and occurs in the thumb and index finger in a pill rolling fashion of frequency 4–5 Hz. PD is unilateral in the beginning but in later stages of disease spreads to the contralateral side.

The parkinsonian patient develops a simian posture with flexion of knees, elbows, wrists; trunk and metacarpophalangeal joints and inadequate defensive postural responses lead to propulsion, retropulsion, and falls. Episodes of freezing can occur during gait initiation, turning, or in front of an obstacle. Approximately 15–20 per cent of patients develop dementia. Non-motor manifestations of PD such as sialorrhoea, depression, apathy, drenching sweats, REM sleep behaviour disorder, urinary frequency and urgency, erectile dysfunction, anxiety, and pain can precede motor symptoms.[15,54–60]

Drugs associated with parkinsonism

Parkinsonism may be induced and be associated with the use of certain drugs such as neuroleptics (phenothiazines, butyrophenones, thioxanthenes), antihypertensive drugs (reserpine, alpha methyldopa, and verapamil), gastrointestinal drugs (antiemetic such as metoclopramide or prochlorperazine), and exposure to carbon monoxide or heavy metals such as cyanide, manganese, and mercury.

Neurodegenerative syndromes associated with parkinsonism

Certain neurodegenerative diseases such as multisystem atrophy, progressive supranuclear palsy, corticobasal ganglionic degeneration, Alzheimer's disease, CJD, and Huntington's disease may present with features of parkinsonism.

A commonly used scale for staging is the Modified Hoehn and Yahr staging and UPDRS (Unified Parkinson's Disease Rating Score). PD is primarily a clinical diagnosis. In cases of diagnostic uncertainty a dopamine transporter-SPECT scan be performed and if a structural lesion is suspected an MRI brain is indicated.

Levodopa is the mainstay of treatment in PD. Other treatment options are dopamine agonists including ergot derivatives (bromocriptine, pergolide, cabergoline) and non-ergots (pramipexole and ropinirole).[61–63] Catechol-O-methyl transferase inhibitors tolcapone and entacapone are used as second-line agents. Monoamine oxidase inhibitors (MAO-B) selegiline and rasagiline, anticholinergic agents such as benztropine and trihexiphenidyl are also used in treating tremor but are poorly tolerated in the elderly due to severe neuropsychiatric manifestations.

Apo-morphine is used as an infusion to treat severe motor fluctuations and on-off syndrome which hasn't responded to other medical therapy. The main side effects are sedation and vomiting.[6] Stereotactic neurosurgery with insertion of deep brain stimulators (DBS) following the principles of high-frequency electrostimulation in the ventral lateral nucleus of the thalamus is the procedure of choice in patients with failed medical therapy or late complications.[64–67] Internal pallidum (GPi) DBS is effective in treatment of dyskinesia in older patients.[67] DBS is, however, associated with a risk of intracerebral haemorrhage, infection, and mechanical failure.

Progressive supranuclear palsy

Progressive supranuclear palsy is a rapidly progressive tauopathy characterized by paresis of vertical gaze and later horizontal (hence the name), proximal axial muscle rigidity, loss of postural reflexes leading to falls, dysarthria, personality change with dementia, during the later stages.[19,21]

Normal pressure hydrocephalus

Normal pressure hydrocephalus is a triad of dementia, 'magnetic gait' or ataxia and urinary incontinence. CT and MRI reveal ventricular enlargement which is out of proportion to the sulci. It is important to recognize this as ventriculoperitoneal shunting may lead to marked improvement of symptoms.[68]

Spinal diseases in the elderly

Spinal disorders in the elderly include osteoarthritis and degenerative disc disease, degenerative deformities, trauma, infections, tumours, and inflammation. Spondylosis, osteoporosis, and malignancy are more common.

Degenerative disc disease, lumbar spinal stenosis, and lumbar spondylosis are also common disorders in the elderly. Nearly 60 per cent of cases of metastatic cause of spinal cord compression are due to breast, prostate, and lung cancer. Extramedullary spread is more common than intramedullary. Other malignant causes include renal cell carcinoma, myeloma, colonic carcinoma, and non-Hodgkin's lymphoma. Pain is the commonest symptom with weakness in up to 75 per cent of cases and sphincter involvement in 50 per cent of cases. X-rays of spine can reveal 'winkling owl sign' which is obliteration of the bony pedicle. MRI is the diagnostic investigation of choice. Treatment is tailored towards ameliorating symptoms and is an oncological emergency.

Conclusion

Neurological disorders are more common in older people and result in a loss of functional independence leading to institutionalization and an increase in carer burden, and have a major impact on society as a whole. Involvement of the appropriate speciality, early diagnosis, investigation, and multidisciplinary management is extremely important.

References

1. Waldemar G, Dubois B, Emre M, Scheltens P, Tariska P, Rossor M. Diagnosis and management of Alzheimer's disease and other disorders associated with dementia. The role of neurologists in Europe. European Federation of Neurological Societies. *Eur J Neurol.* 2000;7(2):133–144.
2. Waldemar G, Dubois B, Emre M, *et al.* Recommendations for the diagnosis and management of Alzheimer's disease and other disorders associated with dementia: EFNS guideline. *Eur J Neurol.* 2007;14(1):e1–e26.
3. Bostrom F, Hansson O, Blennow K, *et al.* Cerebrospinal fluid total tau is associated with shorter survival in dementia with Lewy bodies. *Dement Geriatr Cogn Disord.* 2009;28(4):314–319.
4. Lowenson JD, Roher AE, Clarke S. Protein aging extracellular amyloid formation and intracellular repair. *Trends Cardiovasc Med.* 1994;4(1):3–8.
5. Braak H, Braak E. Evolution of neuronal changes in the course of Alzheimer's disease. *J Neural Transm Suppl.* 1998;53:127–140.
6. Braak H, Braak E. Development of Alzheimer-related neurofibrillary changes in the neocortex inversely recapitulates cortical myelogenesis. *Acta Neuropathol.* 1996;92(2):197–201.
7. Mattsson N, Zetterberg H, Hansson O, *et al.* CSF biomarkers and incipient Alzheimer disease in patients with mild cognitive impairment. *JAMA.* 2009;302(4):385–393.
8. Seeley WW, Bauer AM, Miller BL, *et al.* The natural history of temporal variant frontotemporal dementia. *Neurology.* 2005;64(8):1384–1390.
9. Rohrer JD, Warren JD, Omar R, *et al.* Parietal lobe deficits in frontotemporal lobar degeneration caused by a mutation in the progranulin gene. *Arch Neurol.* 2008;65(4):506–513.
10. Rohrer JD, McNaught E, Foster J, *et al.* Tracking progression in frontotemporal lobar degeneration: serial MRI in semantic dementia. *Neurology.* 2008;71(18):1445–1451.
11. Sharp SI, Aarsland D, Day S, Sonnesyn H, Ballard C. Hypertension is a potential risk factor for vascular dementia: systematic review. *Int J Geriatr Psychiatry.* 2011;26(7):661–669.
12. O'Sullivan M, Jarosz JM, Martin RJ, Deasy N, Powell JF, Markus HS. MRI hyperintensities of the temporal lobe and external capsule in patients with CADASIL. *Neurology.* 2001;56(5):628–634.
13. Adib-Samii P, Brice G, Martin RJ, Markus HS. Clinical spectrum of CADASIL and the effect of cardiovascular risk factors on phenotype: study in 200 consecutively recruited individuals. *Stroke.* 2010;41(4):630–634.
14. Aarsland D, Bronnick K, Fladby T. Mild cognitive impairment in Parkinson's disease. *Curr Neurol Neurosci Rep.* 2011;11(4):371–378.
15. Chaudhuri KR, Schapira AH. Non-motor symptoms of Parkinson's disease: dopaminergic pathophysiology and treatment. *Lancet Neurol.* 2009;8(5):464–474.
16. Olin JT, Aarsland D, Meng X. Rivastigmine in the treatment of dementia associated with Parkinson's disease: effects on activities of daily living. *Dement Geriatr Cogn Disord.* 2010;29(6):510–515.
17. de Lau LM, Schipper CM, Hofman A, Koudstaal PJ, Breteler MM. Prognosis of Parkinson disease: risk of dementia and mortality: the Rotterdam Study. *Arch Neurol.* 2005;62(8):1265–1269.
18. Chaudhuri KR, Odin P. The challenge of non-motor symptoms in Parkinson's disease. *Prog Brain Res.* 2010;184:325–341.
19. Williams DR, de Silva R, Paviour DC, *et al.* Characteristics of two distinct clinical phenotypes in pathologically proven progressive supranuclear palsy: Richardson's syndrome and PSP-parkinsonism. *Brain.* 2005;128(Pt 6):1247–1258.
20. Williams DR, Holton JL, Strand C, *et al.* Pathological tau burden and distribution distinguishes progressive supranuclear palsy-parkinsonism from Richardson's syndrome. *Brain.* 2007;130(Pt 6):1566–1576.
21. Silveira-Moriyama L, Gonzalez AM, O'Sullivan SS, *et al.* Concomitant progressive supranuclear palsy and multiple system atrophy: more than a simple twist of fate? *Neurosci Lett.* 2009;467(3):208–211.
22. Wenning GK, Colosimo C, Geser F, Poewe W. Multiple system atrophy. *Lancet Neurol.* 2004;3(2):93–103.
23. Geser F, Seppi K, Stampfer-Kountchev M, *et al.* The European Multiple System Atrophy-Study Group (EMSA-SG). *J Neural Transm.* 2005;112(12):1677–1686.
24. Albers GW, Caplan LR, Easton JD, *et al.* Transient ischemic attack—proposal for a new definition. *N Engl J Med.* 2002;347(21):1713–1716.
25. Burn J, Dennis M, Bamford J, Sandercock P, Wade D, Warlow C. Long-term risk of recurrent stroke after a first-ever stroke. The Oxfordshire Community Stroke Project. *Stroke.* 1994;25(2):333–337.
26. Dennis M, Bamford J, Sandercock P, Molyneux A, Warlow C. Computed tomography in patients with transient ischaemic attacks: when is a transient ischaemic attack not a transient ischaemic attack but a stroke? *J Neurol.* 1990;237(4):257–261.
27. Dennis M, Bamford J, Sandercock P, Warlow C. Prognosis of transient ischemic attacks in the Oxfordshire Community Stroke Project. *Stroke.* 1990;21(6):848–853.
28. Sandercock P, Bamford J, Dennis M, *et al.* Atrial fibrillation and stroke: prevalence in different types of stroke and influence on early and long term prognosis (Oxfordshire community stroke project). *BMJ.* 1992;305(6867):1460–1465.
29. Collins R, Peto R, MacMahon S, *et al.* Blood pressure, stroke, and coronary heart disease. Part 2, Short-term reductions in blood pressure: overview of randomised drug trials in their epidemiological context. *Lancet.* 1990;335(8693):827–838.

30. MacMahon S, Peto R, Cutler J, *et al*. Blood pressure, stroke, and coronary heart disease. Part 1, Prolonged differences in blood pressure: prospective observational studies corrected for the regression dilution bias. *Lancet.* 1990;335(8692):765–774.

31. Hopps S, Marcy TR. Warfarin versus aspirin: using CHADS2 to guide therapy for stroke prevention in nonvalvular atrial fibrillation. *Consult Pharm.* 2009;24(11):841–844.

32. Cairns JA. ACP journal club. CHA2DS2-VASc had better discrimination than CHADS2 for predicting risk for thromboembolism in atrial fibrillation. *Ann Intern Med.* 2011;154(10):JC5–JC13.

33. Park JH, Joung B, Son NH, *et al*. The electroanatomical remodelling of the left atrium is related to CHADS2/CHA2DS2VASc score and events of stroke in patients with atrial fibrillation. *Europace.* 2011;13(11):1541–1549.

34. International Carotid Stenting Study investigators. Carotid artery stenting compared with endarterectomy in patients with symptomatic carotid stenosis (International Carotid Stenting Study): an interim analysis of a randomized controlled trial. *Lancet.* 2010;375:985–997.

35. Mas J-L, Trinquart L, Leys D, et al. for the EVA-3S investigators. Endarterectomy Versus Angioplasty in Patients with Symptomatic Severe Carotid Stenosis (EVA-3S) trial: results up to 4 years from a randomised, multicentre trial. *Lancet Neurol.* 2008;7:885–892.

36. Jager HR. Diagnosis of stroke with advanced CT and MR imaging. *Br Med Bull.* 2000;56(2):318–333.

37. Albers GW, Clark WM, Madden KP, Hamilton SA. ATLANTIS trial: results for patients treated within 3 hours of stroke onset. Alteplase Thrombolysis for Acute Noninterventional Therapy in Ischemic Stroke. *Stroke.* 2002;33(2):493–495.

38. Qureshi AI, Mendelow AD, Hanley DF. Intracerebral haemorrhage. *Lancet.* 2009;373(9675):1632–1644.

39. Prasad K, Mendelow AD, Gregson B. Surgery for primary supratentorial intracerebral haemorrhage. *Cochrane Database Syst Rev.* 2008;4:CD000200.

40. Mendelow AD, Unterberg A. Surgical treatment of intracerebral haemorrhage. *Curr Opin Crit Care.* 2007;13(2):169–174.

41. Duncan JS. Idiopathic generalized epilepsies with typical absences. *J Neurol.* 1997;244(7):403–411.

42. Tatum WOt, Husain AM, Benbadis SR, Kaplan PW. Normal adult EEG and patterns of uncertain significance. *J Clin Neurophysiol.* 2006;23(3):194–207.

43. Menon B, Shorvon SD. Ischaemic stroke in adults and epilepsy. *Epilepsy Res.* 2009;87(1):1–11.

44. Shorvon S, Trinka E. Nonconvulsive status epilepticus and the postictal state. *Epilepsy Behav.* 2010;19(2):172–175.

45. Duncan JS. Imaging and epilepsy. *Brain.* 1997 Feb;120 (Pt 2):339–377.

46. Duncan JS. Interictal focal activity in temporal lobe epilepsy. *J Neurol Neurosurg Psychiatry.* 1998;65(2):149.

47. Benbadis SR, Tatum WO 4th. Advances in the treatment of epilepsy. *Am Fam Physician.* 2001;64(1):91–98.

48. Johannessen CU, Johannessen SI. Valproate: past, present, and future. *CNS Drug Rev.* 2003;9(2):199–216.

49. Benbadis SR, Tatum WO 4th, Gieron M. Idiopathic generalized epilepsy and choice of antiepileptic drugs. *Neurology.* 2003;61(12):1793–1795.

50. French JA. Is the epilepsy responsive or resistant? Only time will tell. *Ann Neurol.* 2009;65(5):489–490.

51. Deuschl G, Bain P, Brin M. Consensus statement of the Movement Disorder Society on Tremor. Ad Hoc Scientific Committee. *Mov Disord.* 1998;13(Suppl 3):2–23.

52. de Lau LM, Breteler MM. Epidemiology of Parkinson's disease. *Lancet Neurol.* 2006;5(6):525–535.

53. Chaudhuri KR, Yates L, Martinez-Martin P. The non-motor symptom complex of Parkinson's disease: a comprehensive assessment is essential. *Curr Neurol Neurosci Rep.* 2005;5(4):275–283.

54. Chaudhuri KR, Healy DG, Schapira AH. Non-motor symptoms of Parkinson's disease: diagnosis and management. *Lancet Neurol.* 2006;5(3):235–245.

55. Chaudhuri KR. The dopaminergic basis of sleep dysfunction and non motor symptoms of Parkinson's disease: evidence from functional imaging. *Exp Neurol.* 2009;216(2):247–248.

56. Chaudhuri KR, Martinez-Martin P. Quantitation of non-motor symptoms in Parkinson's disease. *Eur J Neurol.* 2008;15(Suppl 2):2–7.

57. Chaudhuri KR, Naidu Y. Early Parkinson's disease and non-motor issues. *J Neurol.* 2008;255(Suppl 5):33–38.

58. Berendse HW, Booij J, Francot CM, *et al*. Subclinical dopaminergic dysfunction in asymptomatic Parkinson's disease patients' relatives with a decreased sense of smell. *Ann Neurol.* 2001;50(1):34–41.

59. Mitra T, Chaudhuri KR. Sleep dysfunction and role of dysautonomia in Parkinson's disease. *Parkinsonism Relat Disord.* 2009;15(Suppl 3):S93–S95.

60. Pavese N, Metta V, Bose SK, Chaudhuri KR, Brooks DJ. Fatigue in Parkinson's disease is linked to striatal and limbic serotonergic dysfunction. *Brain.* 2010;133(11):3434–3443.

61. Naidu Y, Chaudhuri KR. Transdermal rotigotine: a new non-ergot dopamine agonist for the treatment of Parkinson's disease. *Expert Opin Drug Deliv.* 2007;4(2):111–118.

62. Horstink M, Tolosa E, Bonuccelli U, *et al*. Review of the therapeutic management of Parkinson's disease. Report of a joint task force of the European Federation of Neurological Societies (EFNS) and the Movement Disorder Society-European Section (MDS-ES). Part II: late (complicated) Parkinson's disease. *Eur J Neurol.* 2006;13(11):1186–1202.

63. Horstink M, Tolosa E, Bonuccelli U, *et al*. Review of the therapeutic management of Parkinson's disease. Report of a joint task force of the European Federation of Neurological Societies and the Movement Disorder Society-European Section. Part I: early (uncomplicated) Parkinson's disease. *Eur J Neurol.* 2006;13(11):1170–1185.

64. Deuschl G, Bain P. Deep brain stimulation for tremor [correction of trauma]: patient selection and evaluation. *Mov Disord.* 2002;17(Suppl 3):S102–S111.

65. Limousin-Dowsey P, Pollak P, Van Blercom N, Krack P, Benazzouz A, Benabid A. Thalamic, subthalamic nucleus and internal pallidum stimulation in Parkinson's disease. *J Neurol.* 1999;246(Suppl 2):II42–II45.

66. Krack P, Batir A, Van Blercom N, *et al*. Five-year follow-up of bilateral stimulation of the subthalamic nucleus in advanced Parkinson's disease. *N Engl J Med.* 2003;349(20):1925–1934.

67. Benabid AL, Krack PP, Benazzouz A, Limousin P, Koudsie A, Pollak P. Deep brain stimulation of the subthalamic nucleus for Parkinson's disease: methodologic aspects and clinical criteria. *Neurology.* 2000;55(12 Suppl 6):S40–S44.

68. Toma AK, Papadopoulos MC, Stapleton S, Kitchen ND, Watkins LD. Systematic review of the outcome of shunt surgery in Normal Pressure Hydrocephalus. *Acta Neurochir.* 2013;155:1977–1980.

CHAPTER 13

Cardiovascular diseases in the elderly

Heinrich Cornelissen, Ivan L. Rapchuk, and John F. Fraser

Introduction

The ageing population of the Western world continues to grow exponentially with cardiovascular disease now the leading cause of morbidity and mortality.[1] Currently in the United Kingdom, 12 million people are pensioners and 1.25 million people are 85 years of age or older.[2] In the United States, more than 15 million people are aged 80 and older. Cardiovascular disease is significantly more prevalent in the elderly population and cardiovascular events related to ageing are the main contributors to overall adverse outcome after surgery. Advanced age is heavily weighted in scoring systems, such as EuroSCORE, logistic EuroSCORE, and Parsonnet score, in predicting the risk of operative mortality from cardiac surgery.[3] Vascular ageing is an independent risk factor for cardiovascular disease in the absence of other traditional risk factors. Anaesthetists in the Western world are faced with an increasing workload of elderly patients in their practice[4] and need a full understanding of the biology of ageing and its effects on the cardiovascular system, as well as having an understanding of the therapies in the elderly. Through a more complete understanding of cardiovascular ageing, the anaesthetist can more effectively plan and manage the perioperative care of the elderly patient. (See also Chapter 6.)

Physiology

The function of the central vasculature is to cushion and dampen the pressure oscillations produced by ventricular ejection. Energy from ventricular ejection is then transferred along the vascular tree. The peripheral pulse that results is due to the pressure wave generated by ventricular ejection and distension of the aorta. During ventricular systole, pressure waves are propagated antegrade. When the pressure wave reaches branch points or when there are abrupt changes in lumen diameter, the waves are reflected back to the central circulation. The resultant wave in the aorta is the sum of the forward and reflected wave (Fig. 13.1). Most reflected waves return to the central circulation during early diastole and augment coronary blood flow.

The healthy arterial tree fulfils the cushioning and conduit function very efficiently, with minimal drop in mean pressures between central and peripheral arteries and minimal energy expenditure. Potential energy is stored in the elastic vessel walls during systole and converted to kinetic energy assisting vascular flow during diastole. Energy is dissipated in the major arteries, so that blood flow is almost continuous and laminar through peripheral arterioles and capillaries, except in brain, kidney, and coronary capillary beds. These vascular beds are similar to central vessels, as they are exposed to pulsatile blood flow and energy. Unlike other organs that are protected by vasoconstriction, small vessels of the brain and kidney are exposed to highly pulsatile flow as they have very low vascular resistance. The vessels in the brain and kidney also have minimal wave reflections, so pressure pulsations may even extend to the venous system.[1]

Systolic blood pressure (SBP) increases with distance from the heart while diastolic blood pressure (DBP) and mean blood pressure decrease slightly (1–2 mmHg). Pulse pressure (SBP − DBP) thus increases to between 10 and 15 mmHg from the aorta to peripheral arteries. This change in pressure allows the left ventricle (LV) to eject against a lower systolic BP and lower afterload.

The neurohumoral cascade of ageing

As has been described, advancing age is the major factor for cardiovascular disease and dysfunction, and is associated with morphological changes in the vasculature that result in atherosclerosis, central aortic dilatation, collagen accumulation, and thickening of the arterial wall.[5,6] These changes produce an increase in vascular stiffness, increased blood pressure (both systolic and pulse pressure), and central blood pressure augmentation.[1,7,8] Investigations into mechanisms of this ageing process now revolve around the recurring theme of age-related perturbations in immune function, and the pro-inflammatory response upregulated with ageing.

The ageing process is associated with a reduced leucocyte telomere length, altered binding of inflammatory cells to the vasculature, and bone marrow progenitor cell depletion or exhaustion—all leading to an inability of the ageing individual to cope with oxidative stress and inflammation.[9,10] The pro-inflammatory state of the ageing individual is caused by an upregulation in the pro-inflammatory cytokines and adhesion molecules, cyclo-oxygenase (COX)-2, and lipoxygenases, and alterations in the production of nitric oxide (NO).[10,11] Accumulated data strongly suggest that continuous (chronic) upregulation of pro-inflammatory mediators (e.g. tumour necrosis factor alpha (TNFα, interleukin (IL)-1β, IL6, COX-2, inducible nitric oxide synthase (iNOS)) is induced during the ageing process due to an age-related redox imbalance that activates many

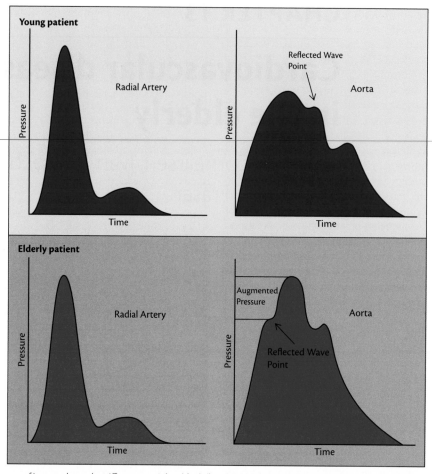

Fig. 13.1 Illustration of the influence of increased vascular stiffness on peripheral (radial) and central (aortic) derived pressures. Note the similarity of peripheral radial pressures in individuals with normal (upper left panel) and increased (lower left panel) vascular stiffness. In young individuals with normal vascular stiffness, central aortic pressures are lower than radial pressures (upper panels). In contrast, in older individuals with increased vascular stiffness, central aortic pressures are increased and can approach or equal peripheral pressures as a result of wave reflection and central wave augmentation during systole (lower panels). Reproduced from Barodka, V.M., et al., 'Review article: implications of vascular aging', *Anaesthesia and Analgesia*, 112, 5, pp. 1048–1060, copyright 2011, with permission from the International Anesthesia Research Society and Wolters Kluwer.

pro-inflammatory signalling pathways, including the nuclear factor kappa B (NF-κB) signalling pathway. These pro-inflammatory molecular events are basic mechanisms underlying ageing and age-related diseases as well as age-related physiological functional declines and the accompanying chronic diseases concomitant with ageing.[10,12] A clear correlation has been identified between inflammation and worse outcomes in heart failure and other cardiovascular diseases with the upregulation of many pro-inflammatory cytokines and a decrease in the anti-inflammatory mediators.[11] Pro-inflammatory mediators (Table 13.1) that are implicated in vascular ageing include: TNFα, which causes necrosis of myocardial cells as well as disturbances in the inducible nitric oxide synthetase system and beta receptor sensitivity; IL6; C-reactive protein (CRP)—an acute phase protein strongly associated with cardiovascular risk; and platelet derived growth factor—involved in endothelial dysfunction and ultimately atherosclerosis.[11,13,14]

The increased understanding of the relevance of the renin–angiotensin–aldosterone system (RAAS) indicates its major role in the neurohumoral control of vascular ageing. Angiotensin-II (AT-II) is the main effector hormone of the RAAS and acts through two receptor subtypes: AT-II receptor 1 (AT$_1$R) when stimulated activates numerous intracellular protein kinases which initiate

vascular remodelling through induction of hyperplasia, hypertrophy, and age-related medial degeneration and sclerosis (ARMDS); and AT-II receptor 2 (AT$_2$R) that acts in a contrary manner to activate the nitric oxide (NO) system and stimulate the release of arachidonic acid.[15,16] AT-II also enhances the production of reactive oxygen species by activating nicotinamide adenine dinucleotide phosphate (NADPH) oxidase and uncoupling endothelial NO synthetase leading to protein and lipid oxidation mainly in the mitochondria.[17] RAAS blockade has an age-retarding effect on the vasculature by slowing the production of reactive oxygen species, decreasing the hypertrophic and apoptotic signals, and blocking fibroblast proliferation and collagen synthesis.[15] The exact molecular mechanism of action of the RAAS on human vasculature is not entirely clear, however a number of pathways have been shown to be affected: the *Klotho* gene, which protects against oxidative stress and ageing changes in renal vasculature, is suppressed by activation of the RAAS; the NAD-dependant protein deacetylases of the Sirtuin family (SIRT1 and SIRT3) have a critical role in DNA repair, stress resistance and longevity, and the activity of these genes is decreased by RAS activation causing vascular angiogenesis and senescence; the gene encoding for the mitochondrial protein p66 has a positive effect on the vasculature by protecting

Table 13.1 Pro-inflammatory and anti-inflammatory agents that are elevated in patients with heart failure

Pro-inflammatory effects			
TNF-α	sTNFR	sTNFR2	sFas
CD40L	TRAIL	Activin A	Pentraxin-3
RANTES	CRP	IL-6	IL8
MCP-1	MIP-1a	Myeloperoxidase	
Cardiotrophin			
Anti-inflammatory effects			
IL-10	IL-13	IL-18	
Pro-inflammatory and anti-inflammatory effects			
Adiponectin	Resistin		

CRP: C-reactive protein; IL: interleukin; MCP: macrophage chemoattractant protein; MIP: macrophage inflammatory protein; RANTES: regulated on activation normally T-cell expressed and secreted; sTNFR1/sTNFR2: soluble TNF receptor 1/2; TNF: tumour necrosis factor; TRAIL: TNF-α related apoptosis-inducing ligand.

Reproduced with permission: Oikonomou, E., et al., 'The role of inflammation in heart failure: new therapeutic approaches', *Hellenic J Cardiol*, 2011; 52(1): 30–40.

against the accumulation of oxidative damage that occurs as we age—however, this gene activation is blocked by action of the RAS; NF-κB is a transcription factor activated in inflammatory processes that controls the expression of many inflammatory cytokines, chemokines, immune receptors, and cell surface adhesion molecules—and it is upregulated by the RAAS causing remodelling and fibroblast proliferation in the vasculature.[10,16,18–22] In animal studies the blocking of RAAS activation protects against neurodegenerative processes and promotes longevity, and it is postulated this action extends to humans.

There is a significantly pleiotropic effect of many of the agents involved in the inflammation and activation of vascular remodelling in the ageing animal. An organism's pro-inflammatory status determines the degree of ageing and hence the progression of age-related diseases. The redox-sensitive transcription factors such as NF-κB, SIRT1 and SIRT3, forkhead transcription factors (FOXOs) play essential roles in the downstream expression of pro-inflammatory mediators and upregulation of pro-inflammatory cytokines and adhesion molecules.[10,22,23] The intricate interplay among the pro-inflammatory factors and the resulting changes in the vasculature to become more sensitive to reactive oxygen species and chronic age-related disease suggest certain inevitability to the ageing process. However, the pliability of these genetic inflammatory factors and their connection with modifiable neurohumoral pathways does point to the potential of therapeutic interventions to significantly retard vascular ageing.

The endothelium is a key modulator of the intravascular coagulation balance, and determinant of atherosclerosis. Endothelium-derived NO generated by endothelial NO synthase (eNOS) is a major regulator of this endothelial protection. Vascular NO relaxes blood vessels, prevents platelet aggregation and adhesion, limits oxidation of low-density lipoprotein (LDL) cholesterol, inhibits proliferation of vascular smooth muscle cells, and decreases the expression of pro-inflammatory genes that advance atherogenesis.[19,24] Oxidative stress—an increased production and/or impaired

inactivation of reactive oxygen species (ROS)—leads to reduced bioactivity of NO. Risk factors for cardiovascular disease—such as ageing, hypertension, diabetes mellitus, hypercholesterolemia, and atherosclerosis, all impair endothelial function. These risk factors lead to dramatic increases in ROS in the vascular wall, a situation that culminates in oxidative stress. ROS include free oxygen radicals, oxygen ions, and peroxides. There are several enzyme systems that can potentially produce ROS in the vessel wall, with four systems being of major importance. These include NADPH oxidase, xanthine oxidase, a dysfunctional eNOS (in which oxygen reduction is uncoupled from NO synthesis), and enzymes of the mitochondrial respiratory chain.[24] Angiotensin-converting enzyme (ACE) activity and local AT-II concentrations are increased in atherosclerotic plaques, as inflammatory cells in the vessel wall can produce these mediators. The stimulating effects of AT-II on the activity of NADPH oxidases suggests that an activated renin–angiotensin system could cause increased vascular O_2 production and thus vascular dysfunction.[16,17,24]

Endothelial dysfunction and oxidative stress have been identified as common denominators of many cardiovascular risk factors as they support pro-inflammatory, prothrombotic, proliferative, and vasoconstrictor mechanisms involved in the initiation, progression, and complications of atherosclerosis.[24,25] The pathophysiological changes that occur with ageing produce inflammation and oxidative stress, and are likely to involve changes in a number of different enzyme systems; most importantly, there is an upregulation of NADPH oxidases and eNOS.[10,24] Together this causes an increased production of peroxynitrite (ONOO) that conveys oxidative damage to eNOS and/or its cofactor BH_4 leading to 'uncoupling' of the enzyme. As a consequence, the uncoupled eNOS most likely leads to an increased production of ROS (Fig. 13.2), which contributes significantly to vascular oxidative stress and endothelial dysfunction.[19,24,26] These changes in NO production and ROS activity are also associated with RAS activation and pro-inflammatory cytokine release. This interaction produces a large and intertwined clinical picture that displays the highly complex nature of ageing and its effect on the vascular system's delicate neurohumoral balance.

Pathophysiology of vascular ageing

Changes that occur in ageing are likely to be the result of both genetic and environmental factors. The hallmark of vascular ageing is vascular stiffening. Vascular ageing and atherosclerosis are often confused with each other, but are two separate entities. The stiffening of the vasculature with vascular ageing chiefly occurs in the media and adventitia, even in the absence of atherosclerosis. Atherosclerosis mainly results in intimal thickening.[27] The change in the media is known as age-related medial degeneration and sclerosis (ARMDS).[28] The rate at which this vascular stiffening develops varies so vascular age, rather than chronological age, is the best predictor of cardiovascular events and mortality.[27] Markers of vascular age are predictive of adverse cardiac, cerebrovascular, and renal outcomes.[27] Vascular changes are not uniform throughout the vascular tree, but are often patchy. The changes of vascular ageing occur in central and conduit vessels, while sparing more peripheral vessels. Age-related dilatation occurs in the ascending and descending thoracic aorta, with dilatation more marked in the ascending aorta. Diseases, such as hypertension, diabetes, atherosclerosis, and renal impairment as well as the effects of smoking

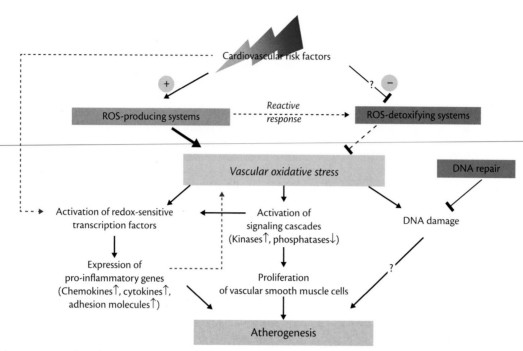

Fig. 13.2 Pictorial representation of vascular oxidative stress as a cause of atherogenesis. Reactive oxygen species (ROS) generation occurs as ageing and/or cardiovascular risk factors predominate. The resulting oxidative stress leads to atherogenesis via activation of redox sensitive transcription factors and activation of signalling cascades. ROS also cause nuclear and mitochondrial DNA damage. The ageing process leads to expression of pro-inflammatory genes that may be the primary process in the activation of oxidative stress (dashed blue lines). Forstermann, U., 'Nitric oxide and oxidative stress in vascular disease', *Pflügers Archiv European Journal of Physiology*, 459, 6, pp. 923–939, copyright 2010. With kind permission from Springer Science and Business Media.

further exacerbate the age-related changes. However, the relative importance of cardiovascular risk factors diminishes with age.[29]

Compliance and stability of the vessel wall is related to the relative proportions of collagen and elastin. The proximal aorta is more elastic and contains relatively more elastin than peripheral arteries and arterioles. The inflammatory process of ageing disturbs the balance between the slow turnover and production of collagen and elastin. This leads to fragmentation of elastin and excessive collagen accumulates due to the slow turnover of elastin (Fig. 13.3). Slow turnover of elastin result in glycation and glyco-oxidative reaction of this protein.[28] This alteration in the metabolism of tissue proteins leads to excessive production of abnormal collagen and diminished quantities of normal elastin. Endothelial cells become abnormal and more permeable in this process. Vascular smooth muscle cells (VSMCs), macrophages and mononuclear cells, matrix metalloproteases (MMPs), transforming growth factor (TGF)-β, intracellular cell adhesion molecules, and cytokines infiltrate the intima of stiffened vessels, further contributing to the increased intimal thickening. MMPs degrade the extracellular matrix (ECM) by their enzymatic action, creating less effective collagen and fragmented elastin molecules.[29] Macroscopically, these changes manifest as a doubling or tripling of intima-media thickness between the ages 20 and 90, as well as a hypertrophied vascular smooth muscle layer.[29]

Collagen provides the tensile strength of the vessel wall and these proteins are enzymatically cross-linked to render them insoluble to hydrolytic enzymes. Non-enzymatic glycation produces cross-linking of collagen by advanced glycation end-products (AGEs), which contributes to the stiffening of the arterial wall. AGEs stimulate inflammatory responses and increase proinflammatory cytokines, radical oxygen species formation, and vascular

adhesion molecules. AGEs accumulate in the media of the aorta with advancing age. All of these processes cause an increase in vascular stiffness via MMPs.

Transglutaminase is also responsible for irreversible cross-link formation between structural proteins. Increased activity of this enzyme contributes to increased vascular stiffness.[27] Disruption of the non-enzymatic cross-linking of elastin also predisposes the vessel wall to increased mineralization by calcium and phosphorous. Calcification occurs in the intimal layer in plaques and in the medial elastic fibre network (medial elastocalcinosis).[30] Microcalcification is frequent in the media of the aorta in elderly people. Ultimately, the age and inflammation related alterations in elastin production and molecular repair mechanisms contribute to the loss of elasticity of the vasculature. Genetic polymorphisms that are reported to increase vascular stiffness have been identified on loci of ACE or AT_1R, endothelin receptors, fibrillin-1, and metalloproteinases.[27]

Effect of ageing on the cardiovascular system

As a consequence of the effects of ageing on the cardiovascular system, cardiovascular reserve becomes markedly reduced and elderly patients are prone to heart failure. The incidence of heart failure rises exponentially with age and heart failure is the most common indication for hospitalization in elderly patients, with a huge cost burden.[31–34]

The increase in vascular stiffness results in the reflected waveform being returned earlier than if it was cushioned in normal vasculature (Fig. 13.1). This effect is due to pressure waves travelling faster in a stiffer medium. The pulse wave velocity (PWV) can be

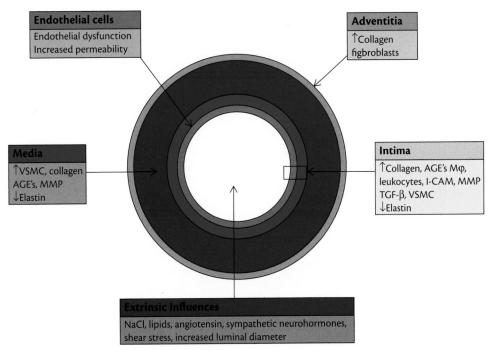

Fig. 13.3 Summary of the multiple causes and locations of arterial stiffness. AGEs: advanced glycation end-products; ICAM: intercellular adhesion molecules; MMP: matrix metalloproteinases; TGF: transforming growth factor; VSMC: vascular smooth muscle cells. Reproduced from Zieman, S.M., et al., 'Mechanisms, pathophysiology, and therapy of arterial stiffness', *Arteriosclerosis, Thrombosis, and Vascular Biology*, 25, 5, pp. 932–943, copyright American Heart Association, with permission.

measured and the velocity increases in parallel with vascular stiffness (Fig. 13.4). Pulse wave velocity can double between ages 20 to 80, and corresponds with a fourfold decrease in aortic distensibility.[1] The resultant pressure waveform shows the reflected waveform occurring in late systole, which imposes increased loading conditions on the LV and causes a decrease in ejection efficiency. The LV afterload is increased by arterial stiffening and by the early return of the reflected wave. Coronary blood flow is also impaired, both as a consequence of loss of augmentation of flow during diastole (because the reflected wave occurs earlier) and due to an increased reliance on flow during systole, causing the heart to be exquisitely sensitive to decline in systolic pressure when coronary ischaemia is present. Vascular stiffening results in elevated SBP, both centrally and peripherally, decreased DBP, a widened pulse pressure (SBP – DBP) and increased arterial wave reflectance.[9] Isolated systolic hypertension is the most common form of hypertension in elderly patients. This, together with increased pulse pressure and increased aortic PWV are markers of significant risks of myocardial events, heart failure, strokes, and mortality in older patients.[35,36]

As discussed previously, the brain and kidneys are exposed to high pulsatile pressure and their degree of protection by vasoconstriction is less than that of other organs. During vascular stiffening, microcirculatory damage occurs in these organs, due to dissipation of excess pulsatile energy. Microcirculatory damage takes the form of micro infarctions and micro haemorrhages, which manifests clinically in the brain as cognitive dysfunction and dementia (small lacunar infarcts and white matter defects).[1]

Ageing affects the heart directly, as well as a consequence of vascular ageing. As early as 1937 Sir Thomas Lewis (in *Diseases of the Heart. Described for Practitioners and Student*) recognized the syndrome of dyspnoea, normal systolic function and absence of histologic myocardial abnormalities at autopsy in elderly patients—a

syndrome we recognize today as diastolic dysfunction. Increased loading conditions result in LV ejection into a stiffer vasculature and greater systolic pressures have to be generated for the same stroke volume. The stroke volume increases with a decreased heart rate to maintain the same cardiac output. In non-compliant vasculature, as occurs in ageing vessels, this causes the central aortic pressures to increase. The increased aortic pressure results in myocardial hypertrophy. Interstitial fibrosis, collagen deposition and remodelling cause increased stiffness in the ventricular wall and although the cardiac myocytes hypertrophy, the total number of cardiac myocytes decrease with age, as a result of cellular senescence and apoptosis.[37] Myocyte hypertrophy is exaggerated in ageing, when myocytes die and are not replaced. This results in both impairment of relaxation during diastole, as well as impairment during systolic contraction. Calcium flux slows, reducing the speed of myocardial contraction and dP/dT, but not diminishing the actual contractile strength. Altered calcium flux (slow uptake by the sarcoplasmic reticulum, as a result of cardiac myocyte hypertrophy) contributes to sustained contraction in systole, as well as delayed and impaired relaxation during early diastole [38]. The sustained contraction prolongs the time for ventricular ejection into the stiffened vasculature, thus maintaining cardiac output and ventricular function. The main effect is a reduction in LV diastolic compliance and filling time and an increase in left atrial (LA) pressures required during late diastolic filling to maintain the same LV filling volume (LVEDV). The elevated LA pressure transmits pressure retrograde to pulmonary veins and capillaries, resulting in interstitial fluid oedema, dyspnoea, and other symptoms of heart failure. Patients with diastolic dysfunction may be asymptomatic at rest, so it is prudent to ask about dyspnoea on exertion. This diastolic dysfunction explains the high incidence of heart failure in elderly patients with normal systolic function. Current

Young patient

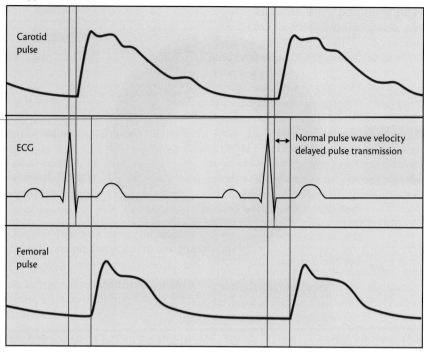

Elderly patient

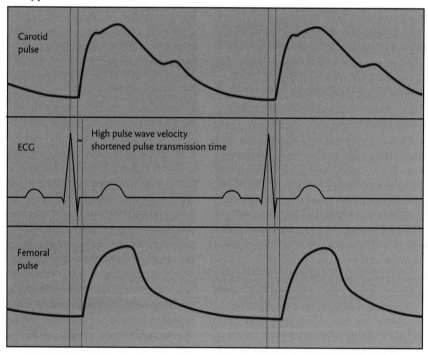

Fig. 13.4 Example of pulse wave velocity measurements in two individuals, one with profoundly increased vascular stiffness (top panel) and the other with high normal vascular stiffness (lower panel). Pulse wave velocity is calculated as the distance (femoral–carotid) divided by time (derived from the electrocardiogram). Reproduced from Barodka, V.M., et al., 'Review article: implications of vascular aging', *Anaesthesia and Analgesia*, 112, 5, pp. 1048–1060, copyright 2011, with permission from the International Anesthesia Research Society and Wolters Kluwer.

estimates are that more than half of all elderly patients with heart failure, have diastolic heart failure (i.e. LV ejection fraction more than 45 per cent, with systolic function unable to account for heart failure).[34] As occurs in systolic heart failure, neurohumoral activation is triggered in diastolic heart failure and it is thus a true heart failure syndrome.[39] The ageing heart is increasingly reliant on the contribution of atrial contraction for late diastolic filling and adequate LVEDV, thus atrial fibrillation and dysrhythmias may have a significant negative effect on cardiac output. The LA size increases with age, reflecting the significance of the contribution of atrial activity to late diastolic filling. LA enlargement from pressure over-load may contribute to atrial fibrillation being the most common dysrhythmia in elderly patients. Atrial fibrillation is also the most common cause of strokes in the elderly (Framingham Heart Study). Similarly, LV preload is important to maintain adequate stroke volume and cardiac output. However these patients are volume sensitive. They easily develop pulmonary oedema or low cardiac output and prerenal failure perioperatively or due to antifailure medication and vigorous diuresis.

Systolic function is maintained, despite an age-related increase in LV systolic stiffness (as measured by increasing end-systolic elastance (Ees)). Comparable increases in arterial elastance maintain the Ea/Ees ratio, but as they are both increased, the ventricular-arterial interaction becomes limited, such that even small changes in ventricular filling can result in large changes in arterial pressure. This phenomenon may contribute to the increased prevalence of hypotension during postural shift and fluid depletion.

Measurements of ageing

Vascular ageing may be undetected in subjects who are normotensive, with no overt cardiovascular disease. Preventative therapy can be targeted at these individuals, to reduce vascular and cardiac remodelling and dysfunction and prevent cardiovascular events.[40] Assessment of vascular stiffness may assist in evaluating risks during anaesthesia.[41]

As pathological changes of vascular ageing affect central and conduit vessels more than peripheral vessels, peripheral blood pressure measurements can be a poor indicator of vascular ageing in asymptomatic individuals. Most arterial stiffness occurs in the aorta and thus indices of aortic stiffness are more accurate predictors of mortality and morbidity from cardiovascular events. Carotid–femoral pulse wave velocity (cfPWV), carotid augmentation index (AIx), and central pulse pressure have predictive value for mortality and morbidity from cardiovascular events and end-stage renal failure. However, other indices are a more accurate reflection of vascular stiffness and therefore vascular ageing. Ascending aortic (AA) strain and distensibility and aortic arch pulse wave velocity determined by magnetic resonance imaging (MRI), are reliable (sensitive and specific) markers of vascular ageing. Of these, AA distensibility in younger individuals less than 50 years of age and aortic arch PWV in older individuals, reflect most accurately subclinical large artery stiffening.[40]

Pulse pressure is a surrogate measure of arterial stiffness and has been shown to have predictive value for cardiovascular events. A raised pulse pressure represents generalized stiffening of the large arteries and more advanced arterial disease.[42]

Carotid-femoral PWV is considered the gold standard measurement of arterial stiffness in an expert consensus document on arterial stiffness from the European Network for Non-invasive Investigation of Large Arteries.[41] Carotid–femoral PWV can be measured non-invasively by applanation tonometry of peripherally acquired waveforms (as velocity is change in distance over change in time, velocity can be calculated if distance and time are known). The distance is measured between the carotid artery and suprasternal notch and the femoral artery and the suprasternal notch and the time interval is measured from the R wave of the electrocardiogram to the start or peak of the pulse wave at each artery, allowing the calculation of the velocity. Obesity or large breasts may overestimate the distance measured and heart rate significantly influences cfPWV. In young people, the velocity is approximately 6 m/s and increases to approximately 10 m/s by age 65 and continues to increase with age. Several commercially available non-invasive devices can be used to determine PWV. A cfPWV greater than 12 m/s is considered to be abnormal.[40]

The degree of aortic stiffness, as measured by cfPWV, is associated with the magnitude of decrease of the systolic arterial pressure, during induction of anaesthesia with propofol/remifentanil.[41] It may be a more useful risk predictor than more commonly used measures, such as age, American Society of Anesthesiologists (ASA) classification of physical state, and drug quantity, and provide additional information in risk assessment for patients with a history of cardiovascular events. It may be particularly useful in assessing risk of haemodynamic instability and cardiovascular events during anaesthesia in patients with undetermined or low risk.

Carotid augmentation index (AIx), a marker of waveform reflection, is analysed, using the right common carotid waveform. Carotid blood pressure is obtained from the carotid waveform, calibrated with the mean and diastolic brachial pressure. Carotid augmentation index is the ratio of the augmented pressure (height above the inflection point to late systolic peak) to the pulse pressure, as a percentage.

Aortic distensibility and aortic strain (together with aortic arch PWV) can be determined by MRI and is determined using maximal and minimal aortic lumen area and relative change in area, respectively. These parameters begin to significantly decrease early in life (from 3rd decade) and are stronger correlates of ageing than more peripheral indices.

Aortic arch PWV is calculated using the transit time of the flow curves and the distance between the ascending and descending aortic locations of the phase-contrast acquisition.

The normal range for aortic arch PWV is still to be determined, but in some studies, the normal range in older individuals is shown to be 9–10 m/s.[40]

Diagnosis of diastolic dysfunction

Diastolic dysfunction is diagnosed by cardiac catheterization and by Doppler assessment using transmitral diastolic filling patterns by pulsed wave Doppler echocardiography. Increased LV diastolic pressures, above 16 mmHg, are seen with normal LV systolic function and volumes during cardiac catheterization.

With normal diastolic transmitral filling patterns, two peaks of filling occur. Early filling, following mitral valve opening when LV pressure falls below LA pressure, and late diastolic filling with atrial contraction. Peak flow velocities can be measured by Doppler echocardiography (Fig. 13.5), the E peak, corresponding with early diastolic filling and the A peak, with atrial contraction. In normal healthy young people, the E/A ratio is greater than 1, due to predominant rapid filling early in diastole and modest additional filling during atrial contraction.

With 'delayed relaxation' (impaired relaxation), the amount and rate of early filling is reduced and the amount of filling during atrial contraction is enhanced, resulting in an E/A ratio of less than 1. This is seen in normal healthy older people, with no overt cardiovascular disease, but also in patients with LV hypertrophy, atrial hypertension and coronary artery disease. This corresponds with a mild degree of diastolic dysfunction.

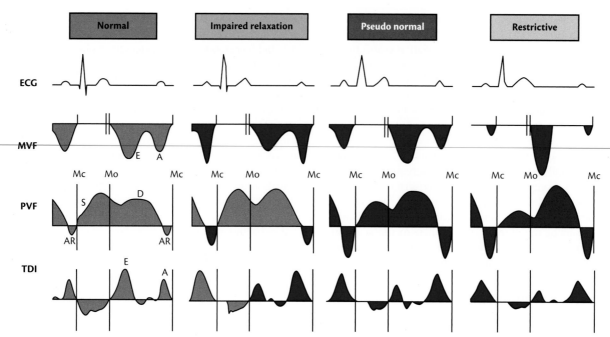

Fig. 13.5 Example of pulsed wave Doppler echocardiography. MVF: transmitral blood flow; PVF: pulmonary vein flow; TDI: tissue Doppler imaging. Light grey, normal pattern and dark grey, abnormal. Reproduced with permission from R. Fenek et al., *Core Topics in Transesophageal Echocardiography*, 2010, © Cambridge University Press.

Two other filling patterns occur, that is always abnormal and corresponds with moderate and severe diastolic dysfunction. 'Pseudonormalization' occurs where the E/A ratio is greater than 1 (as in normal subjects), yet there is still diastolic dysfunction. Here the LA pressure is increased and restores the diastolic pressure gradient between the LA and LV. The increased LA size and pressure seen is a compensatory response to impaired relaxation of the LV. Pseudonormalization can be differentiated from normal filling patterns by obtaining mitral annular velocities via tissue Doppler, or by preload reduction using the Valsalva manoeuvre or nitroglycerine infusions- two manoeuvres that uncover the underlying E/A pattern.

The other abnormal filling pattern is 'restrictive', whereby early filling is abnormally increased due to high LA pressures. Reduced atrial contraction leads to a reduction in atrial filling and the E/A ratio may be greater than 2. This restrictive pattern is indicative of severe diastolic dysfunction.

Therapies to prevent or retard vascular ageing

Advancing age has been shown to be the major risk factor for the development of disease in the cardiovascular system. At the macroscopic level an intimal thickening and increased vascular calcification produce a generalized stiffening of the arterial tree.[9] The mechanisms by which this happen include mechanical shear stress on the intravascular structures; a reduction in endothelium dependant dilation of the peripheral arteries in response to either chemical or mechanical stress; a reduction in the bioavailability of the molecule NO as production decreases due to ageing endothelium; and an upregulation of pro-inflammatory cytokines and pathways.[26,43] These mechanisms all lead to either oxidative stress or the inability to deal with normal levels of oxidative stress, and cause a reduction in the ability of ageing arterioles to undergo adequate endothelium dependant dilation.[9,26] The various mechanisms of intravascular ageing, and the signalling pathways relevant to the ageing process are all potential targets of vascular anti-ageing treatments that hope to reduce oxidative damage or enhance cellular defences.[16] The treatments that follow are either pharmacological, non-pharmacological and lifestyle related, or emerging therapies based on fighting the inflammation of ageing that occurs within the vascular system.

Angiotensin-converting enzyme inhibitors and angiotensin receptor blockers

The RAAS has been recognized to have a functional role in the treatment of blood pressure for over 50 years. ACE generates AT-II, which then acts through two receptor subtypes—AT_1R and AT_2R (Table 13.2).[15] Binding of AT-II to AT_1R activates a cascade of intracellular protein kinases that result in vascular remodelling through induction of hypertrophy, hyperplasia and alterations in smooth muscle cells.[15] AT_2R, when stimulated by AT-II exerts an opposite effect including anti-inflammatory, anti-proliferative, and anti-apoptotic actions.[15] With ageing, upregulation of AT_1R occurs with a similar decrease in the expression of AT_2R, and there is evidence that this altered ratio of AT_1R to AT_2R results in elevated blood pressure and inflammation.[15,44]

Recent studies have now lent molecular credence to this concept by pointing to anti-atherosclerotic, anti-inflammatory, antiproliferative, and antioxidant properties that occur with blockade of the RAAS.[45] AT-II also enhances the production of reactive oxygen species by activating NADPH oxidase and uncoupling eNOS—this increases protein and lipid oxidation and results in vascular ageing.[17] RAAS blockade has an age-retarding effect by protecting against the neurodegenerative and pro-inflammatory processes that generate reactive oxygen species and damage tissue by causing mitochondrial dysfunction.[17,44] A number of studies have shown a large benefit for patients taking angiotensin receptor blockers and

Table 13.2 Opposing functions of AT$_1$R and AT$_2$R which might be linked to ageing

AT$_1$R	AT$_2$R
Vasoconstriction	Vasodilatation
Cell growth	Antigrowth
Cell proliferation	Cell differentiation
Antinatriuresis	Natriuresis
Production of O$_2^-$	Production of nitric oxide
Stimulation of fibroblast proliferation and collagen synthesis	Inhibition of fibroblast proliferation
Apoptosis	Anti-apoptosis

Reprinted from *Clinics in Geriatric Medicine*, 27, 1, Abadir, P.M., 'The frail renin-angiotensin system', pp. 53–65, copyright 2011, with permission from Elsevier.

ACE inhibitors in treatment of hypertension, diabetic nephropathy, cerebrovascular disease and heart failure.[46–48] Additionally, both ACE inhibitors and AT-II receptor blockers have been definitively shown to reduce arterial stiffness, wave reflections and central pulse pressure independent of the blood pressure lowering effect.[49–51]

β-blockers

β-blockers have been shown to reduce blood pressure to an equivalent extent as diuretics, ACE inhibitors, calcium channel blockers, and angiotensin receptor blockers.[52] However, treatment with β-blockers has been shown to be less effective at reducing cardiovascular events—especially stroke—when compared with these other therapies.[51,52] It has been postulated that β-blocker therapy may lead to a reduction in blood pressure, but the slowing of the heart rate induced by this medication maintains the disturbed wave reflections and augments central aortic systolic pressure.[53,54] The studies performed on atenolol demonstrate that β-blocker therapy may have little effect on the micro and macrovascular structure of arteries, and does not enhance endothelial function or the endothelium's ability to handle oxidative stress.[53] Newer β-blockers such as nevibolol and carvedilol—endowed with the additional vasodilating activity mediated by endothelial NO release—may produce a more favourable metabolic profile, beneficial effects on arterial stiffness, and antioxidant and endothelial protective properties.[53] This theoretical effect however, has yet to be borne out in human clinical trials.

Statins

There has been significant interest in the utilization of 3-hydoxy-3-methylglutaryl-coenzyme A reductase inhibitors (statins) as a treatment for both cardiovascular disease and the stiffening of the arteries that occurs as we age.[55] Treatment with statins can significantly reduce cardiovascular events and mortality in patients at risk, and the relative risk reduction is even greater in the elderly because the event rate is that much higher.[56,57] Clinical trials such as JUPITER, AURORA, EUROASPIRE, and GALAXY provide further evidence that early treatment with a statin (and possibly the specific drug rosuvastatin) achieves great benefit not only in lipid lowering, but also in decreasing the low-grade systemic inflammation that characterizes ageing and leads to negative vascular changes in the elderly.[58–60] The anti-inflammatory, antiproliferative, and immunomodulatory actions of statins lead to a reduction in arterial stiffness in middle-aged and older adults independent of baseline cardiometabolic risk factors, and it has been suggested that statin treatment equates to reversing 15 years of age-related arterial stiffening.[55,61]

Physical activity

The cardiovascular benefits of exercise are well known, with many studies delineating that habitual moderate to vigorous intensity physical activity attenuates arterial stiffening. Endurance trained individuals demonstrate a lower large elastic artery stiffness and greater endothelial-dependant dilation as they increase in age in comparison with sedentary peers.[62, 63] The exact mechanisms of this effect on the endothelium and elasticity of large and medium arteries is still largely unknown, however there is putative evidence of why it occurs.

The ageing individual that is physically active has an increased bioavailability of nitric oxide and increased expression and activity of eNOS allowing for greater endothelial dilation.[26] These active individuals have decreased oxidative damage in their arterial tree associated with an increased activity of the antioxidant enzyme superoxide dismutase.[64] Additionally, active elderly individuals have a reduction in the activity of the oxidant enzyme NADPH oxidase, an increased release of tissue-type plasminogen activator allowing for greater intrinsic fibrinolytic capacity, and an increase in the release of endothelial progenitor cell number and function over their sedentary peers.[64–66] Although much progress has been made, current research is still ongoing to elucidate the exact mechanisms by which individuals who regularly perform aerobic exercise mitigate the functional changes that occur in the cardiovascular system with advancing age—changes that decrease the incidence of cardiovascular events and strokes, frailty, functional decline, and cognitive impairment over sedentary individuals.[67,68]

Lifestyle modification

Alterations in lifestyle such as smoking cessation, caloric restriction, and stress avoidance have been shown to slow the ageing process within the vascular tree.[9,16] Caloric restriction significantly reduces ageing-related deaths in both rhesus monkeys and rats; and humans on low-calorie diets have lower levels of the pro-inflammatory cytokines TNFα and CRP.[16] The pathophysiology of smoking-related hastening of vascular damage has been linked, at least in part, to cigarette-induced increases in oxidative stress. By enhancing the production of superoxide and other reactive oxygen species, cigarette smoke inactivates NO within the vasculature, thereby disrupting endothelial function.[69] Cigarette smoking has been shown to definitively hasten vascular ageing.

High dietary salt intake increases vascular stiffness with advancing age. Vascular smooth muscle cell (VSMC) tone is increased and there is a marked increase in the medial layer with hypertrophy of VSMCs. The production of NO is reduced by the effect of sodium on the endothelium and the stimulation of ROS results in arterial stiffening. Arterial compliance is improved by low dietary sodium intake in older subjects.[29,70]

The moderate consumption of alcohol is associated with significantly lower PWV. The protective effect of alcohol appears to be related to increased cellular cholesterol efflux and reverse cholesterol transport.[29]

Emerging therapies

Vascular ageing can now be viewed as having a pathogenetic mechanism that includes neurohumoral deregulation, with disturbance of the sympathetic and parasympathetic balance, disruption of the renin–angiotensin system, and excessive inflammation.[11] There are many cytokines implicated in the pathogenesis of vascular ageing and heart failure such as TNFα, TRAIL, CRP, IL6, IL8, sFas.[11,15,28] The signalling pathways and molecular inflammation involved are under extensive investigation as potential targets for protection of the vasculature against the ageing process.

Inhibition of the pro-inflammatory cytokines and inflammatory genes, or upregulation of the anti-inflammatory cytokines and anti-inflammatory genes may lead to reduced oxidative stress and a lessening of the effect that ageing has on the vasculature (Fig. 13.6). There are a number of pathways currently being investigated.[28] For example, the genetic deletion of the p66Shc protein—which plays a role as a redox enzyme implicated in mitochondrial ROS generation and activation of apoptosis—leads to an extended lifespan via protection from ageing-dependant endothelial dysfunction.[16] This and other therapies are currently being applied only in animal models; however, they may hit at the heart of the process that leads to endothelial ageing and stiffening of the arteries in the aged.

Conclusion

Although the Western world has an ageing population, the health burden is less than expected as the health of the elderly has improved.

In addition to stiffening of the vasculature and myocardium, blunted β-adrenergic responses and impaired autonomic reflex control of heart rate seen in advanced age, contribute to the increased perioperative risk seen in the elderly.[15] Changes in the cardiovascular system related to ageing, may affect cardiovascular performance in the perioperative period or in periods of cardiovascular stress. Even in the absence of overt clinical disease, resting organ function declines with advancing age (e.g. impaired respiratory gas exchange and decline in renal capacity to conserve and eliminate water and sodium), which further increases cardiovascular risk. Parameters of vascular ageing, rather than chronological age, may be the best predictors of adverse outcome following surgery as biological and chronological age may differ considerably. Rather than using chronological age as a measure of old age, the use of other parameters of vascular ageing, such as diastolic dysfunction and pulse wave analysis may be more useful, especially in asymptomatic individuals. Subclinical large artery stiffening is reliably detected using ascending aorta distensibility in patients younger than 50 years of age and aortic arch PWV in older patients. Utilization of these tests may be useful in risk stratification and improving patient outcome, with complex surgical or anaesthetic procedures.

Vascular ageing is associated with upregulation of pro-inflammatory mediators, a generalized pro-inflammatory state, and an altered neurohumoral response to stress. Therapeutic measures, such as blockade of the RAAS, avoidance of smoking, and maintaining physical activity, mitigate the changes of ageing on vasculature.

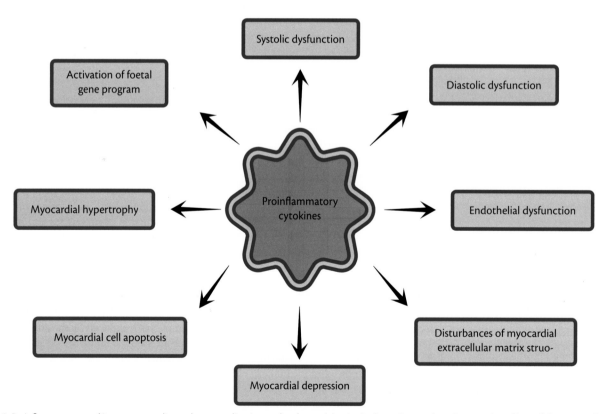

Fig. 13.6 Proinflammatory cytokines act on cardiac and extra-cardiac tissues, thereby participating in the pathogenesis and progression of heart failure. Reproduced with permission: Oikonomou, E., et al., 'The role of inflammation in heart failure: new therapeutic approaches', *Hellenic J Cardiol*, 2011; 52(1): 30–40.

Acknowledgement

Dr Jonathon Fanning for redrawing all illustrations through this chapter.

References

1. Barodka VM, Joshi BL, Berkowitz DE, Hogue CW Jr, Nyhan D. Review article: implications of vascular aging. *Anesth Analg.* 2011;112(5):1048–1060.

2. National Confidential Enquiry into Patient Outcome and Death. *An age old problem. A review of the care received by elderly patients undergoing surgery.* London: NCEPOD, 2010.

3. Silvay G, Castillo JG, Chikwe J, Flynn B, Filsoufi F. Cardiac anesthesia and surgery in geriatric patients. *Semin Cardiothorac Vasc Anesth.* 2008;12(1):18–28.

4. Tonner PH, Kampen J, Scholz J. Pathophysiological changes in the elderly. *Best Pract Res Clin Anaesthesiol.* 2003;17(2):163–177.

5. Benetos A, Buatois S, Salvi P, *et al.* Blood pressure and pulse wave velocity values in the institutionalized elderly aged 80 and over: baseline of the PARTAGE study. *J Hypertens.* 2010;28(1):41–50.

6. Safar ME. Arterial aging—hemodynamic changes and therapeutic options. *Nat Rev Cardiol.* 2010;7(8):442–449.

7. Chowienczyk P. Pulse wave analysis: what do the numbers mean? *Hypertension.* 2011;57(6):1051–1052.

8. Choi CU, Kim EJ, Kim SH, *et al.* Differing effects of aging on central and peripheral blood pressures and pulse wave velocity: a direct intraarterial study. *J Hypertens.* 2010;28(6):1252–1260.

9. Kovacic JC, Moreno P, Nabel EG, Hachinski V, Fuster V. Cellular senescence, vascular disease, and aging: part 2 of a 2-part review clinical vascular disease in the elderly. *Circulation.* 2011;123(17):1900–1910.

10. Chung HY, Lee EK, Choi YJ, *et al.* Molecular inflammation as an underlying mechanism of the aging process and age-related diseases. *J Dent Res.* 2011;90(7):830–840.

11. Oikonomou E, Tousoulis D, Siasos G, Zaromitidou M, Papavassiliou AG, Stefanadis C. The role of inflammation in heart failure: new therapeutic approaches. *Hellenic J Cardiol.* 2011;52(1):30–40.

12. Chung HY, Cesari M, Anton S, *et al.* Molecular inflammation: underpinnings of aging and age-related diseases. *Ageing Res Rev.* 2009;8(1):18–30.

13. Mizuno Y, Jacob RF, Mason RP. Inflammation and the development of atherosclerosis. *J Atheroscler Thromb.* 2011;18(5):351–358.

14. Chen W, Frangogiannis NG. The role of inflammatory and fibrogenic pathways in heart failure associated with aging. *Heart Fail Rev.* 2010;15(5):415–422.

15. Abadir PM. The frail renin-angiotensin system. *Clin Geriatr Med.* 2011;27(1):53–65.

16. Camici GG, Shi Y, Cosentino F, Francia P, Lüscher TF. Anti-aging medicine: molecular basis for endothelial cell-targeted strategies—a mini-review. *Gerontology.* 2011;57(2):101–108.

17. de Cavanagh EM, Inserra F, Ferder L. Angiotensin II blockade: a strategy to slow ageing by protecting mitochondria? *Cardiovasc Res.* 2011;89(1):31–40.

18. Yoon HE, Ghee JY, Piao S, *et al.* Angiotensin II blockade upregulates the expression of Klotho, the anti-ageing gene, in an experimental model of chronic cyclosporine nephropathy. *Nephrol Dial Transplant.* 2011;26(3):800–813.

19. Ota H, Ghee JY, Piao S, *et al.* SIRT1/eNOS axis as a potential target against vascular senescence, dysfunction and atherosclerosis. *J Atheroscler Thromb.* 2010;17(5):431–435.

20. Lakshminarasimhan M, Steegborn C. Emerging mitochondrial signaling mechanisms in physiology, aging processes, and as drug targets. *Exp Gerontol.* 2011;46(2–3):174–177.

21. Csiszar A, Wang M, Lakatta EG, Ungvari Z. Inflammation and endothelial dysfunction during aging: role of NF-kappaB. *J Appl Physiol.* 2008;105(4):1333–1341.

22. Li M, Fukagawa NK. Age-related changes in redox signaling and VSMC function. *Antioxid Redox Signal.* 2010;12(5):641–655.

23. Kovacic JC, Moreno P, Hachinski V, Nabel EG, Fuster V. Cellular senescence, vascular disease, and aging: part 1 of a 2-part review. *Circulation.* 2011;123(15):1650–1660.

24. Forstermann U. Nitric oxide and oxidative stress in vascular disease. *Pflugers Arch.* 2010;459(6):923–939.

25. Herrera MD, Mingorance C, Rodríguez-Rodríguez R, Alvarez de Sotomayor M. Endothelial dysfunction and aging: an update. *Ageing Res Rev.* 2010;9(2):142–152.

26. Seals DR, Jablonski KL, Donato AJ. Aging and vascular endothelial function in humans. *Clin Sci (Lond).* 2011;120(9):357–375.

27. Barodka VM, Joshi BL, Berkowitz DE, Hogue CW Jr, Nyhan D. Implications of vascular aging. *Anesth Analg.* 2011;112(5):1048–1060.

28. Sawabe M. Vascular aging: from molecular mechanism to clinical significance. *Geriatr Gerontol Int.* 2010;10(Suppl 1):S213–S220.

29. Zieman SM, Melenovsky V, Kass DA. Mechanisms, pathophysiology, and therapy of arterial stiffness. *Arterioscler Thromb Vasc Biol.* 2005;25:932–943.

30. Atkinson J. Age-related medial elastocalcinosis in arteries: mechanisms, animal models, and physiological consequences. *J Appl Physiol.* 2008;105(5):1643–1651.

31. Jugdutt BI. Heart failure in the elderly: advances and challenges. *Expert Rev Cardiovasc Ther.* 2010;8(5):695–715.

32. Robinson T, Smith A, Channer KS. Reversible heart failure: the role of inflammatory activation. *Postgrad Med J.* 2011;87(1024):110–115.

33. Yazdanyar A, Newman AB. The burden of cardiovascular disease in the elderly: morbidity, mortality, and costs. *Clin Geriatr Med.* 2009;25(4):563–577, vii.

34. Wake R, Iida H, Shimodozono S, *et al.* The recent concept of heart function in elderly patients. *Clin Med Geriatr.* 2009;3:9–11.

35. Alecu C, Labat C, Kearney-Schwartz A, *et al.* Reference values of aortic pulse wave velocity in the elderly. *J Hypertens.* 2008;26:2207–2212.

36. Paini A, Boutouyrie P, Calvet D, Tropeano AI, Laloux B, Laurent S. Discrepancies between carotid and aortic stiffness. *Hypertension.* 2006;47:371–376.

37. Wong LS, van der Harst P, de Boer RA, Huzen J, van Gilst WH, van Veldhuisen DJ. Aging, telomeres and heart failure. *Heart Fail Rev.* 2010;15(5):479–486.

38. Rooke GA. Cardiovascular aging and anesthetic implications. *J Cardiothorac Vasc Anesth.* 2003;17(4):512–523.

39. Sanders D, Dudley M, Groban L. Diastolic dysfunction, cardiovascular aging, and the anesthesiologist. *Anesthesiol Clin.* 2009;27(3):497–517.

40. Redheuil A, Yu WC, Wu CO, *et al.* Reduced ascending aortic strain and distensibility: earliest manifestations of vascular aging in humans. *Hypertension.* 2010;55(2):319–326.

41. Alecu C, Cuignet-Royer E, Mertes PM, *et al.* Pre-existing arterial stiffness can predict hypotension during induction of anaesthesia in the elderly. *Br J Anaesth.* 2010;105(5):583–588.

42. Dolan E, Thijs L, Li Y, *et al.* Ambulatory arterial stiffness index as a predictor of cardiovascular mortality in the Dublin outcome study. *Hypertension.* 2006;47:365–370.

43. Duprez DA. Is vascular stiffness a target for therapy? *Cardiovasc Drugs Ther.* 2010. 24(4):305–310.

44. Benigni A, Cassis P, Remuzzi G. Angiotensin II revisited: new roles in inflammation, immunology and aging. *EMBO Mol Med.* 2010;2(7):247–257.

45. Montecucco F, Mach F. Statins, ACE inhibitors and ARBs in cardiovascular disease. *Best Pract Res Clin Endocrinol Metab.* 2009;23(3):389–400.

46. Gradman AH. Role of angiotensin II type 1 receptor antagonists in the treatment of hypertension in patients aged ≥65 years. *Drugs Aging.* 2009;26(9):751–767.

47. Shah R, Wang Y, Foody JM. Effect of statins, angiotensin-converting enzyme inhibitors, and beta blockers on survival in patients ≥65 years of age with heart failure and preserved left ventricular systolic function. *Am J Cardiol*. 2008;101(2):217–222.

48. Protogerou AD, Papaioannou TG, Lekakis JP, Blacher J, Safar ME. The effect of antihypertensive drugs on central blood pressure beyond peripheral blood pressure. Part I: (Patho)-physiology, rationale and perspective on pulse pressure amplification. *Curr Pharm Des*. 2009;15(3):267–271.

49. Nichols WW, Epstein BJ. Actions of selected cardiovascular hormones on arterial stiffness and wave reflections. *Curr Pharm Des*. 2009;15(3):304–320.

50. Safar ME, Smulyan H. Atherosclerosis, arterial stiffness and antihypertensive drug therapy. *Adv Cardiol*. 2007;44:331–351.

51. Logan AG. Hypertension in aging patients. *Expert Rev Cardiovasc Ther*. 2011;9(1):113–120.

52. Aronow WS. Current role of beta-blockers in the treatment of hypertension. *Expert Opin Pharmacother*. 2010;11(16):2599–2607.

53. Agabiti-Rosei E, Porteri E, Rizzoni D. Arterial stiffness, hypertension, and rational use of nebivolol. *Vasc Health Risk Manag*. 2009;5(1):353–360.

54. Arif SA, Mergenhagen KA, Del Carpio RO, Ho C. Treatment of systolic heart failure in the elderly: an evidence-based review. *Ann Pharmacother*. 2010;44(10):1604–1614.

55. Orr JS, Dengo AL, Rivero JM, Davy KP. Arterial destiffening with atorvastatin in overweight and obese middle-aged and older adults. *Hypertension*. 2009;54(4):763–768.

56. Long SB, Blaha MJ, Blumenthal RS, Michos ED. Clinical utility of rosuvastatin and other statins for cardiovascular risk reduction among the elderly. *Clin Interv Aging*. 2011;6:27–35.

57. Berthold HK, Gouni-Berthold I. Lipid-lowering drug therapy in elderly patients. *Curr Pharm Des*. 2011;17(9):877–893.

58. Barrios V, Escobar C. Rosuvastatin along the cardiovascular continuum: from JUPITER to AURORA. *Expert Rev Cardiovasc Ther*. 2009;7(11):1317–1327.

59. Candore G, Caruso C, Jirillo E, Magrone T, Vasto S. Low grade inflammation as a common pathogenetic denominator in age-related diseases: novel drug targets for anti-ageing strategies and successful ageing achievement. *Curr Pharm Des*. 2010;16(6):584–596.

60. Kones R. Rosuvastatin, inflammation, C-reactive protein, JUPITER, and primary prevention of cardiovascular disease—a perspective. *Drug Des Devel Ther*. 2010;4:383–413.

61. Hsia J, MacFadyen JG, Monyak J, Ridker PM. Cardiovascular event reduction and adverse events among subjects attaining low-density lipoprotein cholesterol <50 mg/dl with rosuvastatin The JUPITER Trial (Justification for the Use of Statins in Prevention: an Intervention Trial Evaluating Rosuvastatin). *J Am Coll Cardiol*. 2011;57(16):1666–1675.

62. Wilson M, O'Hanlon R, Basavarajaiah S, et al. Cardiovascular function and the veteran athlete. *Eur J Appl Physiol*. 2010;110(3):459–478.

63. Gando Y, Yamamoto K, Murakami H, et al. Longer time spent in light physical activity is associated with reduced arterial stiffness in older adults. *Hypertension*. 2010;56(3):540–546.

64. Seals DR, Walker AE, Pierce GL, Lesniewski LA. Habitual exercise and vascular ageing. *J Physiol*. 2009;587(Pt 23):5541–5549.

65. Seals DR, Desouza CA, Donato AJ, Tanaka H. Habitual exercise and arterial aging. *J Appl Physiol*. 2008;105(4):1323–1332.

66. Donato AJ, Eskurza I, Silver AE, et al. Direct evidence of endothelial oxidative stress with aging in humans: relation to impaired endothelium-dependent dilation and upregulation of nuclear factor-kappaB. *Circ Res*. 2007;100(11):1659–1666.

67. Heckman GA, McKelvie RS. Cardiovascular aging and exercise in healthy older adults. *Clin J Sport Med*. 2008;18(6):479–485.

68. Sattelmair JR, Pertman JH, Forman DE. Effects of physical activity on cardiovascular and noncardiovascular outcomes in older adults. *Clin Geriatr Med*. 2009;25(4):677–702, viii–ix.

69. Schmidt AC, Flick B, Jahn E, Bramlage P. Effects of the vasodilating beta-blocker nebivolol on smoking-induced endothelial dysfunction in young healthy volunteers. *Vasc Health Risk Manag*. 2008;4(4):909–915.

70. Lakatta EG, Levy D. Arterial and cardiac aging: Major shareholders in cardiovascular disease enterprises. *Circulation*. 2003;107:139–146.

CHAPTER 14

Respiratory diseases in the elderly

Irwin Foo

Introduction

Respiratory diseases are a major feature in elderly patients presenting for surgery. In the 2010 National Confidential Enquiry into Patient Outcome and Death (NCEPOD) report entitled *An Age Old Problem* which reviewed care received by elderly patients undergoing surgery, respiratory disease was the third commonest (28 per cent) comorbidity present at the time of admission[1]. A substantial proportion of postoperative morbidity and mortality is due to respiratory complications postoperatively. This excess risk is due to the interaction between functional changes with ageing of the respiratory system (e.g. changes in the mechanical properties of the lung leading to decreased vital capacity, increased residual volume, and changes in gas exchange parameters) and common respiratory diseases found in this age group resulting in reduced reserve and respiratory insufficiency. This chapter will focus on the common respiratory diseases found in the elderly surgical patient that contribute to postoperative morbidity and which are amenable to preoperative optimization therefore excluding pulmonary malignancies and interstitial lung diseases.

Chronic obstructive pulmonary disease

Chronic obstructive pulmonary disease (COPD) is a preventable and treatable disease which is slowly progressive and characterized by airflow obstruction that is not fully reversible. The disease is associated with an inflammatory response due to inhalation of noxious gases. COPD affects mainly the lungs but also has significant systemic effects.[2] In most patients, cigarette smoking is responsible for the inflammatory response but other factors such as chronic exposure to indoor airborne pollutants, e.g. cigarette smoke and house dust, and fumes and smoke generated from burning biomass fuel also play a part in the pathogenesis of the disease. COPD is a major health burden worldwide and affects more than 5 per cent of the adult population in the United States. It is the third leading cause of death and the 12th leading cause of morbidity.[3] Unlike other chronic diseases which are projected to decrease in prevalence, the diagnosis of COPD is expected to increase worldwide.[4]

COPD diagnosis

A diagnosis of COPD is confirmed when patient has symptoms of dyspnoea, chronic cough with or without sputum production, wheezing and poor exercise tolerance with airflow obstruction as demonstrated by spirometry. The obstructive ventilatory defect in this case is defined as forced expiratory volume in 1 s (FEV_1)/forced vital capacity (FVC) ratio of less than 70 per cent on postbronchodilator spirometry. Using this definition, the prevalence of COPD is age dependent. In one population-based study, the prevalence of COPD in patients aged 75–80 years was 41.7 per cent compared with 16.8 per cent in patients aged between 50 and 54 years.[5] This doubling in the number of patients may be related to the increase in survival of patients with COPD and the increase in new cases detected due to ageing itself.

However, as ageing of the respiratory system is associated with a natural decrease in FEV_1/FVC, this may represent on overdiagnosis in the elderly. In a cross-sectional population-based study, the increase in the rate of airflow obstruction in asymptomatic non-smoking elderly population was such that in the over 80s 50 per cent met the COPD criteria.[6] For this reason, the authors proposed different cut-off points for diagnosing COPD in the elderly (Table 14.1)

This acknowledges that there are several similarities in the histological appearances of the lung between an elderly non-smoking adult and in patients with COPD. For example, there is increased bronchial thickening and dilatation of alveoli with an enlargement of airspaces and a reduction in the gas exchange surface area coupled with a loss of supporting tissue for peripheral airways (senile emphysema). This results in a decrease in elastic recoil of the lung and increased residual volume and functional residual capacity. This loss of elastin is similar to the loss of skin elasticity and wrinkling of the skin which occurs in ageing. The major difference between the changes in lung ageing and COPD is the presence of active alveolar wall destruction in COPD.[7]

In patients unable to perform spirometry adequately, the use of high-resolution computed tomography (HRCT) might provide useful information in the diagnosis of COPD, e.g. the combination of the extent of emphysema as seen on HRCT and lung function measurements (lung diffusion capacity) provided good physiological information for the assessment and diagnosis of COPD patients.[8] The related term chronic bronchitis is a clinical diagnosis describing the presence of cough and sputum production for at least 3 months in each of two consecutive years. Although useful as a clinical and epidemiological term, not all patients with chronic bronchitis will have or will develop chronic airflow obstruction.[9]

Table 14.1 FEV_1/FVC ratio cut-off points for the diagnosis of COPD in different age groups

Age	FEV_1/FVC ratio
<70 years	<70%
70–80 years	<65%
>80 years	<60%

Data from Hardie JA, Buist AS, Vollmer WM, et al. Risk of over-diagnosis of COPD in asymptomatic elderly never-smokers. *European Respiratory Journal* 2002;20: 1117–1122.

Pathology and pathogenesis of COPD

The pathological changes of COPD can be usefully divided up into the four different lung compartments:

- Central airways—mucous gland hyperplasia leading to mucous hypersecretion and ciliary dysfunction (responsible for the chronic cough).

- Peripheral airways—chronic inflammation and fibrosis, characterized by macrophage, neutrophil, and CD8 lymphocyte infiltration (responsible for airflow limitation).

- Lung parenchyma—alveolar wall destruction resulting in irreversible enlargement of air spaces distal to the terminal bronchioles (emphysema). Different patterns have been described, e.g. panacinar emphysema (dilated air spaces evenly distributed across acinii), proximal emphysema (dilated air spaces mainly in the respiratory bronchioles), and paraseptal emphysema (dilated air spaces abutting the pleura or blood vessels). This alveolar destruction gives rise to hyperinflation, decrease in elastic recoil, expiratory flow limitation due to dynamic compression and gas exchange abnormalities.

- Pulmonary vasculature—thickened arteriolar walls and remodelling (especially with hypoxia) resulting in increased pulmonary vascular resistance and pulmonary hypertension and gas exchange impairment.

The most convincing evidence for a direct causal link in COPD is for cigarette smoke. Many epidemiological studies have shown that cigarette smoking is by far the most important risk factor for the development of COPD.[10] A history of greater than 40 pack-years of smoking is the single best predictor for airflow obstruction consistent with a diagnosis of COPD[11] and smoking causes a greater annual rate of decline of FEV_1 than do non-smokers. Stopping smoking slows the decline in FEV_1.[12]

Worldwide, indoor air pollution may be a significant factor especially with the use of heating and cooking with biomass fuel in poorly ventilated dwellings. This leads to a high level of particulate matter indoors.[13] Intense occupational exposure to dust, gases and fumes have also been implicated in the development of COPD and the effects of occupational exposure and smoking is additive.[14]

Although cigarette smoke and other inhaled noxious particles causes the inflammatory response seen, an imbalance of proteinases and antiproteinases in the lungs and oxidative stress are also involved in the pathogenesis.[15] This results in a variable natural history and not all individuals follow the same course. This may well explain why not all smokers develop clinically significant COPD. Genetic factors certainly play a role with the best known

genetic factor being a deficiency of the serine protease α1 antitrypsin which affects 1–3 per cent of patients with COPD.[16] Other genetic factors have been implicated, e.g. genes coding for transforming growth factor β1[17], microsomal epoxide hydrolase 1[18] and tumour necrosis factor-alpha (TNFα)[19] however, results were inconsistent.

It is often quoted that between 15 and 20 per cent of smokers develop clinically significant COPD but this may be an underestimation as the criteria for COPD diagnosis has changed since the classic study by Fletcher and colleagues (1976).[20] It may be as high as 50 per cent.[21] Furthermore, it has been shown that the distribution of FEV_1 shifts as a function of smoking dose in a population study and the conclusion reached was that with enough smoking, almost all smokers will have measurably reduced function but only some will be severely affected.[22]

Systemic effects of COPD

Although COPD principally affects the lungs, it also produces significant systemic consequences. The cardiovascular and the musculoskeletal systems are frequently affected and there is an increase in the diagnosis of the metabolic syndrome (defined as the presence of three of the following factors: abdominal obesity, elevated triglycerides, reduced high-density lipoproteins, hypertension and hyperglycaemia).[23] As COPD is regarded as an inflammatory disease, it is likely that circulating cytokines and other inflammatory mediators may contribute to the development of these extrapulmonary manifestations. Systematic reviews have identified a relationship between COPD and increased levels of C-reactive protein, fibrinogen, circulating leucocytes and the pro-inflammatory cytokine TNFα.[24] It has even been suggested that the term chronic systemic inflammatory syndrome be incorporated into the diagnosis of COPD to emphasize the systemic nature of the disease.[25] Cigarette smoking which is the major risk factor for COPD may be the common link between COPD and systemic inflammation as it causes both lung and systemic inflammation, systemic oxidative stress, marked changes in vasomotor and endothelial function and increased procoagulant factors.

A high prevalence of cardiovascular complications is found in COPD patients. A twofold increase in hypertension, ischaemic heart disease, cardiac arrhythmias and congestive cardiac failure was found in a population-based study comparing COPD patients and an age-matched control group of smokers without COPD.[26] Furthermore, in two large studies on therapeutic agents in moderate to severe COPD patients, nearly one-third of all-cause mortality in the trial population was accounted for by cardiovascular causes.[27, 28]

Skeletal muscle wasting and dysfunction are recognized as important features of COPD and are important causes for disability.[29] Low exercise tolerance leads to physical deconditioning and a reduction in quality of life. It is postulated that muscle mass depletion is caused by mitochondrial abnormalities and loss of contractile proteins with muscle malfunction of the remaining muscle. Apart from the role of pro-inflammatory cytokines in the development of peripheral muscle weakness, other factors, e.g. deconditioning, oxidative stress, imbalance in protein metabolism, use of systemic corticosteroids, hypoxaemia, hypercapnia, electrolyte disturbances, and cardiac failure, have all been implicated.

Reduced bone mineralization and osteoporosis is highly prevalent in COPD patients with estimates ranging from 35–60 per cent.[30] Systemic inflammation is associated with loss of bone mineral density although there are other contributory factors include smoking, corticosteroid use, and low body mass index (BMI). A serious consequence is the increase in the rate of pathological vertebral fractures which further contribute to immobility, pain, and reduced sputum clearance.[31]

Nutritional depletion in COPD is well recognized. Body weight is directly related to the severity of lung function as determined by the FEV_1 and mortality is increased as the body weight decrease irrespective of lung function. Low body weight is therefore an independent marker of poor outcome.[32] Malnutrition affects approximately 10–15 per cent of patients with mild-to-moderate disease and 50 per cent of patients with advanced-stage disease and chronic respiratory failure.[33] Weight loss has been postulated to be the result of a high metabolic rate that is not compensated for by increased dietary intake. The raised basal metabolic rate is in part due to systemic inflammation but other factors include medications used to treat COPD (β-2 agonists and theophylline), increased catecholamines and the oxygen cost of breathing.[28]

What is less well recognized is the high prevalence of obesity among patients with mild-to-moderate COPD particularly in males. Recent reports suggest that fat mass contributes to systemic inflammation in COPD and is postulated to compound the systemic adverse effects.[34] However, this theory is at odds with the observation of lower mortality in COPD patients with a high body mass index compared to those with a low BMI (also known as the obesity paradox).[35]

A threefold increase in the prevalence of the metabolic syndrome was found in patients with COPD.[22] Insulin resistance was also found to be higher in COPD patients and these authors found a correlation between insulin resistance and circulating interleukin-6 and TNFα suggesting that glucose homeostasis may be another systemic complication of COPD.[36]

Psychosocial factors

Psychosocial factors, e.g. cognitive function, mood status, self-sufficiency (confidence to perform activities of daily living) and social support play a role in determining the health status of COPD patients. For example, cognitive impairment may interfere with self-management and is an under-recognized problem amongst patients.[37] There is even a specific pattern of cognitive dysfunction involving verbal memory impairment, attention and deductive thinking in patients with severe COPD with hypoxia and hypercapnia which is only partially reversible with oxygen therapy.[38]

The prevalence of depression is high in COPD patients independent of both age and disability and is associated with an increased symptom burden, poorer physical and social functioning, increased healthcare utilization, longer hospital stay and poorer survival.[39,40] In one study in elderly patients with disabling COPD, almost half of them showed symptoms of a depressed mood compared to 11 per cent of age-matched non-COPD controls.[41]

Social environment is also important. COPD patients who live alone have a higher risk for a prolonged hospital stay and lower family support and care was found to be a risk for depression among patients hospitalized with an exacerbation of COPD.[40]

Assessment and management of the elderly COPD patient

COPD severity is graded according to the severity of airflow obstruction (Table 14.2) as mild, moderate, severe, and very severe according to the National Institute for Health and Clinical Excellence 2010 clinical guideline.[42]

It is useful for guiding management but is less predictive of the risk of hospitalization and mortality when compared with the BODE index[43] (Table 14.3). The BODE index is a multidimensional grading system using BMI, airflow Obstruction, Dyspnoea and Exercise capacity as its scoring variables. Patients are scored between 0 and 10, with higher scores indicating a higher risk of death.

However, even this scoring system may be inadequate in assessing the impact of pulmonary systemic effects and psychosocial factors on the health status of elderly patients as discussed earlier. Therefore, the multidimensional assessment in the form of the comprehensive geriatric assessment (CGA) tool has been advocated in elderly COPD patients.[44] This approach in the older COPD patients is appropriate as apart from underestimating their own level of disability, their quality of life and functional status are poorer compared with similarly aged persons.[45] They are also more at risk of becoming frail and once hospitalized are less likely to return to independent living.[46] The CGA tool is an effective instrument for minimizing disability and loss of independence in older patients.

The management of COPD consists of assessment of severity, reduction of risk factors, management of the stable disease and accompanying comorbidities, and prevention of exacerbations. The management of COPD in the elderly is similar to their younger counterparts with regards to pharmacological treatment but a more

Table 14.2 Gradation of severity of airflow obstruction

Post-bronchodilator FEV_1/FVC	FEV_1 % predicted	Severity of airflow obstruction
<0.7	≥80%	Stage 1: mild (+ symptoms)
<0.7	50–79%	Stage 2: moderate
<0.7	30–49%	Stage 3: severe
<0.7	<30%	Stage 4: very severe(or FEV_1 <50% with respiratory failure)

National Clinical Guideline Centre (2010) Chronic obstructive pulmonary disease: Management of chronic obstructive pulmonary disease in adults in primary and secondary care. Clinical guideline 101. Published by the National Clinical Guidelines Centre at The Royal College of Physicians, 11 St Andrews Place, Regent's Park, London, NW11 4LE. Copyright © NCGC. *Reproduced by permission.*

Table 14.3 BODE index

Variable	Points on BODE index			
	0	1	2	3
FEV_1 (% of predicted)	≥65	50–64	36–49	≤35
Distance walked in 6 min (m)	≥350	250–349	150–249	≤149
MMRC dyspnoea scale	0–1	2	3	4
Body mass index	>21	≤21		

From *New England Journal of Medicine*, Celli BR, Cote CG, Marin JM et al., 'The Body-Mass Index, airflow obstruction, dyspnea, and exercise capacity index in chronic obstructive pulmonary disease', 350, 10, pp. 1005–1012, Copyright © 2004 Massachusetts Medical Society. Reprinted with permission from Massachusetts Medical Society.

holistic approach is required. For example, achieving independence in activities of daily living should be regarded to be more important than improvement in FEV_1.

Smoking cessation remains the only intervention that is proven to decrease the smoking-related decline in lung function[12] and should be offered to all patients regardless of age. All elderly COPD patients should be offered influenza and pneumococcal vaccines to prevent precipitating an exacerbation of the disease.

Pharmacological management consists of short-acting bronchodilators (either β agonist or muscarinic agonist) for breathlessness and exercise limitation. If breathlessness persists, long-acting bronchodilators are added or alternatively combination long-acting and inhaled corticosteroids depending on FEV_1 status. Triple therapy may be considered for persistent breathlessness. In the elderly, extra care should be taken in the assessment of adverse effects of these pharmacological agents, e.g. with inhaled corticosteroids, there is an increased risk of cataracts, fragility fractures and an excess of severe pneumonia.[47]

Furthermore, in this age group, the correct inhaler technique is essential as even with the most competent inhaler technique, only 15–30 per cent of each actuation is deposited at the site of action.[48] It has been established that cognitive impairment and loss of manual dexterity are barriers to effective inhaler technique and the delivery of bronchodilator and corticosteroid therapy. An Abbreviated Mental Test Score of less than 7 out of 10 and a Mini Mental State Examination score of less than 24 out of 30 were predictive of an inadequate inhaler technique.[49] These global cognition tests should be performed to evaluate suitability of elderly patients to use inhalers and whether alternative methods, e.g. nebulizers should be used. Inhaler therapy, especially inhaled corticosteroids should not be interrupted as an observational study found that there was a ninefold increase in the rate of exacerbations on interruption of inhaled corticosteroids in stable moderate to severe COPD patients.[50] Apart from treatment targeted at the lungs, the future may lie in the treatment of the chronic systemic inflammation, e.g. limited evidence suggests the use of statins to treat systemic inflammation reduces morbidity and mortality in patients with COPD.[51]

Pulmonary rehabilitation programmes are individually tailored and are designed to optimize physical and social performance and autonomy. In particular, elderly patients will benefit from targeted muscle training. Exercise training has been shown to improve exercise capacity in COPD patients.[52] Apart from exercise training, pulmonary rehabilitation programmes offers education, psychosocial/behavioural interventions, nutritional therapy, and outcome assessment.

Avoidance of exacerbations is important in the elderly as their frequency is increased with age and the outcome poorer when compared to younger patients. Connors and colleagues found that the mortality rate of acute exacerbation increased by 30 per cent for every 10 years.[53] COPD exacerbations in older patients were also more likely to be associated with bronchial infections: evidence of pathogens were seen in 78 per cent of patients over 70 years.[54] Optimizing treatment for stable COPD helps to reduce exacerbations, e.g. maintaining high levels of physical activity in daily life.

Preoperative optimization of elderly COPD patients include:

◆ Counselling and pharmacotherapy for smoking cessation. Even a short period of abstinence (12–72 hours) is beneficial for carbon monoxide elimination, normalization of cardiovascular parameters and improvement in bronchotracheal ciliary function.[55]

◆ Preoperative physiotherapy using incentive spirometry and inspiratory muscle training. A short 2-week training programme

in the elderly using an inspiratory threshold-loading device reduced the incidence of atelectasis postoperatively.[56]

◆ Drug therapy optimization—substitution of inhalers for nebulized therapy.

◆ Assessment and management of systemic effects, e.g. concomitant cardiovascular disease.

◆ Detection of drug interactions from polypharmacy.

◆ Involvement of care of the elderly team early for additional management.

This is important as patients with a diagnosis of COPD have a 2.7–4.7-fold increased risk of postoperative pulmonary complications and the further away the surgery is from the diaphragm, the lower the complication rate.[57]

Asthma

Asthma is a chronic airway inflammatory disorder associated with airflow obstruction and bronchial hyper-responsiveness in which many cells and cellular elements play a role. Airflow obstruction is variable in severity and is reversible either spontaneously or with treatment but may become irreversible over many years. A history of recurrent episodes of wheezing, chest tightness, breathlessness and cough especially at night and in the early morning is suggestive of asthma but in the elderly, these symptoms may be poorly recognized. For example, elderly asthmatics experience less intense respiratory distress during histamine bronchoprovocation challenge compared to their younger counterparts[58] and there may be cough impairment secondary to the presence of other comorbidities such as Parkinson's disease.[59] This contributes to the underdiagnosis of asthma in the elderly.

Prevalence and diagnosis

As asthma is a chronic and generally incurable disease, its prevalence should be similar in both the older and younger population. However, asthma is less recognized in the elderly as it is considered a disease of childhood and adolescence. Apart from reduced perception of asthma symptoms, other reasons for underdiagnosis include dyspnoea due to physiological ageing, self-limitation of activities, social isolation, the misconception that adult-onset asthma is rare and comorbid conditions, e.g. congestive cardiac failure.[60] The prevalence of asthma in the over-65s has been estimated to be between 3.8–7.1 per cent[61]—this may well be an underestimate due to equivocal criteria for diagnosis and the partial loss of reversibility which complicates diagnosis and makes distinction from COPD difficult. Nevertheless, it is important to try to distinguish the two conditions as although both are characterized by the presence of airway obstruction, they have distinct pathogenesis and different treatment goals. In a population-based study, the overall age and sex-adjusted incidence of asthma in the elderly is 95 per 100 000 (declining from 103 per 100 000 in subjects aged 65–74 years to 58 per 100 000 in subjects aged >85 years).[62] Risk factors for asthma in the elderly include atopy (genetic tendency to mount abnormal responses to common allergens), airway hyper-responsiveness (bimodal distribution: early and late phases of life), smoking, environmental pollution, and gastro-oesophageal reflux.[63]

Although asthma is mainly a clinical diagnosis, it should be supported by objective measurements. Either clinical spirometry or pulmonary function tests demonstrating airflow obstruction that improves significantly in response to bronchodilators (12 per

Table 14.4 Levels of asthma control

A. Assessment of current clinical control (preferably over 4 weeks)			
Characteristic	**Controlled (All of the following)**	**Partly Controlled (Any measure present)**	**Uncontrolled**
Daytime symptoms	None (twice or less/week)	More than twice/week	Three or more features of partly controlled asthma*†
Limitation of activities	None	Any	
Nocturnal symptoms/awakening	None	Any	
Need for reliever/rescue treatment	None (twice or less/week)	More than twice/week	
Lung function (PEF or FEV$_1$)‡	Normal	<80% predicted or personal best (if known)	
B. Assessment of Future Risk (risk of exacerbations, instability, rapid decline in lung function, side-effects)			
Features that are associated with increased risk of adverse events in the future include:			
Poor clinical control, frequent exacerbations in past year*, ever admission to critical care fore asthma, low FEV$_1$, exposure to cigarette smoke, high dose medications			

* Any exacerbation should prompt review of maintenance treatment to ensure that it is adequate

† By definition, an exacerbation in any week makes that an uncontrolled asthma week

‡ Without administration of bronchodilator

Lung function is not a reliable test for children 5 year and younger

FEV$_1$: forced expiratory volume in 1 s; PEF: peak expiratory flow. Global Initiative for Asthma, 2008.

From the Global Strategy for Asthma Management and Prevention 2012, © Global Initiative for Asthma (GINA), all rights reserved. Available from http://www.ginasthma.org.

cent or 200 ml improvement in FEV$_1$). In the majority of elderly patients, FEV$_1$ measurements are acceptable and reproducible as shown in the SARA study with the patients' mean age of 73 years.[64] To further distinguish between asthma and COPD in the elderly, it has been suggested that assessment of the carbon monoxide diffusing capacity (DLCO) be undertaken in equivocal cases as there is a significant difference in DLCO values between the two. COPD patients tend to have lower DLCO values due to the loss of alveolar–capillary surface area that is associated with alveolar destruction.[65] Specialist tests such as airway response to methacholine may also help to diagnose asthma. The severity of asthma is classified by clinical features and lung function (Table 14.4).[66]

Natural history of asthma in the elderly

Airway inflammation in asthma is a multicellular process involving eosinophils, T-helper 2 lymphocytes and mast cells. Apart from a reduced eosinophil degranulation response to interleukin-5 stimulation, older asthmatics (55–80 years) had similar eosinophil adhesion and chemotaxis responses to stimulation when compared with younger asthmatics (20–40 years).[67] Over a prolonged time, there is basement membrane thickening, collagen deposition, increased smooth muscle mass, and mucous gland hypertrophy leading to a thickened airway wall and a reduced airway calibre. This is termed airway remodelling and is believed to be responsible for the non-reversible component seen in long-standing chronic asthma including elderly asthmatics. One of the hallmarks of a prolonged asthma duration is an accelerated decline in lung function. In the 15-year follow-up study of ventilatory function in adults with asthma performed in Copenhagen, the decline in lung function was quantified as 38 ml/year in asthmatics compared with 22 ml/year in normal individuals even after adjustments for height and sex.[68] Furthermore, long-standing asthma and ageing is associated with reduced acute responsiveness to bronchodilators.[69]

Two distinct patterns of asthma are found in the elderly: early and late onset asthma. They have different clinical presentations and responses to treatment. The differences are shown in Table 14.5. Elderly patients with early-onset asthma complain less about asthma symptoms but tend to have more impairment of

lung function and a poorer response to bronchodilators. This poor response to bronchodilators is related to airway remodelling and diminished responsiveness of airway β$_2$-adrenoceptors.[69]

The importance of recognizing asthma in the elderly cannot be over-emphasized as this patient group is associated with more frequent and severe attacks which increases the number of episodes of hospitalization and emergency department visits.[70] Furthermore, asthma deaths in older patients account for greater than 50 per cent of asthma fatalities annually due to underdiagnosis, undertreatment, and the presence of other comorbidities.[71] In one study of elderly asthmatics, only 6 per cent of subjects with a peak expiratory flow rate lower than 70 per cent predicted were on any respiratory medications.[72]

Management of asthma in the elderly

Treatment goals in the elderly are no different from that of the younger asthmatics which include symptom control, prevention of exacerbations and hospital admissions, maintenance of pulmonary function as close to normal levels as possible, improving quality of life, avoidance of side effects from medications, and prevention of the development of irreversible airflow limitation. However, with elderly asthmatics, the response to bronchodilators may be suboptimal, other comorbidities may increase side effects of therapy,

Table 14.5 Main differences between early- and late-onset asthma

	Early-onset asthma	**Late-onset asthma**
Atopy	More frequent	Less frequent
Pulmonary function	Marked impairment	More accelerated FEV$_1$ decline
Obstruction reversibility	Less reversible obstruction	More frequent response to bronchodilators
Airway hyper-responsiveness	More related to lung function	More related to airway inflammation

Reproduced with permission of the European Respiratory Society. Bellia V, et al., 'Asthma in the Elderly', *European Respiratory Society Monograph* 2009; 43 (Respiratory Diseases in the Elderly): 56–76; DOI: 10.1183/1025448x.00043005.

cognitive impairment may preclude an adequate inhaler technique, and polypharmacy may increase the likelihood of drug interactions.

Non-pharmacological management should be optimized in the elderly asthmatic. The withdrawal of medications that can aggravate asthma, e.g. non-selective β-blockers, non-steroidal anti-inflammatory drugs, should be considered. All elderly asthmatics should be offered influenza and pneumococcal vaccines and encouraged to stop smoking and to lose weight if obesity is an issue. Before inhaler therapies are offered, it is essential to ensure that elderly patients are able to use the devices and are not cognitively impaired. Other alternative devices such as nebulizers should be used if patients are unable to use the inhaler correctly. Recommended pharmacological medications are divided into controllers or relievers. Controllers are taken daily on a long-term basis to keep asthma under clinical control predominantly through their anti-inflammatory effects. These include inhaled corticosteroids, leukotriene modifiers, long acting β$_2$-agonists, sustained-release theophyllines and oral corticosteroids while relievers are medications used on an as-needed basis, to relieve bronchoconstriction (short acting β$_2$-agonists).

Inhaled corticosteroids are the cornerstone of treatment for persistent asthma. Although inhaled corticosteroids were demonstrated in the elderly to reduce the risk of rehospitalization and mortality from all causes, this therapy remained underused in this population.[73] This is probably related to the side effects seen with inhaled corticosteroids. One of the most common being pain and dysphagia caused by oropharyngeal and oesophageal mycotic infections, usually due to *Candida albicans*. Hoarseness and cough are also more frequently reported in the elderly due to oral deposition of steroids as a consequence of faulty inhaler technique. All this may be reduced by the use of a spacer device and by teaching patients to rinse their mouth after each inhalation. Furthermore, corticosteroids may induce an increase in β- adrenoceptor density which would partially offset the diminished responsiveness of airway β$_2$-adrenoceptors seen in older asthmatics.[74]

Long-acting inhaled β$_2$-agonists (LABA) including formoterol and salmeterol have been demonstrated to be efficacious and safe in the elderly. They have a steroid sparing effect when added to a moderate dose of inhaled corticosteroids and should be considered before raising the dose of the inhaled corticosteroid. The use of anticholinergic drugs (ipratropium bromide and tiotropium) may be used as an alternative to β$_2$-agonists in selected patients who are not responsive to β$_2$-agonists although there are conflicting results regarding their efficacy.[75,76]

Close monitoring for adverse reactions to asthma drugs should be undertaken as the number of comorbid conditions increase with age especially cardiovascular disease. β$_2$-agonists may induce tachyarrhythmias, hypokalaemia, and hypertension whilst theophylline may induce potentially fatal ventricular arrhythmias in the elderly especially as its pharmacokinetics are different compared to younger individuals.[77] Corticosteroids apart from local adverse side effects from the inhaled route may worsen osteoporosis if administered systemically.[78]

As with COPD patients, preoperative optimization includes minimizing symptoms and airway hyper-responsiveness by smoking cessation and avoidance of wheeze-inducing medications. Regular nebulizer therapy and a short course of systemic corticosteroids (prednisolone 40 mg orally for 1 week) may be required prior to surgery.

Obstructive sleep apnoea

Obstructive sleep apnoea (OSA) is defined by the occurrence of more than five obstructive respiration events per hour of sleep associated with nocturnal or daytime symptoms (loud snoring, nocturnal choking, nocturia, daytime sleepiness, and poor concentration) or by the occurrence of more than 15 obstructive respiratory events per hour of sleep.[79]

The prevalence of OSA increases with age and ranges from 30–80 per cent depending on the chosen threshold for diagnosis using the apnoea/hypopnoea index (calculated from the number of apnoea and hypopnoea periods lasting 10 s or more per hour of sleep (apnoea/hypopnoea index: AHI): AHI >5 or AHI >15 commonly chosen in studies).[80] It affects older men and women equally. Age-related alterations in respiratory anatomy and physiology may be a contributory factor in the increased prevalence. There is some evidence of increased upper airway adipose tissue deposition, structural bony changes of the pharynx leading to narrowing of the airway, sleep-induced changes in upper airway muscle activity and ventilatory control instability in this age group although these changes are not universally seen. There appears to be no specific pathophysiological mechanism responsible for the increased incidence.[81]

Clinical presentation in the elderly may be classical (history of snoring in an overweight male, associated with nocturnal choking, nocturia, daytime sleepiness and a witnessed apnoea during sleep) or non-typical, modified by comorbidities and general health status. In some patients, the presence of nocturia, mild cognitive dysfunction, accidental falls, driving accidents, glaucoma, and non-arteritic anterior ischaemic optic neuropathy may be suggestive of OSA which can be easily missed. Diagnosis should follow referral to a formal sleep medicine unit and may be based on full polysomnography which will allow discrimination between obstructive and central events, other sleep disorders (e.g. periodic leg movements) as well as an assessment of the amount and quality of sleep.[81] The AHI cut-off value to diagnose OSA in elderly patients is usually greater than five events per hour of sleep although some studies have used higher cut-off values of 10–20 events per hour. There is as yet no universal agreement for an age-adjusted threshold for the diagnosis of OSA.

Epidemiological studies have suggested that OSA increases the risk of arterial hypertension, stroke, and ischaemic disease.[82] However, studies have indicated that middle-aged patients are more at risk of cardiovascular morbidity than older adults.[83] One possible explanation is an age-related resistance to oxidative stress in the myocardium and this would explain a greater tolerance to OSA in older patients.[84] Nevertheless, apart from cardiovascular morbidity, excessive daytime sleepiness is commonly reported and may contribute to cognitive impairment, poor quality of life and depression in the elderly which may be improved with treatment.[85]

Treatment of OSA in the elderly is no different from the younger patient. Continuous positive airway pressure (CPAP) remains the gold standard treatment although in older patients a lower level of CPAP is needed to abolish the apnoeas and hypopnoeas.[86] Studies examining compliance in older patients with CPAP found no difference compared to younger patients therefore should not be withheld.[87] However, 'living alone' is a factor associated with poor compliance. In obese patients, weight management should be encouraged. Treatment of OSA in elderly patients apart from reversing neuropsychological impairment also reverses the nocturia which can be troublesome in this age group.

As the presentation of OSA in the elderly may be atypical and often missed, at preoperative assessment, a high index of suspicion is required. The importance of recognizing OSA is the increased risk for partial or total airway obstruction in the elderly especially when sedative and opioid analgesics are given. A monitored postoperative placement is warranted and CPAP use may be necessary. Referral to a sleep medicine unit for diagnosis is required.

Conclusion

An understanding of these common respiratory diseases in elderly patients presenting for surgery is required to optimize and to minimize complications. As with other comorbidities, a multidisciplinary approach is necessary for achieving the best outcomes for the older patient.

References

1. National Confidential Enquiry into Patient Outcome and Death (NCEPOD). *An age old problem: a review of the care received by elderly patients undergoing surgery.* <http://www.ncepod.org.uk/2010eese.htm>.

2. Celli BR, MacNee W, Agusti A, *et al.* Standards for the diagnosis and treatment of patients with COPD: a summary of the ATS/ERS position. *Eur Respir J.* 2004;23:932–946.

3. National Heart, Lung, and Blood Institute. *Data fact sheet: chronic obstructive pulmonary disease.* Report no. 03-5229. Bethesda, MD: National Heart, Lung, and Blood Institute, 2003.

4. World Health Organization. *Global surveillance, prevention and control of chronic respiratory disease. A comprehensive approach.* Geneva: WHO Publications, 2007.

5. Celli BR, Halbert RJ, Isonaka S, *et al.* Population impact of different definitions of airway obstruction. *Eur Respir J.* 2003;22:268–273.

6. Hardie JA, Buist AS, Vollmer WM, *et al.* Risk of over-diagnosis of COPD in asymptomatic elderly never-smokers. *Eur Respir J.* 2002;20:1117–1122.

7. Ito K and Barnes PJ. COPD as a disease of accelerated lung ageing. *Chest.* 2009;135:173–180.

8. Cerveri I, Dore R, Corsico A, *et al.* Assessment of emphysema in COPD: a functional and radiological study. *Chest.* 2004;125:1714–1718.

9. Vestbo J, Lange P. Can GOLD stage 0 provide information of prognostic value in chronic obstructive pulmonary disease? *Am J Respir Crit Care Med.* 2002;166:329–332.

10. US Department of Health and Human Services. *The health consequences of smoking: A report of the Surgeon General.* Atlanta, GA: US Department of Health and Human Services, Centers for Disease Control and Prevention, National Center for Chronic Disease Prevention and Health Promotion, Office on Smoking and Health, 2004.

11. Holleman DR, Simel DL. Does the clinical examination predict airflow limitation? *JAMA.* 1995;273:313–319.

12. Anthonisen NR, Connett JE, Murray RP. Smoking and lung function of lung health study participants after 11 years. *Am J Respir Crit Care Med.* 2002;166:675–679.

13. Smith KR. Inaugural article: national burden of disease in India from indoor air pollution. *Proc Natl Acad Sci USA.* 2000;97:286–293.

14. Kaufmann F, Drouet D, Lellouch J, *et al.* Occupational exposure and 12 year spirometric changes among Paris area workers. *Br J Ind Med.* 1982;39:221–232.

15. Repine JE, Bast A, Lankhorst I. Oxidative stress in chronic obstructive pulmonary disease. Oxidative Stress Study Group. *Am J Respir Crit Care Med.* 1997;156:341–347.

16. Stoller JK and Aboussouan LS. α1-antitrypsin deficiency. *Lancet.* 2005;365:2225–2236.

17. Celedon JC, Lange C, Raby BA, *et al.* The transforming growth factor—beta1 (TGFB1) gene is associated with chronic obstructive pulmonary disease (COPD). *Hum Mol Genet.* 2004; 13: 1649–1656.

18. Cheng SL, Yu CJ, Chen CJ, *et al.* Genetic polymorphism of epoxide hydrolase and glutathione S-transferase in COPD. *Eur Respir J.* 2004;23:818–824.

19. Keatings VM, Cave SJ, Henry MJ, *et al.* A polymorphism in the tumour necrosis factor—alpha gene promoter region may predispose to a poor prognosis in COPD. *Chest.* 2000;118:971–975.

20. Fletcher C, Peto R, Tinker C, *et al. The natural history of chronic bronchitis and emphysema.* Oxford: Oxford University Press, 1976.

21. Lundback B, Lindberg A, Lindstrom L, *et al.* Not 15 but 50% of smokers develop COPD? Report from the Obstructive Lung Disease in Northern Sweden Studies. *Respir Med.* 2003;97:115–122.

22. Burrows B, Knudson RJ, Cline MG, *et al.* Quantitative relationship s between cigarette smoking and ventilatory function. *Am Rev Respir Dis.* 1977;115:195–205.

23. Marquis K, Maltais F, Duguay V, *et al.* The metabolic syndrome in patients with chronic obstructive pulmonary disease. *J Cardiopulm Rehabil.* 2005;25:226–232.

24. Gan WQ, Man SF, Senthilselvan A, *et al.* Association between chronic obstructive pulmonary disease and systemic inflammation: a systematic review and a meta-analysis. *Thorax.* 2004;59:574–580.

25. Fabri LM, Rabe KF. From COPD to chronic systemic inflammatory syndrome? *Lancet.* 2007;370:797–799.

26. Curkendall SM, DeLuise C, Jones JK, *et al.* Cardiovascular disease in patients with chronic obstructive pulmonary disease, Saskatchewan, Canada. *Ann Epidemiol.* 2006;16:63–70.

27. Calverley PMA, Anderson JA, Celli B, *et al.* Salmeterol and fluticasone proprionate and survival in chronic obstructive pulmonary disease. *N Engl J Med.* 2007;356:775–789.

28. Tashkin DP, Celli B, Senn S, *et al.* A 4 year trial of tiotropium in chronic obstructive pulmonary disease. *N Engl J Med.* 2008;359:1543–1554.

29. Decramer M, De Benedetto F, Del Ponte A, *et al.* Systemic effects of COPD. *Respiratory Medicine* 2005;99:S3–S10.

30. Biskobing DM. COPD and osteoporosis. *Chest.* 2002;121:609–620.

31. McEvoy CE, Endsrud KE, Bender E, *et al.* Association between corticosteroid use and vertebral fractures in older men with chronic obstructive pulmonary disease. *Am J Respir Crit Care Med.* 1998;157:704–709.

32. Wilson DO, Rogers RM, Wright EC, *et al.* Body weight in chronic obstructive pulmonary disease. The National Institutes of Health Intermittent Positive-Pressure Breathing Trial. *Am Rev Respir Dis.* 1989;139:1435–1438.

33. Ferreira IM, Brooks D, Lacasse Y, *et al.* Nutritional support for individuals with COPD: a meta-analysis. *Chest.* 2000;117:672–678.

34. Poulain M, Doucet M, Drapeau V, *et al.* Metabolic and inflammatory profile in obese patients with chronic obstructive pulmonary disease. *Chron Respir Dis.* 2008;5:35–41

35. Rutten EPA, Wouters EFM. New modalities of nutritional aspects of pulmonary disease in the elderly. *Eur Respir Monogr.* 2009;43:240–255.

36. Bolton CE, Evans M, Ionescu AA, *et al.* Insulin resistance and inflammation—A further systemic complication of COPD. *COPD.* 2007;4:121–126.

37. Antonelli-Incalzi R, Corsonello A, Trajano L, *et al.* Screening of cognitive impairment in chronic obstructive pulmonary disease. *Dement Geriatr Cogn Disord.* 2007;23:264–270.

38. Antonelli-Incalzi R, Gemma A, Marra C, *et al.* Verbal memory impairment in COPD. Its mechanisms and clinical relevance. *Chest.* 1997;112:1506–1513.

39. Coultas DB, Edwards DW, Barnett B, *et al.* Predictors of depressive symptoms in patients with COPD and health impact. *COPD.* 2007;4:23–28.

40. Ng T-P, Niti M, Tan W-C, *et al.* Depressive symptoms and chronic obstructive pulmonary disease. *Arch Intern Med.* 2007;167:60–67.

41. Yohannes AM, Roomi J, Waters K, *et al.* Quality of life in elderly patients with COPD: measurement and predictive factors. *Respir Med.* 1998;92:1231–1236.

42. National Institute for Health and Clinical Excellence. *Chronic obstructive pulmonary disease (updated).* CG101. London: NICE, 2010. <http://www.nice.org.uk/guidance/CG101>.

43. Celli BR, Cote CG, Marin JM, *et al.* The body-mass index, airflow obstruction, dyspnea, and exercise capacity index in chronic obstructive pulmonary disease. *N Engl J Med.* 2004;350:1005–1012.

44. Antonelli-Incalzi R, Pedone C, Pahor M. Multidimensional assessment and treatment of the elderly with COPD. *Eur Respir Monogr.* 2009;43:35–55.

45. Yohannes AM, Roomi J, Baldwin RC, *et al.* Depression in elderly outpatients with disabling chronic obstructive pulmonary disease. *Age Ageing.* 1998;27:155–160.

46. Cydulka RK, McFadden ER, Emerman CL, *et al.* Patterns of hospitalisation in elderly patients with asthma and chronic obstructive pulmonary disease. *Am J Respir Crit Care Med.* 1997;156:1807–1812.

47. Ernst P, Wilchesky M, Suissa S. Are current treatment recommendations suited to elderly patients with asthma or COPD? *Eur Respir Monogr.* 2009;43:267–285

48. Newman SP, Moren F, Pavia D, *et al.* Deposition of pressurised aerosols in the human respiratory tract. *Thorax.* 1981;63:52–55.

49. Allen SC. Practical aspects of inhaler therapy in frail elderly patients. *Eur Respir Monogr.* 2009;43:256–266.

50. Jarad NA, Wedzicha JA, Burge PS, *et al.* An observational study of inhaled corticosteroid withdrawal in stable chronic obstructive pulmonary disease. ISOLDE study group. *Respir Med.* 2009;93:161–166.

51. Soyseth V, Brekke PH, Smith P, *et al.* Statin use is associated with reduced mortality in COPD. *Eur Respir J.* 2007;29:279–283.

52. O'Donnell DE, McGuire M, Samis L, *et al.* General exercise training improves ventilatory and peripheral muscle strength and endurance in chronic airflow limitation. *Am J Respir Crit Care Med.* 1998;157:1489–1497.

53. Connors AF, Dawson NV, Thomas C. Outcomes following acute exacerbation of severe chronic obstructive pulmonary disease. *Am J Respir Crit Care Med.* 1996;154:959–967.

54. Papi A, Bellettato CM, Braccioni F, *et al.* Infections and airway inflammation in chronic obstructive pulmonary disease severe exacerbations. *Am J Respir Crit Care Med.* 2006;173:1114–1121.

55. Gracey DR, Divertie MB, Didier EP. Preoperative pulmonary preparation of patients with chronic obstructive pulmonary disease: a prospective study. *Chest.* 1979;76:123–129.

56. Dronkers J, Veldman A, Hoberg E, *et al.* Prevention of pulmonary complications after upper abdominal surgery by preoperative intensive inspiratory muscle training: a randomised controlled pilot study. *Clin Rehabil.* 2008;22:134–142.

57. Arozullah AM, Khuri SF, Henderson WG, *et al.* Development and validation of a multifactorial risk index for predicting postoperative pneumonia after major non-cardiac surgery. *Ann Intern Med.* 2001;135:847–857.

58. Ekici M, Apan A, Ekici A, *et al.* Perception of bronchoconstriction in elderly asthmatics. *J Asthma.* 2001;38:691–696.

59. Ebihara S, Saito H, Kanda A, *et al.* Impaired efficacy of cough in patients with Parkinson disease. *Chest.* 2003;124:1009–1015.

60. Slavin RG. The elderly asthmatic patient. *Allergy Asthma Proc.* 2004;25:371–373.

61. Burrows B, Barbee RA, Cline MG, *et al.* Characteristics of asthma among elderly adults in a sample of the general population. *Chest.* 1991;100:935–942.

62. Bauer BA, Reed CE, Yunginger JW, *et al.* Incidence and outcomes in asthma in the elderly. A population-based study in Rochester, Minnesota. *Chest.* 1997;111:303–310.

63. Bellia V, Scichilone N, Battaglia S. Asthma in the elderly. *Eur Respir Monogr.* 2009;43:56–76.

64. Bellia V, Battaglia S, Catalano F, *et al.* Aging and disability affect misdiagnosis of COPD in elderly asthmatics: the SARA study. *Chest.* 2003;123:1066–1072.

65. Sciurba FC. Physiologic similarities and differences between COPD and asthma. *Chest.* 2004;126:117S–124S.

66. Global Strategy for Asthma Management and Prevention. *The Global Initiative for Asthma Management (GINA).* Updated 2012.

67. Mathur SK, Schwantes EA, Jarjour NN, *et al.* Age-related changes in eosinophil function in human subjects. *Chest.* 2008;133:412–419.

68. Lange P, Parner J, Vestbo J, *et al.* A 15-year follow up study of ventilatory function in adults with asthma. *N Engl J Med.* 1998;339:1194–1200.

69. Bellia V, Cibella F, Cuttitta G, *et al.* Effect of age upon airway obstruction and reversibility in adult patients with asthma. *Chest.* 1998;114:1336–1342.

70. Braman SS, Hanania NA. Asthma in older adults. *Clin Chest Med.* 2007;28:685–702.

71. Mannino DM, Homa DM, Akinbami LJ, *et al.* Surveillance for asthma—United States, 1980-1999. *MMWR Surveill Summ.* 2002;51:1–13.

72. Banerjee DK, Lee GS, Malik SK, *et al.* Underdiagnosis of asthma in the elderly. *Br J Dis Chest.* 1987;81:23–29.

73. Sin DD, Tu JV. Underuse of inhaled steroid therapy in elderly patients with asthma. *Chest.* 2001;119:720–725.

74. Takayanagi I, Kawano K, Koike K. Effect of ageing on the response of guinea pig trachea to isoprenaline. *Jpn J Pharmacol.* 1990;53:359–366.

75. van Schayck CP, Folgering H, Harbers H, *et al.* Effects of allergy and age on responses to salbutamol and ipratropium bromide in moderate asthma and chronic bronchitis. *Thorax.* 1991;46:355–359.

76. Kradjan WA, Driesner NK, Abuan TH, *et al.* Effect of age on bronchodilator response. *Chest.* 1992;101:1545–1551.

77. Ohnishi A, Kato M, Kojima J, *et al.* Differential pharmacokinetics of theophylline in elderly patients. *Drugs Aging.* 2003;20:71–84.

78. Walsh LJ, Wong CA, Oborne J, *et al.* Adverse effects of oral corticosteroids in relation to dose in patients with lung disease. *Thorax.* 2001;56:279–284.

79. American Academy of Sleep Medicine. *International classification of sleep disorders. Second edition. Diagnostic and coding manual.* Westchester, IL: American Academy of Sleep Medicine, 2005.

80. Young T, Peppard PE, Gottlieb DJ. Epidemiology of obstructive sleep apnea: a population health perspective. *Am J Respir Crit Care Med.* 2002;165:1217–1239.

81. Launois SH, Pepin J-L, Levy P. Sleep apnea in the elderly: a specific entity? *Sleep Med Rev.* 2007;11:87–97.

82. Shamsuzzaman AS, Gersh BJ, Somers VK. Obstructive sleep apnea: implications for cardiac and vascular disease. *JAMA.* 2003;290:1906–1914.

83. Marin JM, Carrizo SJ, Vicente E, *et al.* Long-term cardiovascular outcomes in men with obstructive sleep apnoea-hypopnoea with or without treatment with continuous positive airway pressure: an observational study. *Lancet.* 2005;365:1046–1053.

84. Bianchi G, Di Giulio C, Rapino C, *et al.* p53 and p66 proteins compete for hypoxia-inducible factor 1 alpha stabilization in young and old rat hearts exposed to intermittent hypoxia. *Gerontology.* 2006;52:17–23.

85. Cohen-Zion M, Stepnowsky C, Marler Shochat T, *et al.* Changes in cognitive function associated with sleep disordered breathing in older people. *J Am Geriatr Soc.* 2001;49:1622–1627.

86. Kostikas K, Browne HA, Ghiassi R, *et al.* The determinants of therapeutic levels of continuous positive airway pressure in elderly sleep apnea patients. *Respir Med.* 2006;100:1216–1225.

87. Russo-Magno P, O'Brien A, Panciera T, *et al.* Compliance with CPAP therapy in older men with obstructive sleep apnoea. *J Am Geriatr Soc.* 2001;49:1205–1211.

CHAPTER 15

Preoperative assessment and optimization of the older surgical patient

Jugdeep Dhesi

Introduction

Over the past 20 years, the number of older people undergoing surgical procedures has increased at a faster rate than the rate of population ageing.[1] This is likely to be related to changes in anaesthetic and surgical techniques, patient expectations, and increasing evidence of improved morbidity and mortality following surgery even in the oldest old.[2] Despite these benefits older people remain more likely to be considered to have a clinical profile that is 'too risky for surgery', potentially reducing access to effective elective procedures. Furthermore, adverse postoperative outcomes, particularly medical complications, remain more common in older people compared to their younger counterparts.[3] This is related in part to age-related changes in physiology resulting in lower physiological reserve and in part to pathological changes secondary to comorbidities. A combination of these factors results in an impaired ability to withstand and respond to the stress of surgery. It is not surprising that functional reserve and comorbidities (particularly the cumulative effect of multiple comorbidities) are consistently identified as independent predictors of poor postoperative outcome. This is important, as some of these predictors of poor outcome are potentially modifiable, suggesting that in the older population, careful preoperative assessment and optimization may be the key to improving outcome.

With these factors in mind, the preoperative assessment process in the older population serves two broad purposes. First, to risk-stratify patients in order that health professionals, patients, and their relatives or carers are fully informed of the inherent risks in undergoing a procedure. Second, to proactively identify and optimize modifiable factors, thus improving the patient's likelihood of a successful outcome.

In older patients therefore the role of preoperative assessment is more extensive than in younger patients. It affords an opportunity to:

♦ Provide baseline assessment; recognize known comorbidity, identify previously unrecognized disease, and assess functional reserve.

♦ Optimize the patient; optimize the medical, functional, psychological and social condition of the patient in order to get the patient as 'fit as possible' for surgery.

♦ Assess capacity to consent for surgery and discuss issues around advanced directives.

♦ Predict postoperative risk to inform discussion regarding risk/benefit ratio of surgery with the patient.

♦ Provide information that will aid decision-making in the intra-operative and immediate postoperative period (including appropriate provision of level 2 and 3 care).

♦ Predict likely postoperative complications and facilitate a collaborative approach towards prompt identification and standardized management of medical complications.

♦ Reduce risk of postoperative complications.

♦ Facilitate multidisciplinary working between surgical, anaesthetic, intensive care, and elderly medicine teams.

♦ Facilitate early discharge planning with identification of those who are most likely to require additional postoperative support and/or rehabilitation.

♦ Reduce in-hospital length of stay through improving quality of care.

Preoperative assessment is equally critical in elective, urgent, and emergency settings (Table 15.1), but should be tailored to the time available. For example, a patient presenting with a hip fracture will need to be risk assessed and optimized within 24 hours for surgery, whereas the same process in a patient undergoing an elective hip replacement will not be so time pressured.

Perioperative risk can be organ specific (e.g. risk of cardiac event) or relate to overall mortality. It is influenced by two distinct factors: (1) risks related to the surgical procedure and (2) risks related to the patient's premorbid condition. The overall perioperative risks should guide the depth of preoperative assessment. For example, a patient undergoing minor surgery, with good functional reserve and no comorbidities will not require the same form of preoperative assessment as the frail older person undergoing major elective surgery or that required by the hip fracture patient. It is important to ensure that preoperative assessment is targeted at intermediate-to high-risk cases to allow effective allocation of resources. The decision to proceed with surgery is then based on perioperative risk, the potential risk related to delaying surgery for investigation

Table 15.1 National Confidential Enquiry into Patient Outcome and Death: definitions for type of surgery, December 2004

Term	Definition
Elective surgery	Carried out at a time to suit the patient and surgeon
Urgent surgery	Carried out within 24 hours of admission
Expedited surgery	Carried out within days of decision to operate
Emergency surgery	Carried out within 2 hours of admission or in conjunction with resuscitation

Data from NCEPOD, December 2004.

or treatment, and the risk of not performing surgery. An individual's life expectancy should also be taken into account.

Risk related to the surgical procedure

Clinical series provide information on risks of postoperative complications and mortality in specific surgical subspecialties. Emergency surgery of any type carries a higher risk of postoperative complications and mortality than elective surgery. Furthermore specific procedures are associated with higher cardiac complication rates and mortality than others (Table 15.2).

It is important to recognize the risk related to the procedure itself, as while it may be non-modifiable, the surgical pathway can be adapted to reduce the overall risk. For example, many experts now advocate routine postoperative critical care in level 2 or 3 facilities in all older patients undergoing high-risk surgery. Furthermore, an alternative surgical procedure that is less risky may be considered in a high-risk patient.

Risk related to the patient: functional reserve, comorbidities, frailty, and health

Patient

Whilst age itself is not a good predictor of perioperative risk, ageing is associated with changes in physiology and an increasing

Table 15.2 30 day risk of MI or cardiac death according to type of surgery

Low risk <1%	Intermediate risk 1-5%	High risk >5%
Breast	Abdominal	Aortic
Dental	Carotid	Major vascular
Endocrine	Peripheral angioplasty	Peripheral vascular surgery
Eye	Endovascular repair	
Gynaecological	Head and neck	
Reconstructive	Pulmonary	
Minor orthopaedic, e.g. knee	Major orthopaedic, e.g. hip	
Minor urological	Major urological	
	Spinal	
	Renal or liver transplant	

Adapted from *The American Journal of Medicine*, 118, 10, Boersma E, et al., 'Perioperative cardiovascular mortality in noncardiac surgery: validation of the Lee cardiac risk index', pp. 1134–1141, Copyright 2005, with permission from Elsevier and the Alliance for Academic Internal Medicine.

prevalence and severity of comorbidities. Both these factors influence the risk related to the patient. More recently the contribution of geriatric syndromes such as frailty to perioperative risk is emerging.[5] At present, none of the instruments routinely used for preoperative assessment of older patients are all-inclusive. They each relate to various aspects of the patient's overall 'condition'. In order to provide a complete picture it may be necessary to use a combination of subjective and objective instruments. In most centres routine preoperative clinical care incorporates self-reporting of comorbidity and American Society of Anesthesiologists (ASA) grading, but this alone is now considered insufficient to identify and manage the high risk older patient.

Functional reserve

Physiological ageing impacts on the resting function of many organs as discussed in other chapters. In particular these physiological changes affect the cardiorespiratory systems, resulting in a lower functional reserve even in the fit older person, causing a reduced ability to deal with physiological stress. When pathology is superimposed on physiological change, then there may be a further reduction in functional reserve. It is that reserve that is called upon during times of stress such as surgery, with increases in metabolic requirements, often in the setting of a catabolic state (i.e. cancer or inflammatory processes).

It is not surprising that poor functional reserve is consistently identified as an independent risk factor for adverse postoperative outcome.[6] On the other hand, a high functional reserve, regardless of age and comorbidity predicts good postoperative outcome. In these cases, perioperative management is unlikely to be altered by further testing and the patient should proceed with surgery, even in the presence of other risk factors. Attention should be focussed on patients with poor functional reserve, where risk factors must be meticulously identified and optimized, and the risk/benefit ratio of surgery be carefully considered.

Describing and measuring functional reserve at preoperative assessment

Over the years various methods for assessment of functional capacity have been developed. The emphasis in all of these measures is on *cardiorespiratory* functional capacity. One of the most commonly used methods is the measurement in metabolic equivalents (METs). One MET is defined as the basal metabolic rate of a 40-year-old male of 70 kg at rest (3.5 ml/kg/min). Although METs can be assessed objectively using exercise testing, they can be estimated from the ability to perform activities of daily living (Table 15.3). A patient who is unable to climb two flights of stairs is considered to have poor functional capacity at less than 4 METs. Poor functional capacity defined by METs has been associated with an increased risk of postoperative cardiac events and mortality in certain surgical specialties, in particular thoracic surgery.[7] However, in other non-cardiac surgery poor functional capacity measured in METs does not appear to add predictive value (to age and ASA) for adverse cardiac outcomes and was not associated with increased mortality.[8] Furthermore, METs can be low for reasons other than cardiorespiratory, for example, arthritis, visual impairment or dementia and many older people fall below the threshold of 4 METs, limiting its use as a discriminating tool.

As an objective measure of functional reserve, cardiopulmonary exercise testing (CPET) (see Chapter 19) has become increasingly popular. It involves exercising a patient on a cycle ergometer

Table 15.3 METS and equivalent activity

METS	Activity
1	Resting basal metabolic rate
2	Walking slow pace
3	House work
4	Climbing two flights of stairs
8	Jogging/swimming

Data from Ainsworth, BE. (2000) 'Compendium of Physical Activities: An update of activity codes and MET intensities', *Medicine & Science in Sports & Exercise*, 32 (9 Suppl): S498–504.

attached to 12-lead electrocardiography whilst measuring oxygen uptake and carbon dioxide production. The data obtained are analysed to assess cardiopulmonary fitness. Various parameters can be measured, but anaerobic thresholds (AT) have been used to triage into high and low risk for major abdominal surgery.[9] This can allow tailored perioperative interventions to help reduce morbidity and mortality, as demonstrated initially in colorectal surgery[10] and more recently in vascular surgery. However, similar to METs, there are concerns that older patients may not be able to complete CPET due to factors other than cardiorespiratory fitness, such musculoskeletal disorders and that this may inadvertently limit access to surgery.

Comorbidities

Comorbidities are defined as 'diseases or medical conditions unrelated in aetiology or causality to the principal diagnosis and that coexist with the disease of interest'. The prevalence of comorbidities increases with advancing age, with more than 60 per cent of those aged 65 years and above having at least one comorbidity. Furthermore with increasing age the multiplicity of comorbidities increases.[11] In the surgical population a clear relationship between multiplicity of comorbidities and postoperative complications, poor postoperative functional outcome, and mortality exists.[12–14] However, it is not purely the presence of a comorbidity which dictates outcome. More important is whether the comorbidity is associated with other risk factors or related complications which may affect postoperative outcome. For example, diabetes mellitus with associated obesity and vascular complications would be a significant comorbidity, in comparison to well-controlled asthma.

Describing and measuring comorbidity at preoperative assessment

There are many ways in which comorbidities can be described and measured. Patient identification and self-reporting of comorbidities is accurate and reliable and is better than reliance on administrative data (coding, insurance documentation).[15] However, some authors do promote specific instruments to aid self-reporting and to allow objective self-recording of medical history (e.g. the Self-Administered Co-morbidity Questionnaire).[16]

Whilst all experts acknowledge the need to account for comorbidities, some elect not to use a formal instrument, merely counting a patient's additional diagnoses.[17] Others advocate the use of comorbidity indices derived from the number of coexistent diseases as well as their individual severity, with this information condensed into a single numeric score.

The most widely used comorbidity indices include the Charlson Index, the Index of Coexistent Disease (ICED), and the Functional Co-morbidity Index (FCI). The Charlson Index has been widely used in large studies based on administrative data to predict functional outcome, mortality, and length of hospital stay and resource use. Although it is a valid and reliable tool, it is less sensitive to functional outcomes[18] and is now considered out of date. In contrast the ICED measures both disease severity and overall functional severity (disability). More specifically, it was developed with physical function as the outcome of interest and unsurprisingly performs better than the Charlson Index in this respect.[19] These comorbidity indices are useful as research tools, allowing for comparison between patient groups and stratification of risk, but are too imprecise to replace clinical judgement for a specific patient.[20] Furthermore they fail to assess for common geriatric syndromes (Fig. 15.1) and their use is limited in the busy clinical setting.

Frailty

In comparison to functional capacity and its emphasis on cardiorespiratory reserve, frailty reflects decreased physiological reserve across *multiple* organ systems. As a consequence the frail person is at increased risk of disability and death from minor external stresses.[21] Studies in various surgical populations have identified frailty as an independent risk factor for major morbidity, mortality, protracted length of stay (LOS), and institutional discharge.[22] The appeal of measuring frailty in an older surgical population lies in its utility both as a tool for preoperative risk stratification and also as a method for identifying potentially modifiable factors that can be optimized preoperatively. (Also see Chapter 30.)

Health

In comparison to comorbidity, health is a state of complete physical, mental, and social well-being and not merely the absence of disease or infirmity. Preoperative health status can be measured generally or specifically. For example, generic instruments, such as the SF-36 cover both physical and mental components of health, whilst tools such as the Hospital Anxiety and Depression Score (HADS) or Hip Osteoarthritis Outcomes Scale (HOOS) are disease or condition specific. Activity scales express actual levels of patient activity, which may change in the event of successful surgery. Both general scales and more specific rating scales may be used postoperatively in order to monitor the effect of treatment. At preoperative assessment implicit assessments of health status are often made, but at present measurement of health is limited to research settings.

Assessing the older surgical patient

The following section will focus on the practicalities of assessing and optimizing an older patient for surgery

History

A thorough history, utilizing the tools described, incorporating medical and surgical history, current symptoms, exercise tolerance, and a full medication list (and drug compliance) is important. Previous anaesthetic history, postoperative complications, and previous postoperative recovery should be noted. Levels of functional dependency should be described and social circumstances be clarified to allow timely discharge. Comprehensive geriatric assessment (CGA) methodology can be utilized to assess across these domains.

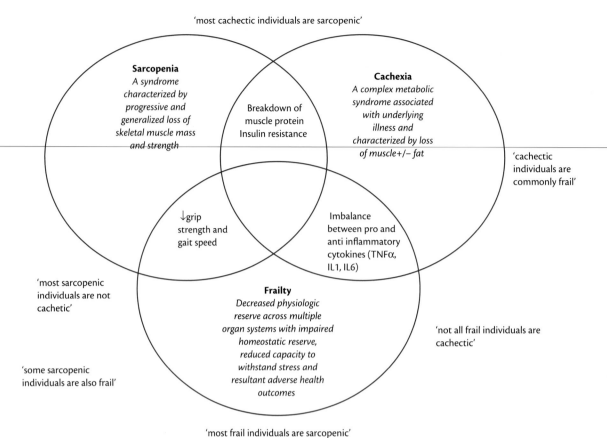

Fig. 15.1 Overlapping geriatric syndromes.

Establishing the history can be difficult for many reasons. Older people are less likely to seek medical advice and medical diagnoses may not have been previously documented. This may be because:

♦ They are less likely to mention symptoms such as decreasing exercise tolerance, incontinence, or becoming more forgetful considering these symptoms to be inevitable consequences of ageing.

♦ Typical symptoms are masked, for example, a patient presenting for arthroplasty may not complain of symptoms of ischaemic heart disease because their exercise level is reduced to such an extent that the classical exertional symptoms of ischaemic heart disease do not occur.

♦ Communication difficulties arising from sensory impairment (impaired hearing), language impairment (e.g. related to cerebrovascular events), and cognitive impairment which may limit the history given by the patient or result in inaccuracies.

Examination

In older patients, the depth and focus of preoperative examination should be guided by the same two factors: risk related to surgery and risk related to the patient. In cases of intermediate- or high-risk surgery and/or if the patient has poor functional capacity, comorbidities, or poor health status the examination must be thorough. In low-risk surgery, in a patient without comorbidities and good functional reserve, the examination may be limited to the area of surgical concern and the cardiorespiratory system.

Investigations

Again, investigations should be guided by the risk related to surgery and risk related to the patient. Blood tests should be performed in all elderly patients undergoing intermediate and high-risk surgery and considered in low-risk procedures. This is not because they are prognostic indicators but because they allow diagnosis and assessment of severity of physiological change, coexisting disease and effect of drugs. Blood tests should include full blood count, renal function, liver function. and bone profile, amongst other more specific tests prompted by the history or examination findings.

Recent guidance has been published for non-cardiac surgery but as a generalization preoperative electrocardiograms (ECGs)[22] should be considered in all patients aged over 65 years other than those having low-risk surgery. If indicated, ECGs should be performed in the 30 days before surgery (Table 15.4).

Further investigations should be considered on a case-by-case basis. See organ-specific chapters for more details.

A structured approach in the older preoperative patient: comprehensive geriatric assessment

Preoperative assessment in older patients is complex. It is important to assess comorbidity, cardiorespiratory reserve, frailty, and health in order to make considered and shared decisions regarding surgery. Routine clinical assessment does not allow this in a systematic manner. In comparison CGA allows objective assessment

Table 15.4 Indications for preoperative ECGs

Definitely required	Consider	Not routinely
High-risk surgery	Intermediate-risk surgery and no risk factors	Low-risk surgery with no risk factors
Intermediate-risk surgery with risk factors for cardiac or peripheral vascular disease (PVD)	Low-risk surgery with risk factors for cardiac or PVD	

Risk factors: ischemic heart disease, heart failure, cerebrovascular disease, diabetes, renal impairment.

Table 15.5 ASA scores

Class	Physical status	Example	Mortality (%)—in general
1	Normal healthy individual	A fit patient	0.05
2	Mild systemic disease that does not limit activity	Essential hypertension, mild diabetes without end-organ damage	0.4
3	Severe systemic disease that limits activity but is not incapacitating	Angina, moderate to severe COPD	4.5
4	Incapacitating systemic disease which is constantly life threatening	Advanced COPD, cardiac failure	25
5	Moribund, not expected to survive 24 hours with or without surgery	Ruptured aortic aneurysm, massive pulmonaryembolism	50

Reproduced from Owens WD, et al., 'ASA physical status classifications: a study of consistency of ratings', *Anesthesiology*, 49, 4, pp. 239–246, copyright 1978, with permission from Wolters Kluwer and the American Society of Anesthesiologists.

across multiple domains (medical, psycho-social, and functional) and differs from standard medical evaluation since it:

- Focuses on elderly individuals with complex problems.

- Allows identification of the so called Geriatric giants or the 'Five I's of Geriatrics' intellectual impairment, immobility, instability, incontinence and iatrogenic disorders. These syndromes affect large numbers of older people, are often unrecognized, unmanaged, cause a significant personal burden to the patient and also impact on short and long term outcomes.

- Emphasizes assessment of functional status and quality of life.

- Uses multidisciplinary skills.

- Allows development of goal orientated interventions.

CGA has been used to good effect in elective orthopaedic patients[23] and in cancer populations.[24] However, in order to be effective it must be targeted at the right patient (i.e. those with complex risk factors), it must involve hands on care and appropriate follow-up of relevant issues. If used in this manner CGA can facilitate case management (including the identification of the most appropriate clinical area), determine long-term care requirements, and make the best use of healthcare resources. However, at present there are no randomized controlled studies providing evidence for this approach in the older general surgical patient.

Preoperative risk assessment

The next step in preoperative assessment is to collate information relating to the risk related to the surgery and the risk related to the patient. This leads to an overall assessment of individual risk of perioperative mortality and morbidity which should be clearly documented, allowing the following:

- An informed discussion with the patient regarding risks and benefits of the proposed surgery.

- Planning for intraoperative care (the use of appropriate devices, e.g. cardiac output monitoring in a patient at risk of cardiac decompensation, or the decision regarding type of anaesthetic, e.g. general or regional).

- Planning for postoperative care (ensuring the patient is monitored in the correct location, e.g. an intensive care bed for the high-risk patient undergoing high-risk surgery).

- Clinical governance, by providing a tool for allowing comparison between units; and appraisal for individual consultant surgeons.

Describing and measuring risk of mortality

A number of risk assessment scores for estimation of risk of perioperative mortality are available. The most frequently encountered is the ASA score. ASA subjectively categorizes patients into five subgroups on the basis of preoperative history and examination, without the need for specific tests (Table 15.5). In population studies ASA is an independent predictor of outcome in terms of intra- and postoperative complications, morbidity, mortality, cost, and length of stay. It is therefore useful as a descriptor of surgical populations for both research and audit purposes. However, it was devised as a statistical tool for retrospective analysis of hospital records and makes no adjustment for age, sex, the nature of the planned surgery, or the relative contributions of comorbidities. Therefore, ASA does not predict risk for an individual patient or a particular operation. Further issues limiting the usefulness of ASA in the clinical setting include its highly subjective nature, its low reliability,[25] and its lack of subtlety especially in the older population who often fall into the ASA 3 or above categories.

An alternative tool is the Physiological and Operative Severity Score for the enUmeration of Mortality and Morbidity (POSSUM). This was also developed as a tool to compare morbidity and mortality for audit purposes. It incorporates six surgical parameters and 12 physiological parameters with each factor weighted to a value of 1, 2, 4, or 8, depending on measurement, to allow for a simplified calculation. Since its conception in 1991, it has been applied to a number of surgical groups including orthopaedics, vascular surgery, head and neck surgery and gastrointestinal and colorectal surgery.[26] The original POSSUM score was thought to over-predict death in certain groups of patients especially in low-risk patients[27] and was therefore modified to the Portsmouth version (P-POSSUM). Subsequently it has become apparent that POSSUM and P-POSSUM predict mortality equally well and that both over-estimate risk. In response more specialty-specific scores, such as V-POSSUM for use in elective vascular surgery, have emerged.[28] Usefulness of POSSUM may be limited at preoperative assessment as not all variables are available at preoperative assessment and estimates will need to be made. In addition it may be difficult to implement in nurse-led preoperative assessment clinics, although web-based tools for POSSUM have made this easier.

In comparison to these general risk assessment tools, organ-specific tools can be used for stratifying organ-specific risk. For example, the Revised Cardiac Risk Index of Lee et al.[29] remains the most commonly used tool for stratifying cardiac risk before non-cardiac surgery. This validated index consists of six independent predictors of postoperative cardiac complications and cardiac-related mortality: high-risk surgery, ischemic heart disease, history of congestive heart failure, history of cerebrovascular disease, insulin-treated diabetes mellitus, and renal disease as measured by preoperative creatinine. The more predictors a patient has, the greater the risk of perioperative cardiac complications. The index can be useful in determining whether a preoperative or perioperative intervention is likely to make a difference to cardiac morbidity or mortality (see Chapter XX). However, the organ-specific nature of these tools is a limiting factor.

Optimizing the older surgical patient

Preoperative assessment often stops at the risk assessment stage. However it should be seen as an opportunity to optimize the patient in order to improve postoperative outcome. This focus on optimization is imperative especially in older people who are at higher risk by virtue of physiological changes, comorbidity and frailty. Although specific guidelines relating to management of individual comorbidities in the preoperative setting exist and are useful, their application should be carefully considered in the context of the older population. The following issues may cause deviation from usual guidelines;

◆ The presence of multiple coexisting comorbidities: e.g. a patient with reversible ischaemic heart disease and postural hypotension associated with Parkinson's disease undergoing vascular surgery may not benefit from beta-blocker therapy.

◆ Medications and problems associated with polypharmacy, drug interactions and compliance: e.g. a patient on numerous drugs may not take additional therapy started for an asymptomatic condition such as hypertension unless clear reasoning is provided.

◆ Practical considerations: e.g. a patient with multiple comorbidities may not want to attend multiple hospital appointments with organ specialists to be optimized for surgery, but may prefer to be seen by a single physician. In this setting a geriatrician with an interest in perioperative medicine may be the most appropriate specialist.

Assessment and optimization of organ-specific disease and commonly encountered comorbidities will be discussed in the relevant chapters elsewhere in this book. In the following section, assessment and optimization of frequently encountered issues more specific to older people and which are often overlooked in routine clinical practice, are discussed.

Dementia

Cognitive impairment and dementia are common in the older population, affecting 10 per cent of those aged over 65 years and 20 per cent of those aged 80 years and above. Despite this, these issues are often unrecognized. This may be because they are accepted as part of normal ageing, or because they have an insidious onset, or because social skills are often preserved until late in the disease process. In the older preoperative patient recognition of cognitive impairment is important as it can impact on:

◆ Preoperative assessment. These patients may provide unreliable or incomplete histories, may be difficult to examine, or non-compliant with investigations.

◆ Capacity to consent to the procedure.

◆ Postoperative complications. Patients with underlying cognitive impairment or dementia are at increased risk of postoperative delirium and postoperative cognitive decline.

All older preoperative patients should be screened for cognitive impairment and dementia. The process and tool used in cognitive assessment needs to be tailored to the individual patient and the time frame to proposed surgery. For example, in emergency surgery the Abbreviated Mental Test (Table 15.6) or even a simple question to the carer or relative such as 'Have you or your carer noticed a change in your memory?' provides a quick and simple approach. In comparison, in high-risk elective surgery detailed assessment may be possible and more appropriate. The Mini Mental Score Examination (MMSE) is the most widely used tool.[30] However, it does not provide an adequate assessment of executive function which is particularly affected by vascular cognitive impairment. For this reason the Montreal Cognitive Assessment tool which examines executive functioning in slightly more detail is being increasingly advocated.[31]

If cognitive impairment is identified then:

◆ The patient should be informed of the finding.

◆ The patient should be referred to either the primary care physician or to specialist services for further assessment and diagnosis.

◆ The implications for the planned surgery should be considered:

• the capacity to consent (whilst recognizing that mental tests assessment per se does not provide assessment of capacity)

• the related perioperative risks in particular postoperative delirium.

Table 15.6 Abbreviated mental test

1. Age
2. Time (to the nearest hour)
42 west street (ask patient to repeat the address to ensure it has been heard correctly)
3. Year
4. Name of hospital
5. Recognition of two persons (e.g. doctor and nurse)
6. Date of birth
7. Year of start of the First World War
8. Name of monarch
9. Count downwards from 20 to 1
10. Recall address

Reproduced from Hodkinson HM, 'Evaluation of a mental test score for assessment of mental impairment in the elderly', *Age and Ageing*, 1972, 1, 4, pp. 233–238, by permission of Oxford University Press and The British Geriatrics Society.

◆ Preoperative strategies to reduce incidence, severity and duration of postoperative delirium should be considered.

◆ The information should be shared across the perioperative team, that is:

- anaesthetic staff, who could consider pharmacological issues (e.g. interactions) and ensure vigilant intraoperative monitoring and management

- surgical ward staff, who could ensure evidence based strategies to reduce the severity, duration, and impact of delirium are implemented

- geriatricians or old age psychiatrists, who could assist in non-pharmacological and pharmacological management of delirium if required.

Delirium

At preoperative assessment in the older patient it is important to consider the risk of postoperative delirium and postoperative cognitive decline (see also Chapter 10.)

Postoperative delirium (POD) is defined using the *Diagnostic and Statistical Manual of Mental Disorders* (DSM)-IV criteria, which describe the acute onset and fluctuating course of a syndrome characterized by a disturbance of cognition and consciousness attributable to an underlying cause. It is thought to occur in a patient who has predisposing factors and is then subjected to precipitants (Table 15.7).

POD should be differentiated from postoperative cognitive dysfunction (POCD), which despite first being described in the 1950s still lacks a universally accepted definition. Most researchers consider POCD to be the syndrome of persistent cognitive change, which occurs after a surgical procedure, and yet research into this ill-defined syndrome is hampered by a lack of consistency in the type and timing of neurocognitive assessment in addition to varying definitions of what actually constitutes a 'change' in neurocognitive score. Given that many of the risk factors for POCD and POD are the same, current debate is considering whether these are in fact two separate syndromes or the same condition represented at different ends of a spectrum of severity.

Postoperative delirium can occur following any surgical procedure but occurs frequently in particular patient groups with an incidence of up to 60 per cent after hip fracture and 35 per cent after certain vascular procedures. Postoperative delirium is associated with increased mortality both in the short term following hospitalization but also at longer-term 12-month follow-up. Furthermore, in those who do survive, delirium is also associated with increased morbidity from postoperative complications and increased rates of institutionalization at hospital discharge.[32]

The pathogenesis of delirium remains incompletely understood, yet it can be useful to think of delirium as occurring due to an insult (in this case, the surgical procedure) in a susceptible individual. Neurochemical changes, neuronal atrophy, and differences in cerebral vasculature in the ageing brain put older patients at increased risk from delirium following the cytokine storm which can result from a surgical procedure. Various cytokines have been implicated in the pathogenesis of delirium including increased levels of interleukin (IL)-6 and IL8 and reduced concentrations of the neuroprotective insulin-like growth factor (IGF)-1 and IL1-receptor antagonist.[33]

The process for identifying and reducing risk of POD should begin at preoperative assessment. Recognition of predisposing factors should occur for two reasons. First, many of these factors are modifiable. Second, non-modifiable risk factors should be actively sought since proactive identification of a patient at risk of delirium can facilitate interventions to reduce the incidence, severity, and/or duration of delirium.

Prevention of delirium is more effective than cure. Prevention strategies can be multi-component interventions or single pharmacological interventions. Multi-component interventions include simple protocols which target the risk factors for delirium. Examples include: optimizing sensory impairments using glasses, magnifiers, hearing aids or amplifiers, maintaining diurnal routines through non-pharmacological promotion of sleep and daytime mobilization, preventing dehydration, and regularly re-orientating patients to time and place. Such simple strategies when systematically employed can significantly reduce the incidence of delirium in high-risk patients groups such as those following hip fracture and have been shown to be cost-effective.[34,35] At present pharmacological prevention of delirium is not mainstream practice, although promising work is ongoing using various medications including haloperidol and melatonin.[36, 37]

Malnutrition

Malnutrition is highly prevalent in the older population and is a strong predictor of postoperative complications and mortality, across different surgical specialties. In particular those undergoing gastrointestinal surgery are at risk due to reduced oral intake and catabolic states induced by carcinoma and surgery in the perioperative period.[38] Although serum albumin is not purely a marker of nutrition (but also of acute phase response), levels <35 g/L are an important predictor of 30-day perioperative morbidity (particularly wound infections) and mortality.[39]

Preoperative assessment in older people should therefore include nutritional assessment. Various nutritional indices are effective at identifying surgical patients at risk, and most incorporate body mass index (BMI) and greater than 5 per cent weight loss in three months. The Malnutrition Universal Screening Tool (MUST) and the Mini-Nutritional Assessment are standard instruments used in

Table 15.7 Examples of predisposing and precipitating factors for postoperative delirium

Predisposing factors	Precipitating factors
Age	Change in environment
Dementia or cognitive impairment	Sleep deprivation
Depression	Loss of sensory aids/clues
History of delirium	Physical restraints
Severe illness or hip fracture	Constipation
Polypharmacy	Urinary retention
Malnutrition/dehydration	Sepsis
Functional dependency	Acute illness (e.g. myocardial infarction)
Sensory impairment	Untreated pain or excess use of analgesics

the older population. Both are screening tools to identify patients who are malnourished, at risk of malnutrition, or obese. They also include management guidelines that can be used to develop care plans across healthcare settings.[40]

It is well recognized that oral nutrition with supplements (if necessary) is the most effective intervention to improve nutritional status. However, there is no clear evidence regarding the impact of timing, duration and type of intervention. If oral nutrition is not possible, enteral nutrition (EN) should be started preoperatively and continued perioperatively. It is more effective than parenteral nutrition (PN), with lower rates of sepsis and shorter length of stay. Meta-analyses have concluded that EN contains immunonutrients that PN lacks, has potential benefits in maintaining gut mucosa and flora, and is cheaper.[41]

Although nutritional assessment tools have not been designed to detect deficiencies of minerals and vitamins, these insufficiencies can impact on outcome. The role of treating subclinical nutritional anaemia preoperatively in elective orthopaedic patients is now accepted as a method of reducing morbidity and mortality in the older surgical group. Current recommendations suggest replacing iron, vitamin B_{12} and folate at least 28 days before scheduled elective surgery.[42] Vitamin D is implicated in the pathogenesis of frailty and sarcopenia, which may affect outcome. Levels should be reviewed and supplementation considered, although at present there is no clear evidence of benefit in older preoperative patients. With a move towards promoting preoperative nutrition as part of enhanced recovery programmes, the potential effect of nutritional supplementation and pharmaconutrients on surgical outcomes in older individuals is being explored.[43]

Preoperative physiotherapy and occupational therapy intervention

There is increasing interest in the use of preoperative multidisciplinary interventions to treat frailty as an independent predictor of poor postoperative outcome in older people. This is particularly relevant as the natural history of frailty shows that it is more common to progress to a state of greater frailty than to improve to a state of lesser frailty and that the transition from one frailty state to another has a resultant impact upon mortality.[44] However, at present there is no conclusive evidence supporting nutritional, therapy, or pharmacological interventions for frailty in older preoperative patients.

In elective surgery, the not atypical 3-month waiting period for surgery such as hip replacement surgery, is associated with significant decline in hip abductor and flexion strength in older people.[45] In these cases preoperative physiotherapy does show some postoperative mobility related gains in elective hip surgery patients, especially with longer (6-week) interventions. Similar benefits were not seen in knee replacement patients across these parameters, but a proactive approach of preoperative assessment with targeted intensive postoperative rehabilitation for higher-risk patients has reduced length of stay in arthroplasty patients.[46] There is also increasing interest in prehabilitation to enhance functional capacity prior to cardiopulmonary and abdominal surgery. Many of the programmes used to date have focussed on education and positive reinforcement, but data on exercise programmes is emerging.[47]

Planning for the surgical admission should commence at preoperative assessment. Preoperative social care needs should be identified and potential postoperative care needs evaluated (e.g. one-level living, need for equipment, or need for postoperative rehabilitation). Coordination with patient, families, carers, and social services should be initiated as soon as possible to reduce in-hospital delays. Although there are few published data on occupational therapy intervention, preoperative home visits with equipment provision can reduce discharge delays from surgical wards.[23] These interventions now form part of enhanced recovery programmes in orthopaedic surgery.

Legal issues

Under the Mental Capacity Act and similar legislation across the developed world, all patients are considered to have capacity to consent unless proven otherwise. In cases where there is doubt regarding capacity to consent the relevant legal framework should be applied, for example the Mental Capacity Act in England and Wales. If the patient is deemed not to have capacity, then advanced directives made by the patient whilst they still had capacity may help to inform the situation or the patient may have appointed a durable power of attorney for health care. In the absence of such directives, the best interests of a patient should be reviewed by all relevant persons (health care professionals, families and carers, advocates) and surgery can proceed if considered to be in the patient's best interest. In cases of emergency surgery, lifesaving treatment can proceed in the best interests of the patient despite the more condensed timeframe. Clear documentation of these issues is paramount. (See also Chapter 36.)

Models of care for preoperative assessment

Many pre-assessment clinics are nurse or junior doctor led and delivered. In most settings these individuals have surgical or anaesthetic backgrounds but very little experience in elderly medicine. In most units preoperative assessment is conducted using proformas and focuses narrowly on the surgical issues or the 'on-table risk'. The patient is identified as being 'fit for surgery' or as requiring further assessment. Further assessment is typically undertaken by primary care practitioners, organ specialists or anaesthetists. There is little formal training for any of these groups in the specific preoperative management of older people. This is illustrated by surveys and case note reviews suggesting that preoperative referrals for medical assessment to organ-specialist physicians rarely results in advice that impacts either on perioperative management or outcome of surgery. In one study, 40 per cent of cardiac consultations made no recommendation other than 'proceed with surgery' or 'cleared for surgery'.[48]

In order to provide a high-quality and cost-effective service, new models of care need to be considered for the high-risk older surgical population. These models should allow the full scope of preoperative assessment, from recognition and optimization of the relevant issues, to formal risk assessment, to shared decision-making and appropriate perioperative planning. This in turn would allow the translation of existing evidence into routine clinical practice, particularly in those with complex comorbidities and functional dependence.

In response, some units have developed anaesthetist led pre-assessment clinics. Often these clinics are for individual patients identified as having complex anaesthetic concerns or specific types of complex surgery. These clinics provide thorough review, risk assessment, and allow informed decision-making, but if optimization is required then the patient may need to attend for further reviews with physicians. In other units general physicians or geriatricians with an interest in perioperative medicine have taken on the role of preoperative assessment. One such model (proactive care of older people undergoing surgery: POPS) (Fig. 15.2) ensures that older patients with medical comorbidities or functional dependence are followed throughout the surgical journey by a multidisciplinary elderly care medicine team. Preoperatively, the team utilizes CGA methodology to assess and optimize the patient for surgery, predict postoperative complications, predict postoperative rehabilitation or care needs, and communicate these issues with health care professionals and families and or carers. The team then follows the patient through to admission and provides regular medical input during the perioperative period. The team aids the surgical team in the early identification and standardized management of medical complications as well as in early, safe, and effective discharge planning. This constitutes a proactive rather than reactive approach. It allows discussion between geriatricians, surgeons, and anaesthetists regarding decisions to proceed with surgery in a patient with complex comorbidities and ethical issues, or whether to withhold treatments, decisions regarding settings for in-hospital care and decisions regarding the discharge destination.[23]

Various models of perioperative care for older surgical patients are emerging, but they all emphasize the need for cross- and multidisciplinary working, utilizing the skills of surgical teams, anaesthetic teams, organ specialists, *and* elderly care medicine teams.

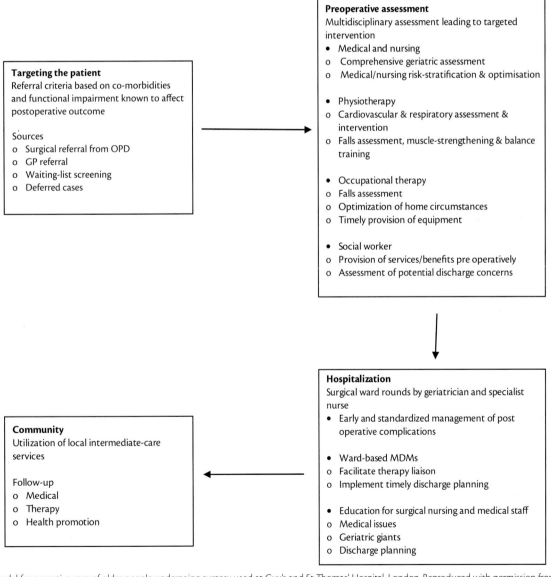

Fig. 15.2 A model for proactive care of older people undergoing surgery used at Guy's and St Thomas' Hospital, London. Reproduced with permission from Jugdeep Dhesi, copyright Guy's and St Thomas' Hospital, London.

Conclusion

The evidence base for improving outcomes in older people having surgery exists and is growing. However, many questions with regards to the clinical management of this population remain unanswered. Amongst many there are questions related to the following:

◆ Geriatric syndromes: for example, whether multi-component preoperative interventions for frailty can improve postoperative outcome?

◆ Specific medical conditions: for example, should iron stores be checked in all older surgical patients and does supplementation improve clinical outcome?

◆ Translation of evidence into the clinical setting: can evidence from comorbidity specific studies be translated into routine clinical practice?

◆ Process and cost-effectiveness of care: for example, what is the most effective way of delivering care, where should it be delivered and by whom, should a new specialty of 'perioperative medicine for the elderly' be considered?

◆ Education and training of the workforce: how should this be delivered across a large multidisciplinary workforce and how can the impact on clinical practice be measured?

References

1. Klopfenstein CE, Herrmann FR, Michel JP, Clergue F, Forster A. The influence of an aging surgical population on the anaesthesia workload: a ten-year survey. *Anesth Analg.* 1998;86:1165–1170.
2. Hamel MB, Henderson WG, Khuri SF, Daley J. Surgical outcomes for patients aged 80 and older: morbidity and mortality from major noncardiac surgery. *J Am Geriatr Soc.* 2005;53(3):424–429.
3. Polanczyk CA, Marcantonio E, Goldman L, et al. Impact of age on perioperative complications and length of stay in patients undergoing non cardiac surgery. *Ann Intern Med.* 2001;134:637–643.
4. Boersma E, Kertai MD, Schouten O, et al. Perioperative cardiovascular mortality in noncardiac surgery: validation of the Lee cardiac risk index. *Am J Med.* 2005;118:1134–1141.
5. Partridge JSL, Harari D, Dhesi JK. Frailty in the older surgical patient. *Age Ageing.* 2012; 41:142–147.
6. Older P, Hall A. Clinical review: how to identify high-risk surgical patients? *Crit Care.* 2004;8:369–372.
7. Biccard BM. Relationship between the inability to climb two flights of stairs and outcome after major non-cardiac surgery: implications for the pre-operative assessment of functional capacity. *Anaesthesia.* 2005;60:588–593.
8. Wiklund RA, Stein HD, Rosenbaum SH. Activities of daily living and cardiovascular complications following elective, noncardiac surgery. *Yale J Biol Med.* 2001;74:75–87.
9. ATS/ACCP statement on cardiopulmonary exercise testing. *Am J Respir Crit Care Med.* 2003;167:211–277.
10. Older P, Smith R, Courtney P, Hone R. Cardiopulmonary exercise testing as a screening test for perioperative management of major surgery in the elderly. *Chest.* 1999;116:355–362.
11. Marengoni A, Angleman S, Melis R, et al. Aging with multimorbidity: a systematic review of the literature. *Ageing Res Rev.* 2011;10(4):430–439.
12. Perka C, Arnold U, Buttgereit F. Influencing factors on perioperative morbidity in knee arthroplasty. *Clin Orthop Relat Res.* 2000;378:183–191.
13. Roche JJ W, Wenn RT, Sahota O, Moran CG. Effect of co-morbidities and postoperative complications on mortality after hip fracture in elderly people: prospective observational cohort study. *BMJ.* 2005;331:1374.
14. Barrett J, Losina E, Baron JA, Mahomed NN, Wright J, Katz JN. Survival following total hip replacement. *J Bone Joint Surg Am.* 2005;87:1965–1971.
15. Katz JN, Chang LC, Sangha O, Fossel AH, Bates DW. Can comorbidity be measured by questionnaire rather than medical record review? *Med Care.* 1996;34:73–84.
16. Sangha O, Stucki G, Liang MH, Fossel AH, Katz JN. The Self-Administered Comorbidity Questionnaire: a new method to assess comorbidity for clinical and health services research. *Arthritis Rheum.* 2003;49:156–163.
17. Groot V, Beckerman H, Lankhorst GJ, Bouter LM. How to measure comorbidity. A critical review of available methods. *J Clin Epidemiol.* 2003;56:221–229.
18. Harse JD, Holman CD. Charlson's Index was a poor predictor of quality of life outcomes in a study of patients following joint replacement surgery. *J Clin Epidemiol.* 2005;58:1142–1149.
19. Groll DL, To T, Bombardier C, Wright JG. The development of a comorbidity index with physical function as the outcome. *J Clin Epidemiol.* 2005;58:595–602.
20. Hall SF. A user's guide to selecting a comorbidity index for clinical research. *J Clin Epidemiol.* 2006;59:849–855.
21. Fried LP, Ferrucci L, Darer J, Williamson JD, Anderson G. Untangling the concepts of disability, frailty, and comorbidity: implications for improved targeting and care. *J Gerontol A Biol Sci Med Sci.* 2004;59(3):255–263.
22. Guidelines for pre-operative cardiac risk assessment and perioperative cardiac management in non-cardiac surgery: the Task Force for Preoperative Cardiac Risk Assessment and Perioperative Cardiac Management in Non-cardiac Surgery of the European Society of Cardiology (ESC) and endorsed by the European Society of Anaesthesiology (ESA). *Eur J Anaesthesiol.* 2010;27:92–137.
23. Harari D, Hopper A, Dhesi J, Babic-Ilman A, Lockwood L, Martin FC. Proactive care of older people undergoing surgery ('POPS'): designing, embedding, evaluating and funding a comprehensive geriatric assessment service for older elective surgical patients. *Age Ageing.* 2007;36:190–196.
24. Pace Group. Shall we operate? Preoperative assessment in elderly cancer patients can help. *Crit Rev Oncol Hematol.* 2008;65:156–163.
25. Haynes SR, Lawler PG. An assessment of the consistency of ASA physical status classification allocation. *Anaesthesia.* 1995;50(3):195–199.
26. Copeland GP, Jones D, Walters M. POSSUM: a scoring system for surgical audit. *Br J Surg.* 1991;78(3):355–360.
27. Prytherch DR, Whiteley MS, Higgins B, Weaver PC, Prout WG, Powell SJ. POSSUM and Portsmouth POSSUM for predicting mortality. Physiological and Operative Severity Score for the enumeration of Mortality and morbidity. *Br J Surg.* 1998;85(9):1217–1220.
28. Prytherch DR, Ridler BM, Beard JD, Earnshaw JJ. The Audit and Research Committee TVSSoGBaI. A model for national outcome audit in vascular surgery. *Eur J Vasc Endovasc Surg.* 2001;21(6):477–483.
29. Guidelines for pre-operative cardiac risk assessment and perioperative cardiac management in non-cardiac surgery. *Eur Heart J.* 2009;30:2769–2812.
30. Mini Mental State Examination, by Marshal Folstein and Susan Folstein, Copyright 1975, 1998, 2001 by Mini Mental LLC, Inc. Published 2001 by Psychological Assessment Resources, Inc. Further reproduction is prohibited without permission of PAR, Inc. The MMSE can be purchased from PAR, Inc. by calling (813) 968–3003.
31. Nasreddine ZS, Phillips NA, Bedirian V, et al. The Montreal Cognitive Assessment, MoCA: a brief screening tool for mild cognitive impairment. *J Am Geriatr Soc.* 2005;53(4):695–699.
32. Noimark D. Predicting the onset of delirium in the post-operative patient. *Age Ageing.* 2009; 38:368–373.
33. Khan BA, Zawahiri M, Campbell NL. Biomarkers for delirium—a review. *J Am Geriatr Soc.* 2011;59:s256–s261.
34. Marcantonio ER, Flacker JM, Wright RJ, Resnick NM. Reducing delirium after hip fracture: a randomized trial. *J Am Geriatr Soc.* 2001;49:516–522.
35. Inouye SK, Bogardus ST Jr, Charpentier PA, et al. A multicomponent intervention to prevent delirium in hospitalized older patients. *N Engl J Med.* 1999;340: 669–676.

36. deJonghe A, Korevaar JC, van Munster BC, de Rooij SE. Effectiveness of melatonin treatment on circadian rhythm disturbances in dementia. Are there implications for delirium? A systematic review. *Int J Geriatr Psychiatry*. 2010;25(12):1201–1208.

37. Kalisvaart KJ, de Jonghe JFM, Bogaards MJ, *et al.* Haloperidol prophylaxis for elderly hip surgery patients at risk for delirium: a randomized, placebo-controlled study. *J Am Geriatr Soc.* 2005;53:1658–1666.

38. Garth AK, Newsome CM, Simmance N, Crowe TC. Nutritional status, nutrition practices and post-operative complications in patients with gastrointestinal cancer. *J Hum Nutr Diet.* 2010;23:393–401.

39. Gibbs J, Cull W, Henderson W, Daley J, Hur K, Khuri SF. Preoperative serum albumin level asa predictor of operative mortality and morbidity:results from the National VA Surgical Risk Study. *Arch Surg.* 1999;134:36–42.

40. Guigoz Y, Lauque S, Vellas BJ. Identifying theelderly at risk for malnutrition. The Mini-Nutritional Assessment. *Clin Geriatr Med.* 2002;18:737–757.

41. Gramlich L, Kichian K, Pinilla J, Rodych NJ, Dhaliwal R, Heyland DK. Does enteral nutrition compared to parenteral nutrition result in better outcomes in critically ill adult patients? A systematic review of the literature. *Nutrition.* 2004;20: 843–848.

42. Goodnough LT, Manaitis A, Earnshaw P. Management of preoperative anaemia in patients undergoing elective surgery. The NATA Consensus Development Working Group. *ISBT Sci Ser.* 2010;5:120–124.

43. Osland EJ, Memon MA. Are we jumping the gun with pharmaconutrition (immunonutrition) in gastrointestinal onoclogical surgery? *World J Gastrointest Oncol.* 2011;3(9):128–130.

44. Gill TM, Gahbauer EA, Allore HG, Han L. Transitions between frailty states among community-living older persons. *Arch Intern Med.* 2006;166(4):418–423.

45. Ackerman IN, Bennell KL. Does preoperative physiotherapy improve outcomes from lowerlimb replacement surgery? A systematic review. *Aust J Physiother.* 2004;50:25–30.

46. Rooks DS, Huang J, Bierbaum BE, *et al.* Effect of preoperative exercise on measures of functional status in men and women undergoing total hip and knee arthroplasty. *Arthritis Rheum.* 2006;55:700–708.

47. Oldmeadow LB, McBurney H, Robertson VJ, Kimmel L, Elliott B. Targeted postoperative care improves discharge outcome after hip or knee arthroplasty. *Arch Phys Med Rehabil.* 2004;85(9):1424–1427.

48. Katz RI, Cimino L, Vitkun SA. Preoperative medical consultations: impact on perioperative management and surgical outcome. *Can J Anaesth.* 2005;52:697–702.

PART 4

Specific Clinical Issues

CHAPTER 16

Prehospital care of the elderly patient

Ross J. Moy and Jeremy Henning

Introduction

Prehospital care is about doing 'just enough' to ensure a patient can be safely delivered to hospital for definitive care. Given that it is generally carried out in austere environments with limited equipment, there has to be a high threshold before doing anything, but when it is done, it has to be done with an absolute eye to detail, in a well-governed system, with crews who are well rehearsed in their drills.

Traditionally prehospital care has focused on trauma care, but as the population ages the requirement to provide a high level of care outside the hospital to the older person will increase. Indeed the elderly have a disproportionate use of ambulance assets; 17 per cent of the UK population is aged over 65, but around 45 per cent of those who arrive in emergency departments (EDs) by ambulance are over 60. Although there is a second peak for trauma-related admissions in the later decades, many of these admissions are for medical reasons, and the prehospital carer will need to be an expert in all areas.

It is, therefore, difficult to discuss prehospital anaesthesia (PHA) in isolation. This chapter will discuss the various presentations that the prehospital carer will encounter, with specific regard to the elderly, but focus on the issues of providing quality anaesthetic care outside the hospital. This is especially difficult in this group of patients, many of whom will have comorbid disease that may not be known to the provider. It is also clear there will be some difficult ethical dilemmas and there must be an awareness that not all possible interventions will be in the best interests of the patient.

Common presentations

The main aim of providing PHA is to secure an airway and/or control ventilation, to enable the safe transfer of a patient to hospital with no further deterioration in their condition (Fig. 16.1). In the majority of cases this is done for victims of trauma, but this almost certainly reflects the tasking that advanced prehospital care teams are given. It is clear that a significant number of elderly patients present to hospital with inadequate airways and poor gas exchange from medical causes, and may benefit from PHA and critical care.

Cardiovascular accident

The outlook for victims of cardiovascular accidents (CVAs) has been transformed by the introduction of thrombolysis, which can result in dramatic improvement of symptoms. However, this is not without its risks, and is therefore usually only carried out in specialist centres. As such these patients may need to be transported considerable distances, which may mean they need airway support in the field.

The first priority, therefore, is recognition of the possible diagnosis. Tools such as the ROSIER score should be useable by all clinicians (Table 16.1), in order to speed the diagnosis. Once diagnosed, a rapid assessment needs to be made to decide if the patient will need further intervention and to get them safely to the correct centre (Fig. 16.1). If anaesthesia is required, special attention is needed to ensure that their cardiovascular parameters are not compromised during induction and maintenance. Hypotension should be avoided in particular, due to the risk of increasing ischaemia in watershed areas. Also note that blood sugar should be measured to exclude hypoglycaemia.

Chest pain

The key decision in the management of the patient with chest pain is to differentiate acute myocardial infarction from other causes. This is principally to identify patients who might benefit from coronary revascularization. Primary percutaneous coronary intervention is often the management of choice although in more rural areas, where this service is not available, thrombolysis is offered, with transfer for rescue angioplasty reserved for those who do not respond to drug therapy.

Should myocardial ischaemia be suspected, glyceryl trinitrate should be given either buccally or sublingually. If no contraindication is present, aspirin 300 mg should be given. Oxygen has been shown to potentially increase myocardial cell death if given too enthusiastically, and should be reserved for patients who are hypoxic.

PHA may be required if the patient is in severe cardiogenic shock, but should be undertaken with great caution as it may worsen the outcome.

Hypothermia

Hypothermia, defined as a core body temperature of less than 35°C, is common in the elderly. It is associated with poverty, isolation, and inadequate heating. It also occurs with falls, poor mobility, or confusion. A particular danger is the elderly person who cannot get up after a fall, and cannot adjust heating or put clothes on.

Hypothermia in the elderly carries a poor prognosis, with mortality as high as 34 percent. There remains considerable debate about the best management of hypothermia in this age group, as rapid warming risks vasodilatation, and reductions in blood

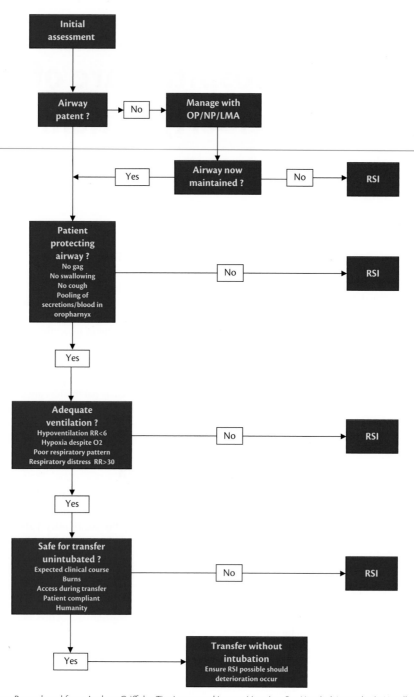

Fig. 16.1 Decision-making process. Reproduced from Andrew Griffiths, Tim Lowes and Jeremy Henning, *Pre-Hospital Anaesthesia Handbook*, 2010, with kind permission from Springer Science+Business Media B.V.

pressure. Also, the high incidence of cardiovascular disease makes rapid infusions of warm fluid dangerous, with the risk of precipitating fluid overload. These complications can be managed in hospital with relative ease, but are potentially very dangerous in the prehospital setting. The mainstay of management should therefore be prevention of further cooling, and rapid transport in a warm ambulance to hospital.

Again, PHA should only be attempted with great caution. There is an incidence of ventricular fibrillation on intubation and maintaining anaesthesia risks worsening the hypothermia. It should be reserved for those deeply unconscious and unable to maintain their airway.

Pulmonary oedema

In the prehospital phase even the most acute, severe pulmonary oedema can usually be managed medically without resorting to positive pressure ventilation. If this is not possible, then continuous positive airway pressure can be attempted, but even with the Bousingac type valves this requires high-flow oxygen, which is

Table 16.1 ROSIER (Recognition of Stroke in the Emergency Room) score

Score new symptoms only	Points
Unilateral facial weakness	+1
Unilateral arm weakness	+1
Unilateral leg weakness	+1
Speech disturbance	+1
Visual field defect	+1
Loss of consciousness/syncope	−1
Any seizures	−1
TOTAL	

Score

>0 = acute stroke likely, take to stroke centre.

−2 to 0 = less likely to be stroke, consider other diagnosis.

Reprinted from *The Lancet Neurology*, 4, 11, Azlisham Mohd Nor, et al., 'The Recognition of Stroke in the Emergency Room (ROSIER) scale: development and validation of a stroke recognition instrument', pp. 727–734, Copyright 2005, with permission from Elsevier.

often limited outside hospitals. In extremis PHA allows for positive pressure ventilation and an improvement in gas exchange.

Acute abdominal pain

This common presentation may result from a number of pathologies. The mainstay of prehospital management is judicious oxygen, analgesia, and fluids. As the elderly tend to have differing inflammatory responses, the classical signs of a surgical abdomen may not be present, even if there is peritonitis.

Abdominal aortic aneurysm dissection or rupture may present with pain or collapse. Should the rupture be contained, the only management is surgical. As the containment may depend on the abdominal muscle tone, any administration of muscle relaxants may precipitate profound hypotension and cardiac arrest. This should therefore only be done if a surgeon is immediately available to quickly cross clamp the aorta, and stop the bleeding. Therefore the only viable option if this is suspected is to get to hospital as soon as possible, avoid anaesthesia until in hospital (even if deeply unconscious), even forgoing intravenous access at scene to expedite transfer.

Exacerbations of chronic obstructive pulmonary disease

Patients with chronic obstructive pulmonary disease may present with infective or non-infective exacerbations. These exacerbations may cause type II ventilatory failure, resulting in CO_2 narcosis. Patients often require non-invasive ventilatory (NIV) support, and this has been shown to improve mortality, and avoid the complications of endotracheal intubation. Many modern prehospital ventilators have settings which allow NIV and it should be employed in preference to invasive ventilation.

However, in extremis, invasive ventilation may be employed to manage pending respiratory arrest. These patients, however, generally have poor prognosis in intensive care, and so this treatment

should only be employed if the patient generally enjoys good health, and is likely to return to an acceptable level of function.

Acute confusion

This is a common presentation to emergency medical services, normally alerted by a concerned friend or carer. The confusion may be as a result of almost any pathology, and may occur *de novo*, or as a result of deterioration in long-standing memory impairment. Common causes include infection, derangement in electrolytes, and abnormalities in blood glucose. Other possibilities include thyroid disease, intracranial pathology, and alcohol abuse. The patient requires careful transfer to hospital for full assessment. As part of this, a judicious use of sedation may be required if the patient is very agitated, especially if the transfer is to be by air. PHA should be avoided if at all possible, as the subsequent sedation required will make in hospital assessment significantly more difficult.

Major trauma in the elderly

The rate of trauma in the elderly is much higher than one might imagine. When one describes trauma, the mind immediately imagines high-speed motor vehicle collisions, shootings, and other such dramatic occurrences. In the elderly population, the majority of trauma is far less spectacular, but all the more life changing. The fall from one's own height, common in the young, and dismissed as quickly, becomes a serious threat to the elderly. So much so that falls are the leading cause of trauma-related death in those over 75. Major trauma also affects the elderly, and age does increase the risk of mortality. This is likely due to the reduction of cardiovascular reserve which occurs with ageing, which makes the patient more susceptible to the effects of haemorrhage. The elderly patient lacks the ability to increase cardiac output in response to stress, making organ hypoxia more likely. They are also likely to have a pre-existing element of age-related organ damage, which the stress of major trauma can exacerbate.

The management of major trauma in the elderly follows standard Advanced Trauma Life Support protocols. In terms of treatable causes of death, they are no different from any other patient. Once the scene is safe, assessment should follow an ABCDE approach, detailed as follows.

Airway

Lack of teeth may make facemask ventilation challenging, and dentures should be left in place if they are well fitting. Tissues in the mouth and nose are more fragile, increasing the risk of bleeding during instrumentation. In addition, oesophageal tone lessens with age, making aspiration more likely. The elderly are also likely to have reduced movement in their necks, producing difficulties in intubation.

If rapid sequence intubation (RSI) is required for airway protection, it should be remembered that age-related cardiovascular changes make hypotension a serious issue. As this can have significant effects on mortality—clinicians should consider the risks and benefits with great care.

Breathing

With age, comes a decline in respiratory function, partly as a result of decreased muscle mass and chest wall compliance. They also have reduced central response to hypoxia and hypercarbia. In addition, the presence of other lung disease may reduce the patient's respiratory reserve. They will require supplemental oxygen and respiratory support at an earlier stage than other patients.

Chest injuries in the elderly should be taken very seriously, as even minor injuries may interfere with the ability to cough, and so place the patient at risk of hypostatic pneumonia, with consequent mortality. Respiratory support should be fairly aggressive in these patients.

Circulation

A degree of atherosclerosis is almost inevitable with ageing, although this may not manifest itself until the stress of trauma reveals it. Similarly, most elderly patients have a degree of primary hypertension, which may or may not be treated. Certain drugs, such as beta-blockers, may mask the physiological response to hypovolaemia. This may mean that an ostensibly normal blood pressure hides a degree of hypotension which may be serious if not treated early. In addition, the elderly patient lacks the ability to increase cardiac output in response to stress. In conjunction with atherosclerosis, this may lead to reduced perfusion of tissues in hypovolaemia.

Along with cardiovascular problems, many elderly patients will have impaired coagulation caused by drugs such as warfarin. Even minor trauma may lead to significant haemorrhage, especially in head-injured patients, and so these patients require hospital admission.

Disability

As the brain shrinks with age, elderly patients are at increased risk of subdural haematoma. This risk is increased considerably in conjunction with anticoagulant medication, and can occur with minimal trauma. As there is generally more space around the brain, there is room for blood to collect, and hence patients may appear well on initial examination. Only a period of observation can identify those who are showing signs of neurological deterioration. Patients taking anticoagulants are at particularly high risk of subdural, from even trivial trauma.

Spinal injuries are more common in the elderly, as deterioration of the intervertebral discs with age forces more of the load onto bone, made more fragile with the osteoporosis of age. They can occur with much lower levels of force than in younger patients, even in falls from the patient's own height.

Exposure

Skin changes and reduction of body fat, along with reduction in the central ability to respond to lower temperatures place the elderly trauma patient at greater risk of hypothermia. As this impairs coagulation, these patients must be protected from the elements, and hypothermia should be looked for and actively managed.

Prehospital anaesthesia

Indications

As intimated earlier, every effort should be made to avoid PHA and intubation, especially in the elderly. As the evidence of benefit is less than clear, it follows that if it is undertaken it must be done effectively, and only if the patient would not survive to hospital (or morbidity increase) without it. Having said that, the threshold to secure

Table 16.2 Indications for prehospital anaesthesia

Unable to safely manage to hospital without intubation/ventilation
Airway problems, not easily resolved by other measures
Respiratory insufficiency, impenVding respiratory collapse
Rapidly falling Glasgow Coma Score
Requirement for sedation to facilitate safe transport
Humanitarian, e.g. profound analgesia
Expected in-hospital course, i.e. to expedite transfer to CT or theatre

the airway in the prehospital arena is often lower than in hospital as factors such as time to definitive care and mode of transport (with associated difficulties in maintaining the airway in cramped spaces) need to be taken into account (see Tables 16.2 and 16.3).

It equally follows that the only real absolute contraindication to PHA is an inability to carry it out safely. This would be the case if there was either inadequate equipment or a poorly trained team.

It can therefore be seen that the decision to undertake PHA is complex. However, as it has been shown that increasing on-scene time may increase mortality, so the decision has to be made quickly. A simple decision-making algorithm is given in (Fig. 16.1).

Conduct

As PHA will be carried out as an emergency drill, a RSI will always be required. Although this is a complex procedure involving over 100 distinct psychomotor skills, it can be broken down into six distinct phases (see Table 16.4).

Phases of rapid sequence induction (the 6 Ps)

Preoxygenation

In the chaotic prehospital environment it can be tempting to abbreviate this phase, however it is a vital safety measure that should never be curtailed. At least 3 minutes of high-flow oxygen needs to be administered whatever the circumstances. This may require careful small doses of sedation such as midazolam to facilitate it if the patient is agitated. If the respiratory rate is low, gentle ventilation via a bag/valve/ mask system may also be required.

Preparation

This is possibly the most important part of the whole process. Normally anaesthesia is carried out in a resuscitation bay or operating theatre with everything to hand. The prehospital team has to work out of their bags, so it is essential that this phase is carried out with an absolute eye to detail. For this reason it is recommended

Table 16.3 Contraindications for prehospital anaesthesia

Untrained team
Not supported by prehospital system
Inadequate equipment
Known anaphylaxis to drugs to be used
Obvious anatomy likely to make intubation impossible
Croup/epiglottitis
Stridor

Table 16.4 The 6 Ps of prehospital anaesthesia

Pre-oxygenation	Use high flow oxygen
	Assist ventilation if respiratory rate low
Preparation	Pre-assessment
	Prepare equipment
	Position patient and team
	Protect C spine/trachea
Pre-medication	If required
Paralyse and sedate	Use sedation and relaxant drugs
Pass the tube	Use a bougie every time
Postintubation care	Maintain safety in transfer

that the team frequently rehearses the drill and uses a checklist to ensure nothing is forgotten. An example checklist is included in Fig. 16.2. This phase can be broken down into five subphases, but can be carried out whilst pre-oxygenation is ongoing.

Pre-assessment

This should be an abbreviated version of the traditional in-hospital pre-anaesthetic assessment, and can follow the ABCDE approach, even in the medical patient. It should be focused on predicting any possible problems that might occur during induction.

Airway

It can be predicted that airway maintenance and intubation will be difficult in this group of patients. It is known that the incidence of poor views of the glottis increases in the trauma patient, and it can be difficult with an edentulous patient to get a good seal with a face mask for ventilation. Quite how difficult the prehospital airway can be is open to debate, some papers have reported intubation failure

rates of up to 25 per cent, whilst others report 100 per cent success. On balance, it would appear that skilled practitioners, using sedation *and* muscle relaxant drugs have a higher success rate.

What is clear is that traditional methods of airway assessment in the prehospital environment are impossible; the Mallampati score is impractical and the thyromental distance is difficult to estimate, therefore, every prehospital airway should be considered 'difficult'.

Breathing

This will have been assessed as part of the decision-making process, but by this time, there will have been some pre-oxygenation carried out. If a pneumothorax is present it may be wise to drain it prior to induction, or, at the very least, get the equipment ready to do soon after. If the patient is to be ventilated, it can be appropriate to perform a thoracostomy without a drain. It is not recommended to transport an intubated, ventilated, and sedated patient with just a needle decompression as this can easily fall out or become occluded.

Circulation

It must be anticipated in this group of patients that their blood pressure will fall on induction, not only will the anaesthetic drugs unmask incipient hypovolaemia, but most of them have direct cardiodepressant effects. Therefore, it is imperative that there is good working access to the circulation, which is well secured. Often it is difficult to achieve this via a peripheral vein, central cannulation is not indicated in the prehospital arena, and peripheral cut-downs take time. It is therefore recommended that after a single attempt at peripheral intravenous cannulation, an intraosseous approach is used. This can be easily achieved using proprietary needles such as the EZIO or FAST.

Equally the team must prepare to counteract hypotension; therefore it is advisable to have a free flowing bag of fluid attached and some vasopressors to hand. Care must be taken in the elderly to not

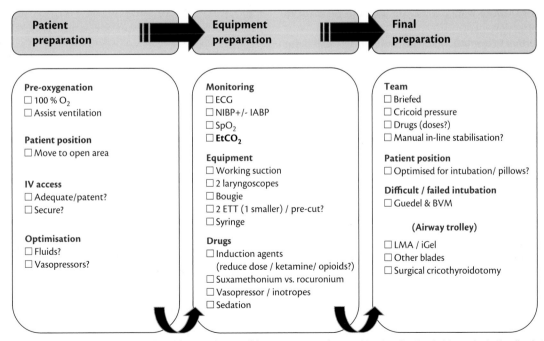

Fig. 16.2 Emergence pre-intubation checklist. Reproduced from Andrew Griffiths, Tim Lowes and Jeremy Henning, *Pre-Hospital Anaesthesia Handbook*, 2010, with kind permission from Springer Science+Business Media B.V.

give too much fluid, but equally not to mask hypovolaemia with vasopressors.

Disability

As the patient is about to be sedated this will be the last opportunity to make a meaningful assessment of consciousness. It is particularly important to note the Glasgow Coma Score (and in particular the motor component), as this may have prognostic significance. This part of the assessment may also guide whether or not the patient should go to a neurosurgical centre.

Exposure

Not only will the patient need to be protected from the elements, driving rain and bright direct sunlight can make laryngoscopy more difficult. It is therefore advisable to either move the patient under cover, or to get a sheet held over the team.

It may be important to also ensure the patient does not get cold. As previously mentioned, the hypothermic patient should be protected from further cold stress, but also it is known that the cold trauma patient has a worse prognosis. Conversely recent evidence suggests that a post-cardiac arrest patient and the head injured may benefit from moderate hypothermia. Local experts should be consulted as to what is right for each specific prehospital system.

Prepare patient, personnel, drugs, and equipment

At this stage all the equipment that may be needed should be put to hand and checked. This can be achieved by either having the kit in a tool roll, or by getting it out of the bags and onto a clean surface (such as a plastic bag) as a kit dump. Laryngoscopes should be inspected and endotracheal cuffs tested. Each system will vary as to how they do this, but it must be as a well-practised drill.

Any drug that may be needed should be drawn up and ready to use. The person giving the drugs must be appropriately briefed as to how much to give and in which order (remembering that the elderly patient may need significantly reduced doses, and require a longer time for them to work). It may be useful to get them to repeat these instructions back.

It is also important to institute vital signs monitoring at this point (if not already started). These should comply with the minimum monitoring standards for in-hospital anaesthesia, although it has to be noted this may not always be possible. Pulse oximetry can be unreliable in the cold, shut down patient and non-invasive blood pressure monitors may not work in a vibrating helicopter. End-tidal carbon dioxide monitoring should, however, be seen as absolutely vital, indeed the absence of it may be considered a contraindication to PHA. Not only does it help confirm endotracheal tube placement, it also gives an indication of cardiac output.

Pre-RSI checklist

Once all of this is complete the checklist must be completed. No matter how experienced the team is, and no matter how well drilled they are, this is another vital safety step and must not be abbreviated. One team member should read out the list (challenge) and the other check and verbally acknowledge the point (response).

Positioning

One of the best ways of ensuring a good view at laryngoscopy is to ensure the patient is in the optimal position, at the intubator's waist height and with their head in the 'sniffing the morning air' position. This is often impossible in the prehospital environment, often the neck will need to be held in the neutral position and the patient will be on the ground.

If it is not possible to bring the patient to waist height, the intubator must change their position to bring their waist to the patient's level. If the patient is put on an ambulance trolley, then the intubator can kneel, if they are on the floor then the same can be achieved if the intubator sits with the patient's head between their knees and ankles in their axilla.

It is also important to have clear all round access to the patient during induction. As they will almost certainly be in extremis, they may need cardiopulmonary resuscitation, and the institution of positive pressure ventilation may reveal a pneumothorax which needs urgent drainage. Therefore the patient should be extricated to an open area before embarking on anaesthesia.

Protection

Cervical spine

There is a clear risk of damage to the cervical spine during trauma, and any patient who has had a significant injury should be treated as at risk. Whilst it is true that much of the damage will be caused during the initial event, when muscle relaxant is given any inherent splinting by the muscles of the neck will be lost. Therefore, at all times the anaesthetized trauma patient must have three-way immobilization (stiff neck collar, head tapes, and blocks) or have someone providing manual in-line stabilization. It should be noted that a well-fitting stiff neck collar with a chin piece will make oral intubation almost impossible, and therefore must be removed prior to laryngoscopy.

Airway and cricoid pressure

This group of patients must be assumed to have a full stomach, and whilst the significance of aspiration is uncertain (it often occurs before anaesthesia, and is a marker of significant disease/injury, rather than caused by anaesthesia), every effort must be taken to avoid it. Therefore, cricoid pressure should be used; however, it must be noted that it will often make the view at laryngoscopy worse and can make face mask ventilation impossible. If this is the case it should be abandoned early, inability to ventilate and failure of oxygenation will always be more significant than aspiration.

Premedication

Once all the equipment has been made ready, the drugs drawn up and the team briefed, pre-medication can be given. This should be aimed at preventing the predictable side effects of the anaesthetic agents to be given, and is usually limited to high-dose opioids (e.g. fentanyl) to obtund the pressor response to laryngoscopy and atropine in children (to prevent bradycardia). Some operators choose to give a small fluid bolus at this point to try to offset hypotension.

Paralysis and sedation

The main aim of this phase is to give drugs to allow safe intubation; as previously discussed, success is markedly increased if both hypnotic agents and muscle relaxants are given.

It is impossible to give clear guidance on the choice of drugs to be used. Essentially the right drugs are the ones that the operators are familiar with, therefore it is important that a narrow range is chosen by each system and the teams are experts in their use.

Traditionally etomidate has been the usual induction agent of choice. It has a relatively wide therapeutic range and is more cardiovascularly stable than many other agents. However, it does decrease adrenal steroid production, and there is increasing evidence that even in a single dose this can affect outcome. Ketamine is becoming more popular, it is also relatively cardiac stable (indeed it may even increase blood pressure) and as a single dose probably does not worsen outcomes from head injuries (as previously thought).

Suxamethonium is the muscle relaxant of choice in most reported systems. It has the advantage of providing profound muscle relaxation quickly with a very clear end point (fasciculations). It also has a place in many 'difficult' airway algorithms as it wears off quickly, allowing spontaneous respirations in the 'can't intubate, can't ventilate' scenario and therefore the potential for the patient to 'wake up' in this difficult situation. It must be noted in the prehospital arena the 'wake up' is not an option—if the patient could make it to hospital without their trachea being intubated, they should never have been anaesthetized in the first place. Therefore, it will be wearing off at just the point when critical desaturation is taking place and alternative airways are being placed. For this reason many systems are now using rocuronium, which, if used in high enough doses, has a similar time to onset, but does not wear off for at least 20 minutes.

Passage of the tube

Clearly this is the whole aim of PHA. A clear view of the glottis is required to do this swiftly yet is rarely achieved, so every technique of maximizing success must be used. As discussed earlier the patient (or intubator) must be in as good a position as possible, and a gum elastic bougie used for every attempt. Traditionally a MacIntosh laryngoscope is used, but there may be some benefit in using other types. The McCoy blade is reported to give better views if the neck is immobilized and there is increasing evidence that other devices (e.g. Airtraq® and Glidescope®) can improve the chances of success. As with the choice of drugs, the choice of laryngoscope will often be down to system and personal preference, but whatever is used the whole team must be practised and familiar with its use.

If it proves impossible to intubate the trachea via the oral route a 'failed intubation' drill must be followed. Each system should have a set drill for use in this circumstance, which again must be regularly practised. The aim of these drills must be to maintain oxygenation, possibly at the expense of not using a 'gold standard' tube. It should be noted that repeated attempts at oral laryngoscopy rarely achieve tracheal intubation, and must be discouraged. Most failed intubation drills will only allow one further attempt before moving on to another technique, and this will only ever be useful if the operator can do something different to their first attempt. An example failed intubation drill is given in Fig. 16.3.

Postintubation care

Many consider that induction of anaesthesia and the successful placement of a tracheal tube as the most difficult part of this procedure. However it is clear that without close attention to detail continuing through the postintubation phase, into hospital there is significant risk of harm. It has been shown that a single episode

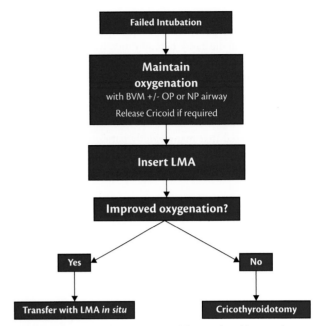

Fig. 16.3 An example of a failed intubation drill. Reproduced from Andrew Griffiths, Tim Lowes and Jeremy Henning, *Pre-Hospital Anaesthesia Handbook*, 2010, with kind permission from Springer Science+Business Media B.V.

of desaturation or hypotension can worsen the prognosis in head injury, and there is no reason to believe this is not the case in other conditions, so postintubation care must be considered just as important. This is the reason why this chapter has referred to the technique of PHA rather than prehospital rapid sequence intubation/induction.

The first part of postintubation care is confirmation of tube placement. Ideally it will have been seen to pass through the vocal cords, and bilateral chest movement seen. Auscultation can be carried out to confirm bilateral breath sounds, but is rarely useful in the noisy prehospital environment. Therefore capnography, with a visible waveform, must also be used to confirm placement.

Once the tube has been confirmed as being in position, drugs must be given to facilitate ventilation and to prevent the patient from waking up. A long-acting muscle relaxant should be given at this point and sedation started. Many systems use a mixture of 1 mg midazolam/1 mg morphine per ml saline, which can either be bolused or used as a continuous infusion. Propofol infusions are also used, however hypotension must be avoided and the careful use of vasopressors may also be required.

Before further onward movement a final check must be undertaken to ensure that all cannulae and tubes are securely in place, and monitors are connected and working. Even in transport it is vital that anaesthesia is maintained and the patient closely supervised. Experience from interhospital transfer of critically ill patients show that many will have a significant deterioration in condition en route, therefore the team must be ready to react. Again this can be set out as a drill and an example algorithm (Fig. 16.4).

Ethical issues

Elder abuse

Regrettably, this is a common and underreported crime. Vulnerable elderly people are at risk of neglect, physical, sexual, and financial abuse. Estimates on frequency vary, and can be as high as 14 per cent, although many patients are unable or unwilling to report it. This abuse can be at the hands of family members, neighbours, professional carers, or strangers. The prehospital carer is in a unique situation to observe the patient in their own environment and must be aware of this possibility.

Futility

It has to be realized that many elderly patients will simply be at the end of their lives if they are in such a critical situation. As such it may be that the burdens of treatment are too much for them

to bear in the face of the fact that whatever the practitioner does they are likely to die. In these circumstances, it may well be better to not intervene and let the patient die with dignity at home. If this is the case, this does not stop the prehospital practitioner from providing care, and close liaison with the patient's normal medical team will be needed. Often it is impossible to ascertain absolute facts in the short time given to make a decision, so the presumption must be made towards full active treatment. Care must however be taken in these circumstances to not give an overly optimistic view of prognosis to friends and relatives who may be with the patient.

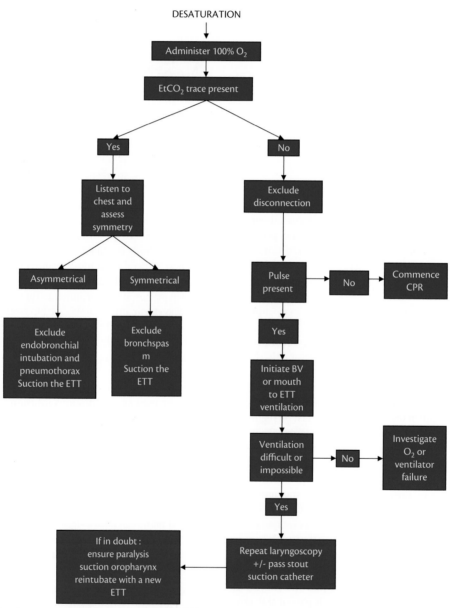

Fig. 16.4 Actions on deterioration en route. Reproduced from Andrew Griffiths, Tim Lowes and Jeremy Henning, *Pre-Hospital Anaesthesia Handbook*, 2010, with kind permission from Springer Science+Business Media B.V.

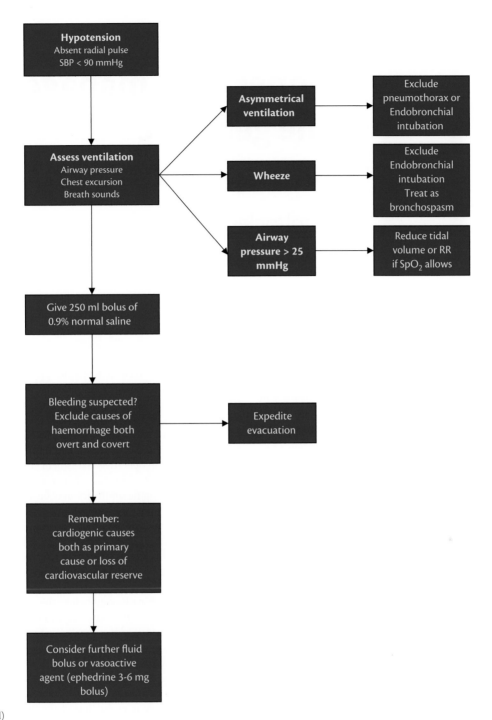

Fig. 16.4 (continued)

Systems issues

From all of the earlier discussions, it can be seen that for PHA to be successful, not only does the individual need to be skilled, but the team has to be practised and this will require the prehospital system they work in to have processes in place to ensure safety. Both the National Association of Emergency Medical Systems in the United States, and the Association of Anaesthetists in the United Kingdom have produced guidance to safely provide this potentially lifesaving procedure, which should be followed closely.

Conclusion

It is clear that PHA, especially in the elderly, is not for the faint hearted. However, it can be provided safely if an absolute eye to detail is maintained and the team doing it is well versed in it, and regularly practises it. As with many controversial areas, only time will tell if it truly saves lives, so in the short term it is vital that any system providing it ensures it does not harm their patients—*primum non nocere.*

CHAPTER 17

Perioperative management of the geriatric trauma patient

Aris Sophocles III and Ashish C. Sinha

Introduction

Trauma is a life-altering event, and a frequent cause of death, among people 65 years of age and older. The elderly have less physiological reserve to tolerate trauma, recover more slowly, and have a higher morbidity and mortality than younger patients with the same level of injury.[1] The elderly are also more predisposed to traumatic accidents from age-related changes in sensation including decreased proprioception, visual field disturbances, impaired auditory acuity, and delayed reaction time. Progressive changes in cardiovascular function place this population at an increased risk for falls and motor vehicle accidents from syncope, cardiac dysrhythmias, and orthostatic hypotension. The most common causes of geriatric traumatic injuries, in order of frequency, are falls, motor vehicle collisions, and pedestrians versus motor vehicle accidents.[2] Falls are responsible for as much as 50 per cent of geriatric trauma.[3] There is a lack of consensus in the geriatric, trauma, and perioperative literature as to what age defines the terms 'elderly' and 'geriatric'. Sixty-five years and older is commonly used to define the lower limit of the geriatric population, and 80 years and older has been used to look for more extreme effects of ageing. For the purpose of this chapter, 'geriatric' and 'elderly' applies to people aged 65 and older. This group represents greater than 12 per cent of the US population, undergoes approximately one-third of the 25 million surgical procedures performed annually, and consume about one-third of all health expenditures and one-half of the $140 billion annual US federal healthcare budget.[4] There is consensus that physiological age, which is affected by lifestyle, luck, and the presence or absence of chronic disease, is a more accurate predictor of morbidity and mortality than chronological age, but with increase in age comes an increase in chronic disease. This chapter focuses on the physiological changes that affect the incidence of, response to, and perioperative management of traumatic injury in the elderly.

A common finding in geriatric trauma literature is that for any given accident the geriatric population sustains more serious injuries and has an increased mortality. Traumatic injuries are often emergency cases. In the geriatric population emergency cases have a significantly increased level of morbidity and mortality compared to the same level of injury in elective cases. A study by Hosking et al. looking at surgical outcomes in 795 elderly patients aged 90

and older found that the mortality rate in the first 48 hours was 7.8 per cent for emergency surgery versus 0.6 per cent in aged-matched patients undergoing similar elective surgery.[5] The increased prevalence of age-related disease and decreased functional reserve hinders the ability to recover from the physiological challenges of trauma, surgery, and anaesthesia, especially in the setting of trauma without the luxury of preoperative optimization.

The geriatric trauma patient is a unique subset of geriatric patients. Paramount to optimal care is having the appropriate questions and differential diagnosis at the forefront of your mind. For example, in the preoperative assessment try to identify 'what preceded the accident'? Was it just a fall or was there an event that preceded the fall? Slipping on the ice may be a reasonable assumption in a young adult, but with the elderly it is important to rule out a preceding cardiac, neurological, pathological fracture, or metabolic event. Elder abuse is a less common cause but must be on all clinicians' list of differential diagnosis. The incidence of elder abuse and neglect may be as high as 25 per cent.[6] Mandatory reporting of elder abuse exists across the United States.[7] It is preferable to diagnose an occult pathology before the operation rather discovering it as a result of an unforeseen intraoperative event or in the post-anaesthesia care unit when the patient fails to return to his or her baseline. Owing to the extent of physiological variability and the increased propensity towards haemodynamic instability, another pressing question in your preoperative assessment is 'what monitoring do I need to safely guide this patient through surgery?'. Further along in your evaluation of the patient you will need to develop anaesthetic and postoperative plans to minimize haemodynamic perturbations and help the patient return to his baseline functional status as quickly as possible.

Geriatric trauma patients have a greater morbidity and mortality from infection and multisystem organ failure than younger adult trauma patients, but with aggressive treatment the outcome differences decrease.[8] By optimizing the perioperative management of geriatric trauma patients we can enhance their ability to regain full function as much as possible and maintain it for the remainder of their lives.

Common thoracic injuries affecting ventilation in geriatric trauma include rib fractures, sternum fractures, and pulmonary contusions. A study by Lee et al.[9] found that motor vehicle accidents in patients 65 years and older had a higher rate of chest injuries (23.4 per cent versus 18.2 per cent in younger patients; p = 0.003) with the most common injuries being rib fractures (23.58 per cent), flail chest (9.55 per cent), and sternal fractures (6.0 per cent). These patients also had nearly twice the mortality of younger patients. A decreased ability to heal fractures and the loss of pulmonary functional reserve make thoracic trauma particularly dangerous in the elderly.

Because no organ system functions independently, changes in one organ system invariably impact upon other organ systems. A central nervous system change that affects the pulmonary system is decreased sensitivity to hypoxia and hypercarbia. Between the ages of 25 and 70 there is approximately a 50 per cent reduction in minute ventilation in response to hypoxia and hypercarbia.[10] One cardiovascular change is decreased diastolic function, which can lead to pulmonary congestion and reduced pulmonary functional reserve.

Decreased functional reserve complicates anaesthetic management. Pedersen et al. examined over 7000 perioperative geriatric patients and found that 10.2 per cent of patients 80 years of age and older developed pulmonary complications.[11] Lui et al. found a similar rate of 7 per cent pulmonary complications in patients 80 years of age and older.[12] The decrease in immune function with ageing predisposes geriatric trauma patients to respiratory failure, acute lung injury, the need for mechanical ventilation, and ventilator-associated pneumonia.[13–15] Avoiding anaesthetic-related pulmonary complications will improve ventilation, increase oxygen delivery to vital organs, and decrease mortality in elderly trauma patients.

Precise fluid management is crucial in patients with decreased renal and cardiovascular reserve. Geriatric patients are less able to tolerate hypovolaemia or fluid overload. Early resuscitation with fluids and inotropes guided by invasive monitoring has been shown to decrease mortality in elderly trauma patients.[16,17] There is evidence from both the orthopaedic and geriatric literature that perioperative fluid deficits are associated with a worse long-term prognosis. Venn et al. found that invasive intraoperative haemodynamic monitoring with fluid challenges during repair of femoral fracture under general anaesthetic shortened the time to becoming medically fit for discharge.[18] Clifton et al., in a retrospective analysis of geriatric traumatic brain injury (TBI), found that a fluid balance deficit greater than 594 ml was associated with an adverse effect on outcome, independent of its relationship to intracranial pressure, mean arterial pressure, or cerebral perfusion pressure.[19] Fluid resuscitation in geriatric trauma should be approached thoughtfully and with caution. For suspected hypovolaemia, a crystalloid bolus of 1 or 2 L can be given gradually. If there is no significant improvement in vital signs, invasive monitoring, blood products, and colloids should be considered.[14,20] Of note, decreased renal reserve makes this population more vulnerable to hyperchloraemic metabolic acidosis with high volume, normal-saline resuscitation.[2]

Elderly trauma patients are at a higher risk of head injury and TBI than younger adults. They also have increased length of hospital stay and an increased mortality rate from head injuries.[21,22] Falls, followed by motor vehicle and pedestrian accidents, are the most common causes of geriatric head injuries. Almost expectedly, age is an independent predictor of worse outcome.[22,23] Structural changes that influence the effect of head injuries include a decrease in brain mass from loss of neurons and a decrease in epidural

space as the dura becomes more adherent to the skull bones. These changes contribute to the threefold increase in the incidence of subdural haematomas.[24] The presentation of subdural haematomas may be more subtle and gradual because of the increase in intracranial space that gives blood more time to collect before compressing the brain or compromising blood flow. Common presenting symptoms include headache, loss of balance, and syncope.

Anaesthetic considerations in the geriatric trauma patient

Preoperative assessment in the geriatric trauma patient

While performing your preoperative assessment and primary survey you should ask yourself, 'What preceded the traumatic event?'. If the injury resulted from a fall or motor vehicle collision, was there a physiological event that preceded the accident? If this is a possibility, was the change cardiac, neurological, or metabolic in origin? Myocardial infarction, transient ischaemic attacks, falls resulting in the slow development of subdural haematomas, and metabolic derangements are all more common in the elderly.

The anaesthetist should perform a modified primary survey in the geriatric trauma patient as part of the preoperative evaluation. The classic ABCD (airway, breathing, circulation, disability) approach to assessment and resuscitation is useful for organizing the physical exam. Common to trauma patients of all ages are the increased risks of full stomach and airway obstruction from direct injury, tissue swelling, or a foreign body. As already mentioned, the elderly are more prone to aspiration and have decreased protective airway reflexes secondary to muscular and neural degenerative changes in the larynx.[25] Pre-emptive preparation should include first-, second-, and third-line difficult airway equipment, and appropriate resources for rapid sequence intubation. There is cadaveric evidence that cricoid pressure worsens cervical spine instability, so the risks of aspiration must be weighted with the risks of worsening a cervical spine injury.[26] Elderly patients have a higher prevalence of fixed and removable dental hardware. The removable ones may be left in the mouth for mask ventilation but should be removed prior to intubation.

An important part of the airway exam in the geriatric trauma patient is assessment of the cervical spine. The cervical spine is the most common location of vertebral fractures in the elderly trauma patient.[2] Central cord syndrome and spinal cord injuries are more common in the elderly because of underlying osteoporosis, narrowed cervical canals, and muscle atrophy.[27,28] Elderly trauma patients with cervical spine injuries have worse outcomes than their younger counterparts.[2] Identifying areas of tenderness and decreased movement will aid with transferring, positioning, and intubation. It is paramount to maintain cervical spine immobilization until cervical spine injury has been ruled out.[24] Degenerative and arthritic changes in the atlanto-occipital joint restrict cervical spine mobility and impair visualization during intubation. Video laryngoscopes and fibreoptic bronchoscopes can be very useful for intubating patients with decreased neck mobility and cervical spine precautions.

Assessment of breathing includes visual inspection, palpation, and auscultation. Common thoracic injuries affecting ventilation in geriatric trauma include rib fractures, sternum fractures, flail chests, and pulmonary contusions. Pulmonary contusion is common in blunt thoracic injuries. Hypoxaemia from pulmonary contusion responds to positive pressure ventilation via mask until a definitive airway is established.[29] Also, as mentioned earlier, geriatric patients have an increased risk of both chronic and acute aspiration.

The effects of ageing on organ systems and the increased prevalence of chronic disease alter the cardiovascular response to trauma. The clinician should have a higher index of suspicion for diagnosing and treating shock, as typical compensatory signs such as tachycardia will be dampened by concurrent age-related cardiovascular changes. A normal or borderline low blood pressure in a geriatric trauma patient may be a sign of imminent decompensation.[14]

Disability assessment includes inspecting for bodily and neurological injuries. Geriatric trauma patients are more susceptible to orthopaedic injuries because of their decreased bone density. Long bone and pelvis injuries are common and place geriatric trauma patients at an increased risk for fat embolism. Signs and symptoms of fat embolism include alterations in mental status, tachypnoea, tachycardia, and petechiae.[30] Abdominal trauma in the elderly has a fourfold increase in mortality compared to younger adults.[2]

Assessing for neurological injuries in the elderly trauma patient may be complicated by the concurrence of sensory deficits and pre-existing neurological conditions such as prior strokes or dementia. It is prudent not to assume that decreased mental status is normal even with a history of dementia because confusion and fluctuations from baseline may be secondary to decreased cerebral perfusion, impending shock, or intracranial pathology. Geriatric trauma patients are more prone to intracranial venous bleeding. Slow intracranial bleeding may manifest as delayed changes in mental status. The Glasgow Coma Scale is a common assessment tool in the emergency department (ED). Using this in the preoperative assessment and comparing the results with those from the ED may be useful to evaluate acute changes in mental status. If a venous bleed is suspected, an emergency head computed tomography scan is necessary.

After the primary survey, every effort should be made to perform a thorough physical examination and obtain a detailed history within the time constraints of the emergency. There is tremendous interindividual variability in health and functional reserve in the geriatric population. The preoperative assessment is an invaluable opportunity to assess functional reserve, by organ system, for each patient to better understand the patient's health status. When elderly trauma patients are unable to appropriately answer questions, friends and family members can offer valuable information about the accident, prior mental and functional status, and past medical history. A thorough preoperative evaluation helps differentiate trauma related injuries from the patient's baseline health status.

Additional areas that deserve attention in the elderly are functional status, nutritional status, and do not attempt resuscitation (DNAR) status. Functional status is different from functional reserve, and refers to behaviours necessary to maintain daily life, also known as activities of daily living (ADL). These include aspects of social and cognitive functioning necessary to function independently. Multiple studies indicate that functional status is as important a predictor for postoperative morbidity and mortality as the burden of chronic disease indices.[31]

Malnutrition is more common in the geriatric population and may be predictive of poor surgical outcomes. One of the more studied markers for nutritional status is the serum albumin. A study by

Gibbs et al. looking at 30-day operative mortality and morbidity in over 50 000 patients found those patients with serum albumin concentrations less than 21 g/L versus greater than 46 g/L had an increase in mortality (29 per cent vs 1 per cent) and morbidity (65 per cent vs 10 per cent).[32]

The preoperative assessment is an opportunity to discuss DNAR preferences and identify a surrogate decision-maker. Relying on family members to make decisions on the patient's behalf when the patient no longer has decision-making capacity is a poor substitute for discussing these preferences with the patient in advance. Studies have shown that family proxy decision-makers come no closer than chance at predicting what a patient would want under hypothetical circumstances.[33] Physicians don't fare much better. A study by Krumholz el al. found that physicians are incorrect in predicting resuscitation preferences in 25 per cent of their patients.[34]

Practical anaesthetic considerations

Also see Chapter 3.

Choosing an induction agent

One of the most common induction agents is propofol, a rapidly acting alkylphenol with a short half-life. Induction doses are approximately 60–70 per cent those for young adults (1.2–1.7 mg/kg versus 2.0–2.5 mg/kg). There is also a decrease in clearance of propofol in the elderly resulting in decreased maintenance requirements.[35,36] A significant adverse effect of propofol is dose-dependent cardiac depression and peripheral vascular dilatation that result in hypotension. This response is exaggerated in the elderly owing to the cardiovascular changes described earlier, and can be minimized with slow administration, reduced loading dose, and vigilant re-dosing with titration to effect.

Etomidate has the advantage of being more cardiovascularly stable than propofol. This is advantageous in elderly patients with little to no cardiovascular functional reserve. Like propofol, induction doses should be reduced in the elderly. Arden et al. found that 80-year-old patients required half the amount of etomidate to reach the same electroencephalographic endpoint correlating with hypnosis and amnesia as 20-year-old patients. Interestingly, they found the increased sensitivity was more likely from age-related changes in redistribution than brain sensitivity. The initial distribution volume for etomidate decreased significantly with increasing age leading to a higher initial blood concentration in the elderly following any given dose of etomidate.[37] Etomidate has its own deleterious side effects including increased postoperative nausea and vomiting and adrenal suppression.

Ketamine is another induction drug that is less likely to decrease systemic vascular resistance and blood pressure than propofol. Potential contraindications for ketamine include its sympathomimetic effects on the cardiovascular system, which can increase myocardial oxygen demand, and have an increased incidence of postoperative delirium, along with an increase in intracranial pressure. Its psychotropic and cardiovascular effects can be attenuated with benzodiazepine premedication.

Analgesia

Of note, transdermal opioids such as fentanyl patches are not easily titratable and are relatively contraindicated in the elderly for acute postoperative pain.[38]

Elderly patients may demonstrate increased sensitivity to opioids.[39] Therefore careful titration and frequent assessment for inadequate pain control or adverse side effects will optimize pain management in the postoperative period and improve patient comfort and satisfaction. Adequate pain decreases postoperative morbidity, shortens hospital stay, and reduces healthcare costs.

Regional anaesthesia

Regional anaesthesia has several potential benefits compared to general anaesthesia in the elderly depending on the surgery. These include: decreased blood loss, decreased endocrine stress response, decreased incidence of postoperative thromboembolic complications, and improved postoperative cognition.[39] Chung et al., however, found similar levels of postoperative cognitive dysfunction when regional anaesthesia was combined with minimal intravenous sedation.[40]

The most significant increased risk of spinal anaesthesia in the elderly is haemodynamic instability.

Monitoring

The anaesthetist should have a low threshold for deciding to use invasive monitoring in the elderly trauma patient. There is evidence for improved survival when early invasive monitoring is used to guide resuscitation in elderly trauma patients.[16] Invasive monitoring allows for detection of occult low flow states, perfusion deficits, and shock that can occur when the patient appears cardiovascularly stable by conventional, non-invasive monitors. Early detection and intervention are crucial in patients with limited functional reserve to reduce the incidence of multisystem organ failure from inadequate tissue perfusion. Candidates for invasive haemodynamic monitoring include those with chronic systemic disease, significant injury, high-risk mechanism of injury, uncertain cardiovascular status, or renal disease.[14]

Blood gas analysis is another important component of intraoperative monitoring. The base deficit may be particularly useful in the elderly as a measure of tissue perfusion, oxygen debt, and adequacy of resuscitation. A study by Davis et al. evaluating the significance of base deficit in trauma patients 55 years and older found that a base deficit of 6 mmol/L or less was associated with increased mortality compared to similar trauma patients under 55 years of age.[41]

Positioning

Despite the urgency to begin the procedure in emergent trauma operations, time and care must be taken to position the patient carefully with adequate padding around pressure areas and bony prominences. Geriatric patients have decreased skin turgor and loss of subcutaneous soft tissues that provide padding to younger adults and are particularly vulnerable to pressure sores. Loss of subcutaneous tissue and decreased elasticity of skin increase the potential for damage to superficial tissues and neural structures. Increased skin fragility also predisposes the elderly to burns from improperly placed electrosurgical dispersive pads.[30] Meticulous attention to detail when transferring and positioning patients will help prevent iatrogenic injury.

Thermoregulation

See Chapter 34. Treating heat loss is especially challenging in the elderly trauma patients. Many are already hypothermic on admission following their injuries and may require aggressive heat management to prevent further loss as they are assessed and resuscitated prior to definitive management. Minimizing exposure during examination and using forced air body warmers, fluid warmers, and increasing all treatment room temperatures to 26.6° Celsius (~80° Fahrenheit) should be routine in this population to minimize preventable heat loss.

Postoperative considerations

A major goal for the perioperative care of the geriatric trauma patient is rapid return to prior functional status. Musculoskeletal injuries are the most common traumatic injury in the elderly and can lead to prolonged periods of immobility and decreased functional status. In turn this leads to a loss of independence, decreased quality of life, and depression. In the geriatric hip fracture literature, early fracture fixation facilitates earlier mobilization, improves ADL scores, and decreases postoperative mortality.[42–44] Delayed ambulation after hip fracture surgery is associated with delirium, postoperative pneumonia, and increased length of hospital stay.[45] Physical therapy helps with early mobilization and may reduce the risk of future falls and fractures.[43,46] A multidisciplinary approach to perioperative management of elderly hip fracture trauma patients is associated with decreased medical complications, decreased surgical delays, and shorter hospital stays.[47]

Conclusion

As the elderly population increases, so too will the incidence of geriatric trauma. Relatively minor trauma can be a life-altering event, transforming a relatively independent member of society to a person requiring prolonged rehabilitation and full time assistance. A thorough understanding of the physiological changes seen in the ageing process and the response to traumatic injury will allow you to tailor an anaesthetic plan that will optimize the patient's recovery.

Common threads addressed in this chapter include the progressive, age-related decrease in functional reserve, the significant variability among elderly trauma patients, and the need for meticulous attention to detail in all stages of perioperative care. Ageing affects all organ systems and decreases the capacity for adaptation to stress and ability to compensate for a perturbation in homeostasis. The variability between patients requires a thorough preoperative assessment and an individualized plan. Finally, meticulous attention to detail in all stages of perioperative care is paramount to avoiding iatrogenic harm and optimizing care.

References

1. McMahon DJ, Schwab CW, Kauder D. Comorbidity and the elderly trauma patient. *World J Surg.* 1996;20:1113–1119.
2. Mandavia D, Newton K. Geriatric trauma. *Emerg Med Clin North Am.* 1998;16:257–274.
3. Mosenthal AC, Livingston DH, Elcavage J, Merritt S, Stucker S. Falls: epidemiology and strategies for prevention. *J Trauma.* 1995;38:753–756.
4. Muravchick S. *Geroanesthesia: principles for management of the elderly patient.* St. Louis, MO: Mosby, 1997.
5. Hosking MP, Warner MA, Lobdell CM, Offord KP, Melton LJ 3rd. Outcomes of surgery in patients 90 years of age and older. *JAMA.* 1989;261:1909–1915.

6. Cooper C, Selwood A, Livingston G. The prevalence of elder abuse and neglect: a systematic review. *Age Ageing*. 2008;37:151–160.

7. Clarke ME, Pierson W. Management of elder abuse in the emergency department. *Emerg Med Clin North Am*. 1999;17:631–644.

8. DeMaria EJ, Kenney PR, Merriam MA, Casanova LA, Gann DS. Aggressive trauma care benefits the elderly. *J Trauma*. 1987;27:1200–1206.

9. Lee WY, Cameron PA, Bailey MJ. Road traffic injuries in the elderly. *Emerg Med J*. 2006;23:42–46.

10. Wahba WM. Influence of aging on lung function—clinical significance of changes from age twenty. *Anesth Analg*. 1983;62:764–776.

11. Pedersen T, Eliasen K, Henriksen E. A prospective study of risk factors and cardiopulmonary complications associated with anaesthesia and surgery: risk indicators of cardiopulmonary morbidity. *Acta Anaesthesiol Scand*. 1990;34:144–155.

12. Liu LL, Leung JM. Predicting adverse postoperative outcomes in patients aged 80 years or older. *J Am Geriatr Soc*. 2000;48:405–412.

13. Yung RL. Changes in immune function with age. *Rheum Dis Clin North Am*. 2000;26:455–473.

14. Lewis MC, Abouelenin K, Paniagua M. Geriatric trauma: special considerations in the anesthetic management of the injured elderly patient. *Anesthesiol Clin*. 2007;25:75–90.

15. Chalfin DB. Outcome assessment in elderly patients with critical illness and respiratory failure. *Clin Chest Med*. 1993;14:583–589.

16. Scalea TM, Simon HM, Duncan AO, et al. Geriatric blunt multiple trauma: improved survival with early invasive monitoring. *J Trauma*. 1990;30:129–134.

17. Soliman IE, Safwat AM. Successful management of an elderly patient with multiple trauma. *J Trauma*. 1985;25:806–807.

18. Venn R, Steele A, Richardson P, Poloniecki J, Grounds M, Newman P. Randomized controlled trial to investigate influence of the fluid challenge on duration of hospital stay and perioperative morbidity in patients with hip fractures. *Br J Anaesth*. 2002;88:65–71.

19. Clifton GL, Miller ER, Choi SC, Levin HS. Fluid thresholds and outcome from severe brain injury. *Crit Care Med*. 2002;30:739–745.

20. Santora TA, Schinco MA, Trooskin SZ. Management of trauma in the elderly patient. *Surg Clin North Am*. 1994;74:163–186.

21. Tieves KS, Yang H, Layde PM. The epidemiology of traumatic brain injury in Wisconsin, 2001. *WMJ*. 2005;104:22–25, 54.

22. Mosenthal AC, Livingston DH, Lavery RF, et al. The effect of age on functional outcome in mild traumatic brain injury: 6-month report of a prospective multicenter trial. *J Trauma*. 2004;56:1042–1048.

23. Mosenthal AC, Lavery RF, Addis M, et al. Isolated traumatic brain injury: age is an independent predictor of mortality and early outcome. *J Trauma*. 2002;52:907–911.

24. Pudelek B. Geriatric trauma: special needs for a special population. *AACN Clin Issues*. 2002;13:61–72.

25. Pontoppidan H, Beecher HK. Progressive loss of protective reflexes in the airway with the advance of age. *JAMA*. 1960;174:2209–2213.

26. Donaldson WF 3rd, Towers JD, Doctor A, Brand A, Donaldson VP. A methodology to evaluate motion of the unstable spine during intubation techniques. *Spine (Phila Pa 1976)*. 1993;18:2020–2023.

27. Schwab CW, Kauder DR. Trauma in the geriatric patient. *Arch Surg*. 1992;127:701–706.

28. Irvine DH, Foster JB, Newell DJ, Klukvin BN. Prevalence of cervical spondylosis in a general practice. *Lancet*. 1965;1:1089–1092.

29. Hurst JM, DeHaven CB, Branson RD. Use of CPAP mask as the sole mode of ventilatory support in trauma patients with mild to moderate respiratory insufficiency. *J Trauma*. 1985;25:1065–1068.

30. Keough V, Letizia M. Perioperative care or elderly trauma patients. *AORN J*. 1996;63:932–937.

31. Inouye SK, Peduzzi PN, Robison JT, Hughes JS, Horwitz RI, Concato J. Importance of functional measures in predicting mortality among older hospitalized patients. *JAMA*. 1998;279:1187–1193.

32. Gibbs J, Cull W, Henderson W, Daley J, Hur K, Khuri SF. Preoperative serum albumin level as a predictor of operative mortality and morbidity: results from the National VA Surgical Risk Study. *Arch Surg*. 1999;134:36–42.

33. Seckler AB, Meier DE, Mulvihill M, Paris BE. Substituted judgment: how accurate are proxy predictions? *Ann Intern Med*. 1991;115:92–98.

34. Krumholz HM, Phillips RS, Hamel MB, et al. Resuscitation preferences among patients with severe congestive heart failure: results from the SUPPORT project. Study to Understand Prognoses and Preferences for Outcomes and Risks of Treatments. *Circulation*. 1998;98:648–655.

35. Schnider TW, Minto CF, Shafer SL, et al. The influence of age on propofol pharmacodynamics. *Anesthesiology*. 1999;90:1502–1516.

36. Peacock JE, Lewis RP, Reilly CS, Nimmo WS. Effect of different rates of infusion of propofol for induction of anaesthesia in elderly patients. *Br J Anaesth*. 1990;65:346–352.

37. Arden JR, Holley FO, Stanski DR. Increased sensitivity to etomidate in the elderly: initial distribution versus altered brain response. *Anesthesiology*. 1986;65:19–27.

38. Beyth RJ, Shorr RI. Principles of drug therapy in older patients: rational drug prescribing. *Clin Geriatr Med*. 2002;18:577–592.

39. Rivera R, Antognini JF. Perioperative drug therapy in elderly patients. *Anesthesiology*. 2009;110:1176–1181.

40. Chung FF, Chung A, Meier RH, Lautenschlaeger E, Seyone C. Comparison of perioperative mental function after general anaesthesia and spinal anaesthesia with intravenous sedation. *Can J Anaesth*. 1989;36:382–387.

41. Davis JW, Kaups KL. Base deficit in the elderly: a marker of severe injury and death. *J Trauma*. 1998;45:873–877.

42. Doruk H, Mas MR, Yildiz C, Sonmez A, Kyrdemir V. The effect of the timing of hip fracture surgery on the activity of daily living and mortality in elderly. *Arch Gerontol Geriatr*. 2004;39:179–185.

43. Tornetta P 3rd, Mostafavi H, Riina J, et al. Morbidity and mortality in elderly trauma patients. *J Trauma*. 1999;46:702–706.

44. Gdalevich M, Cohen D, Yosef D, Tauber C. Morbidity and mortality after hip fracture: the impact of operative delay. *Arch Orthop Trauma Surg*. 2004;124:334–340.

45. Kamel HK, Iqbal MA, Mogallapu R, Maas D, Hoffmann RG. Time to ambulation after hip fracture surgery: relation to hospitalization outcomes. *J Gerontol A Biol Sci Med Sci*. 2003;58:1042–1045.

46. Gregg EW, Pereira MA, Caspersen CJ. Physical activity, falls, and fractures among older adults: a review of the epidemiologic evidence. *J Am Geriatr Soc*. 2000;48:883–893.

47. Khasraghi FA, Christmas C, Lee EJ, Mears SC, Wenz JF, Sr. Effectiveness of a multidisciplinary team approach to hip fracture management. *J Surg Orthop Adv*. 2005;14:27–31.

CHAPTER 18

The elderly and intensive care medicine

Richard Keays and Neil Soni

Introduction

The populations of the Western world are becoming older. Their expectations are rising, in part by changing health technology and pharmacology that has altered the management of disease, and part by the evolution of a societal perspective that suggest that both old age and disease can overcome by a combination of individual choice and the application of resources. Both are only partially correct and the result is an ageing population often with significant acquired comorbidities presenting to intensive care with an acute illness. Neither the acute presentation nor the comorbidities are peculiar to the elderly and the management of the problems are the same as in the rest of the population. It has been said that intensive care medicine is becoming a specialty largely focused on care of the elderly. In spite of the present and increasing predominance of elderly patients in critical care units both in sheer numbers and in total bed days this remains a relatively understudied area. This chapter seeks to look at the implications of managing the elderly presenting to critical care.

Definitions

Intensive care has the nursing ratios, usually one to one, medical input, and technological capability to provide supportive and therapeutic care to the critically ill. The intention is to restore health but, as the World Health Organization (WHO) has described, health is a state of complete physical, mental, and social well-being and not merely the absence of disease and infirmity (WHO Constitution). Even approaching this goal is a huge challenge. Inevitably, in a proportion, it will fail but in doing so may subject the patient and their families to unnecessary discomfort and physical and emotional hardship. In some of these cases the prolongation of dying is not a justifiable goal. This is a relevant concept across the entirety of the critically ill population but it is often more so in the elderly, where life expectancy may be limited and comorbidities most prevalent, where the balance can be most difficult. The term old or elderly is easily used but hard to define.

There is no clear or agreed definition of elderly. It has been defined by chronology, social role or status, capabilities, and physical status. It has also been defined as when the population life expectancy is less than 10 years or in some cultures 'when active contribution is no longer possible'.[1] Most commonly it is taken as the national pension age, 60 for females and 65 for males, although this is now a more fluid end point. It has varied with time so that in 1875 it was over 50, currently around 65, and the 'over 80s' also seem to be becoming an 'identifiable' group. There are the additional problems; even the simple device of using pension age is confounded by the paradox that longevity in females reverses the pension age position. Beyond the Western world, the country's socioeconomic situation impacts heavily on age demographics.

In medicine the position is more complex. To all clinicians it is quite clear that in later life there is increasingly poor correlation between chronological and physiological age. The medical literature has no common definition and uses a wide range of arbitrary values from 67 to 70, over 70s, and more recently over 80s to describe population groups.[2]

Demographics of ageing in the intensive care unit

In a classic paper[3] the United States and the United Kingdom were compared in terms of the elderly and hospitalization. In the over-85-year-old population, 47 per cent died in hospital in the United Kingdom, whilst it was only 31 per cent in the United States. So a larger proportion of this population died in hospital in the United Kingdom but only 1.3 per cent received intensive care in the United Kingdom compared with 11 per cent in the United States.[3] If only surgical patients are considered then 1.9 per cent of those over 85 died in the intensive care unit (ICU) in the United Kingdom compared to 31.5 per cent in the United States. There are similar hospital mortalities between countries but very different locations at time of death, with more patients dying in the ICU in the United States.

From a different perspective, of all hospital discharges in the United Kingdom only 2.2 per cent had been in the ICU while in the United States it was 19.3 per cent. This may be in part because of the available facilities. It is changing but in 2005 the United Kingdom had 3.3/100 000 population ICU beds, Australia 7.8/100 000, Germany 24/100 000 and 20/100 000 in the United States.[4]

The pattern of admission is also evolving; in Australia and New Zealand 13 per cent of ICU admissions were older than 80 years and the numbers increased by about 5 per cent per annum between 2000 and 2005.[5]

Of those patients dying in the ICU only 10–20 per cent died through unsuccessful resuscitation and the rest died through some form of limitation of treatment.[6]

Approaching the problem from a different direction is to consider what happens to a whole cohort of elderly people. One such longitudinal study from America following over 1 million patients (mean age 79 years) over a 5-year follow up period found that over one-half were admitted to ICU at some point. Admission rates are known to be higher in the USA but nevertheless, contrary to expectations, only a third of these critical care admissions happened in the final 6 months of life and over two-thirds of elderly patients were still alive 6 months after the initial ICU admission.[7] However, 3 per cent of the cohort were multiple users and accounted for 23 per cent of total ICU admissions and 15 per cent of the total cost (approximately $3 billion).

The ageing process

See also Chapter 1.

Profound physiological changes accompany ageing but they are both extremely variable and relatively unpredictable across any population. What is clear and of far greater importance is that with age most individuals accumulate a range of comorbidities with pathophysiological implications. Hence ageing is the combination of both inevitable physiological change and accumulated pathophysiology.

The influence of factors other than age is best illustrated by epidemiological studies. A good example is cardiovascular risk in males. In 55-year-olds who are relatively fit and well the risk of dying from cardiovascular disease by age 80 is about 4.7 per cent, so there is clearly an intrinsic risk. If, however, they had any two of the following risk factors—smoking, diabetes, poor blood pressure control, or high cholesterol—the risk increases to 29.6 per cent. This significant change in the predicted risk of mortality is only the tip of the morbidity iceberg.[8] Clearly, these risks arise from an individual's genotype, evidenced by their family history, but long-term environmental factors such as nutrition or occupational exposures are also crucial. It is extremely hard to separate out those changes that are solely age related.

Functional capacity

See also Chapter 15.

This should be considered in terms of both physical and intellectual function. One aspect of physical functionality is exercise capability. The current way of looking at this is with metabolic equivalents (METs). One MET is the oxygen consumption by the aerobic demand of a 70 kg male in a resting state and approximates to 3.5 ml/kg/min. As activity increases so do the METs and so different types of activity can be looked at in terms of the METs they need. In general terms moderate exercise would be 4–7 METs.

This approach has been widely used in assessing surgical risk as an overall measure of respiratory and cardiovascular function and hence reserve. It should be a good indicator of ageing if ageing were predictable and if no other factors were present. Even advanced age, which is often associated with reduced functionality, may also be relatively normal. Nevertheless the concept of METs can be used as a global assessment of functionality. It is only one measure. Musculoskeletal capability may be limited by arthritis, body shape or neurological deficits and all these will impinge on METs as an accurate indicator of true functionality. Likewise neurological and psychological functions are important in terms of activity, responsiveness, and motivation and so these are important in a global assessment that must go beyond simply METs. Age is relevant but

rarely is the sole limiting factor on functionality, which is more often associated with the acquired comorbidities.

The organ systems

It is impossible to separate age-related changes and the pathophysiology accrued over the years. Nevertheless age carries with it physiological decline and the likelihood of comorbidity so patients present as a variable combination of the two. As each organ system has defined changes associated with age it seems relevant to describe these briefly (as they have been described in earlier chapters) and to then look at the impact of the commoner comorbidities and the net effect. It cannot be comprehensive.

In the assessment of the patient both components need to be integrated and therefore in terms of probability, age carries potential morbidity and mortality. As with every other population presenting to ICU determining what is recoverable and what is futile, poses significant problems.

Cardiovascular

See also Chapter 6.

There are some well recognized changes to the cardiovascular system with the main ageing changes being myocardial and vascular stiffening, with impaired cardiac and vascular compliance. The blunted sympathetic responses produce the 'hyposympathetic heart' with a tendency to increased end-diastolic volume (see Table 18.1). This is in addition to the age-related reduction in cardiac contractility. Overall cardiac reserve and flexibility of response is reduced, but is usually more than able to deal with the normal physical requirements of the elderly—but not with more excessive demands.[9–11]

Table 18.1 Cardiovascular ageing

Cellular changes; reduced excitation contraction coupling, calcium homeostasis, myocyte function and increased atrial natriuretic peptide
Decrease in myocytes, altered connective tissues, increased ventricular wall size
Reduction in conductive tissues and numbers of sinus node cells
Decreased contractility, reduced ventricular compliance, increased ventricular filling pressure, blunting of beta adrenoreceptor responsiveness, reduced coronary flow reserve
Stiffer arteries, reduced elasticity. Thicker media and intima
Alterations in autonomic tone with reduced beta adrenoreceptor mediated vasodilatation. Reduced nitric oxide activity
Reduced heart rate, increase end diastolic volume, increased stroke volume, reduced peak values for ejection fraction, cardiac output
Impaired conduction, atrial fibrillation
Reduced preload reserve, reduced overall cardiac reserve and predisposition to cardiac failure
Clinical effects
More arrhythmias, hypertension, reduced exercise tolerance, dyspnoea and heart failure

In the critically ill, it is probably the general reduction in cardiac reserve reducing the patient's ability to cope with the stress of illness that is the greatest concern. Arrhythmias such as chronic atrial fibrillation are common in the elderly but often new-onset atrial fibrillation develops in the postoperative patient. In one study of non-cardiac surgery, 22 per cent of over-70-year-olds developed atrial fibrillation in the postoperative period.[12] When it does occur reduced reserve means that there is more likelihood of cardiac compromise so they may be more at risk from hypotension, cardiac failure, and then ischaemia. In the postoperative population over 85 years old the commonest cause of death is myocardial infarction.[13,14]

Cardiac surgery exemplifies the age problem. If patients are selected on the basis of lack of comorbidity and good functional status, then there is little difference between octogenarians and younger populations. Those with risk factors such as previous bypass grafts, heart failure, chronic airways disease, and renal disease tend to do badly, as do those presenting as emergencies. Interestingly, long-standing problems such as diabetes, hypertension, and vascular disease are of lesser importance.[15]

Respiratory

See also Chapter 7.

There is a less compliant chest wall, with reduced gas exchange and impaired reflexes to both hypoxia and hypercapnia. These factors alone make it more likely that weaning will be problematic but there is also evidence of diminished antioxidant defences,[16] and bronchial lavage sampling shows changes in both immunoglobulin and CD4/CD8 ratios implying chronic antigenic stimulation.[17] Additionally, there is an increasing burden of age-associated, non-pulmonary problems such as nocturnal gastro-oesophageal reflux, kyphosis and vertebral collapse, and sleep apnoea. Far more important across the entire population is that time related deterioration in lung function associated with environmental exposure and in particular smoking which will tend to accrue. These added comorbidities are of far greater consequence than the effects of ageing.

The associations with ageing are clear but what is cause and what is effect? The chances of requiring ventilation increases with age and an American study put this likelihood at approaching 10 per cent in the over 75s ([18]). Several studies of patients requiring ventilation demonstrate an association between mortality and an age greater than 70. Esteban quantified mortality in age bands such that for those less than 40 years it was 21 per cent; between 40 and 70 years, 30 per cent; and for greater than 70 it was 36 per cent.[19] Going beyond ICU to discharge there is a high 3-year mortality in the elderly and 57 per cent of those deaths occur early after discharge.[20] It is extremely variable but for those requiring prolonged ventilation, greater than 21 days, there is also a clear association with ongoing chronic illness and a high 1-year mortality.[21] In summary old age and prolonged ventilation result in higher mortality both in and beyond ICU but also more chronic ongoing illness.

The issue is somewhat confounded by the ventilation of those with known chronic obstructive airways disease. In this group acute exacerbations tend to do well and have a lower mortality at 28 per cent, which is lower than other causes of respiratory failure. Despite doing relatively well, there is a strong correlation between both subsequent mortality and the severity of lung disease.[19] This is

significantly influenced not only by the extent of pre-existing problems but also their need for ongoing care at the time of hospital discharge. If they were not fit to go directly home, then post-discharge mortality was increased.[22] At 5 months a high proportion will need assistance with at least one aspect aspects of daily living. Twenty-seven per cent will score a low quality of life although similar to their pre-existing state. The rest will do well with minimal impairment.[22]

The main considerations are the factors present at admission in terms of acute illness by severity score, and also the pre-morbid functional state of the patient. In those who have severe acute respiratory failure not only will the outcome be worse but also the likelihood of ongoing chronicity is increased, especially if ventilation is prolonged. Under these circumstances the physiological reserve of the patient will be important in determining the likelihood of a successful outcome both in the short and in the longer term.

Renal

See also Chapter 8.

The likelihood of renal failure increases with age (see Table 18.2). Against this background there is definite association between acute renal failure and mortality and hence, as the incidence rises, mortality increases.[23] The actual attributable mortality to acute kidney injury (AKI) itself remains similar between old and young.[24] The mortality in the elderly is quoted variously between 15 and 40 per cent, although in those requiring renal replacement therapy it has been quoted at 62 per cent.[25]

The increased risk of AKI is associated with acquired preconditions that accumulate with age. Risks such as renovascular disease, congestive cardiac failure, the increased use of drugs that might impair renal function, such as non-steroidal analgesics, invasive interventions and surgery all increase with age.[26,27] The causes of acute renal failure are ill defined but a third are obstructive in origin and of course prostatic disease is prevalent. Of the implicated drugs; non-steroidal analgesics, angiotensin-converting enzyme inhibitors and contrast medium have all been implicated, although a time-honoured cause, contrast medium was not a risk

Table 18.2 Acute renal failure in the elderly

Pre-renal causes
Hypovolaemia
Hypoperfusion, cardiac failure, shock such as sepsis.
Pharmacological, e.g. non-steroidal anti-inflammatory drugs (NSAIDS)
Renovascular, hepatorenal syndrome
Renal causes
Acute glomerulonephritis
Interstitial nephritis, drugs, e.g. NSAIDS, antibiotics-penicillins, allopurinol
Acute tubular necrosis
Toxicity-contrast medium, rhabdomyolysis. Gentamicin
Post-renal causes
Prostatic disease, stones, malignancy

factor in elderly trauma patients in a recent study.[28] Surgery provides additional risk, not just because of changes in volume status and blood pressure, but also the possibility of abdominal hypertension. Sepsis is also implicated and as the risk of sepsis rises with age so does the mortality although, again, age is not the independent risk factor. In one study only three out of 23 biopsies of AKI of unknown cause showed evidence of acute tubular necrosis.[29] The cause of death in this population was multiple organ failure 29 per cent, disseminated infection 41 per cent, gastrointestinal bleeding in 16 per cent, myocardial infarction 5 per cent, and stroke in 1.9 per cent.[29]

The outcome from acute renal failure is determined by the underlying cause and the functional status rather than the disease severity (see Table 18.2).[30] Drug related AKI does better than most other causes.

The relationship between age renal failure and outcome is complex. Age itself has little effect on acute renal failure.[31] However long-term effects may be significant and the mean survival of octogenarians after an episode of acute renal failure was 19 months.[29,32] Schiffl reported a mortality of 18 per cent in the first year, 4 per cent the next year, and then about 2 per cent per year.[33] This is similar to a study of 700 patients with a mortality of 41 per cent at 28 days, 57 per cent at 1 year, and 70 per cent by 5 years. The quality of life was lower in these patients than in the general population but not dependent on age.[34] The likelihood of needing ongoing dialysis has also been reported. Schiffl and colleagues looked at 226 survivors (47 per cent survived) and none was dependent on RRT at discharge. About half had complete recovery of renal function. Even at 5 years very few needed dialysis.[33]

Chronic renal failure

Patients with chronic renal failure tend to be older and are more prone to acute kidney injury. But when they get renal failure it tends to be with a lower severity of illness and hence has shorter stay and lower mortality.[35] As the elderly are more likely to have worse baseline creatinine clearance due to comorbidities, such as diabetes and cardiac failure, they tend to have worse recovery rates.[33,35,36] They are more likely to need longer-term dialysis and the risk may be increased by up to seven times.[32] The issue again is that although chronic renal failure is more common in the elderly the age itself is not really directly related.

A secondary but important effect is that in the elderly there is often a reduced ability to excrete drugs. The consequence may be prolonged half-life (by a factor of 1.4), altered volumes of distribution (+24 per cent) and reduced clearance.[37] This is probably a source of excess morbidity in the elderly.

Liver

See also Chapter 9.

This is relatively unaffected and has huge intrinsic reserve so that a reduced mass of up to 30 per cent at 80 years probably has little effect, other than loss of reserve. There is a tendency to reduced liver blood flow by up to 40 per cent at 80 years and also reduced metabolic function, in particular demethylation and the production of cholinesterase. It may have some effect on drug handling.[38] These rarely translate into clinical relevance.

It is acquired liver disease, cirrhosis, that is the potent predictor of mortality and this is relatively independent of age.[39]

Central nervous system

See also Chapter 12.

Deterioration in the central nervous systems may be massive, minimal, or anything in between, but frequently there is some decline in cognitive performance with age, though this is contentious. There are many postulated mechanisms and there are even some semi-specific changes that can be identified on magnetic resonance imaging.[40] Amongst these are cerebrovascular disease associated with atherosclerosis and the secondary effects of hypertension. There is some linkage between the decline of the sex steroids and neural function but also a wide range of neurochemical alterations including melatonin levels have also been demonstrated.[1,41,42] There are alterations in the blood–brain barrier and changes in the ability of the brain to adapt to circumstances such as the loss of the mild hypoxia acclimatizing effect.[43,44] Another area of interest is the influence of sleep disorders which are more common in the elderly and neurocognitive dysfunction.[45]

Specific features include memory loss which is apparent in at least 10 per cent over the age of 70 and about 50 per cent of these have some variant of Alzheimer's disease. This increases by doubling each decade.[46] These patients are especially vulnerable to developing delirium in the ICU. There is age-related decline in hearing in 25 per cent of patients at around 65 but this increases to over 70 per cent in those over 75.[3] Likewise there is a decline in the sensory modalities such as touch.[38]

Acquired neurological deterioration is common. Some cognitive decline is almost inevitable and probably irrelevant but it is dementia that causes more concern. It is multifactorial and while cerebrovascular pathology and a strong association with strokes, small and large, is important as is a previous head injury amongst many other factors.[47] Often deemed irreversible in ICU there are now potential interventions on the horizon which may alter the ICU perspective. At present delirium is the bigger issue with up to 70 per cent of elderly patients (> 65 years) experiencing delirium while in hospital. A third are admitted with it and another third develop delirium while in ICU.[48] Delirium is 'an acute confusional state that occurs in the face of an underlying organic aetiology'. It is different from dementia in that the onset level of inattention is rapid as is the change in level of consciousness. Clinically it has a broad spectrum of presentation from inattention, disorientation and agitation through to apathy, immobility, and depression.[49] Coma, sedatives, and infection are risk factors but other pharmacological agents, noise, light, and other sleep disturbing factors may all be important.[50] Immobility and bed rest is also associated with disturbed sleep patterns and loss of diurnal rhythms.[51] Pre-existing impairment whether from alcohol or drug dependency or previous cognitive impairment are obviously predisposing factors.[52] It is common after major surgery and in particular hip fracture with rates of up to 60 per cent of patients.[53,54] Up to 80 per cent of ventilated patients are delirious.[55] Following cardiac surgery it is very common but tends to show improvement fairly rapidly after discharge in about half of these patients but in the remainder neurocognitive decline can persist for years. This is common in ICU and on discharge many elderly patients still have delirium much of which will persist as cognitive dysfunction.[52] This would translate into longer hospital stay and likely a higher mortality. Delirium is an independent predictor of 6-month mortality.[56] Part of this is post-traumatic stress disorder which is seen in all age groups, when searched for, and influences mental health related quality of life.[57] Age is a risk factor for persistent psychological issues.[42,58] Despite this, Stoll et al. showed a high level of life satisfaction in the elderly.[58] What is obvious is that the psychological assessment of the elderly post intensive care is in its infancy. The occurrence of delirium is common and often persistent. The existing tools for assessing delirium are the confusion assessment method for ICU (CAM-ICU) and intensive care delirium screening checklist (ICDSC). ICDSC score of more than 4 correlates with both increased mortality and in survivor's persistent cognitive dysfunction.[59] More recently the ten risk factor assessment tool for the prediction of delirium in ICU (PRE-DELIRIC) which has been validated for ICU.[60] Awareness of the problem should lower the threshold for diagnosis and then these scores, which have been hard to implement, may be used more widely. Anecdotally, the families of elderly patients discharged home often report behavioural and other changes which imply long-lasting sequelae.

The literature on formal follow-up and assessment is in its infancy but it is the authors' belief that the optimistic statistics in the literature belie a significant underestimated problem that should be the focus of proper investigation in the immediate future.

Gastrointestinal

The elderly often complain of issues with gut motility. From an intensive care perspective conditions such as diverticulitis are common. Immobility and bed rest might affect absorption and this might include vitamin B_{12} or D. Both should be considered. Poor nutrition may also influence other potential deficiencies.

Skin

Ageing skin has characteristic changes. There is a decrease in elastin fibres, and thinning of both dermis and epidermis. Mechanically this leads to a reduced cohesion between the skin layers. Some of these changes in the skin may be associated with the reduction is the sex steroids.[61] There is very little literature on the effects of healing and the skin in the elderly in critical care.

Endocrine

There may be non-specific alterations in endocrine function. Impaired thyroid function is common. The incidence of type 2 diabetes increases with increasing age. Adrenal activity is rarely affected but obviously does occur, often in association with other comorbidities. In males both testosterone and adrenal androgens decrease with age and this is associated with loss of muscle strength and mass. In women the reduction in oestrogen post menopause has various effects although the overall impact appears to be one of sarcopenia. This can be partially reversal by hormone replacement therapy but is best counteracted by exercise. Physical activity is fundamental to muscle functionality and the declining activity often found in the elderly results in reduced mass and increased likelihood of disability.[62]

Metabolic

Over the age of about 70 there is a tendency for weight loss associated with a general change in body composition with increased fat and reduced muscle mass. There is less protein turnover and less fat oxidation.[63] It has been estimated that there is a 2 per cent decrease in basal metabolic rate per decade and there is a reduced

requirement for calories as one ages however protein requirements stay the same.[64] Despite reduced calorific requirements malnutrition and inadequate calorific intake is common. This 'anorexia of ageing' is multifactorial including the social impact of eating alone, the time taken to eat, and psychological states such as depression. There are also some fundamental changes physiologically. Early satiation is common particularly after larger meals. Delayed gastric emptying is partly due to reduced gastric fundal compliance with impaired smooth muscle relaxation. The consequent feeling of fullness suppresses ghrelin which also reduces appetite. There are also raised levels of cholecystokinin in the elderly inducing satiation.[63] Dehydration and micronutrient deficiencies are also common; loss of water-soluble vitamins such as thiamine with diuretic therapy, folate and vitamins A, C, and E deficiency, and vitamin B_{12} deficiency due to atrophic gastritis and reduced intrinsic factor secretion.[64]

Ageing is associated with changes in muscle mass, muscle composition, and hence in strength and functionality termed sarcopenia. The main muscle groups' strength are reduced by about 30 per cent by the 7th decade and continue to decrease to over 50 per cent in octogenarians.[65] There is a real reduction in motor unit numbers which curiously does not affect strength until a critical point is reached.[66]

With less musculoskeletal activity there is less energy use and hence heat production. This is associated with altered heat regulation and although the elderly often die with either hyperthermia or hypothermia the tolerance to either is not significantly compromised.[62] The old may be more susceptible to extremes of temperature.[40,67,68]

The relevance to this physiology in ICU is that sarcopenia in the elderly needs to be taken in the context of the chronic disease which may accentuate the negative energy balance, such as chronic heart failure or chronic obstructive pulmonary disease (COPD). These patients have reduced nutritional reserve. There is a close association between weight loss and frailty, and thereby functionality. That is related to both complications and mortality. This aspect of functionality may be a very significant phenomenon in the recovery phase and may determine the ability of a patient to regain independence.[65]

Pharmacology

See also Chapter 3.

There are marked changes in pharmacokinetics and pharmacodynamics in the elderly with those influenced more by renal than liver changes predominating. The impaired ability of the kidneys to excrete drugs influences half-life which may be prolonged. The volume of distribution may also either increase or decrease depending on the drug and changes in body composition.[37,69] There may be changes in sensitivity to drugs partly through altered pharmacokinetics as described, or interaction with physiology such as the decline in sensitivity to beta-adrenergic agonists and antagonists with age. By a similar mechanism the incidence of orthostatic hypotension with anti hypertensives increases. The central nervous system however becomes more sensitive to centrally acting drugs.[67,70]

Fluid management must incorporate some general considerations. These include the potential presence of both cardiovascular and renal impairment, a reduced flexibility in cardiac output and an increasing dependence on alterations in systemic vascular resistance. This and other changes in muscle and fat may alter fluid redistribution. This is unpredictable across the population but should be assessed in the individual.

The biggest single problem in the pharmacology of the elderly is the polypharmacy which is rife. Many elderly patients will be on a panoply of different medications depending on their chronic health problems. Most drugs have side effects and interactions and as the number of medications increases so does the likelihood of complications from their use especially when the patient is ill. The classic example is antihypertensives in the elderly causing postural hypotension. There is a literature relating to the role of polypharmacy in hospital and ICU admission with two very different mechanisms. The drugs being the source of the problem and the inadvertent discontinuation of important medications also has implications.[38,41,43,47,71] It is not a minor issue and is an important part of the assessment of the elderly should be rationalization of medication.

Infection

See also Chapter 35.

Nutritional reserve, immobility, and comorbidities may all predispose to infection so it is not surprising that *Clostridium difficile* is more common in the elderly accounting for 50 per cent of all admissions with *C. difficile*. This may also be related to their normal place of residence with institutionalized care being a further predisposition. The associated 30-day mortality is higher than in younger patients and is particularly high in those older than 75 years old, or those who have chronic respiratory disease, a high APACHE score, or septic shock.[39]

The incidence of nosocomial bloodstream infection is relatively low but in the elderly the impact is very high,[72] with a reported 90-day mortality of 26 per cent compared with 15 per cent in a younger population.[73] In the elderly severe infection is more common and has a higher mortality both in and out of hospital so that at 2 years the standardised mortality ratio for the elderly was 2.56 compared to the young.[74,75] In these studies age is a surrogate for functional state immobility and comorbidity.

Surgery outcome

More elderly patients are having increasingly complex surgery. Both operative mortality and postoperative complications are higher in the elderly and again relate to lack of reserve and more comorbid illnesses. This is true for both cardiac and non-cardiac surgery.[76–78] After cardiac surgery only 47 per cent of octogenarians returned straight back home. One set of mortality figures for coronary artery bypass are 8 per cent in the elderly versus 3 per cent in the younger group and for coronary artery plus mitral valve, 19.6 per cent versus 12.2 per cent. The elderly had twice the incidence of stroke and renal failure. The complications correlate with the comorbidities present and if the patient is fit the results are similar to the young.[15,79,80] Of the common comorbidities type 1 diabetes, hypertension, and COPD are all known risk factor across age groups.[81]

In the over 80s, medical and orthopaedic patients had far greater mobility and self-care problems than either abdominal surgical patients or age-matched controls.[82] This study also demonstrated that mortality rates at 6 months after ICU discharge was 76 per cent for unplanned emergency surgical patients against 30 per cent for planned surgical patients. Orthopaedic surgical patients had 6-month mortality somewhere in between these quoted figures.

Emergency surgery poses major problems with higher complication rates.[80,83] The elderly presenting as emergencies have been eloquently described as 'a heterogeneous cohort of both potentially treatable patients and those who are dying'.[84] This defines a very significant issue that impacts on intensive care. Identifying the treatable from the futile is difficult across all age groups but in the elderly with limited life expectancy and severe comorbidity the difference may be committing the patient and their family to emotional and physical hardship and this is clearly justifiable with a good outcome but far harder to defend if the outcome was never likely to be good. The patient's wishes or preferences should ideally be taken into account but frequently that is not possible. It is one of the few circumstances where 'acting in a patient's best interest' is actually the line of least resistance and not in their interest at all. Important decisions need to be taken at appropriate times, and usually this is before embarking on heroic actions, futile surgery which, once started, are difficult to stop. This is an area of practice that has not been studied but anecdotally is very poorly managed.

See also Chapter 36.

ICU outcome

Given the lack of clarity of what constitutes the elderly the general picture would suggest survival at discharge of around 75 per cent falling a further 10 per cent by 6 months.[44] One study[74] suggests that, for the over 80s, half will not survive ICU but half the survivors will be alive 2 years later. There is also some lack of clarity over whether age itself, the severity of the acute illness or the accumulated comorbidities and declining functional status that accompany the ageing process affects ICU outcome. APACHE scoring attributes only 7 per cent of the outcome predictive power to age alone. Nevertheless, in some studies of ICU admissions, increasing age does appear to be independently associated higher 30-day hospital mortality.[72,85,86] Intuitively, the pre-morbid functional status and presence of comorbidities should significantly affect ICU outcome. In patients over 85 years of age there is a higher mortality but this appears to be somewhat predicated by the pre-morbid state.[42,87] In a study of over 15 000 elderly patients compared to non-elderly ICU admissions, the elderly were more likely to have greater comorbid illnesses and higher illness severity scores which led to a higher ICU mortality and these patients were more likely to be discharged to either rehabilitation or long-term care.[5] Even supposedly soft indicators such as coming from a care home was associated with higher in-hospital mortality and the medium term mortality at 6 months is also increased if discharged to care facilities.[20] Conversely, other studies have failed to find an association between outcome and pre-existing comorbidities or functional status.[88,89] Amongst those discharged from ICU but who went on to die most were predictable at the time of discharge and tended to die in the first 3 months.[87]

If age itself is not an indicator then its use as a surrogate for general status is also unpredictable.[90] Nevertheless, it is possible to conclude that the outcome for elderly patients admitted to ICU for medical indications or after emergency surgery is poor and that outcome relates to the pre-morbid state, the severity of the acute illness and the presence of an underlying fatal illness, as in other populations.[74,91,92] In general elderly ICU patients tend to have a worse long-term outcome.[40] The role of the pain and anxiety experienced in ICU, which is probably important, has not been evaluated in terms of outcome.[93]

A focus on mortality evades the more relevant question of the quality of life after ICU. At ICU discharge most patients have significant functional disability when evaluated against activities of normal daily living.[94] This will improve and subsequent recovery is more relevant but the evidence is hard to interpret. It is a generalization but those with major acute events with little comorbidity often report a substantially lower quality of life afterwards while those with significant pre-existing comorbidity, and hence relatively lower expectations notice less of an impact on their quality of life.[40,67]

A very common finding in the elderly is that the functional status is clearly worse, often considerably worse, but that the 'feeling of well-being was good'.[95-98] This is a contentious area with some studies showing no real impairment in quality of life. Probably the best indicators of real outcome for the elderly are measures such as returning home which has rarely been assessed but is often a very important consideration for the individual. Conti and colleagues assessed this with the results seen in Table 18.3. This approach is probably more relevant than mortality figures.[99]

In the future there needs to be more focus on both physical and mental functionality as an outcome measure. Patients need to be not only alive but have reasonable functional status and ideally capable of returning home.[5,8,44,65,99–101]

Assessment for admission

A knowledge of pre-morbid functionality and the severity of comorbid illnesses is a prerequisite to deciding on suitability for admission. This is taken in the context of the acute insult and an analysis of whether the disease process is reversible and if the patient is salvageable. If not then the application of intensive care is likely to impose a physical and mental burden on the patient and their family that cannot be justified by the likely negative outcome. It is worth stating that physicians may overestimate the mental and functional status of patients accepted for admission and underestimate it for those whose admission is rejected.[102]

Age has little role to play in this decision other than its association with physiological decline and the acquisition of comorbidity. It is also worth noting that many elderly patients will have one form or another of advanced directive.

History

This should involve speaking to the patient or, if impossible, to their relatives to make an assessment of their previous functionality physically and mentally (see Table 18.4).[103] Establish if comorbidities are present and if so how severe. Determine whether the patient is living at home or in a home and how independent they are. Living in a nursing home may sometimes but not always be a surrogate for significant functional impairment.[5] In the elderly nursing home population anaemia, cancer, heart failure, renal failure, and COPD are all related to poor 1-year outcome.[104] For those with previous hospital admissions a history of supported ventilation is also a potentially important feature. There is a need to know the physical and mental trajectory over the last few months or years that may indicate significant functional decline. Details relating to level of activity—house-, room-, chair-, or bed-bound—are powerful indicators.

Clinical signs

The general habitus is useful. Posture, muscle bulk or more often wasting, and the condition of the skin all help indicate physical well-being or otherwise. In the long-term ill health is a potent cause for self-neglect and so the state of the teeth, the lower legs and the feet are very important indicators. Peripheral oedema and infection indicate potential comorbidities, while chest wall shape may suggest chronic airways disease.

Movement and agility is less easily evaluated in acute conditions but again some impressions can be gained by the previous factors. All of these provide a picture of the level of their functionality and the degree to which comorbidity exists.

Table 18.3 Factors that influence elderly patients getting home from ICU[99]

Important factors
Over 75 years of age
Neoplasia
Chronic heart failure
Neurological or neurosurgical cause for admission
Trauma
Respiratory failure
Cardiology
Neurological complication
Cardiological complication
Haematological complication
Surgical complication.
Less important
Planned surgery
Visceral surgery
Chronic renal disease
Living alone

Table 18.4 History

Where do they live—at home or in care
Independence—how much support
Mobility—shopping, walking
Memory, confusion sleeping pattern
Previous hospital admissions in particular ventilation or chronic renal failure
Comorbidity respiratory, cardiology and neurology but also arthritis and mobility
Drugs
Patient's preferences if known

The physiological changes with age correlate poorly with actual age, and it is the acquired comorbidities that accumulate with age that influence functionality. Then the acute nature of the presentation needs to be evaluated and its reversibility taken in the context of the other problems. The patient's preferences either declared or previously informed are a very important part of this assessment. Most importantly no individual part of this should overwhelm all other considerations. Examination should try to integrate the physiological changes of age with the comorbidities and assess these in the context of the acute insult that has necessitated admission.

Treatment intensity

Over the last decade the average SAPS score on admission to ICU for patients over 80 years, has increased. These patients tend to have a more severe acute illness but with less pre-existing functional disability. Consistent with this has been and a general increase in treatment intensity with more renal replacement therapy and more vasopressors. This has been accompanied by a step-wise change in the odds of survival.[95,105] A similar approach but with less ventilation, fewer tracheostomies, less renal support, and a lower ICU cost but similar outcome has also been reported. The suggestion from both studies is that this is due to better patient selection.[106] The ELDICUS study looked at the benefit of intensive care in reducing mortality across different age groups by comparing patients who were triaged to receive intensive care or not. Mortality was highest in patients rejected for intensive care as compared with those who were accepted and this difference was largest in the elderly population.[107]

The conclusion is that with careful patient selection, high-intensity treatment is appropriate and can produce good results but selection is important.

Expectations and preferences

An important consideration at the time of admission is the likely expectation in terms of the outcome. This will in large part be related to the quality of life before admission, as this will have a significant effect on physical and mental capabilities in the aftermath of intensive care. As age is frequently associated with a reduction in physical reserve so lifestyle is an accommodation to these circumstances. Hence the accepted physical limitations of the elderly prior to admission may be an easier goal to achieve following ICU than in the young where full recovery to the pre-morbid state may be more difficult and the loss of reserve more obvious. Issues about quality must be geared to the expectations of the patient both physically and psychologically.

Despite the growing likelihood that end of life is increasingly a hospital death, 86 per cent of patients wanted to die at home. Only 16 per cent would take life-prolonging drugs if they made them feel worse and most would want palliation even if it shortened life. Most would not want to be put on a ventilator to gain a week of life and the numbers were similar if it were for a month of extra life.[108] Of those octogenarians who survive ICU half declared they would not want ICU treatment again if it were required.[98] However, one must be careful about making assumptions in this group of patients. The SUPPORT study showed a poor understanding by physicians of patients' preferences[109] and further declared that, despite the fact that more than half of over 70-year-olds would want CPR most

physicians substantially underestimated this.[110] In 1999, Singer and his colleagues[111] identified the following as being most important to patients:

♦ Receiving adequate pain and symptom management.

♦ Avoiding inappropriate prolongation of dying.

♦ Achieving a sense of control.

♦ Relieving burden on others.

♦ Strengthening their relationship with loved ones.

Key to acting on patients' preferences means ensuring the patient has a clear understanding about their acute illness and its ramifications including prognosis so they can make a personal cost/benefit analysis not just about survival but about the implications of the treatment.[92]

End of life

Death in ICU is usually through some form of withdrawal. Only 10 per cent of patients dying in ICU die through failed cardiopulmonary resuscitation.[6] Limitation of life support is very common as is either withdrawing or withholding treatment. Active shortening of the dying process, defined by a circumstance in which someone performed an act with the specific intention of shortening the dying process, is rare in most countries. There is huge variation in practice between countries not only in the decision process but in the issuing of 'do not attempt resuscitate' orders and the modes of withdrawal and withholding treatment.[112]

Patient preferences are very important as is physician recognition of medical futility. Key to this area of management is a clear view of what ICU is intended to provide. An understanding of whether the goals are achievable and acceptance that subjecting a patient and their family to the unpleasant rigours of ICU in the sure knowledge that it will achieve no useful outcome is unacceptable. These determinations must be made objectively. Although age itself is not a strong risk factor for treatment withdrawal, a physician's opinion that the outcome was probably going to be poor and that intensive care treatment was not wanted by the patient did significantly increase the likelihood of treatment withdrawal.[113] Increasingly advance directives are likely to be present and there is an obligation to seek these out early and to respect patient preference.

Conclusion

In developing the APACHE score Knaus showed that most predictive power for outcome was derived from the acute physiological condition, a much smaller component was the admission disease, 13.6 per cent, but age only constituted about 7 per cent. In the elderly the physiological changes of ageing are not contraindications in their own right. The comorbidities present are far more important but need to be assessed in company with the acute condition and the reversibility of the combination of all three components. In this approach it is the same as for any patient of any age. It is more likely that an older patient will have advance directives and so will have already voiced their personal preferences.

A simplistic view might be to suggest intensive care enables an acute episode to be reversed with the intention of returning the patient to the position they were in before that episode or close to it. There needs to be recognition that majority of treatment is supportive, and provides the physiological reserve they have lost until it can be regained. Those with less reserve will need more support. The patient will invariably need a certain amount of physical reserve to meet the challenges of the treatment and the recovery. The decision to use ICU requires acknowledgement that ICU has negative as well as positive aspects and that it can be a very unpleasant experience with far reaching sequelae both physical and mental, for both patients and relatives. Justification is provided by a good outcome so it is implicit that the opinion at the time of admission is that full recovery is possible or indeed probable. As in every other population appropriate use of intensive care can produce impressive results but inappropriate use can be disastrous for the patient and their family. Age itself is not a contraindication.

References

1. Gorman M. *Development and rights of older people.* London: Earthscan Publications Ltd, 1999.

2. Roebuck J. When does old age begin? The evolution of the English definition. *J Soc History.* 1979;12(3):416–428.

3. Wunsch H, Linde-Zwirble WT, Harrison DA, Barnato AE, Rowan KM, Angus DC. Use of intensive care services during terminal hospitalizations in England and the United States. *Am J Respir Crit Care Med.* 2009;180(9):875–880.

4. Wunsch H, Angus DC, Harrison DA, *et al.* Variation in critical care services across North America and Western Europe. *Crit Care Med.* 2008;36(10):2787–2793, e1–e9.

5. Bagshaw SM, Webb SA, Delaney A, *et al.* Very old patients admitted to intensive care in Australia and New Zealand: a multi-centre cohort analysis. *Crit Care.* 2009;13(2):R45.

6. Sprung CL, Cohen SL, Sjokvist P, *et al.* End-of-life practices in European intensive care units: the Ethicus Study. *JAMA.* 2003;290(6):790–797.

7. Iwashyna TJ. Critical care use during the course of serious illness. *Am J Respir Crit Care Med.* 2004;170(9):981–986.

8. Berry JD, Dyer A, Cai X, *et al.* Lifetime risks of cardiovascular disease. *N Engl J Med.* 2012;366(4):321–329.

9. O'Rourke MF, Hashimoto J. Mechanical factors in arterial aging: a clinical perspective. *J Am Coll Cardiol.* 2007;50(1):1–13.

10. Priebe HJ. The aged cardiovascular risk patient. *Br J Anaesth.* 2000 Nov;85(5):763–778.

11. Suttner SW, Piper SN, Boldt J. The heart in the elderly critically ill patient. *Curr Opin Crit Care.* 2002;8(5):389–394.

12. Vaporciyan AA, Correa AM, Rice DC, *et al.* Risk factors associated with atrial fibrillation after noncardiac thoracic surgery: analysis of 2588 patients. *J Thorac Cardiovasc Surg.* 2004;127(3):779–786.

13. Djokovic JL, Hedley-Whyte J. Prediction of outcome of surgery and anesthesia in patients over 80. *JAMA.* 1979;242(21):2301–2306.

14. Menaker J, Scalea TM. Geriatric care in the surgical intensive care unit. *Crit Care Med.* 2010;38(9 Suppl):S452–S459.

15. Alexander KP, Anstrom KJ, Muhlbaier LH, *et al.* Outcomes of cardiac surgery in patients ≥80 years: results from the National Cardiovascular Network. *J Am Coll Cardiol.* 20001;35(3):731–738.

16. Kelly FJ, Dunster C, Mudway I. Air pollution and the elderly: oxidant/antioxidant issues worth consideration. *Eur Respir J Suppl.* 2003;40:70s–5s.

17. Meyer KC, Ershler W, Rosenthal NS, Lu XG, Peterson K. Immune dysregulation in the aging human lung. *Am J Respir Crit Care Med.* 1996;153(3):1072–1079.

18. Behrendt CE. Acute respiratory failure in the United States: incidence and 31-day survival. *Chest.* 2000;118(4):1100–1105.

19. Esteban A, Anzueto A, Frutos F, *et al.* Characteristics and outcomes in adult patients receiving mechanical ventilation: a 28-day international study. *JAMA.* 2002;287(3):345–355.

20. Wunsch H, Guerra C, Barnato AE, Angus DC, Li G, Linde-Zwirble WT. Three-year outcomes for Medicare beneficiaries who survive intensive care. *JAMA.* 2010;303(9):849–856.

21. Cox CE, Carson SS, Lindquist JH, Olsen MK, Govert JA, Chelluri L. Differences in one-year health outcomes and resource utilization by definition of prolonged mechanical ventilation: a prospective cohort study. *Crit Care.* 2007;11(1):R9.

22. Garland A, Dawson NV, Altmann I, *et al.* Outcomes up to 5 years after severe, acute respiratory failure. *Chest.* 2004;126(6):1897–1904.

23. Boumendil A, Somme D, Garrouste-Orgeas M, Guidet B. Should elderly patients be admitted to the intensive care unit? *Intensive Care Med.* 2007;33(7):1252–1262.

24. Pascual J, Liano F. Causes and prognosis of acute renal failure in the very old. Madrid Acute Renal Failure Study Group. *J Am Geriatr Soc.* 1998;46(6):721–725.

25. Metnitz PG, Krenn CG, Steltzer H, *et al.* Effect of acute renal failure requiring renal replacement therapy on outcome in critically ill patients. *Crit Care Med.* 2002;30(9):2051–2058.

26. Coca SG. Acute kidney injury in elderly persons. *Am J Kidney Dis.* 2010;56(1):122–131.

27. Sacanella E, Perez-Castejon JM, Nicolas JM, *et al.* Mortality in healthy elderly patients after ICU admission. *Intensive Care Med.* 2009;35(3):550–555.

28. McGillicuddy EA, Schuster KM, Kaplan LJ, *et al.* Contrast-induced nephropathy in elderly trauma patients. *J Trauma.* 2010;68(2):294–297.

29. Akposso K, Hertig A, Couprie R, al. Acute renal failure in patients over 80 years old: 25-years' experience. *Intensive Care Med.* 2000;26(4):400–406.

30. Iribarren-Diarasarri S, Aizpuru-Barandiaran F, Munoz-Martinez T, *et al.* Health-related quality of life as a prognostic factor of survival in critically ill patients. *Intensive Care Med.* 2009;35(5):833–839.

31. Feest TG, Round A, Hamad S. Incidence of severe acute renal failure in adults: results of a community based study. *BMJ.* 1993;306(6876):481–483.

32. Ishani A, Xue JL, Himmelfarb J, *et al.* Acute kidney injury increases risk of ESRD among elderly. *J Am Soc Nephrol.* 2009;20(1):223–228.

33. Schiffl H, Fischer R. Five-year outcomes of severe acute kidney injury requiring renal replacement therapy. *Nephrol Dial Transplant.* 2008;23(7):2235–2241.

34. Ahlstrom A, Tallgren M, Peltonen S, Rasanen P, Pettila V. Survival and quality of life of patients requiring acute renal replacement therapy. *Intensive Care Med.* 2005;31(9):1222–1228.

35. Khosla N, Soroko SB, Chertow GM, *et al.* Preexisting chronic kidney disease: a potential for improved outcomes from acute kidney injury. *Clin J Am Soc Nephrol.* 2009;4(12):1914–1919.

36. Wald R, Quinn RR, Luo J, Li P, *et al.* Chronic dialysis and death among survivors of acute kidney injury requiring dialysis. *JAMA.* 2009;302(11):1179–1185.

37. Aymanns C, Keller F, Maus S, Hartmann B, Czock D. Review on pharmacokinetics and pharmacodynamics and the aging kidney. *Clin J Am Soc Nephrol.* 2010;5(2):314–327.

38. Woodhouse K, Wynne HA. Age-related changes in hepatic function. Implications for drug therapy. *Drugs Aging.* 1992;2(3):243–255.

39. Zilberberg MD, Shorr AF, Micek ST, Doherty JA, Kollef MH. Clostridium difficile-associated disease and mortality among the elderly critically ill. *Crit Care Med.* 2009;37(9):2583–2589.

40. Ridley S, Plenderleith L. Survival after intensive care. Comparison with a matched normal population as an indicator of effectiveness. *Anaesthesia.* 1994;49(11):933–935.

41. Olivier P, Bertrand L, Tubery M, Lauque D, Montastruc JL, Lapeyre-Mestre M. Hospitalizations because of adverse drug reactions in elderly patients admitted through the emergency department: a prospective survey. *Drugs Aging.* 2009;26(6):475–482.

42. Jandziol AK, Ridley SA. Validation of outcome prediction in elderly patients. *Anaesthesia.* 2000;55(2):107–112.

43. Malhotra S, Karan RS, Pandhi P, Jain S. Drug related medical emergencies in the elderly: role of adverse drug reactions and non-compliance. *Postgrad Med J.* 2001;77(913):703–707.

44. Khouli H, Astua A, Dombrowski W, *et al.* Changes in health-related quality of life and factors predicting long-term outcomes in older adults admitted to intensive care units. *Crit Care Med.* 2011;39(4):731–737.

45. Malhotra RK, Desai AK. Healthy brain aging: what has sleep got to do with it? *Clin Geriatr Med.* 2010;26(1):45–56.

46. Martin JE, Sheaff MT. The pathology of ageing: concepts and mechanisms. *J Pathol.* 2007;211(2):111–113.

47. Cooper B. Thinking preventively about dementia: a review. *Int J Geriatr Psychiatry.* 2002;17(10):895–906.

48. McNicoll L, Pisani MA, Zhang Y, Ely EW, Siegel MD, Inouye SK. Delirium in the intensive care unit: occurrence and clinical course in older patients. *J Am Geriatr Soc.* 2003;51(5):591–598.

49. Marquis F, Ouimet S, Riker R, Cossette M, Skrobik Y. Individual delirium symptoms: do they matter? *Crit Care Med.* 2007;35(11):2533–2537.

50. Page V. Delirium in intensive care patients. *BMJ.* 2012;344:e346.

51. Vernikos J, Schneider VS. Space, gravity and the physiology of aging: parallel or convergent disciplines? A mini-review. *Gerontology.* 2010;56(2):157–166.

52. van den Boogaard M, Schoonhoven L, Evers AW, van der Hoeven JG, van Achterberg T, Pickkers P. Delirium in critically ill patients: impact on long-term health-related quality of life and cognitive functioning. *Crit Care Med.* 2012;40(1):112–118.

53. Berggren D, Gustafson Y, Eriksson B, *et al.* Postoperative confusion after anesthesia in elderly patients with femoral neck fractures. *Anesth Analg.* 1987;66(6):497–504.

54. Gustafson Y, Berggren D, Brannstrom B, *et al.* Acute confusional states in elderly patients treated for femoral neck fracture. *J Am Geriatr Soc.* 1988;36(6):525–530.

55. Ely EW, Inouye SK, Bernard GR, Gordon S, Francis J, May L, *et al.* Delirium in mechanically ventilated patients: validity and reliability of the confusion assessment method for the intensive care unit (CAM-ICU). *JAMA.* 2001;286(21):2703–2710.

56. Ely EW, Shintani A, Truman B, Speroff T, Gordon SM, Harrell FE, Jr., *et al.* Delirium as a predictor of mortality in mechanically ventilated patients in the intensive care unit. *JAMA.* 2004;291(14):1753–1762.

57. Wood KA, Ely EW. What does it mean to be critically ill and elderly? *Curr Opin Crit Care.* 2003;9(4):316–320.

58. Stoll C, Schelling G, Goetz AE, Kilger E, Bayer A, Kapfhammer HP, *et al.* Health-related quality of life and post-traumatic stress disorder in patients after cardiac surgery and intensive care treatment. *J Thorac Cardiovasc Surg.* 2000;120(3):505–512.

59. Ouimet S, Riker R, Bergeron N, Cossette M, Kavanagh B, Skrobik Y. Subsyndromal delirium in the ICU: evidence for a disease spectrum. *Intensive Care Med.* 2007;33(6):1007–1013.

60. Boogaard M, Pickkers P, Slooter AJ, *et al.* Development and validation of PRE-DELIRIC (PREdiction of DELIRium in ICu patients) delirium prediction model for intensive care patients: observational multicentre study. *BMJ.* 2012;344:e420.

61. Makrantonaki E, Schonknecht P, Hossini AM, *et al.* Skin and brain age together: The role of hormones in the ageing process. *Exp Gerontol.* 2010;45(10):801–813.

62. Doherty TJ. Invited review: aging and sarcopenia. *J Appl Physiol.* 2003;95(4):1717–1727.

63. Wilson MM, Morley JE. Invited review: aging and energy balance. *J Appl Physiol.* 2003;95(4):1728–1736.

64. Elmadfa I, Meyer AL. Body composition, changing physiological functions and nutrient requirements of the elderly. *Ann Nutr Metab.* 2008;52(Suppl 1):2–5.

65. Berger MJ, Doherty TJ. Sarcopenia: prevalence, mechanisms, and functional consequences. *Interdiscip Top Gerontol.* 2010;37:94–114.

66. McNeil CJ, Doherty TJ, Stashuk DW, Rice CL. Motor unit number estimates in the tibialis anterior muscle of young, old, and very old men. *Muscle Nerve.* 2005;31(4):461–467.

67. Krstic G. Apparent temperature and air pollution vs. elderly population mortality in Metro Vancouver. *PloS One.* 2011; 6(9):e25101.

68. Robbins AS. Hypothermia and heat stroke: protecting the elderly patient. *Geriatrics.* 1989;44(1):73–77, 80.

69. Jerkic M, Vojvodic S, Lopez-Novoa JM. The mechanism of increased renal susceptibility to toxic substances in the elderly. Part I. The role of increased vasoconstriction. *Int Urol Nephrol.* 2001;32(4):539–547.

70. Lin YK, Ho TJ et al. Mortality risk associated with temperature and prolonged temperature extremes in elderly populations in Taiwan. *Environmental Research.* 2011;111(8):1156–1163.

71. Bittner EA, Yue Y, Xie Z. Brief review: anesthetic neurotoxicity in the elderly, cognitive dysfunction and Alzheimer's disease. *Can J Anaesth.* 2011;58(2):216–223.

72. Blot S, Cankurtaran M, Petrovic M, *et al.* Epidemiology and outcome of nosocomial bloodstream infection in elderly critically ill patients: a comparison between middle-aged, old, and very old patients. *Crit Care Med.* 2009;37(5):1634–1641.

73. Lee CC, Chen SY, Chang IJ, Chen SC, Wu SC. Comparison of clinical manifestations and outcome of community-acquired bloodstream infections among the oldest old, elderly, and adult patients. *Medicine (Baltimore).* 2007;86(3):138–144.

74. Roch A, Wiramus S, Pauly V, *et al.* Long-term outcome in medical patients aged 80 or over following admission to an intensive care unit. *Crit Care.* 2011;15(1):R36.

75. Cuthbertson BH, Roughton S, Jenkinson D, Maclennan G, Vale L. Quality of life in the five years after intensive care: a cohort study. *Crit Care.* 2010;14(1):R6.

76. Hamel MB, Henderson WG, Khuri SF, Daley J. Surgical outcomes for patients aged 80 and older: morbidity and mortality from major noncardiac surgery. *J Am Geriatr Soc.* 2005;53(3):424–429.

77. Lawrence VA, Hazuda HP, Cornell JE, *et al.* Functional independence after major abdominal surgery in the elderly. *J Am Coll Surg.* 2004;199(5):762–772.

78. Schurr P, Boeken U, Litmathe J, Feindt P, Kurt M, Gams E. Predictors of postoperative complications in octogenarians undergoing cardiac surgery. *Thorac Cardiovasc Surg.* 2010;58(4):200–203.

79. Rady MY, Johnson DJ. Cardiac surgery for octogenarians: is it an informed decision? *Am Heart J.* 2004;147(2):347–353.

80. Liu LL, Leung JM. Predicting adverse postoperative outcomes in patients aged 80 years or older. *J Am Geriatr Soc.* 2000;48(4):405–412.

81. Bochicchio GV, Joshi M, Bochicchio K, Shih D, Meyer W, Scalea TM. Incidence and impact of risk factors in critically ill trauma patients. *World J Surg.* 2006;30(1):114–118.

82. Pavoni V, Gianesello L, Paparella L, Buoninsegni LT, Mori E, Gori G. Outcome and quality of life of elderly critically ill patients: An Italian prospective observational study. *Arch Gerontol Geriatr.* 2012;54(2):e193–198.

83. Keller SM, Markovitz LJ, Wilder JR, Aufses AH, Jr. Emergency and elective surgery in patients over age 70. *Am Surg.* 1987;53(11):636–640.

84. Fassier T, Duclos A, Comte B, Tardy B. Decision to forgo life-sustaining therapies for elderly critically ill patients is a multidisciplinary challenge. *Intensive Care Med.* 2011;37(1):175–176.

85. Farfel JM, Franca SA, Sitta Mdo C, Filho WJ, Carvalho CR. Age, invasive ventilatory support and outcomes in elderly patients admitted to intensive care units. *Age Ageing.* 2009;38(5):515–520.

86. Sligl WI, Eurich DT, Marrie TJ, Majumdar SR. Age still matters: prognosticating short- and long-term mortality for critically ill patients with pneumonia. *Crit Care Med.* 2010;38(11):2126–2132.

87. Somme D, Maillet JM, Gisselbrecht M, Novara A, Ract C, Fagon JY. Critically ill old and the oldest-old patients in intensive care: short- and long-term outcomes. *Intensive Care Med.* 2003;29(12):2137–2143.

88. Barnato AE, Albert SM, Angus DC, Lave JR, Degenholtz HB. Disability among elderly survivors of mechanical ventilation. *Am J Respir Crit Care Med.* 2011;183(8):1037–1042.

89. Yende S, Angus DC, Ali IS, et al. Influence of comorbid conditions on long-term mortality after pneumonia in older people. *J Am Geriatr Soc.* 2007;55(4):518–525.

90. Kleinpell RM, Ferrans CE. Factors influencing intensive care unit survival for critically ill elderly patients. *Heart Lung.* 1998;27(5):337–343.

91. Rivera-Fernandez R, Sanchez-Cruz JJ, Abizanda-Campos R, Vazquez-Mata G. Quality of life before intensive care unit admission and its influence on resource utilization and mortality rate. *Crit Care Med.* 2001;29(9):1701–1709.

92. Marik PE. Management of the critically ill geriatric patient. *Crit Care Med.* 2006;34(9 Suppl):S176–S182.

93. Jeitziner MM, Hantikainen V, Conca A, Hamers JP. Long-term consequences of an intensive care unit stay in older critically ill patients: design of a longitudinal study. *BMC Geriatr.* 2011;11:52.

94. van der Schaaf M, Dettling DS, Beelen A, Lucas C, Dongelmans DA, Nollet F. Poor functional status immediately after discharge from an intensive care unit. *Disabil Rehabil.* 2008;30(23):1812–1818.

95. Montuclard L, Garrouste-Orgeas M, Timsit JF, Misset B, De Jonghe B, Carlet J. Outcome, functional autonomy, and quality of life of elderly patients with a long-term intensive care unit stay. *Crit Care Med.* 2000;28(10):3389–395.

96. Hennessy D, Juzwishin K, Yergens D, Noseworthy T, Doig C. Outcomes of elderly survivors of intensive care: a review of the literature. *Chest.* 2005;127(5):1764–1774.

97. Kaarlola A, Tallgren M, Pettila V. Long-term survival, quality of life, and quality-adjusted life-years among critically ill elderly patients. *Crit Care Med.* 2006;34(8):2120–2126.

98. Garrouste-Orgeas M, Timsit JF, Montuclard L, et al. Decision-making process, outcome, and 1-year quality of life of octogenarians referred for intensive care unit admission. *Intensive Care Med.* 2006;32(7):1045–1051.

99. Conti M, Friolet R, Eckert P, Merlani P. Home return 6 months after an intensive care unit admission for elderly patients. *Acta Anaesthesiol Scand.* 2011;55(4):387–393.

100. Daubin C, Chevalier S, Seguin A, et al. Predictors of mortality and short-term physical and cognitive dependence in critically ill persons 75 years and older: a prospective cohort study. *Health Qual Life Outcomes.* 2011;9:35.

101. Maillet JM, Somme D, Hennel E, Lessana A, Saint-Jean O, Brodaty D. Frailty after aortic valve replacement (AVR) in octogenarians. *Arch Gerontol Geriatr.* 2009;48(3):391–396.

102. Rodriguez-Molinero A, Lopez-Dieguez M, Tabuenca AI, de la Cruz JJ, Banegas JR. Physicians' impression on the elders' functionality influences decision making for emergency care. *Am J Emerg Med.* 2010;28(7):757–765.

103. Hofhuis J, Hautvast JL, Schrijvers AJ, Bakker J. Quality of life on admission to the intensive care: can we query the relatives? *Intensive Care Med.* 2003;29(6):974–979.

104. van Dijk PT, Mehr DR, Ooms ME, et al. Comorbidity and 1-year mortality risks in nursing home residents. *J Am Geriatr Soc.* 2005;53(4):660–665.

105. Lerolle N, Trinquart L, Bornstain C, et al. Increased intensity of treatment and decreased mortality in elderly patients in an intensive care unit over a decade. *Crit Care Med.* 2010;38(1):59–64.

106. Boumendil A, Aegerter P, Guidet B. Treatment intensity and outcome of patients aged 80 and older in intensive care units: a multicenter matched-cohort study. *J Am Geriatr Soc.* 2005;53(1):88–93.

107. Sprung CL, Artigas A, Kesecioglu J, Pezzi A, Wiis J, Pirracchio R, et al. The Eldicus prospective, observational study of triage decision making in European intensive care units. Part II: Intensive care benefit for the elderly. *Crit Care Med.* 2012;40(1):132–138.

108. Barnato AE, Herndon MB, Anthony DL, et al. Are regional variations in end-of-life care intensity explained by patient preferences?: A Study of the US Medicare Population. *Med Care.* 2007;45(5):386–393.

109. A controlled trial to improve care for seriously ill hospitalized patients. The study to understand prognoses and preferences for outcomes and risks of treatments (SUPPORT). The SUPPORT Principal Investigators. *JAMA.* 1995;274(20):1591–1598.

110. Hamel MB, Teno JM, Goldman L, et al. Patient age and decisions to withhold life-sustaining treatments from seriously ill, hospitalized adults. SUPPORT Investigators. Study to Understand Prognoses and Preferences for Outcomes and Risks of Treatment. *Ann Intern Med.* 1999;130(2):116–125.

111. Singer PA, Martin DK, Kelner M. Quality end-of-life care: patients' perspectives. *JAMA.* 1999;281(2):163–168.

112. Yaguchi A, Truog RD, Curtis JR, et al. International differences in end-of-life attitudes in the intensive care unit: results of a survey. *Arch Intern Med.* 2005;165(17):1970–1975.

113. Cook D, Rocker G, Marshall J, et al. Withdrawal of mechanical ventilation in anticipation of death in the intensive care unit. *N Engl J Med.* 2003;349(12):1123–1132.

CHAPTER 19

Vascular surgery in the elderly

Sameer Somanath and Elke Kothmann

Introduction

With an increasingly ageing population, the number of vascular procedures performed on elderly patients is rising globally. Around 95 per cent of vascular procedures in the United Kingdom are performed on the elderly, and a fifth of these operations are in individuals over the age of 80.[1] Vascular surgery is classified as high-risk surgery and has an overall perioperative mortality of 5 per cent.[2] Also, an age greater than 74 was shown to be one of the key factors predicting a fivefold increase in the likelihood of death following vascular surgery.[3] Despite the upward trend for minimally invasive vascular surgery, the older patient with multiple comorbidities requires the same degree of perioperative care as would be offered for an open procedure.

Preoperative assessment and optimization

See also Chapter 15.

Ideally all patients should be seen in a pre-assessment clinic (PAC) by an anaesthetist with an interest in vascular anaesthesia. This assessment should happen as soon as possible after the surgery is scheduled to provide sufficient time to screen for various comorbidities and optimize any newly diagnosed conditions. Preoperative evaluation allows the clinician to risk stratify the patient and provides a window of opportunity to medically optimize the patient prior to surgery. It also ensures the appropriate level of care is available after the surgery.

Coexisting medical diseases and management

Patients presenting for vascular surgery generally have a host of comorbidities as a consequence of genetic predisposition and lifestyle factors such as smoking. The diseases commonly associated with vascular patients are coronary artery disease (CAD), diabetes mellitus, renal insufficiency, cerebrovascular disease, and smoking-related lung disease. The basic pathophysiology in patients with vascular disease is atherosclerosis which is a generalized inflammatory disorder affecting medium to large arteries with associated endothelial dysfunction. Atherosclerosis commonly involves the coronary arteries, the carotid circulation, abdominal aorta, and the peripheral arterial tree. The implication of the systemic nature of atherosclerosis is that patients with arterial disease in the aorta or carotid arteries are at a very high risk of having significant CAD.

Ischaemic heart disease

The emphasis of pre-assessment in vascular surgery pertains to the cardiovascular system as cardiac events account for the majority of perioperative morbidity and mortality.[2,3] Less than 10 per cent of vascular patients have normal coronary arteries and over 50 per cent have severe disease.[4]

A robust pre-assessment should encompass a thorough clinical history and examination combined with functional capacity assessment. Recently published European guidelines segregate clinical risk factors into three categories; major, intermediate, and minor (Table 19.1).[5] Major risk factors are a threat to life and should be treated prior to elective surgery. Intermediate risk factors are the same as the risk factors in the Revised Cardiac Risk Index and have a high predictive value for perioperative cardiac events.[6] Current American College of Cardiology (ACC)/American Heart Association (AHA) recommendations state that patients with three or more intermediate risk factors and an unknown or poor functional capacity presenting for vascular surgery may benefit from non-invasive testing for CAD if it will alter the management.[5] Patients with two or fewer clinical risk factors can safely proceed to surgery with heart rate control (Fig. 19.1).

Testing for ischaemic heart disease

Amongst the various stress tests for diagnosing CAD, dobutamine stress echo (DSE) has the highest sensitivity (85 per cent) and specificity (70 per cent) for perioperative cardiac events. Although the positive predictive value is low, the negative predictive value of DSE for perioperative cardiac events ranges from 90–100 per cent, which is reassuring in patients with negative tests.[7–9] Alternative methods of non-invasive testing include myocardial perfusion scanning, cardiac magnetic resonance angiography (MRA) and computed tomography (CT). Although stress electrocardiography (ECG) has a lower sensitivity and specificity, it has the additional benefit of providing an assessment of functional capacity.

Coronary angiography remains the gold standard for diagnosing CAD and is reserved for patients who are symptomatic or who have strongly positive non-invasive tests.

Table 19.1 Categorization of clinical risk factors

Major risk factors	• Unstable coronary syndromes 　• Unstable or severe angina 　• Recent MI (within 1 month) • Significant arrhythmias • Severe valvular disease • Decompensated heart failure
Intermediate risk factors	• History of ischaemic heart disease • History of compensated or prior heart failure • Cerebrovascular disease • Renal insufficiency (creatinine >170 μmol/L or Cr clearance <60 ml/min) • Diabetes mellitus requiring insulin
Minor risk factors	• Age >70 • Abnormal ECG • Rhythm other than sinus • Uncontrolled systemic hypertension

Fleisher LA, Beckman JA, Brown KA, Calkins H, Chaikof E, Fleischmann KE, Freeman WK, Froehlich JB, Kasper EK, Kersten JR, Riegel B, Robb JF. 'ACC/AHA 2007 guidelines on perioperative cardiovascular evaluation and care for noncardiac surgery: a report of the American College of Cardiology/American Heart Association Task Force on Practice Guidelines (Writing Committee to Revise the 2002 Guidelines on Perioperative Cardiovascular Evaluation for Noncardiac Surgery)'. *Circulation*. 2007;116;17:e418–e499. © 2007 by the American College of Cardiology Foundation and the American Heart Association, Inc. Reproduced with permission.

Functional capacity

Assessment of functional capacity is an essential component of the pre-assessment process. Traditionally, functional capacity has been ascertained based on history and is expressed as metabolic equivalents (METs). One MET corresponds to oxygen consumption at rest and represents basal metabolic rate which equates to 3.5 ml/kg/min of oxygen consumption at rest. A history of being unable to climb two sets of stairs equates to less than 4 METs and is representative of poor functional reserve, which is a predictor for poor postoperative outcome. However, subjective assessment of functional capacity may be unreliable and it is preferable to have an objective test to accurately quantify exercise tolerance.

Cardiopulmonary exercise testing

Cardiopulmonary exercise testing (CPET) is the gold standard for assessing functional capacity. It is a safe, non-invasive investigation which provides a global assessment of the oxygen delivery system and provides an integrated assessment of the cardiac, respiratory, haematological, neurological, and musculoskeletal systems. It is invaluable in the risk stratification of patients prior to major surgery and now there is an increasing body of evidence supporting its use to predict short- and medium-term outcomes in vascular surgical patients. During a test, patients perform a ramped work effort either on a cycle ergometer or on a treadmill

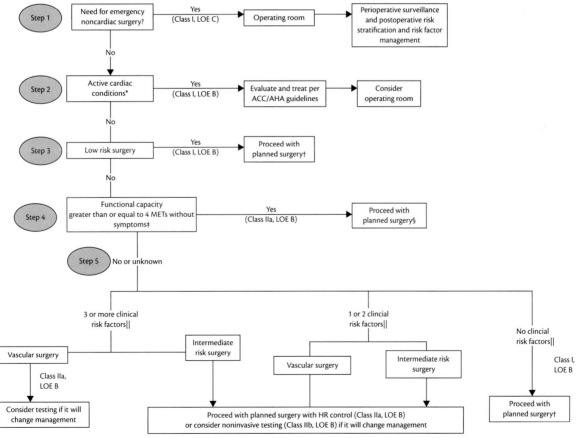

Fig. 19.1 ACC/AHA cardiac evaluation algorithm for non-cardiac surgery. Fleisher LA, Beckman JA, Brown KA, Calkins H, Chaikof E, Fleischmann KE, Freeman WK, Froehlich JB, Kasper EK, Kersten JR, Riegel B, Robb JF. 'ACC/AHA 2007 guidelines on perioperative cardiovascular evaluation and care for noncardiac surgery: a report of the American College of Cardiology/American Heart Association Task Force on Practice Guidelines (Writing Committee to Revise the 2002 Guidelines on Perioperative Cardiovascular Evaluation for Noncardiac Surgery)'. *Circulation*. 2007;116;17:e418–e499. © 2007 by the American College of Cardiology Foundation and the American Heart Association, Inc. Reproduced with permission.

until maximal or sub maximal exertion. The oxygen consumption (VO_2) and the carbon dioxide production (VCO_2) are the two vital parameters measured throughout the test. Anaerobic threshold (AT) refers to the point in the exercise where the metabolic demand exceeds the oxygen supply and marks the onset of anaerobic metabolism. The commonly interpreted and reported variables are VO_2 peak /max (maximal oxygen consumption for the duration of the test), VO_2 AT (oxygen consumption at anaerobic threshold) and VE/VCO_2 at AT. VE/VCO_2 is a marker of ventilatory efficiency and values above 34 suggest a degree of ventilatory impairment secondary to either heart failure or lung disease. Snowden et al. demonstrated that an anaerobic threshold below 10.1 ml/kg/min was an independent predictor of increased postoperative complications and length of stay.[10] A poor performance during CPET also translates into lower medium-term survival rates despite successful aneurysm repairs. In the presence of risk factors, a VE/VCO_2 value above 42 was shown to be a strong predictor of a lower early and late survival following successful open aortic surgery.[11]

Medical optimization

Beta-blockers

The perioperative use of beta-blockers has been the subject of much recent controversy with the pendulum now swinging against the routine institution of beta-blockers in patients presenting for major surgery. POISE, which is the largest randomized controlled trial to date on perioperative beta blockade, concluded that beta-blockers offered a cardioprotective effect with a significant reduction in cardiac events; however this was achieved at a higher overall mortality and stroke rate.[12] Previous studies have shown a positive effect of perioperative beta blockers. Mangano et al. demonstrated a survival improvement from perioperative beta blockers which lasted up to 2 years after major surgery.[13] We need to take this line out as the author has now been discredited for fraudulent research in this trial. Please remove the reference as well.

The updated American College of Cardiology Foundation (ACCF)/American Heart Association (AHA) guidelines on the perioperative cardiac evaluation for non-cardiac surgery recommend that patients already on beta-blockers should remain on them in the perioperative period (Class Ic). Prior to major vascular surgery, it is considered reasonable to institute beta-blockers (titrated to heart rate and blood pressure) in patients with known IHD or at high cardiac risk as defined by the presence of more than one clinical risk factor (Class IIb). The benefits of starting beta-blockers in patients at low cardiac risk (≤1 clinical risk factor) are uncertain and it may be potentially harmful.[5]

When implemented, therapy should be ideally initiated 7–30 days before surgery and should be titrated to achieve heart rates of between 60 and 80 beats/min with the absence of hypotension.

Statins

In addition to cholesterol lowering effects, statins also have powerful anti-inflammatory effects. They improve endothelial function and also have plaque stabilizing properties. Current guidelines suggest that it is reasonable to initiate statin therapy prior to high-risk surgery in patients at cardiac risk.[5] Patients who are already on statin therapy should remain on them as abrupt discontinuation is associated with an increased postoperative cardiac risk.[15]

Angiotensin-converting enzyme inhibitors

Angiotensin-converting enzyme inhibitors (ACEIs) have been shown to improve long-term survival in high-risk patients with or without evidence of left ventricular (LV) systolic dysfunction.[16] Patients already on ACEI for heart failure should continue it perioperatively. It is also recommended that patients with LV dysfunction who are not already on ACEI may benefit from initiation of treatment preoperatively.[17]

Aspirin

Aspirin has been shown to reduce the incidence of stroke in patients undergoing carotid endarterectomy (CEA).[18] Current European guidelines recommend that patients on low dose aspirin should remain on them throughout the perioperative period.[17]

The role of the earlier mentioned medication as therapy to prevent or retard vascular ageing is described in Chapter 13.

Role of multidisciplinary teams

A multidisciplinary team (MDT) is a fundamental part of the patient care pathway for vascular surgery and should aim to deliver an integrated care package based on the best available evidence. The Abdominal Aortic Aneurysm Quality Improvement Programme (AAAQIP) recommends that the MDT should consist of a vascular surgeon, interventional radiologist, specialist vascular nurse, and a clinical vascular scientist.[19] The input from a vascular anaesthetist is an essential component of the decision-making process between an endovascular aneurysm repair (EVAR) and open repair as a proportion of patients might not be physiologically 'fit enough' to survive an open repair.

Abdominal aortic aneurysm and the elderly

The prevalence of abdominal aortic aneurysms (AAAs) is increasing due to an ageing population and an improved awareness, due to the introduction of screening programmes. The introduction of the AAAQIP has led to a marked reduction in the morbidity and mortality of AAA in the United Kingdom.[20]

The National Health Service (NHS) AAA Screening Programme was introduced in 2010, following research and analysis of data from existing screening programmes, which showed a reduction in mortality from AAA when men were offered ultrasound screening in their 65th year.[21] Surgery is considered when an AAA has reached 5.5 cm or greater.

There are two surgical options, either open or endovascular repair. The choice of procedure depends on patient, anaesthetic, surgical, and radiological factors. EVAR is associated with an initial early advantage of lower morbidity and mortality, but this may be offset by an increasing long-term morbidity including re-intervention.[22] Despite the outcome from the EVAR 2 trial, EVAR tends to be the option offered more frequently for high-risk patients, providing the anatomy of the aneurysm is suitable for a stent. Improvements in stent technology have made more aneurysms amenable to stenting including suprarenal AAA. However, if the risk profile from the comorbidities exceed the risk of rupture per year significantly, conservative management may be appropriate. It is vital that the patient is involved in the decision-making process and fully understands the risk and nature of the disease process.[23]

Preoperative care

Pre-assessment forms a vital tool for the assessment of this high-risk group of patients, and should ideally occur in a multi-disciplinary vascular pre-assessment clinic. In England, the development of the Quality Improvement Programme for AAA has aimed to improve and standardize the care received. This should include assessment of comorbidities, especially focusing on cardiovascular and respiratory limitations, other systemic disease processes, and impact on functional capacity. The development of CPET has helped in this evaluation and stratification.[10,11,24] Specialist referral may be required for optimization of cardiovascular or respiratory disease. The UK Small Aneurysms study showed poor preoperative lung and renal function to strongly associate with the risk of postoperative death.[25] At the end of the pre-assessment process a decision should be reached about fitness to proceed to surgery or a decision to delay surgery to improve patient fitness.

Intraoperative care for elective endovascular aneurysm repair

There are several anaesthetic options available for the management of elective EVARs, depending on patient factors, surgical and radiological preferences, and expected duration of procedure. The duration of an infrarenal procedure makes them amenable to local infiltration, central neuraxial blockade (spinal or combined spinal-epidural) or a general anaesthetic technique. Sedation may improve patient satisfaction with the infiltration or central neuraxial technique, as patients with multiple comorbidities such as respiratory or arthritic disease may find it uncomfortable or impossible to lie flat on a narrow radiology table for a couple of hours. The duration of procedure for a suprarenal, fenestrated stent makes it more amenable to a general anaesthetic technique.

The recommended monitoring for any of the discussed techniques is basic monitoring with the addition of five-lead ECG with ST-segment analysis, invasive blood pressure and urine output monitoring. The major periods of haemodynamic stress occur during stent expansion and if an intra-aortic balloon is used to assist in stent placement. This has the same effect on the left ventricle, as brief aortic clamping.

The patient's temperature must be monitored and active warming is usually required despite the minimally invasive procedure. Blood loss is usually less than 500 ml in an uncomplicated stent procedure.

Postoperatively high dependency/level 2 care is required to ensure maintenance of haemodynamic stability.

Anaesthetic management for elective open AAA surgery

The focus of anaesthetic management is to maintain cardiovascular stability, minimize respiratory complications and provide renal protection. An acceptable technique would be a general anaesthetic with a thoracic epidural, however intraoperatively remifentanil may be useful.

Monitoring should include basic monitoring with the addition of five-lead ECG monitoring with ST-segment analysis, invasive blood pressure monitoring, central venous line, urine output, and temperature monitoring. Cardiac output monitoring may be useful but there is no evidence that it improves outcomes or which technique is superior. But it is useful if the patient has known LV dysfunction, as assessment of volume status allows for better prediction of volume status prior to aortic clamping and unclamping.

Cell-salvage techniques have minimized the requirement for exogenous blood transfusion and should be available for open aortic surgery. Temperature monitoring is vital and patients should be actively warmed as hypothermia increases the risk of coagulopathies, increases oxygen requirements postoperatively and wound infection rates.

If there are no contraindications, a thoracic epidural provides good postoperative analgesia and can be used for intraoperative management. The level of epidural insertion should be optimized depending on whether a transverse or vertical incision is planned.

There is limited evidence to support the role of drugs for renal protection during the clamping phase.

Meticulous attention to fluid management is required to minimize cardiovascular stress during clamping and unclamping of the aorta. In the pre-clamp phase, the induction drugs, the technique used for maintenance (whether it be a volatile or total intravenous anaesthesia technique) and the local anaesthetic used for the epidural, will all cause a reduction in the systemic vascular resistance (SVR) and hence the blood pressure. Maintenance of blood pressure is vital to ensure perfusion, however excessive fluids prior to aortic clamping will strain a full ventricle when the clamp is applied, so judicious use of fluid and a vasoconstrictor is recommended prior to aortic clamp application. The vasoconstrictor can then be titrated prior to clamp application; a slightly under filled ventricle is better able to manage the sudden increase in SVR, when the clamp is applied.

During the 'clamp phase', the focus is on optimizing the fluid status to facilitate clamp release and return of the lower limbs into the circulation. Fluid resuscitation during this period can be guided by the arterial line trace, the central venous pressure, and/or cardiac output monitoring. By the time of clamp release the circulation should be optimally full to minimize the acute re-entry of each limb into the circulation. Regular assessment of arterial and venous blood gas analysis will assist in fluid management. A combination of crystalloid and colloid fluids is usually required depending on the amount of blood lost. An acceptable transfusion trigger (around 8–9 g/dl) should be decided upon depending on comorbidities and rate of blood loss. All cell-salvaged blood should be re-transfused and banked blood and products given as required. If there is extensive blood loss near patient coagulation tests (e.g. TEG*) may assist in guiding which clotting products are required.

The re-entry of blood from the limbs after iliac clamp release will have a negatively inotropic effect on the heart. Even if filling has been optimized a positive inotrope may be required to assist the heart during this period. Depending on the preoperative ventricular function this may be small incremental doses (e.g. ephedrine) or may require an infusion (e.g. dobutamine or low-dose adrenaline). The heart should be given time to recover, and fluid re-optimized prior to the other limb being released.

The epidural if not used intraoperatively should be topped-up to establish a block above the incision, prior to attempting to wake the patient. The preoperative assessment and risk scoring will assist in the decision about level 2 or level 3 care postoperatively. Intraoperative difficulties and extent of blood loss need to be considered. If at the end of the procedure the patient is warm, well perfused with an acceptable blood gas and haemoglobin level, and on no or only a small degree of inotropic support, extubation should be aimed for.

Postoperative care

Patients are cared for in a critical care environment. The commonest complications are cardiac in origin and can range from benign arrhythmias to fatal myocardial infarctions. Patients with pre-existing respiratory disease are at a higher risk of developing complications such as atelectasis and pneumonia. Renal failure is a potential complication, especially in cases where there is a prolonged period of clamping around the renal artery. One should also be watchful for rare but serious complications such as colonic ischaemia which may manifest as bloody diarrhoea in the postoperative period.

Ruptured abdominal aortic aneurysms

Ruptured AAA still represents a considerable challenge and has a very high morbidity and mortality rate. The morbidity is high because of the acute physiological insult of major blood loss with vital organ hypoperfusion and increased cardiovascular stress in an attempt to compensate.

Open surgery was traditionally the only surgical option, but specific cases based on CT findings may be suitable for an emergency EVAR procedure. This requires considerable expertise and logistics and is not an option available in all centres. Ongoing trials are investigating how this option compares with open repair for improving patient outcomes.

The management of an open repair of ruptured AAAs still poses major logistical challenges. Effective early communication between all members of the team minimizes delays. The patient should initially be resuscitated cautiously, aiming for a systolic blood pressure of around 100 or lower provided the patient maintains consciousness with that blood pressure. A high blood pressure may cause further bleeding from the rupture site. Time should be taken to discuss with the patient about the anaesthetic and surgical plans. The patient should be anaesthetized on the operating table. Minimal monitoring is acceptable at this stage, i.e. blood pressure, pulse oximetry and ECG. An arterial line is not essential, as it may delay the surgery. Large-bore intravenous access will be required to facilitate rapid fluid infusion during the surgical procedure. A urethral catheter is usually placed prior to induction. The patient is prepped and draped whilst awake, and only when the surgeon is scrubbed and ready next to the operating table, should the anaesthetic induction occur. During the preparation process it is useful to preoxygenate the patient as a rapid sequence induction is usually required. There are several choices for induction drugs, however cardiac stability should be aimed for with a combination that the anaesthetist is familiar with using. Once the induction drugs and the muscle relaxant are given the patient will lose their abdominal tamponade effect and their SVR will decrease, together with a drop in their catecholamine production. Cumulatively, this leads to a rapid fall in blood pressure and cardiac output. Cautious fluid resuscitation and inotrope use should be employed until the aortic clamp is applied, as a

rapid increase in blood pressure will encourage further bleeding from the rupture site. Once the aorta is clamped, full resuscitation of the circulation is required. When a period of cardiac stability is achieved after clamp application, an arterial line and central venous access can be inserted.

The development of major haemorrhage protocols and the use of cell-salvaged blood have assisted in optimizing the resuscitation intraoperatively. A rapid infusion device assists in the delivery fluids at the appropriate temperature. Hypothermia should be actively treated. The transfusion of blood should be guided by estimated initial blood loss and ongoing losses. Regular assessment of the haemoglobin and arterial blood gas analysis should assist in fluid management and blood transfusion. Near patient clotting tests may help in correcting clotting abnormalities and should be used to guide blood product usage.

The preoperative condition of the patient, the complexity of the repair, the extent of blood loss and the physiological state of the patient at the end of the repair usually necessitate level 3 care at the end of the procedure.

Carotid endarterectomy

Carotid endarterectomy (CEA) is beneficial in reducing the incidence of stroke and mortality in patients with severe ipsilateral carotid artery stenosis (50–99 per cent), with the greatest benefit being available to patients who are symptomatic.[26] CEA does not provide any benefit to asymptomatic patients with moderate ipsilateral carotid artery stenosis (30–49 per cent) and is harmful to patients with only mild stenosis (0–29 per cent).[27]

The benefits of CEA are only evident after a period of 2 years due to the inherent stroke rate associated with the procedure. A perioperative mortality in excess of 3 per cent eliminates the long-term benefits gained by CEA performed on asymptomatic individuals. Therefore, CEA should only be performed in institutions with a combined perioperative mortality of less than 3 per cent.

Investigations

Angiography is considered the gold standard for estimating the severity of carotid artery stenosis. However, due to its invasive nature and associated costs, most institutions routinely use non-invasive tests such as carotid duplex ultrasound, CT angiography or MRA. When compared to cerebral angiography, carotid duplex ultrasound was shown to have a sensitivity and specificity greater than 0.8 to diagnose severe carotid artery disease.[28]

Medical therapy

Low-dose aspirin has shown to significantly reduce the incidence of postoperative stroke following CEA.[26] There is recent evidence that low-dose clopidogrel (75 mg) commenced the night before surgery significantly reduces the number of periprocedural embolic events without a significantly increased risk of bleeding complications.[29]

Statins have shown to be beneficial in improving outcomes following CEA[30,31] and should be started on all patients undergoing CEA in the absence of contraindications.

Risk factors

Traditionally, the presence of the following factors has been considered as high risk for undergoing CEA:[32]

◆ Age > 80 years.

◆ Stroke as an indication for CEA.

◆ Contralateral carotid artery stenosis (> 50 per cent).

◆ Coronary artery disease.

◆ Diabetes mellitus on insulin.

With advances in perioperative care, this has been challenged as the perioperative complication rate for high-risk patients has been demonstrated to be similar to the low-risk patients.[33,34] However, patients with multiple comorbidities may not benefit from CEA due to a reduced 5-year survival and this should be considered when deciding to operate on them.

Intraoperative care

The primary aim of the anaesthetic care is to minimize any potential ischaemic cerebral and cardiac injury. All patients should have been appropriately pre-assessed, with a series of blood pressure and heart rate recordings obtained to estimate baseline values. Blood pressure recordings should be obtained from both arms preoperatively to account for possible vascular disease in the subclavian and brachial arteries. Intra operative haemodynamic parameters should ideally be within 15 per cent of baseline recordings.

The anaesthetic options for CEA are either general anaesthesia (GA) or a regional anaesthetic (LA) technique. Previously, there has been weak evidence suggesting that a regional anaesthetic technique, with the patient kept awake during surgery, was possibly better for overall outcomes.[35] However, the GALA trial, which is the largest randomized controlled trial comparing GA versus LA for CEA, failed to demonstrate any significant difference in outcomes between the two anaesthetic techniques.[36] Therefore, the choice of anaesthetic technique for the procedure should be decided on an individual basis following discussions between the patient, surgeon, and anaesthetist.

Regional anaesthesia

Regional anaesthesia can be provided by performing deep cervical plexus blocks, superficial cervical plexus blocks, subcutaneous infiltration by the surgeon, or various combinations of these techniques. Current evidence has shown deep cervical plexus blocks to have higher complication rates when compared to superficial and intermediate cervical plexus blocks, with no added analgesic benefit.[37]

General anaesthesia

GA is usually provided via an endotracheal tube and controlled ventilation. There have been case reports of CEA performed using a laryngeal mask airway,[38] but this is uncommon and not recommended in the majority of cases. It is a standard practice in many institutions to maintain anaesthesia with the use of volatile anaesthetic agents in combination with a remifentanil infusion. The use of remifentanil may necessitate the use of a vasopressor infusion to maintain blood pressure, but overall a stable intraoperative haemodynamic profile is achieved. This also ensures a rapid, good quality wake up following cessation of the anaesthetic to allow for immediate neurological assessment in the postoperative period.

Surgical technique

Following a standard neck incision, the internal carotid artery is identified through meticulous dissection. Following systemic heparinization, clamps are placed both proximal and distal to the diseased arterial segment, which is commonly the carotid bifurcation. During this period, blood supply to the ipsilateral hemi-brain is reliant on collateral supply via the circle of Willis. There are a number of modalities available for estimating the adequacy of the collateral blood supply. Any evidence of cerebral ischaemia is an indication for a shunt across the clamped arterial segment.

The diseased segment, which is commonly the carotid bifurcation, is opened via an arteriotomy incision and the plaque is meticulously cleared. The arteriotomy is then closed employing a patch which has been shown to be superior when compared to primary closure. It is common practice to leave drains *in situ* for 24 hours.

Monitoring

In addition to standard monitoring, it is paramount to monitor 'beat to beat' blood pressure with an arterial line due to the intraoperative haemodynamic lability which can persist for the first 12–24 hours postoperatively. Invasive arterial monitoring should be instituted in the awake patient to observe and expediently treat any precipitous drops in blood pressure that may occur during induction of anaesthesia.

Neurological monitoring

The 'gold standard' for monitoring intraoperative neurological monitoring is considered to be the awake patient undergoing surgery under a loco-regional technique. This allows for continuous monitoring for cerebral ischaemia and is easy to perform, reliable, and inexpensive.

However, for patients undergoing surgery under GA, there are a variety of other options available for neurological monitoring.[39]

Transcranial Doppler (TCD) employs ultrasound waves to estimate the mean velocity of blood in the middle cerebral artery (VMCAi). Absolute values below 30cm/s or a relative reduction of more than 50 per cent following application of the clamp are indications for performing a shunt. TCD also offers the additional benefit of detecting embolization in the intra and postoperative period.

Stump pressures can be measured in the carotid stump after application of the carotid clamp. Pressures in excess of 30 mmHg are indicative of an adequate collateral circulation. Near-infrared spectroscopy (NIRS) is a non-invasive method to measure regional oxygen saturation in the brain and reduction below a certain threshold is used as a trigger to selectively place a surgical shunt.

Other modalities include electroencephalography, somatosensory evoked potentials, and jugular oxygen saturation.

Current evidence suggests that although these modalities have very high sensitivity approaching 100 per cent, the specificity is low and ranges from 43–86 per cent.[40]

Postoperative care and complications

Wound haematomas are one of the most common postoperative complications with the majority responding to manual compression.

Any evidence of airway compromise or significant bleeding is an indication for prompt surgical exploration and evacuation.

Hypertension and hypotension are common postoperative complications in the first few postoperative hours, but this usually does not persist beyond the first 24 hours. Blood pressure should be maintained within pre-determined parameters (typically between systolic blood pressures of 100–160 mmHg) according to local protocols. This might require the use of pharmacological agents such as labetalol or phenylephrine as infusions. It is important to exclude common causes of hypertension such as pain, bladder distension, hypoxia, and hypercapnia.

Cardiac morbidity is the most common cause of postoperative morbidity and mortality and the importance of a thorough preoperative cardiac workup cannot be overemphasized. Perioperative strokes are the second most common cause of mortality commonly occurring due to cerebral hypoperfusion during the period of clamping and/or embolization. Less common causes include carotid artery thrombosis and cerebral hyperperfusion syndrome.

Historically, patients have been managed in a critical care environment postoperatively. However, this has been questioned with an increasing number of institutions having an extended stay in the recovery room (6–8 hours) as this is when most acute complications manifest themselves. If they remain stable over this period, they are discharged to the ward. High dependency care is reserved for high-risk patients with multiple comorbidities.

Peripheral arterial disease

Lower limb peripheral arterial disease (PAD) is associated with significant morbidity and mortality and results in a reduced quality of life due to reduced mobility.[41]

There are a number of risk factors for the development of PAD which include smoking, diabetes, hypertension, dyslipidaemia, chronic renal impairment, increasing age, and male gender. Of these, smoking and diabetes are the strongest etiologic risk factors with a relative risk in excess of 2.

Diagnosis

Although intermittent claudication is the classical symptom in patients with PAD, it may not be present in a substantial proportion of patients suffering from the disease and a high index of suspicion is required. The ratio of the systolic pressure at the ankle and the brachial artery is called the ankle–brachial index (ABI). Normal values lie between 1 and 1.29 and a ratio less than 0.9 confirms the diagnosis of PAD. Values less than 0.4 are suggestive of severe PAD and an ABI of 1.3 or higher is indicative of a calcified incompressible artery. ABI has been shown to be an independent predictor of increased cardiovascular risk and can be used for risk stratification.[42]

Diagnostic methods to delineate the anatomical obstruction include Duplex imaging, MRA and CT angiography, and contrast angiography.

Management

Most patients are initially managed with a combination of medical therapy and lifestyle modification (smoking cessation, exercise therapy). Unfortunately, 10–15 per cent of patients progress towards critical limb ischaemia (CLI) despite best medical therapy.[41] CLI with severe claudication, rest pain, or gangrene is an indication for surgery. Options for revascularization include minimally invasive endovascular techniques, open surgical exploration, or combined approaches.

Elective revascularization procedures

The choice of technique for restoring perfusion to the limb is dependent on the site and extent of thrombosis.

Endovascular techniques such as angioplasty and stenting are well established for short (≤3 cm) stenotic lesions in the iliac arteries. With recent advances in endovascular techniques, more complex lesions are increasingly being managed via the endovascular route.

For stenosis not amenable to endovascular treatment, surgery remains the only option and the type of surgery is dependent on the anatomical site of lesion and the overall fitness of the patient.

Aorto bi-femoral grafts are recommended for patients with significant inflow disease (aorto-iliac occlusive disease) with significant lifestyle limitations due to the disease. However this is a high-risk operation on a par with an open aortic repair and may not be suitable for patients with significant comorbidities. An axillo-femoral graft is a less stressful alternative as it does not involve surgery on the thoracic or abdominal aorta. Despite having a lower long-term graft patency rate when compared to aorto-bifemoral grafting, it remains a reasonable alternative in high-risk patients with limited life expectancy who develop limb-threatening ischaemia.[43] Infrainguinal or outflow disease is treated by femoro-popliteal bypass, femoro-femoral crossovers, or femoro-distal depending on the level of obstruction.

Anaesthesia

Infrainguinal revascularization procedures may be performed under regional anaesthetic techniques such a combined spinal epidural (CSE) which provides an option for extending the duration of anaesthesia if required. It also provides effective postoperative analgesia and minimizes systemic opiate requirements. There are several theoretical benefits to using regional anaesthetic techniques. However, a recent Cochrane review failed to demonstrate significant differences in mortality or morbidity between regional and general anaesthesia for lower limb arterial reconstruction, but there was a trend towards a reduced incidence of pneumonia in the regional anaesthesia group.[44]

Aortic reconstruction is a major surgical undertaking and requires the same degree of perioperative care as one would offer an open abdominal aneurysm repair. Epidural anaesthesia is generally provided for postoperative pain relief.

Postoperative care

In view of the accompanying co-morbidities, all major reconstruction work should be nursed in a critical care environment. Following revascularization, it is essential to regularly monitor pulses to ensure graft patency as graft occlusion is an indication for emergency re-exploration.

Lower limb amputation

Lower limb amputations are performed for severely ischaemic limbs which are not amenable to surgical revascularization. Diabetes mellitus with refractory local sepsis is the other major indication for amputation. Lower limb amputations are very high-risk procedures with 30-day mortality approaching 20 per cent.[45]

Patients presenting for lower limb amputation suffer from multiple comorbidities. In a significant proportion of patients, there are acute derangements of coagulation, fluid, or electrolyte status, all of which should be corrected prior to surgery.

Anaesthesia

For below-knee or above-knee amputations, anaesthesia can be provided by GA or regional anaesthesia. Postoperative pain relief can be provided by LA infusions through a surgically placed sciatic nerve catheter which has an opioid-sparing effect. The general condition of the patient may dictate the need for high-dependency care postoperatively.

Phantom pain can be a significant problem following limb amputations. Unfortunately, there is no convincing evidence for any interventions (pre-emptive analgesia, ketamine, gabapentin) to reduce the incidence of this debilitating complication. Early involvement of the pain team is recommended.

Acute limb ischaemia

Acute limb ischaemia is a surgical emergency and warrants treatment as soon as possible to ensure limb survival. The cause is either embolization in a previously well patient or thrombosis in an already diseased vascular tree. It may be possible to differentiate between the two clinically, but angiography is almost always performed to confirm the diagnosis and establish the extent of the obstruction. In cases of small emboli, perfusion may be restored by catheter embolectomy via a femoral arteriotomy performed under LA. However, in extensive thrombosis and cases not amenable to catheter embolectomy, GA is required for immediate surgical revascularization via either an arterial thrombectomy or a bypass procedure. A non-survivable limb is an indication for amputation.

Conduct of anaesthesia

Patients are generally commenced on anticoagulation once the diagnosis is made, and this precludes the use of regional anaesthetic techniques. Despite the high prevalence of coronary and cerebral vascular disease, clinical urgency limits the extent of preoperative evaluation and optimization that can be performed.

It is common to have significant electrolyte derangements in the perioperative period as a consequence of the ongoing cell death and release of intracellular ions into the circulation, most importantly potassium. Postoperatively, it is important to be watchful for reperfusion injury following successful revascularization. Compartment syndrome requiring fasciotomies has been reported in up to 5 per cent of patients and up to 20 per cent of patients demonstrate biochemical evidence of rhabdomyolysis.[46]

Conclusion

The increase in the need for vascular surgery due to the ageing of the population is not likely to fall for some decades. Although social changes such as population reductions in smoking and better control of hypertension and diabetes may reduce the absolute incidence of major vascular disease there will be continue to be a progressive rise in the number of patients who require surgical intervention to preserve and restore their circulation. Better

understanding of the demands such surgery places on patients has informed the process of perioperative management including intensive preoperative assessment, modification of surgical and endovascular techniques, and the provision of skilled anaesthetic and intensive care. This chapter has covered current practice but this will need constant review as future research provides a clearer basis for practical management of these challenging patients.

References

1. Task Force for Preoperative Cardiac Risk Assessment and Perioperative Cardiac Management in Non-cardiac Surgery; European Society of Cardiology (ESC), Poldermans D, et al. ESC Guidelines for pre-operative cardiac risk assessment and perioperative cardiac management in non-cardiac surgery. *Eur Heart J.* 2009;30:2769–2812.
2. Nowygrod, R, Egorova N, Greco G, et al. Trends, complications, and mortality in peripheral vascular surgery. *J Vasc Surg.* 2006;43(2):205–216.
3. Bayly PJM, Matthews JN, Dobson PM, Price ML, Thomas DG. In-hospital mortality from abdominal aortic surgery in Great Britain and Ireland: Vascular Anaesthesia Society audit. *Br J Surg.* 2001;88(5):687–692.
4. Hertzer NR, Beven EG, Young JR, et al. Coronary artery disease in peripheral vascular patients. A classification of 1000 coronary angiograms and results of surgical management. *Ann Surg.* 1984;199(2):223–233.
5. Fleisher LA, Beckman JA, Brown KA, et al. ACCF/AHA focused update on perioperative beta blockade incorporated into the ACC/AHA 2007 guidelines on perioperative cardiovascular evaluation and care for noncardiac surgery. *Circulation.* 2009;24;120(21):e169–276. <http://circ.ahajournals.org/cgi/reprint/CIRCULATIONAHA.109.192690>.
6. Lee TH, Marcantonio ER, Mangione CM, et al. 1999. Derivation and prospective validation of a simple index for prediction of cardiac risk of major noncardiac surgery. *Circulation.* 1999;100(10):1043–1049.
7. Poldermans D, Fioretti PM, Forster T, et al. Dobutamine stress echocardiography for assessment of perioperative cardiac risk in patients undergoing major vascular surgery. *Circulation.* 1993;87(5):1506–1512.
8. Raux M, Godet G, Isnard R, et al. Low negative predictive value of dobutamine stress echocardiography before abdominal aortic surgery. *Br J Anaesth.* 2006;97(6):770–776.
9. Poldermans D, Arnese M, Fioretti PM, et al. Improved cardiac risk stratification in major vascular surgery with dobutamine-atropine stress echocardiography. *J Am Coll Cardiol.* 1995;26(3):648–653.
10. Snowden CP, Prentis JM, Anderson HL, et al. Submaximal cardiopulmonary exercise testing predicts complications and hospital length of stay in patients undergoing major elective surgery. *Ann Surg.* 2010;251(3):535–541.
11. Carlisle J, Swart M. Mid-term survival after abdominal aortic aneurysm surgery predicted by cardiopulmonary exercise testing. *Br J Surg.* 2007;94(8):966–969.
12. POISE Study Group, Devereaux PJ, Yang H, et al. Effects of extended-release metoprolol succinate in patients undergoing non-cardiac surgery (POISE trial): a randomised controlled trial. *Lancet.* 2008;371(9627):1839–1847.
13. Mangano DT, Layug EL, Wallace A, Tateo I. Effect of atenolol on mortality and cardiovascular morbidity after noncardiac surgery. Multicenter Study of Perioperative Ischemia Research Group. *N Engl J Med.* 1996;335(23):1713–1720.
14. Poldermans D, Boersma E, Bax JJ, et al. The effect of bisoprolol on perioperative mortality and myocardial infarction in high-risk patients undergoing vascular surgery. Dutch Echocardiographic Cardiac Risk Evaluation Applying Stress Echocardiography Study Group. *N Engl J Med.* 1999;341(24):1789–1794.
15. Le Manach, Y, Godet G, Coriat P, et al. The impact of postoperative discontinuation or continuation of chronic statin therapy on cardiac outcome after major vascular surgery. *Anesth Analg.* 2007;104(6):1326–1333.

16. Yusuf S, Sleight P, Pogue J, Bosch J, Davies R, Dagenais G. Effects of an angiotensin-converting-enzyme inhibitor, ramipril, on cardiovascular events in high-risk patients. The Heart Outcomes Prevention Evaluation Study Investigators. *N Engl J Med.* 2000;342(3):145–153.

17. Poldermans D, Bax JJ, Boersma E, et al. Guidelines for pre-operative cardiac risk assessment and perioperative cardiac management in non-cardiac surgery. Guidelines for pre-operative cardiac risk assessment and perioperative cardiac management in non-cardiac surgery. The Task Force for Preoperative Cardiac Risk Assessment and Perioperative Cardiac Management in Non-cardiac Surgery of the European Society of Cardiology (ESC) and endorsed by the European Society of Anaesthesiology (ESA). *Eur Heart J.* 2009;30:2769–2812.

18. Lindblad B, Persson N, Bergqvist D. Does low-dose acetylsalicylic acid prevent stroke after carotid surgery? A double-blind, placebo-controlled randomized trial. *Stroke.* 1993;24:1125–1128.

19. Earnshaw J, Beard J. *The vascular MDT: an essential element in the treatment of patients with vascular disease.* 2011. <http://www.aaaqip.com/files/vascular-mdt-bulletin-arcse-2011.pdf>.

20. http://www.aaaqip.com/files/vascular_society_mortality_report_final-copy_printers-v2-plymmarch2012.pdf.

21. Thompson SG, Ashton HA, Gao L et al. Screening men for abdominal aortic aneurysm: 10 year mortality and cost effectiveness results from the randomised Multicentre Aneurysm Screening Study. *BMJ.* 2009;338:b2307–b2307.

22. The United Kingdom Evar Trial Investigators. Endovascular versus open repair of abdominal aortic aneurysm. *N Engl J Med.* 2010;362(20):1863–1871.

23. Berman L, Dardik A, Bradley EH, Gusberg RJ, Fraenkel L. Informed consent for abdominal aortic aneurysm repair: assessing variations in surgeon opinion through a national survey. *J Vasc Surg.* 2008;47(2):287–295.e2.

24. Older P, Hall A, Hader R. Cardiopulmonary exercise testing as a screening test for perioperative management of major surgery in the elderly. *Chest.* 1999;16(2):355–362.

25. Brady AR, Fowkes FG, Greenhalgh RM, Powell JT, Ruckley CV, Thompson SG. Risk factors for postoperative death following elective surgical repair of abdominal aortic aneurysm: results from the UK Small Aneurysm Trial. *Br J Surg.* 2000;87(6):742–749.

26. Anon. Beneficial effect of carotid endarterectomy in symptomatic patients with high-grade carotid stenosis. North American Symptomatic Carotid Endarterectomy Trial Collaborators. *N Engl J Med.* 1991;325(7):445–453.

27. Rothwell PM, Eliasziw M, Gutnikov SA, et al. Analysis of pooled data from the randomised controlled trials of endarterectomy for symptomatic carotid stenosis. *Lancet.* 2003;361(9352):107–116.

28. Wardlaw JM, Chappell FM, Best JJ, et al. Non-invasive imaging compared with intra-arterial angiography in the diagnosis of symptomatic carotid stenosis: a meta-analysis. *Lancet.* 2006;367(9521):1503–1512.

29. Payne DA, Jones CI, Hayes PD, et al. Beneficial effects of clopidogrel combined with aspirin in reducing cerebral emboli in patients undergoing carotid endarterectomy. *Circulation.* 2004;109(12):1476–1481.

30. Kennedy J, Quan H, Buchan AM, Ghali WA, Feasby TE. Statins are associated with better outcomes after carotid endarterectomy in symptomatic patients. *Stroke.* 2005;36(10):2072–2076.

31. Chaturvedi S. Statins are associated with better outcomes after carotid endarterectomy in symptomatic patients. *Perspect Vasc Surg Endovasc Ther.* 2006;18(1):79–80.

32. Halm EA, Tuhrim S, Wang JJ, et al. Risk factors for perioperative death and stroke after carotid endarterectomy: results of the New York Carotid Artery Surgery Study. *Stroke.* 2009;40(1):221–229.

33. Reed AB, Gaccione P, Belkin M, et al. Preoperative risk factors for carotid endarterectomy: defining the patient at high risk. *J Vasc Surg.* 2003;37(6):1191–1199.

34. Flanigan DP, Flanigan ME, Dorne AL, et al. Long-term results of 442 consecutive, standardized carotid endarterectomy procedures in standard-risk and high-risk patients. *J Vasc Surg.* 2007;46(5):876–882.

35. Tangkanakul C, Counsell CE, Warlow CP. Local versus general anaesthesia in carotid endarterectomy: a systematic review of the evidence. *Eur J Vasc Endovasc Surg.* 1997;13(5):491–499.

36. Anon. General anaesthesia versus local anaesthesia for carotid surgery (GALA): a multicentre, randomised controlled trial. *Lancet.* 2008;372(9656):2132–2142.

37. Pandit JJ, Satya-Krishna R, Gration P. Superficial or deep cervical plexus block for carotid endarterectomy: a systematic review of complications. *Br J Anaesth.* 2007;99(2):159–169.

38. Costa E Silva L, Brimacombe JR. The laryngeal mask for carotid endarterectomy. *J Cardiothorac Vasc Anesth.* 1996;10(7):972–973.

39. Bacuzzi A, Cantore G, Del Bosco A, et al. Cerebral monitoring during CEA: review of the literature. *New Technol Surg.* 2009;1(1). <http://www.newtechnologiesinsurgery.org/Surgery/Surgery.nsf/docCat?OpenForm&Section=teleretina&Action=Papers&ActionSec=Articles&Language=EN&Cat=&Start=1&Count=100&uniiddoc=C43C3C1D1F07F17FC12575CE0061216E#19>.

40. Moritz S, Kasprzak P, Arlt M, Taeger K, Metz C. Accuracy of cerebral monitoring in detecting cerebral ischaemia during carotid endarterctomy. *Anaesthesiology.* 2007;107:563–569.

41. Hirsch AT, Haskal ZJ, Hertzer NR, et al. ACC/AHA 2005 practice guidelines for the management of patients with peripheral arterial disease (lower extremity, renal, mesenteric, and abdominal aortic). *Circulation.* 2006;113(11):e463–e465.

42. Diehm, C, Lange S, Darius H, et al. Association of low ankle brachial index with high mortality in primary care. *Eur Heart J.* 2006;27(14):1743–1749. <http://eurheartj.oxfordjournals.org/content/early/2006/06/16/eurheartj.ehl092.abstract> (accessed 20 July 2011).

43. Passman MA, Taylor LM, Moneta GL, et al. Comparison of axillofemoral and aortofemoral bypass for aortoiliac occlusive disease. *J Vasc Surg.* 1996;23(2):263–271.

44. Barbosa FT, Cavalcante JC, Jucá MJ, Castro AA. Neuraxial anaesthesia for lower-limb revascularization. *Cochrane Database Syst Rev.* 2010;1:CD007083.

45. Ploeg AJ, Lardenoye JW, Vrancken Peeters MP, Breslau PJ. Contemporary series of morbidity and mortality after lower limb amputation. *Eur J Vasc Endovasc Surg.* 2005;29(6):633–637.

46. Norgen, L, Hiatt WR, Dormandy JA, et al. Inter-Society Consensus for the Management of Peripheral Arterial Disease (TASC II). *Eur J Vasc Endovasc Surg.* 2007;33:S1–S70.

CHAPTER 20

Orthopaedic anaesthesia in the elderly

Richard Griffiths

Introduction

Orthopaedic procedures in the elderly can be broadly split into emergency and elective operations. Over the past 20 years more information has been collected in some European countries that makes the analysis of both urgent and planned operations much easier. These reveal that more procedures are being carried out on the elderly and on the very elderly. The success of the orthopaedic prostheses has also meant that more patients are returning for 'revision' operations, sometimes many years after the initial operation was performed.

There are two main disease processes that may lead to an orthopaedic operation in those who are older. These are osteoarthritis and osteoporosis. A rather oversimplified approach to these diseases dictates that osteoarthritis leads to elective joint replacements and osteoporosis leads to emergency or urgent operations for the consequences of fragility fractures.

The elective section will deal mainly with lower limb procedures, knee, and hip replacements. These operations are now routine and more time will be spent on revision operations. Upper limb surgery will also be mentioned.

Emergency orthopaedic surgery in the elderly will be focused on the consequences of fragility fractures. For the upper limb this usually involves a forearm fracture. For the lower limb fractured femur predominates and for the vertebral column operations to restore vertebral body height have gained popularity.

Elective surgery

Lower limb

Arthroplasty registries

The first national registry of elective orthopaedic procedures was started in Sweden in the 1970s[1,2] where hip and knee arthroplasties are kept on separate databases. The Swedish knee registry has been published since 1975[2] and they comment that the incidence has probably not yet peaked. In Sweden most joints are put in for those who are aged 65 to 84.

In England & Wales, The National Joint Registry (NJR) was started in 2003 and the eighth report was recently published.[3] There are many other countries with records for joint replacements, including Canada, Denmark, and Australia.

Examination of the NJR can inform the anaesthetic community of the changing demographic pattern of the patients over the past decade. This includes types of operations performed and also the ages of the patients. There is a separate registry for Scotland,[4] which also has a useful section on the complications of anaesthesia. The NJR does not collect data on type of anaesthesia performed but the demographic information, which does include body mass index and American Society of Anesthesiologists (ASA) grade, does point to an ageing population, which is getting sicker and fatter.

Initially the NJR was a voluntary register but since 2011/2012 NJR reporting is a mandated dataset for acute hospitals in England & Wales. Since 2003 information has been collected on hip and knee operations and since 2010, ankle replacement data has been collected. There are plans to collect information on the upper limb, which is already the case in Scotland.

In 2010, of the almost 77 000 primary and hip revision operations, over 31 per cent of the procedures were in patients who were over 75. 6 per cent of the primary hip operations in women were for those over 85. Almost 11 per cent of the operations were for revision surgery and 86 per cent of these were single-stage operations. Since 2009 more cement-less prostheses have been used, but this is not the case for older patients. Bone cement does pose a few problems[5] but the revision rate is lower for these operations and in those over 75, cemented hip replacements are more popular. As time progresses the revision rate increases and 7 years following the primary operation there is an almost 1 in 20 chance that a revision will be needed. The commonest indication is aseptic loosening of one of the components.

There were almost 82 000 knee procedures carried out in England & Wales in the latest NJR report [3]. The demographics are very similar to the hip data, although the average body mass index for a knee arthroplasty is now clinically obese at 30.6. 33 per cent of the primary knee procedures were carried out in those over 75, with 5 per cent in those over 85.

The NJR does highlight how safe primary hip and knee arthroplasty are. The 30-day death rate for a hip is 0.6 per cent and for a knee is 0.2 per cent. By the end of 7 years, 17 per cent of hip replacements are dead. There is no comparable data for those who have under gone revision procedures. It can only be assumed that they will be older and have more comorbidities than those undergoing the primary operation.

Before any elective orthopaedic operation meticulous preoperative assessment and preparation are needed. The risks of the primary procedure are relatively low and the quality of life benefits are considerable.

Hip arthroplasty

Hip arthroplasty is now a very common surgical intervention that has helped many individuals lead a more active and pain-free life. The primary operation is relatively safe[3] and there are many different anaesthetic and analgesic techniques that can be used to treat these patients.

For the primary operation the emphasis is on good quality preoperative preparation and optimization before surgery. Regional or general anaesthetic techniques, often combined with a variety of peripheral nerve blocks, are the main stay of anaesthesia practice for these cases. The operation is mostly performed in the lateral position, which can become uncomfortable after 60 minutes or more. Care should be taken to pad the lower arm and ensure that the shoulder of the dependant arm is not in an unusual position. For most patients over 75, cemented prostheses are used. Surgical technique has improved and the problems of bone cement are now infrequent in elective cases.[5]

20per cent of primary hip arthroplasties performed in NHS hospitals in England & Wales are classified as ASA 3 or 4. These are the group who may need more invasive monitoring or a period on a level 2-facility postoperatively.

There is very little published data on sub groups of the older patient. The average ages of patients in studies that claim to have elderly patients are often quite young.[6] This study examines the predictors of cognitive decline in elective joint replacements. In the group that developed postoperative delirium there was no evidence of any functional decline 3 months after the surgery. The type of anaesthesia had no effect on the outcome, although there was a non-significant trend towards a greater incidence of postoperative delirium in the general anaesthesia group. The title of this study includes the word elderly but the mean age was less than 75.

A group of European experts, entitled Prospect, short for specific systematic review and consensus recommendations for postoperative analgesia, have published articles on lower limb arthroplasty.[7] For hip surgery they recommend general anaesthesia combined with a peripheral nerve block or spinal anaesthesia supplemented with an opioid.

Blood loss can be a problem during primary hip arthroplasty and there is conflicting advice on whether anaemia impedes functional recovery and outcome from the operation. A large observational series on all types of non-cardiac surgery showed the detrimental effect of letting haematocrit drop or rise, leading to increased 30-day mortality and cardiac morbidity. This happened when the haematocrit fell below 39 per cent or rose above 51 per cent.[8] This study is part of the US Veterans Administration's National Surgical Quality Improvement Programme. Over 300 000 patients were included in this retrospective case series. Most of the patients were male but the fourth and sixth most frequent operation performed in the whole group were total knee arthroplasty and total hip arthroplasty.

The adverse effect of low haemoglobin preoperatively has not been proven in other case series. A much smaller study, involving only 391 patients failed to detect if anaemia was a risk factor for myocardial infarction or mortality in lower limb joint replacement.[9]

Knee arthroplasty

Knee arthroplasty can be a painful postoperative experience. The Prospect consensus group, mentioned earlier, published guidelines on analgesia following knee arthroplasty in 2008.[10]

The knee recommendations, which are less than 4 years old are already being succeeded by centres that focus on 'fast track' surgical programmes for lower limb joint arthroplasties.[11,12] In some countries these novel techniques are called 'enhanced recovery', which is a misleading label, as it does not reflect the total surgical experience. Peripheral nerve blocks are being replaced by local anaesthesia infiltration and infusions. There is some evidence that femoral nerve blocks may delay mobilization and a personal observation is that nerve blocks can cause significant quadriceps weakness in patients over 80, which may delay mobilization.

A large series from Scotland[13] emphasizes the benefits of spinal anaesthesia in combination with the local anaesthetic infiltration. Spinal anaesthesia is favoured by the Scandinavian clinicians in a number of publications highlighting 'fast track surgery'.[11,12] Preoperatively patients are given gabapentin and selective cyclo-oxygenase 2 (COX-2) inhibitors, to help with pain management. The use of any non-steroidal anti-inflammatory agent in the older patient[14] should be viewed with caution. The COX-2 inhibitors do not appear to be devoid of problems. The mean age of the patients in the Scottish study was 70. There does not appear to be many large series with the over 75s undergoing this type of surgery.

Gabapentin has been shown to be beneficial for analgesia in knee arthroplasty[15] but has limited value for hip arthroplasty.[16] There should be some caution exercised with the use of gabapentin to the older patient who is receiving the drug for the first time. Gabapentin may cause chorea and ataxia and this may make the older patient susceptible to falls, which may hinder mobilization from the surgical procedure.[17] There does not appear to be very large series of primary arthroplasties that focus solely on those over 80. Gabapentin and COX-2 inhibitors should be used with caution in patients in this age range.

Primary operations are now routine, but with the population ageing and patients becoming more active joint revisions are increasing in frequency.

Revision arthroplasty for hips and knees

A quick glance at the NJR report for England, Wales, and Northern Ireland from 2010[3] reports that there were 5082 revision knee operations, of which 76 per cent were single stage with an average age of 70. In the same report there were 7852 hip revision operations, 86 per cent of these were single stage and the average age was the same as for knee revisions. The complexity of these operations varies considerably, depending on the reason for the failure of the joint.

Early revisions may be for infected primary prostheses and usually take place shortly after the first operation. Eradication of infection may take a while and can result in two- or even three-stage operations. Close communication with surgical colleagues determines the type of anaesthesia employed. Knee revisions can be done under spinal anaesthesia but any procedure over 2 hours may need a general anaesthetic. The 'fast track' approach to primary knee arthroplasty has now been applied to knee arthroplasty revisions.[18] There were only 29 patients in this study with ages ranging from 34 to 84, all received spinal anaesthesia. The real applicability of spinal anaesthetic and local infiltration analgesia has not been fully explored in a significant group of patients over the age of 80.

Later revisions are often for failure of one of the components of the joint replacement. Knee revisions have the advantage of being performed under a lower limb tourniquet, which may limit the blood loss at operation.

Hip revision arthroplasty

Hip revisions can be lengthy operations with the potential for considerable blood loss, especially from the femoral component. Every precaution should be taken to be able to react to any massive blood loss. Direct arterial monitoring should be considered, which enables beat-to-beat blood pressure variation and the ability to sample frequently for blood gas and haematocrit estimations. Non-invasive cardiac output monitoring should also be considered, although there is a paucity of data on older patients having hip revision surgery with this technology to guide fluid replacement.[19] All fluids should be warmed and temperature monitoring instituted, with warming devices used to reduce any sources of heat loss.

Level 2 care should also be considered for at least 24 hours providing the opportunity for more intensive monitoring because significant blood loss can continue from drainage sites.

Upper limb surgery

Shoulder surgery

Upper limb joint arthroplasty procedures are soon to be collected by the NJR. The success of these operations has improved the quality of life of many older patients. For shoulders the usual position is the 'beach chair' sitting position, which has theoretical disadvantages for cerebral circulation. There is a reduction in cerebral oxygen saturation, as measured by a near-infrared spectroscopy (NIRS).[20] The significance of this finding for the older patient should not be ignored and appropriate advice given regarding the possibility of neurological morbidity, with appropriate positioning which is not so upright.

Ultrasound-guided inter-scalene local anaesthetic blocks are effective analgesia for shoulder operations[21] and avoid the need for opioids in the immediate post-operative period. There is an incidence of phrenic nerve paralysis,[21] although this problem is reduced by using smaller volumes of local anaesthetic.

Joint replacement procedures can now be performed on the elbow, wrist, and joints of the hand. Regional analgesic techniques have become more specific depending on the location of the surgery with the advent of ultrasound guided nerve blocks. Any reduction in systemic analgesics such as opioids and non-steroidal anti-inflammatory drugs is welcomed in the older patient.

Emergency surgery

Emergency orthopaedic surgery in the older patient is often the result of either falls or the consequences of osteoporosis. These latter fractures can be termed 'fragility fractures' and include lesions of the vertebrae, proximal femur, and forearm.

In 2000 there were 9.0 million osteoporotic fractures worldwide.

Vertebroplasty

In 2000 there were 1.4 million vertebral fractures worldwide, and with the population ageing this number is likely to increase.[22] Vertebral fractures are part of the osteoporotic spectrum and the frequency increases, as patients get older. Most happen spontaneously and until the last 10 years they were treated conservatively.

There are two interventional techniques for trying to restore the height and integrity of the fractured vertebra, these are called *vertebroplasty* and *kyphoplasty*.

Vertebroplasty is a procedure that is performed by radiologists in X-ray suites and involves the percutaneous placement of a needle into the fractured vertebra. The patient is supine for this procedure. Once the vertebra has been punctured by the needle, bone cement, polymethylmethacrylate, is injected into the affected vertebral body.

Balloon *kyphoplasty* is a similar procedure to vertebroplasty but involves the placement of a balloon, percutaneously, into the fractured vertebral body. The balloon is inflated so that the end plates of the vertebra are pushed apart before the space created by the balloon is filled with bone cement.

In one large study of kyphoplasty involving 138 patients in the active treatment arm, almost all of the patients were given a general anaesthetic for this procedure.[23] A small number in this study did receive conscious sedation with local anaesthetic adjuvant injected by the radiologist performing the procedure.

Initially the results of small observational studies and case reports were encouraging and pain relief and better function was seen following these limited studies.

In the author's experience vertebroplasty procedures are performed under conscious sedation. This can be via a propofol infusion or with benzodiazepines. Small amounts of opioids are also administered, as these procedures can be painful, despite the use of local anaesthesia to place the needles into the vertebral bodies. All the precautions for delivering safe anaesthesia in a remote environment, a radiology suite, should be undertaken including the presence of a suitably trained anaesthetic assistant. If general anaesthesia is used all the precautions for a prone patient must also be followed.

There is still some debate as to whether types of vertebroplasty are cost effective treatments for vertebral fractures. There is conflicting evidence about the efficacy of these interventions. The debate concerns patient selection, the natural history of a vertebral fracture and the design of the studies that have been performed to evaluate the procedures.

In a multinational trial of kyphoplasty,[23] patients were randomized to an active surgical intervention group or a non-surgical care. The primary outcome measure in this study was a validated global quality of life measure, the SF-36. The kyphoplasty group did show an improvement in this scale compared to the non-surgical group but a lack of blinding and the lack of a true control group limit the interpretation of the data.

An Australian study, which did have a control arm that included a sham vertebroplasty procedure, showed no benefit from vertebroplasty at 3 months. The main outcome was a reduction in pain.[24] The patients selected for this trial had painful lesions before randomization.

There have been other studies which point to a benefit from these invasive procedures[25] but there is still doubt as to whether it truly benefits patients compared to letting the natural history of the condition progress. Only better designed studies will answer these questions and determine whether anaesthetists will be asked to provide continued services for repair of vertebral fractures.

Fractures of the proximal femur

Demographics of Hip Fracture

Robust audit data has been collected in some European countries for a number of years. Sweden had the first hip fracture database[26] in 1988 and although there were some small projects, such as in Peterborough, it was not until 2008 that there has been a National Hip Fracture Database in England & Wales, termed the NHFD.[27] This collects some important information but to date has only recorded very limited information that may be of use to anaesthetists. This is likely to change in the near future. There is a real possibility that important questions, such as, does spinal anaesthesia offer any advantages over general anaesthesia and do nerve blocks contribute to faster rehabilitation, may be answered.

Every anaesthetist will face the challenges of the fractured femur patient during their career. It is probably a benchmark operation that shows the quality of healthcare that is delivered to older patients, if this is done well it is very likely that other procedures in older patients are also done well.

In contrast to elective hip replacement surgery there are very few ASA 1 and 2 patients who present with a hip fracture. The latest NHFD report[27] reports that 65 per cent of all the patients were either ASA 3 (54 per cent) or ASA 4 (11 per cent). This contrasts with 20 per cent ASA 3 and 4 for elective hip replacement[3] in NHS hospitals and only 7 per cent in independent hospitals. The average age of a hip fracture patient in England & Wales is now 84 and despite reservations about the completeness of the data from the NHFD, the latest report has data on over 50 000 hip fractures in England, Wales, and Northern Ireland. There was a slight increase in the mortality figures reported, from 7.7 per cent in 2010 to 8.4 per cent in 2011, but the latter report did have 20 000 more patients included, so this figure is almost certainly a truer reflection of the mortality of hip fractures patients.

There are a number of publications that have guided the clinical management of hip fracture patients, with variable input from anaesthesia organizations.[28–30] Guidelines for anaesthetists have recently been published by the Association of Anaesthetists of Great Britain and Ireland[31] and the reader should refer to these for a comprehensive account of the pre-, intra-, and postoperative management of hip fractures.

Anaesthesia Technique for Hip Fracture

Some important 'pearls' about hip fractures. There is very little evidence that regional or general anaesthesia offer any significant advantages over each other.[32] Surgery is the best form of analgesia, but initial analgesia should be with paracetamol, which can be administered immediately the patient is seen by a healthcare professional. Treatment can be escalated, with opioids and nerve blocks, but with constant assessment.[30] Non-steroidal anti-inflammatory drugs are best avoided in the elderly, although there is a paucity of research with these drugs in this patient group.[33]

Surgery should be planned as soon as possible, on a daytime fully staffed trauma list. There is evidence that delaying surgery may increase morbidity and even mortality.[34,35] Planning for surgery and optimization is a dynamic process, and no time should be lost in sorting out any medical conditions before surgery.

There are some controversial areas of management in these patients, which are also relevant to all patients with 'fragility fractures'.

A comprehensive medical assessment is key to understanding the important medical issues. Close liaison with orthogeriatrics is the key to successful multidisciplinary management of hip fracture. All anaesthetists should be familiar with the abbreviated mental test

score (AMTS)[36] and this should be included in the preoperative assessment.

One-third of hip fracture patients have cognitive impairment and assessment of pain in these patients is particularly difficult. Many of the drugs used to alleviate pain are associated with delirium so the advice should be to administer simple analgesics such as paracetamol. A French study[37] showed that for the post-operative pain associated with hip fracture surgery, intravenous proparacetamol was as effective as morphine or a continuous femoral catheter. There is no reason not to extrapolate these findings to the preoperative phase. Proparacetamol is metabolized to paracetamol and is effectively the same drug.[38]

There are a number of important clinical pointers that should be looked for in the history and examination. Has the patient had a history of recent falls? Is there a heart murmur? Comprehensive falls assessment should follow the acute episode and is conducted by the orthogeriatrics team, but acutely the presence of falls may highlight the possibility of cardiac arrhythmias or an aortic valve lesion. Anaesthetists should be aware of the history of any fall and the possible medical reasons why it has happened.

The Cardiac Murmur

The presence of a heart murmur should highlight the possibility that the patient may have aortic stenosis/sclerosis. A retrospective analysis of patients, who underwent echocardiography because of a previously undetected cardiac murmur following a hip fracture[39] in a busy UK hospital, revealed that approximately 30 per cent of these patients had aortic stenosis/sclerosis. These patients were older and more likely to have a lower AMTS. As the severity of the valve lesion increased general anaesthesia and invasive arterial blood pressure monitoring was more likely. However, some with severe stenosis received regional anaesthesia and with careful monitoring and the use of lower doses of intrathecal local anaesthetic agents this is a viable alternative to general anaesthesia.

Over all, in this retrospective study the incidence of undiagnosed aortic stenosis was in the region of 7 per cent. The investigations in this study did take a number of days to complete and evidence suggests that any delay in optimization and surgery is detrimental to hip fracture patients.[34,35]

When all eligible patients are given a bedside echocardiogram, during the weekdays, the following information was discovered from a large UK hospital: 2 per cent had severe aortic stenosis, 6 per cent had moderate disease, and 30 per cent had mild stenosis or sclerosis.[40] 31 per cent of this cohort, with no murmur detected clinically had aortic stenosis on echocardiography. Conversely, of the patients who had a murmur preoperatively, 30 per cent of these had a normal echocardiogram. Don't abandon the stethoscope, as if a murmur is heard it is more likely to be moderate or severe. Where does all this leave the anaesthetists faced with an older patient, with a painful hip and a murmur? A pragmatic approach is needed, surgery is the best form of analgesia, get an echo, if it will not delay surgery, but do not wait for days for cardiac investigations.[41] Use invasive arterial monitoring if at all worried, the ability to be able to sample frequently for estimations of haematocrit and blood analysis is invaluable.

Blood Loss From Hip Fracture

Blood loss from a proximal femoral fracture can be considerable. It is likely to be greater from extracapsular and sub-trochanteric fractures, than intracapsular fractures. Haemoglobin should be assessed preoperatively, ideally intraoperatively and also monitored in the postoperative period. Blood loss can be 'hidden' in hip fracture and the finding of a much lower postoperative haemoglobin level than expected is not a surprise.[42,43] The Cochrane review on transfusion triggers[44] does contain information from a couple of hip fracture studies but most of the information comes from either intensive care or paediatric patients. A liberal transfusion approach throughout the perioperative period does appear to be beneficial.[45]

The much awaited FOCUS study[46] has just added to the confusion around transfusion strategies in hip fracture. The authors have claimed that there is no difference between a liberal and restrictive transfusion policy in over 2000 patients randomized to the transfusion policy within 3 days of surgery. They did not see a difference in their outcome variables, which were death at 60 days or the ability to walk across a room at 60 days. The patients recruited were supposed to have cardiovascular disease, although, the recruitment criteria were changed during the study. This study had a negative outcome but it failed to answer the important question of whether a high haemoglobin is beneficial during an acute hip fracture episode. It is surprising that the authors did not comment upon the obvious findings of the study. They confirmed that hidden blood loss is a problem, with an average of a 2.5 g drop in haemoglobin, despite only a moderate amount of blood loss recorded at operation. The cardiovascular complications were also three times more frequent in the restrictive group, which was also not highlighted.

Blood loss is a problem; it can hinder rehabilitation and every anaesthetist should be aware that the haemoglobin may fall more than anticipated. The haematocrit or haemoglobin should be measured more frequently around the perioperative period, at least after surgery and the following day.

Drugs that inhibit the action of platelets are important for treating cardiovascular and thromboembolic diseases. Aspirin poses no problems and should be continued throughout the perioperative period. General or regional anaesthesia are safe.

Clopidogrel

Clopidogrel is a prodrug that is metabolized into an active constituent and irreversibly inhibits platelet activity. The drug should be continued throughout the perioperative period and there is evidence that blood loss at operation is only marginally increased.[47] A retrospective analysis of patients with hip fracture, in which, clopidogrel was stopped showed a detrimental effect and an increased mortality.[48] The drug should be continued, the only caution is with the application of regional anaesthesia. There is no need to delay surgery, administer general anaesthesia and measure the blood loss accurately.

Post Surgery Care

There is very little evidence for the use of level 2 or level 3 care in hip fracture. Patients may benefit form a period of intense monitoring although there are no studies on the effectiveness of this intervention.

Hip Fracture Peri-Operative Network

There is a very effective network of anaesthetists and orthogeriatricians in the United Kingdom[49] that aims to improve the care of hip fracture patients. The network has been renamed 'Hip Fracture Peri-Operative Network', to reflect the growing contribution of orthogeriatrics to the acute hospital episode. Team working and the involvement of senior doctors, nurses, and other healthcare professionals are essential for rapid assessment, treatment and rehabilitation of hip fracture patients. Anaesthesia has a key part to play in this process.

Features of emergency care are transferable into elective care. The concern about bone cement implantation syndrome,[5] have been alleviated by vigilance, better surgical technique and close attention to monitoring. However, despite the increasing use of cemented hemiarthroplasties and total hip replacements for hip fractures,[50] great care should be exercised when using cement in the very old and frail hip fracture patient.

Conclusion

Orthopaedic procedures are common in the older patient and following good basic medical principles and constant vigilance are essential features of anaesthesia for these patients, whether the operation is elective or urgent. More patients will be out living their primary joint replacements and needing revision surgery. This is likely to be a growth market, in which anaesthetists will be providing comprehensive assessment, anaesthesia, and analgesia.

References

1. Swedish Hip Arthroplasty Register. <http://www.shpr.se/en/default/aspex>.
2. Swedish Knee Arthroplasty Register. <http://www.knee.nko.se>.
3. National Joint Registry. *8th Annual Report 2010–2011*. <http://www.njrcentre.org.uk/NjrCentre/Portals/0/Documents/NJR%208th%20Annual%20Report%202011.pdf>.
4. The Scottish Arthroplasty Project. <http://www.arthro.scot.nhs.uk/>.
5. Donaldson AJ, Thomson HE, Harper NJ, Kenny NW. Bone cement implantation syndrome. *Br J Anaesth*. 2009;102(1):12–22.
6. Jankowski CJ, Trenerry MR, Cook DJ, *et al*. Cognitive and functional predictors and sequelae of postoperative delirium in elderly patients undergoing elective joint arthroplasty. *Anesthes Analg*. 2011;112:1186–1193.
7. Fischer B, Simanski C, on behalf of the PROSPECT Working Group. A procedure-specific systematic review and consensus recommendations for analgesia after total hip replacement. *Anaesthesia*. 2005;60:1189–1202.
8. Wu W-C, Schifftner TI, Henderson WG, *et al*. Preoperative haematocrit levels and postoperative outcomes in older patients undergoing noncardiac surgery. *JAMA*. 2007;297:2482–2488.
9. Mantilla CB, Wass CT, Goodrich KA, *et al*. Risk for perioperative myocardial infarction and mortality in patients undergoing hip or knee arthroplasty: the role of anemia. *Transfusion* 2011;51:82–91.
10. Fischer HB, Simanski CJ, Sharp C, *et al*. A procedure-specific systematic review and consensus recommendations for postoperative analgesia following total knee arthroplasty. *Anaesthesia*. 2008;63(10):1105–1123.
11. Andersen LO, Husted H, Kristensen BB, Otte KS, Gaarn-Larsen L, Kehlet H. Analgesic efficacy of intracapsular and intra-articular local anaesthetic for knee arthroplasty. *Anaesthesia*. 2010;65:904–911.
12. Andersen LO, Gaarn-Larsen L, Kristensen BB, Husted H, Otte KS, Kehelt H. Analgesic efficacy of local anaesthetic wound administration in knee arthroplasty: volume versus concentration. *Anaesthesia*. 2010;65:984–990.
13. McDonald DA, Siegmeth R, Deakin AH, Kinninmonth AWG, Scott NB. An enhanced recovery programme for primary total knee arthroplasty in the United Kingdom—follow up at one year. *Knee*. 2012;19(5):525–529.
14. Aneja A, Farkouh ME. Non-steroidal anti-infammatory drugs and the heart. *Heart*. 2011;97:517–518.

15. Clarke H, Pereira S, Kennedy D, Gilron I, Gollish J, Kay J. Gabapentin decreases morphine consumption and improves functional recovery following total knee arthroplasty. *Pain Res Manag*. 2009;14(3):217–222.

16. Clarke H, Periera S, Kennedy D, et al. Adding gabapentin to a multimodal regimen does not reduce acute pain, opioid consumption or chronic pain after total hip arthroplasty. *Acta Anaesthesiol Scand*. 2009;53(8):1073–1083.

17. Attupuratgh R, Aziz R, Wollman D, Muralee S, Tampi RR. Chorea associated with gabapentin use in an elderly man. *Am J Geriatric Pharmacother*. 2009;7:220–224.

18. Husted H, Otte KS, Kristensen BB, Kehlet H. Fast-track knee revision arthroplasty—a feasibility study. *Acta Orthop*. 2011;82(3):438–444.

19. Ceccomi M, Fasano N, Langiano N, et al. Goal directed haemodynamic therapy during elective total hip arthroplasty under regional anaesthesia. *Crit Care*. 2011;15:R132.

20. Moerman AT, De Hert SG, Jacobs TF, De Wilde LF, Wouters PF. Cerebral oxygen desaturation during beach chair position. *Eur J Anaesthesiol*. 2012;29(2):82–89.

21. Riazi S, Carmichael N, Awad I, Holtby RM, McCartney CJL. Effect of local anaesthetic volume (20 *vs* 5 ml) on the efficacy and respiratory consequences of ultrasound-guided interscalene brachial plexus block. *Br J Anaesth*. 2008;101(4):549–556

22. Johnell O, Kanis A. An estimate of the worldwide prevalence and disability associated with osteoporotic fractures. *Osteoporosis Int*. 2006;17:1726–1733.

23. Wardlaw D, Cummings SR, Meirhaeghe JV, et al. Efficacy and safety of balloon kyphoplasty compared to non surgical care for vertebral compression fracture (FREE): a randomised controlled trial. *Lancet*. 2009;373:1016–1024.

24. Buchbinder R, Osborne RJ, Ebeling PR, et al. A randomized trial of vertebroplasty for painful osteoporotic vertebral fractures. *N Engl J Med*. 2009;361:557–568.

25. Klazen CAH, Lohle PNM, de Vries J, et al. Vertebroplasty versus conservative treatment in acute osteoporotic vertebral compression fractures (Vertos II): an open-label randomised trial. *Lancet*. 2010;376(9746):1085–1092.

26. Nationella höftfrakturregistret. <http://www.vardhandboken.se/Lankbibliotek/Kvalitetsregister/Rikshoft/>

27. National Hip Fracture Database. <http://www.nhfd.co.uk/>.

28. British Orthopaedic Association and British Geriatrics Society. *The care of patients with fragility fracture*. 2007. <http://www.nhfd.co.uk/>.

29. Scottish Intercollegiate Guidelines Network. *Management of hip fracture in older people*. Edinburgh: SIGN, 2009. <http://www.sign.ac.uk/pdf/sign111.pdf>.

30. National Institute for Health and Clinical Excellence. *The management of hip fracture in adults*. London: NICE, 2011. <http://www.nice.org.uk/nicemedia/live/13489/54918/54918.pdf>.

31. Griffiths R, Alper J, Beckingsdale A, et al. Management of proximal femoral fractures 2011. *Anaesthesia*. 2012;67(1):85–98.

32. Parker MJ, Handoll HHG, Griffiths R. Anaesthesia for hip fracture surgery in adults. *Cochrane Database Syst Rev*. 2004;(4):CD000521.

33. Abou-Setta AM, Beaupre LA, Rashiq S, et al. Comparative effectiveness of pain management interventions for hip fracture: a systematic review. *Ann Intern Med*. 2011;155:234–245

34. Shiga T, Wajima Z, Ohe Y. Is operative delay associated with increased mortality of hip fracture patients? Systematic review, meta-analysis and meta-regression. *Can J Anaesth*. 2008;55:146–154.

35. Khan SK, Kalra S, Khanna A, Thiruvengada MM, Parker MJ. Timing of surgery for hip fractures: a systematic review of 52 published studies involving 291,413 patients. *Injury*. 2009;40:692–697.

36. Hodkinson, HM. Evaluation of a mental test score for assessment of mental impairment in the elderly. *Age Ageing*. 1972;1(4):233–238.

37. Cuvillon P, Ripart J, Debureaux S, et al. Analgesia after hip fracture repair in elderly patients: the effect of a continuous femoral nerve block: a prospective and randomised study. *Annales francaises d'anesthesie et de reanimation*. 2007;26:2–9.

38. McNicol ED, Tzortzopoulou A, Cepeda MS, et al. Single-dose intravenous paracetamol or propacetamol for prevention or treatment of postoperative pain: a systematic review and meta-analysis. *Br J Anaesth*. 2011;106:764–775.

39. McBrien ME, Heyburn G, Stevenson M, et al. Previously undiagnosed aortic stenosis revealed by auscultation in the hip fracture population—echocardio- graphic findings, management and outcome. *Anaesthesia*. 2009; 64: 863–870.

40. Loxdale SJ, Sneyd JR, Donovan A, Werrett G, Viira DJ. The role of routine pre-operative bedside echocardiography in detecting aortic stenosis in patients with a hip fracture. *Anaesthesia*. 2012;67(1): 51–54

41. Ricci WM, Rocca GJD, Combs C, Borrelli J. The medical and economic impact of pre-operative cardiac testing in elderly patients with hip fractures. *Injury Int J Care Injured*. 2007;38S3:S49–S52.

42. Foss NB, Kehlet H. Hidden blood loss after hip fracture surgery. *JBJS Br*. 2006;88:1053–1059.

43. Smith GH, Tsang J, Molynuex SG, White To. The hidden blood loss after hip fracture. *Injury*. 2011;42(2);133–135.

44. Carless PA, Henry DA, Carson JL, Hebert PPC, McClelland B, Ker K. Transfusion thresholds and other strategies for guiding allogeneic red blood cell transfusion. *Cochrane Database Syst Rev*. 2010;(10):CD002042.

45. Foss NB, Kristensen MT, Jensen PS, Palm H, Krasheninnikoff M, Kehlet H. The effects of liberal versus restrictive transfusion thresholds on ambulation after hip fracture surgery. *Transfusion*. 2009;49:227–234.

46. Carson JL, Terrin ML, Noveck H, et al. Liberal or restrictive transfusion in high-risk patients after hip surgery. *N Engl J Med*. 2011;365:2453–2462.

47. Chechik O, Thein R, Fichman G, Hain A, Tov TB, Steinberg EL. The effect of clopidogrel and aspirin on blood loss in hip fracture surgery. *Injury*. 2011;42:1277–1287.

48. Collyer TC, Reynolds HC, Truyens E, Kilshaw L, Corcoran T. Perioperative management of clopidogrel therapy: the effects on in-hospital cardiac morbidity in older patients with hip fractures. *Br J Anaesthes*. 2011;107:911–915.

49. The Hip Fracture Perioperative Network. <http://www.networks.nhs.uk/hipfractureanaesthesia>.

50. Costa M, Griffin XL, Pendleton N, Pearson, N, Parsons N. Does cementing the femoral component increase the risk of peri-operative mortality for patients having replacement surgery for a fracture of the neck of the femur. *J Bone Joint Surg Br*. 2011;93B:1405–1410.

CHAPTER 21

Cardiac anaesthesia in the elderly

Ivan L. Rapchuk, Pragnesh Joshi, and John F. Fraser

Introduction

Life expectancy is steadily increasing, with the number of individuals over the age of 75 growing at a faster rate than any other demographic. European population projections estimate that all Member States of the European Union (EU) can expect an increase in the median age without exception due to persistently low fertility and continuously increasing numbers of survivors to higher ages.[1] The percentage of persons aged 65 years and over in the EU is expected to increase from 17.1 per cent in 2008 to 30.5 per cent in 2060—constituting a real number of 151.5 million individuals. In particular, the population aged 80 years and over is projected to increase the most in relative terms for all countries.[1] These changes affect the workload for anaesthetic providers—especially those involved in anaesthesia for cardiac surgery and cardiovascular procedures.

Coronary artery disease (CAD) is an organ specific manifestation of the systemic process of atherosclerosis and the incidence of CAD increases with age. The reported incidence of cardiovascular disease is 63 per cent in people over 75 years in Australia (<http://www.abs.gov.au>). Autopsy studies of octogenarians reveal that 60 per cent of patients have significant CAD and the most common cause of death is myocardial infarction.[2] The discussion surrounding the provision of healthcare resources, medical economics, and medical ethics for this demographic is complex, and places great demands on individual healthcare practitioners and those making larger sociopolitical decisions on who to offer high levels of care. Data suggest that case selection rather than chronological age determines the success of cardiac procedures. In fact, cardiac surgery in the elderly patient can be performed with low operative mortality, excellent long-term survival, and postoperative quality of life exceeding that of the general elderly population if selection of patients is appropriate.[3] Preoperative planning for the elderly patient undergoing cardiac surgery optimizes outcomes and maximizes the chance for success, while decreasing the likelihood of a complicated and prolonged postoperative course (see Figs 21.1–21.3).[4]

The physiological changes of ageing

There are significant changes in the physiology of the elderly patient that occur with increasing chronological age. These changes are ubiquitous across all organ systems and will only be summarized here as they are covered by other chapters in this textbook. Fig. 21.4 highlights a number of the changes.[5]

The cardiovascular system undergoes well-documented changes due to ageing that occur even in apparently healthy and unaffected older individuals (see also Chapter 6). Thickening and stiffening of large and medium-sized arteries causes an increase in systolic blood pressure and decrease in diastolic blood pressure concomitant with every increase in decade after age 60.[6] These changes are due to the loss of elastic fibres, calcium deposition, and collagen build-up in the medial layer of the arteries.[6] Oxidative stress and inflammation increase with advancing age leading to inflammation and impaired vascular function—a morphological change that is distinct and additive to the arteriosclerotic changes.[7] Ventricular systolic function is relatively preserved, however concentric wall thickening occurs due to cellular hypertrophy and diastolic function declines by up to 50 per cent from the 3rd to 9th decades.[7] There is an age-related decline in aerobic capacity, and deficits in both number and efficiency of β-adrenergic receptors and signalling contribute to this reduced cardiovascular performance.[6]

The ageing thoracic system is compromised both in parenchymal tissue and chest wall—characterized by a significant reduction in lung elasticity, compliance of the chest wall, respiratory muscle strength, and an overall small reduction in diffusing capacity.[8] Forced vital capacity (FVC) begins to decline later than forced expiratory volume in 1 s (FEV_1) and at a slower rate—this natural fall in the FEV_1/FVC ratio may result in over-diagnosis of chronic obstructive pulmonary disease (COPD) in the elderly.[8] The diminished response to hypoxia in the elderly heightens vulnerability to ventilatory failure during the high-demand states seen in the perioperative setting, and increases the likelihood of worse outcomes.[8] This ventilatory failure can be exacerbated by the decreased ciliary function and force of cough in this cohort.[9]

Poor nutritional status and cognitive impairment decrease the elderly cardiac patient's ability to deal with perioperative stress. The major central nervous system diseases in the elderly are depression, dementia, delirium, and Parkinson's disease; and the ageing of the autonomic nervous system is characterized by progressively limited capacity to adapt to stress and other changes.[4] The ageing process results in changes in the kidney that are both anatomical and functional, and cause the increased propensity of the elderly to develop acute renal failure in times of physiological

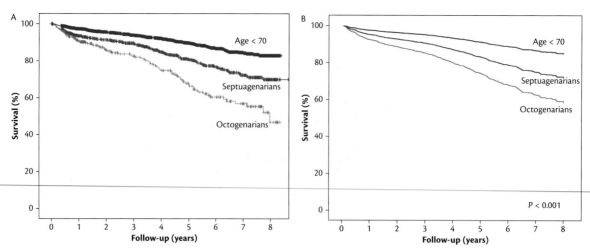

Fig. 21.1 Unadjusted (A) and adjusted (B) Kaplan–Meier survival curves after coronary artery bypass grafting surgery for octogenarians. After a mean follow-up of 4.0 ± 2.5 years, 1-year and 5-year survival rates were 90.7% ± 1.8% and 66.3% ± 3.6% for octogenarians versus 96.2% ± 0.4% and 86.8% ± 0.8% for younger patients. Predictors of late death in octogenarians included extensive aortic calcification, concomitant CABG, previous renal failure or stroke and low body mass index. Silvay G, Castillo JG, et al., 'Cardiac anesthesia and surgery in geriatric patients', *Seminars in Cardiothoracic and Vascular Anesthesia*, 12, 1, pp. 18–28, copyright © 2008 by Sage Publications, reprinted by Permission of SAGE Publications.

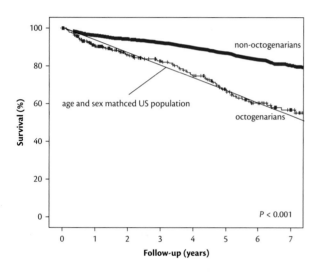

Fig. 21.2 2 Kaplan–Meier survival for of octogenarians after coronary artery bypass grafting compared with the survival of an age-matched and gender-matched US population. Late survival of octogenarians undergoing CABG was similar to the expected survival of an age and sex matched population according to actuarial data from the 2003 US population. Silvay G, Castillo JG, et al., 'Cardiac anesthesia and surgery in geriatric patients', *Seminars in Cardiothoracic and Vascular Anesthesia*, 12, 1, pp. 18–28, copyright © 2008 by Sage Publications, reprinted by Permission of SAGE Publications.

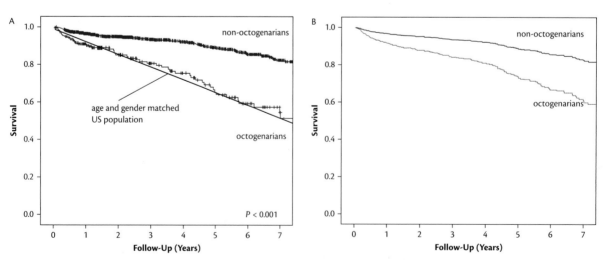

Fig. 21.3 Unadjusted (A) and adjusted (B) survival curves after aortic valve replacement for octogenarians compared with non-octogenarians. Our analysis revealed that after a mean follow-up time of 3.6 ± 2.5 years, 1-year and 5-year survival rates were 90.3% ± 2.1% and 63.8% ± 4.8% for octogenarians versus 96.3% ± 0.6% and 88.8% ± 1.3% for younger patients (Figure 3B) (P < .001). These figures suggest the burden of comorbidity in this elderly patient group may negate any benefit on long-term survival gained by improvements in early outcome. Silvay G, Castillo JG, et al., 'Cardiac anesthesia and surgery in geriatric patients', *Seminars in Cardiothoracic and Vascular Anesthesia*, 12, 1, pp. 18–28, copyright © 2008 by Sage Publications, reprinted by Permission of SAGE Publications.

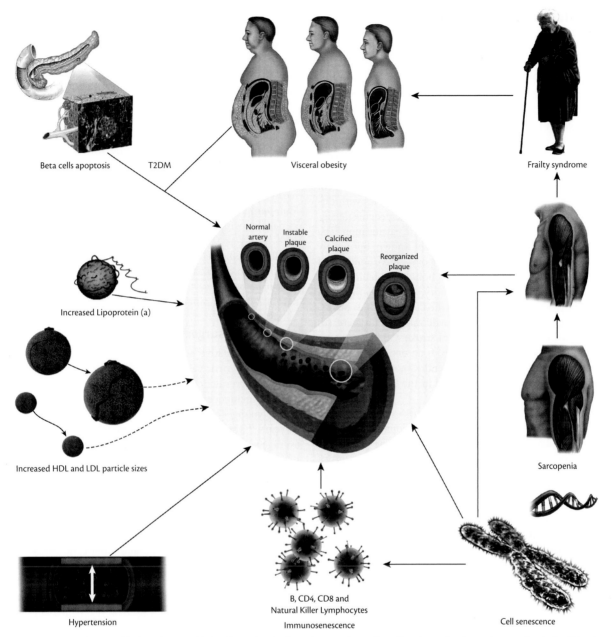

Fig. 21.4 Atherogenesis in the very elderly. In the very elderly, atherosclerotic disease is not only manifested by plaques in advanced stage of evolution (fibrotic, calcified), but also by the growing number of plaques of recent onset and with an unstable phenotype. The emergence of these new lesions occur as a result of persistence and changes in traditional risk factors such as hypertension, dyslipidemia and diabetes mellitus, but also by the emergence of potentially anti-atherogenic mechanisms related to aging. Among these sarcopenia, cellular senescence, frailty syndrome and immunosenescence stand out. Together, new and traditional atherogenic mechanisms provide the acceleration of atherogenesis and increased cardiovascular risk in the very old. Reprinted from *Atherosclerosis*, 225, 2, Freitas WM, Carvalho LS, et al., 'Atherosclerotic disease in octogenarians: a challenge for science and clinical practice', pp. 281–289, Copyright 2012, with permission from Elsevier and the European Atherosclerosis Society.

challenges. A drop in glomerular filtration and changes in glomerular haemodynamics decrease the ability of the kidney to cope with alterations in renal sodium and potassium handling, which negatively affects diluting and concentrating ability.[10] The incidence of, and susceptibility to, type 2 diabetes increases with age, as the proliferative and regenerative capacity of beta cells and beta cell mass decrease.[11] Ageing is characterized by progressive impairment in homeostatic mechanisms which influences both pharmacokinetics and pharmacodynamics. Elderly patients are susceptible to the effects of frequently prescribed drugs acting on central nervous system (e.g. benzodiazepines) with a

high potential for adverse drug reactions, and there is reduced effectiveness of conventional doses of cardiovascular drugs (e.g. diuretics and β-blockers).[12] Anaemia is more common in the elderly.[13] The most common cause is idiopathic anaemia with increased inflammatory markers and relatively low erythropoietin levels, next most common being iron deficiency anaemia and myelodysplastic syndromes.[14]

Physiological changes in the elderly are highly variable depending on the individual patient and it is critically important to assess older patients using a range of individualized clinical and physiological parameters rather than on the basis of age alone.

Cardiac surgical perspectives in the elderly

Ischaemic heart disease in the elderly

Coronary arteries in the elderly are commonly tortuous with diffuse atherosclerosis and calcification in the arterial wall. Coronary calcification is quite difficult to negotiate at the time of surgical anastomosis which increases the likelihood of incomplete revascularization and complications such as plaque separation, distal embolization, dissection, or inadvertent endarterectomy. It is common practice to identify the segment of coronary artery with the least disease for grafting, and to avoid grafting an artery that is of small calibre with poor distal run-off. Coronary arteries with diffuse disease and poor distal flow likely have little prognostic significance. The elderly also have increased aortic calcification. The exact mechanism of aortic calcification is not known, but widely accepted theories include active model theory—incorporation of autologous cell type cytokines, similar to bone remodelling—and the passive physiochemical model theory.[14] The Framingham study showed that the prevalence of calcified atheromatous plaque doubles with each decade of age.[14,15] Aortic calcification increases the complexity of surgery and the risk of stroke. Off-pump aortic coronary artery bypass grafting (OPCAB) is an option for surgical revascularization with calcification of ascending aorta but is a challenging task for surgeons not experienced in the technique and is equivocal in benefit.

Atherosclerosis is a systemic process with risk factors, such as advancing age, that are identical for the development of coronary, cerebrovascular, and carotid atherosclerosis. The prevalence of carotid stenosis in patients undergoing CABG is reported to be between 6.1 per cent and 38 per cent,[16–18] and the prevalence of severe carotid stenosis is reported to be 4.1–13.3 per cent.[19,20] Carotid artery disease is a risk factor for postoperative cerebrovascular attack (CVA).[16,21,22] Elderly patients undergoing coronary artery bypass grafting (CABG) should be screened for carotid artery disease with a duplex scan or computed tomography (CT) angiogram.[20] The timing and approach for treating carotid and coronary artery disease varies among surgeons and institutions. Symptomatic carotid artery disease should be treated as a staged, reversed staged or synchronous procedure with CABG depending on the severity of CAD. Carotid artery stenting is another option, however the International Carotid Stenting Study favoured endarterectomy over stenting due to unacceptable early stroke risk in the stent group.[23]

It is well known that the left internal mammary artery (LIMA) provides the best long-term patency rate.[24] Saphenous vein grafts (SVGs) are totally occluded in about 30 per cent of patients after 10 years, and a further 30 per cent of the patent SVGs show varying degrees of graft disease.[24, 25] It is not common for octogenarians to undergo re-operative CABG due to advances in percutaneous technology. The main goal of CABG is to provide symptomatic relief rather than prognostic benefits, except for those who present with tight left main CAD. Despite the lack of evidence of long-term benefit of LIMA in octogenarians, it is quite common to utilize this conduit for grafting the left anterior descending artery. It is likely to provide long-term benefit and also removes the need for aorto-coronary bypass. There is a risk of sternal wound infection in diabetic patients when IMA is utilized, however age has not shown to be a risk factor for sternal wound complication.[26, 27] The radial artery is used only if the veins in the lower limb are not available or affected by varicosities. In such situations the radial artery should be assessed with preoperative ultrasound to exclude calcification—a not uncommon finding in the elderly.

Urgent and emergent operations are associated with higher morbidity and mortality across all age groups. Elderly patients are affected greatly by urgent/emergent status of the operation compared to younger patients, with resultant higher morbidity and mortality.[28–30] If possible, preoperative status should be optimized to reduce morbidity and mortality, and patients should be medically stabilized to delay surgery from emergent to urgent or to elective status. Patients presenting with ST-elevation myocardial infarction (STEMI) should be delayed for at least a week, and patients presenting with stable left main CAD or those who have received clopidogrel should be delayed a few days. Intra-aortic balloon pump (IABP) can be utilized to achieve and maintain stability in patients with high-risk features.[29] Elderly patients who present with high-risk features, and are not amenable to optimization, should be considered for percutaneous intervention or a hybrid approach. In complex patients a multidisciplinary approach involving cardiologists, cardiac surgeons, intensivists, and geriatricians is necessary for planning appropriate treatment.

Aortic valve surgery

Senile degenerative aortic stenosis (AS) is the most frequently encountered aortic valve pathology in the elderly.[31] In the Helsinki study, the prevalence of moderate aortic stenosis was 5 per cent, and the incidence of critical AS increased from 1–2 per cent in people younger than 76 years of age to 6 per cent in people above 86 years.[31] The natural history of symptomatic AS is very poor with average survival of 5 years, 3 years, and 2 years after development of angina, syncope, and heart failure respectively.[32] A multivariate analysis of almost 6000 patients showed that the five most important predictors of mortality after aortic valve surgery (AVR) were age greater than 80 years, NYHA class more than or equal to III, ejection fraction (EF) less than 30 per cent, emergency AVR, and concomitant bypass surgery.[33] The hospital mortality after AVR in octogenarians varies between 5 and 7 per cent.[34,35] Mortality figures after AVR in the elderly are quite high compared to younger patients but still better than medical management. Varadarajan et al., in a comparison of 5 years survival with and without AVR in octogenarians, showed that survival was 68 per cent in patients who underwent surgery compared to 22 per cent for those who did not have surgery.[36] Current evidence suggests that age is not a contraindication for AVR and there is considerable functional and symptomatic improvement after surgery (see Fig. 21.5).[34,37–40]

Calcification in the aorta makes the aortic wall rigid and impenetrable—features that make closure of the aorta challenging. Aggressive approaches include decalcification of the aorta and endarterectomy or replacement of the ascending aorta. These additional procedures increase cardiopulmonary bypass (CPB) time, add complexity to the operation and significantly increase the risk of stroke and mortality in the elderly group.[35,38] There should be a low threshold to perform CT scans to assess the aorta in elderly patients, as it shows calcification and provides guidance for surgeons to avoid localized calcific areas during application of cross clamp or aortic cannulation.

Increasing numbers of patients are being referred for AVR who have had previous CABG, and many have patent grafts, which makes redo surgery quite complex. A patent, anteriorly located SVG or LIMA graft requires isolation and occlusion during the operation. Handling of previously placed venous grafts makes them

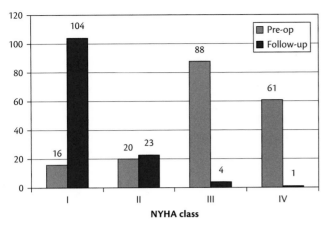

Fig. 21.5 Patients New York Heart Association (NYHA) class distribution preoperatively (pre-op) and at follow-up. At follow-up, one hundred and twenty-seven patients were in NYHA class I or II. The 4-year actuarial survival was 70.5%, the event-free survival was 60.6%, and almost all (97.5%) of the interviewed patients thought that they had benefited from the operation. Reproduced from Cerillo AG, Assal Al Kodami A, et al., 'Aortic valve surgery in the elderly patient: a retrospective review', *Interactive CardioVascular Thoracic Surgery*, 6, 3, pp. 308–313, copyright 2007 by permission of Oxford University Press, European Association for Cardio-Thoracic Surgery, and The European Board of Cardiovascular Perfusion.

vulnerable to injury or coronary embolization, and 'no touch' or minimal handling is necessary to avoid dislodgement and embolization of atheroma to coronary arteries. The aortotomy needs to be tailored according to the position of the previous SVG on the aorta, and closure of aortotomy should be performed without compromising the aorto-venous anastomosis. The mortality rate of redo AVR in the setting of previous CABG varies between 5 and 16.6 per cent to as high as 32 per cent.[41–43] Five-year survival following redo-AVR with CABG has been reported to be 40.2 per cent in one study.[43] Although the outcome of primary AVR in octogenarians are quite good, the mortality and morbidity following redo AVR remains quite high. The role of percutaneous aortic valve replacement is expanding, and an institutional and multidisciplinary approach should be adopted when considering redo AVR in an elderly patient with comorbidities.

Most elderly patients have associated cardiac pathologies including CAD, mitral valve disease, or aortic root dilation/calcification. The addition of any other procedure contributes to increased CPB time, and an increased risk of complications. Although Brunvand et al.[44] showed no difference in outcome following isolated AVR compared to AVR with CABG in octogenarians, a more recent meta-analysis of more than 40 studies revealed mortality of 9.7 per cent—significantly higher than the mortality and morbidity of isolated AVR in octogenarians.[45,46] Moderate mitral regurgitation (MR) or mitral stenosis (MS) due to degenerative mitral calcification is not uncommon in the elderly. MR from moderate functional lesions is best left alone as the addition of a mitral procedure can increase perioperative risk substantially.[47] However, if the MR is due to intrinsic valve pathology then surgical correction should be considered for more than moderate degrees of MR. Baumgartner et al. reported that the presence of moderate organic MR has an adverse impact on survival in the elderly undergoing aortic valve replacement.[47] Mitral valve repair in a patient with a calcified mitral annulus can be quite challenging. The technique of Alfieri repair when suitable is a good option to minimize complexity of the procedure.[47] For a dilated aortic root, supracoronary replacement of the ascending aorta can be undertaken with relatively lower morbidity compared to aortic root

replacement. Tailoring aortoplasty of the dilated ascending aorta, by excising a longitudinal ellipse of aorta instead of aortic replacement is also a reasonable option in high-risk elderly.[48,49] Patients with a contraindication to sternotomy or a porcelain aorta should be considered for aortic valve bypass surgery or percutaneous AVR. Left ventricle apico-aortic conduit (aortic valve bypass surgery) has been performed in high risk patients. This procedure utilizes a valved Dacron conduit whereby inflow is attached to the apex of the left ventricle, outflow is connected to the descending thoracic aorta, and the procedure is carried out via left thoracotomy without CPB.[50] It is an alternative for high risk or inoperable patients not suitable for sternotomy. Main indications are porcelain aorta, previous multiple sternotomies/AVRs complicated by infection and severe patient prosthesis mismatch, and advantages of on-pump AVB include the avoidance of aortic cannulation, cross-clamping, and cardioplegic cardiac arrest.[1,50]

Aortic valve replacement by upper hemi-sternotomy has been done for quite a few years but has not received widespread acceptance. Minimally invasive AVR by right mini-thoracotomy with peripheral cannulation for CPB is another alternative to AVR via sternotomy. Glower et al. published the experience of mini-thoracotomy AVR in 306 patients including all age groups, reporting early mortality of 1.5 per cent and a return to preoperative activity within 2 weeks of operation.[51] The role of minimally invasive methods to replace the aortic valve in elderly is yet to be fully explored.

Mitral valve surgery in elderly

The most common mitral valve lesion in the elderly is MR.[52] The most common causes of MR in the elderly are degenerative or ischaemic heart disease, with less frequent causes being rheumatic valvular disease and endocarditis.[52] MS is much less common than MR in this cohort. Severe symptomatic MR in the absence of contraindications requires surgical treatment and guidelines for the same are well established.[37] Chronic severe MR associated with pulmonary hypertension, right heart failure, and coronary atherosclerosis is a high-risk group.[53,54] Patients with such risk factors should be investigated thoroughly with cardiac catheterization and MRI to assess right ventricular function. Limited data is available about the outcome of elderly patients with poor right ventricular function. Management of moderate MR coexisting with aortic valve disease or ischaemic heart disease is controversial. The surgical approach to address the mitral valve with other coexisting cardiac lesions should be based on multidisciplinary discussions and individualized patient assessment.

Mitral valve surgery is challenging in the elderly. A database registry showed mortality increased from 4.1 per cent in patients less than 50 years to 17 per cent in patients more than 80 years undergoing mitral valve replacement.[53] Even more striking was the finding that the major postoperative complications increased from 13.5 per cent to 35.5 per cent.[53] This was a database analysis rather than randomized study, yet reflects the facts of current practice. Although mitral repair is the gold standard for treatment of MR, a trend of decreasing mitral valve repair with increasing age is seen in a study analysis of the STS database.[55] A non-randomized study with adjusted propensity scores comparing mitral valve repair to mitral valve replacement in the elderly showed that repair was better than replacement.[54] In this study, 30-day mortality for mitral repair was 11 per cent while it was 18.9 per cent for valve replacement.[54] Isolated segmental prolapse of the posterior mitral leaflet, or MR due to annular dilation, is highly likely to result in a durable repair and would be a reasonable procedure to attempt. However, mitral valve repair (MVR) for more complex mitral pathology frequently results in prolonged cross-clamp time. MVR with preservation of subvalvar apparatus is often a more appropriate choice in complex pathology. MVR for moderate ischaemic MR is a controversial issue. No randomized trials compare repair versus replacement for ischaemic MR in any age group. The likelihood of good short and long-term outcomes after MVR need to be balanced against the higher perioperative risks and increased complexity of surgery when considering repair versus replacement in the elderly patient. Surgery for ischaemic MR is associated with higher immediate mortality and poor long-term outcome in the elderly.[56] The need for any other procedures (CABG or valve procedure) further increases the risk and reduces long-term survival.[54] A multidisciplinary approach should be adopted in complex patients.

Degenerative mitral annular calcification (MAC) is common in the elderly. Diabetes mellitus, hypertension, hyperlipidaemia and female gender are implicated in the development/progression of MAC.[57] MAC presents a significant challenge to the surgeon. The most aggressive approach is to decalcify the annulus by detaching the posterior leaflet, reconstructing the atrio-ventricular junction with a pericardial patch, and reattaching the posterior leaflet or implanting a prosthetic valve. This procedure is complex, requiring both experience and a prolonged cross clamp time. The other approaches include a repair of leaflet pathology with neo-chordae, or edge-to-edge repair if technically suitable (Alfieri technique). For MS, valve sutures can be passed through the tough portion of posterior leaflet or left atrial wall without removing calcium from the annulus. Minimally invasive mitral valve surgery has been shown to result in shorter hospital stays and improved early recoveries in a general population.[58] In this technique, a small anterolateral thoracotomy is performed and CPB is instituted with femoral arterial and venous cannulation. A large retrospective study by Vollroth et al.,[59] and a subgroup analysis in the series of Iribarne et al., showed that minimally invasive mitral surgery in the elderly was as safe and effective as standard sternotomy with equivalent long-term survival.[58,60] Minimally invasive mitral surgery has an associated learning curve that results in prolonged bypass and cross-clamp time early in the experience.

Aortic surgery in elderly

Commonly seen aortic pathologies in the elderly are degenerative aneurysms and aortic dissections, and it is not uncommon to see coexistent aortic valve disease or CAD.[61] An aortic aneurysm is a dilatation of the aorta 50 per cent more than expected for that individual. The natural history of untreated ascending aortic aneurysms shows a 5-year survival of 13 per cent compared to 75 per cent in patients without aneurysms.[61] As aortic diameter grows, the risk of dissection also increases. A retrospective review by Shah et al. showed no significant difference in early mortality following repair of ascending aortic aneurysms in patients over 80 years of age versus less than 80 years; however, stroke rate was significantly higher in the older age group.[62] When survival was compared with an age-matched population of octogenarians at 1 year, it was significantly lower in patients operated on for aortic aneurysms.[62] The prognostic benefit of the operation is not clear in the elderly, and major aortic surgery in octogenarians requires careful patient selection to ensure ascending aortic aneurysm repair can be undertaken with acceptable mortality.

Surgical management of dissection is indicated if the entry tear is located in ascending aorta or arch (Stanford type A). If the entry tear is located distal to the origin of subclavian artery (Stanford type B), medical management or endovascular stenting is offered first. It is well known that the mortality of an untreated type A dissection is more than 50 per cent in 48 hours.[63] Due to the high mortality of non-surgical management, surgery is an obvious choice in type A dissection. Data from the International Registry of Acute Aortic Dissection (IRAD) reported a mortality of 26 per cent after surgical repair of type A dissection.[64] According to IRAD data 83.8 per cent of patients were alive at median follow up of 2.8 years, however the outcomes were substantially worse in octogenarians.[65] Although operative mortality increases with age, it is less than the mortality of medically treated type A aortic dissections in octogenarians, which was 58 per cent as reported by IRAD.[64] A multicentre study on post-surgical outcome of type A dissection by Piccardo et al. reported an in-hospital mortality 45.6 per cent and complication in 69.2 per cent for patients older than 80 years.[66] A similar mortality was observed in patients older than 70 years undergoing type A dissection repair by IRAD.[67] Although age has been identified as an independent risk factor for mortality, it alone should not be used as a criteria to exclude patients from being a surgical candidate for treatment of type A dissection.[66,67] The presence of high risk features such as cardiogenic shock, cerebrovascular stroke, coma, myocardial infarction, and multiple organ malperfusion syndrome are associated with very high morbidity and mortality.[68,69] The higher incidence of prolonged hospitalization, CVA, institutional discharge, and morality after repair of type A dissection in the elderly brings into question the role of surgical treatment.[70] Judicious use of resources is advocated due to dismal short- and long-term outcomes, but it is also important to consider ethical and moral issues, legislation, culture, and the accepted standard of practice in each institution. A multidisciplinary approach involving intensive care specialists, surgeons, and family is helpful in decision-making.

Preoperative preparation for cardiac surgery

The ageing process is characterized by an increased potential for failure to maintain homeostasis under conditions of physiological stress (outlined in Chapter 6). Increasing age independently predicts morbidity and mortality; however, it is not the only important factor. Appropriate testing such as echocardiography, pulmonary function testing, angiography and other imaging is essential. A dental examination is critical in the geriatric population as advanced caries, oral/gingival infection, and other dental pathology must be identified and addressed prior to elective cardiac surgery.[4] Preoperative chest radiographs document the baseline appearance of the lungs, and allow for recognition of a deviated trachea and left main stem bronchus which may complicate the placement of single- or double-lumen endotracheal tubes (and lead to the need for fibreoptic guidance to prevent tracheal trauma).[4] The history and preoperative workup prior to cardiac surgery in the elderly patient should assess physiological parameters and functional status, including assessment of the cardiovascular reserve sufficient to withstand a very stressful operation. Elderly patients who are otherwise acceptable surgical candidates should not be denied surgery based solely on their age. Several scores are currently available to assess the perioperative risk of cardiac patients—the two most widely used are the *European system for cardiac operative risk evaluation* (EuroSCORE) and the Society of Thoracic Surgeons (STS) score.[71] These commonly used scores focus on medical diagnoses and medical comorbidities as the main variables in assessing and predicting risk, but take very little into account relating to the biological status of the patient. To improve risk assessment in the elderly it is important to integrate this biological status—focussing on the geriatric syndrome of frailty (see also Chapter 30). Frailty is an emerging concept and poorly incorporated into the risk assessment of the cardiac surgical patient. Frailty and disability in the elderly include such variables as the Fried criteria (weight loss, weakness assessed by grip strength, self-reported exhaustion, gait speed and activity level for instrumental activities of daily living), physical performance (balance tests, body control tests), and a visible estimate of patient frailty by two independent physicians skilled in this area.[71] A number of newer studies that include a comprehensive assessment of frailty, in addition to clinical features and laboratory measurements, seem to better predict outcomes for patients at this extreme of age.[71,72] A simple and commonly used method to assess frailty is the Katz index of independence in the activities of daily living (Katz ADL).[73] In a multicentre cohort, the addition of frailty over the Parsonnet or STS PROM (Predicted Risk Of Mortality) alone provided incremental value and improved model discrimination.[72] A single-centre study found frailty to be an independent predictor of in-hospital mortality, institutional discharge, and mid-term survival.[74] Clinicians should use an integrative approach combining frailty, disability and pre-existing validated risk scores to better characterize elderly patients referred for cardiac surgery, and identify those at increased risk of perioperative complications (see Fig. 21.6).

Cardiac surgery in the elderly is not just about surgical success or discharge from ICU, but returning the patient to a fully functional postoperative state. The comprehensive, multidisciplinary, and proactive preoperative assessment to detect the multiple risk factors and comorbidities common in older patients requires more resources to complete compared with the conventional assessment; yet is justified by the benefits of identifying high-risk patients, improving communication between surgeon and patient, and preventing perioperative adverse events by optimizing physical and mental reserve. The American Geriatrics Society and American College of Surgeons have recently completed a position paper on the optimal preoperative assessment of the geriatric surgical patient.[75] Although not specific to cardiac surgery, the recommendations can be viewed as universal for this patient population (see Table 21.1).[75]

Depression is more common in the elderly, and should actively be screened for, as preoperative depression has been associated with increased mortality after CABG and longer postoperative length of stay after both CABG and valve operations.[76] Delirium is known to complicate surgery in the elderly and has an association with higher mortality, higher rates of institutionalization, greater costs and use of hospital resources, longer lengths of stay, and compromised functional recovery in many types of surgery.[77] Risk factors for delirium should be identified and modified. Postoperative pulmonary complications (PPCs) incur the highest total hospital cost compared with infectious, thromboembolic, and cardiac adverse events, require the longest median length of stay, and predict long-term mortality in elderly patients (≥70 years) undergoing non-cardiac surgery.[75] Strategies to decrease the

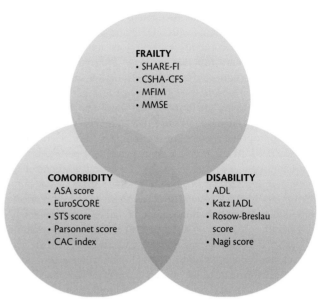

Fig. 21.6 Cardiac surgery risk is better described by an intersection of the risks outlined by frailty, disability and comorbidity. SHARE-FI: Survey of health, aging and retirement in Europe—frailty index; CSHA-CFS: Canadian Society of Health and Aging Clinical Frailty Score; MFIM: modified functional independence measure; MMSE: modified mini-mental state exam; ASA: American Society of Anesthesiologists; CAC: Charlson Age-Comorbidity Index; ADL: activities of daily living; IADL: instrumental activities of daily living.

Table 21.1 Checklist for the optimal preoperative assessment of the geriatric surgical patient

In addition to conducting a complete history and physical examination of the patient, the following assessments are strongly recommended:
• Assess the patient's **cognitive ability** and **capacity** to understand the anticipated surgery
• Screen the patient for **depression**
• Identify the patient's risk factors for developing postoperative **delirium**
• Screen for **alcohol** and other **substance abuse/dependence**
• Perform a preoperative **cardiac** evaluation according to the American College of Cardiology/American Heart Association algorithm for patients undergoing non-cardiac surgery
• Identify the patient's risk factors for postoperative **pulmonary** complications and implement appropriate strategies for prevention
• Document **functional status** and history of **falls**
• Determine baseline **frailty** score
• Assess patient's **nutritional status** and consider preoperative interventions if the patient is at severe nutritional risk
• Take an accurate and detailed **medication history** and consider appropriate perioperative adjustments. Monitor for **polypharmacy**
• Determine the patient's **treatment goals** and **expectations** in the context of the possible treatment outcomes
• Determine patient's **family** and **social support system**
• Order appropriate preoperative **diagnostic tests** focused on elderly patients

Reprinted from *Journal of the American College of Surgeons*, 215, 4, Chow WB, et al., 'Optimal preoperative assessment of the geriatric surgical patient: a best practices guideline from the American College of Surgeons National Surgical Quality Improvement Program and the American Geriatrics Society', pp. 453–466, Copyright 2012, with permission from Elsevier and the American College of Surgeons.

likelihood of PPCs include preoperative optimization of pulmonary function in patients with COPD and asthma, smoking cessation, preoperative intensive inspiratory muscle training, and selective pulmonary function testing.[75] Pharmacological review and documentation of the patient's complete medication lists, including use of non-prescription agents and herbal products is essential. Identifying medications that should be discontinued or avoided perioperatively, and dose-reducing or substituting potentially inappropriate medications, minimizes the risk for adverse drug reactions. Avoid benzodiazepines and using pethidine for the treatment of pain (yet ensure that pain is adequately controlled as excess pain is a risk for postoperative delirium), and use caution when prescribing antihistamine H_1 antagonists and other medications with strong anticholinergic effects—all to decrease the risk of postoperative delirium.[75] Regarding other medications: maintain β-blockade if already initiated; maintain or consider starting perioperative statin therapy; adjust doses of medications based on glomerular filtration rate (GFR) not on serum creatinine; and monitor for polypharmacy and potential adverse interactions, discontinuing nonessential medications when possible.[75] Monitor renal function, as preoperative renal dysfunction measured by creatinine and estimated GFR is an independent predictor of interval to death for cardiac surgical patients (see Fig. 21.7).[78]

Carotid angiography or duplex studies are appropriate in elderly patients. Cerebral imagining using CT or magnetic resonance imaging (MRI) remains the gold standard for defining cerebral pathology.[4] As physicians ultimately responsible for the surgical patient, the referring cardiologist, surgeon and anaesthetist must advocate for the patient to receive all the appropriate preoperative evaluations and interventions to ensure the patient can make informed decisions and receive the highest quality care.

Cardiopulmonary bypass and the elderly

Beside surgical trauma and ischaemia, blood contact with the non-physiological surfaces of the extracorporeal circuit is a major trigger of the so-called systemic inflammatory response syndrome occurring after cardiac surgery—an inflammatory reaction associated with CPB that has been recognized for more than three decades. Despite enormous efforts to understand the complex mechanisms underlying this phenomenon, and to avoid its related systemic deleterious effects, it is still quite poorly understood.[79] The incidence and severity of complications increases with length of time spent on CPB, as many of the deleterious effects are secondary to blood exposure to non-endothelial surfaces (contact activation) and the consequent activation of the coagulation, kallikrein, fibrinolytic, and complement systems.[80,81] Miniaturized CPB systems—a closed CPB with a shorter circuit line, and without cardiotomy suction and venous reservoir thus avoiding air–blood contact—have been evaluated as a promising alternative to conventional CPB by reducing the inflammatory response, postoperative organ complications and blood transfusion.[79,82]

Animal studies have shown that the cardioprotection afforded by cardioplegia is modulated by age and gender, and is significantly decreased in the aged female.[83] Specific pathways in the mitochondrion modulate cardioprotection on CPB in the aged (particularly in the elderly female), and alterations in these pathways significantly contributes to decreased myocardial functional recovery and increased myonecrosis following ischaemia.[83] Autoregulation of cerebral blood flow (CBF) ensures delivery of oxygenated blood to the brain commensurate with cerebral O_2 demand. Impaired cerebral autoregulation may predispose patients to cerebral hypoperfusion during CPB, and disturbed autoregulation is independently associated with mortality after brain injury.[84] Impaired CBF autoregulation might contribute to brain ischaemic injury when the arterial pressure is low (such as during CPB), and by leading to brain hyperaemia with high arterial pressure increasing cerebral embolic load and promoting cerebral oedema in the setting of the systemic inflammation from CPB.[84] Increased age predisposes to impaired cognition after cardiac surgery, however cognitive dysfunction after CPB in the elderly cannot be explained by impaired CBF autoregulation as autoregulation is not affected by increases in age.[84,85] Use of IABP perioperatively does not adversely affect cerebral autoregulation, but reductions in the inflation ratio during counterpulsation weaning can progressively worsen the efficiency of cerebral autoregulation and increase the risk for cerebral hypoperfusion.[86]

Cognitive deficits after cardiac surgery were thought to be caused by the physiological disturbances associated with CPB, and that 'off-pump' coronary revascularization (OPCAB) may potentially be associated with improved outcomes. However, long-term follow-up studies have failed to demonstrate a significant reduction in the incidence of postoperative cognitive dysfunction with OPCAB versus 'on-pump' CABG.[87] It is important to note that there are relatively few trials that compare the various options for myocardial revascularization in the elderly and high-risk patient, and it is difficult and inappropriate to extrapolate the results of trials including younger, low-risk patients to the high-risk groups.[88] Demaria et al.[89] (125 octogenarians, observational study) reported significantly lower operative mortality and stroke after OPCAB; Ricci et al.[90] (269 octogenarians, observational study) reported significantly lower perioperative stroke and a higher freedom from major perioperative complications—however, the patients also required a higher need for re-operation and had a non-significant trend towards higher operative mortality in the OPCAB group. Another study found that OPCAB and CABG had similar rates of operative mortality but a significant reduction in major complications occurred in the OPCAB group except for a higher rate of perioperative myocardial infarction.[91] For octogenarians OPCAB offers a safe and effective alternative to CABG which confers a number of short-term benefits, but may have adverse differences in mortality or outcomes in the long term. A recent meta-analysis summarized that OPCAB in patients over 80 years of age is associated with significantly lower postoperative stroke and with a trend toward better early survival; however, suboptimal quality of the available studies, particularly the lack of comparability of the study groups, prevents conclusive results.[45] Additionally, a Cochrane Database systematic review of 86 trials did not demonstrate any significant benefit for OPCAB regarding mortality, stroke, or MI; and in contrast observed better long-term survival in patients undergoing on-pump CABG (see Figs. 21.8 and 21.9)[91,92]

Stroke is a significant cause of the high morbidity and mortality in elderly patients undergoing CABG. However, the focus is starting to shift from CPB towards factors common to both on and off-pump techniques such as surgery, anaesthesia, postoperative critical care, and patient-related predisposing factors. Priming of the immune system by ageing and atherosclerosis may result in an exaggerated systemic and cerebral inflammatory response to cardiac surgery and

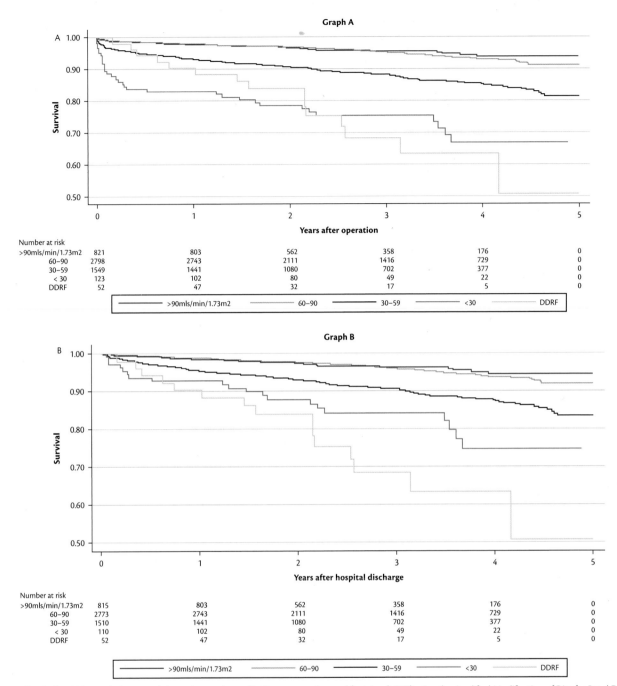

Fig. 21.7 The Kaplan-Meier survival curves of the study sample stratified by preoperative renal function (eGFR) using the simplified Modification of Diet for Renal Disease (MDRD) formula with follow-up data obtained from the National Death Index. The greatest early mortality occurred in the severe renal dysfunction group; however, the DDRF group showed increased mortality over time compared with the other groups. An eGFR of approximately 90 mL/min/1.73 m² was associated with the best survival outcomes. A, The sample from the time of surgery. B, The actuarial survival for those discharged alive from the hospital. DDRF, Dialysis-dependent renal failure. Reprinted from *The Journal of Thoracic and Cardiovascular Surgery*, 146, 1, Dhanani J, Mullany DV, et al., 'Effect of preoperative renal function on long-term survival after cardiac surgery', pp. 90–95, Copyright 2012, with permission from Elsevier, The American Association for Thoracic Surgery, and The Western Thoracic Surgical Association.

anaesthesia, causing neuronal loss or dysfunction resulting in cognitive dysfunction independent of any affects from CPB.[87]

Intraoperative management and the elderly

Appropriate selection of the elderly patient for cardiac surgery generally means that intraoperative management does not differ significantly from comparative younger patients. There are, however, certain practices that pertain to this age group that yield improved results and outcomes.

The main complication of cardiac surgery in the elderly patient compared with the younger patient is the increased incidence of cerebrovascular damage and stroke.[90] One explanation is increased atherosclerosis of the ascending aorta, which correlates significantly with the age of the patient and may be a good predictor of early

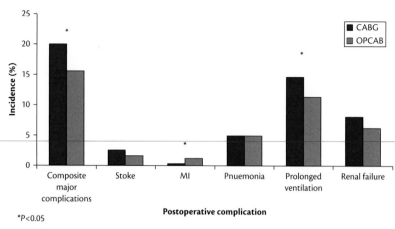

Fig. 21.8 Incidence of postoperative outcomes contributing to composite incidence of major complications for patients undergoing primary, isolated CABG or OPCAB operations. Compared with OPCAB, conventional CABG incurred more postoperative atrial fibrillation (28.4% vs 21.5%; P = .003), prolonged ventilation (14.7% vs 11.4%; P = .05), and major complications (P = .04). Importantly, postoperative stroke (2.6% vs 1.7%; P = .21) and renal failure (8.1% vs 6.2%; P = .12) rates were no different between groups. Despite more complications in CABG patients, operative mortality was similar after both CABG (5.1%) and OPCAB (5.9%; P =.53) operations. Moreover, patients had similar total hospital (P = .75) and postoperative (P = .41) lengths of stay as well as similar total costs (P = .43). MI, Myocardial infarction; CABG, conventional coronary artery bypass grafting; OPCAB, off-pump coronary artery bypass grafting. Reprinted from *The Journal of Thoracic and Cardiovascular Surgery*, 141, 1, LaPar DJ, Castigliano M, et al., 'Is off-pump coronary artery bypass grafting superior to conventional bypass in octogenarians?', pp. 81–90, Copyright 2011, with permission from Elsevier, The American Association for Thoracic Surgery, and The Western Thoracic. Surgical Association.

postoperative cognitive dysfunction (POCD) and stroke due to the resultant cerebral emboli.[93,94] Epiaortic ultrasound scanning is strongly recommended in the elderly to ensure an appropriate site of aortic cannulation and cross-clamping, and can lead to consideration of OPCAB or an aortic no-touch surgical procedure.[95,96] Intraoperative epiaortic ultrasound scanning changes the operative planning in 4 per cent of patients, improving neurological outcome in a large series of 6051 patients by reducing the rate of postoperative stroke, and is superior to transoesophageal echocardiography (TOE) for aortic assessment.[97,98] In addition to aortic atheroma, microvascular disease and impaired cerebral autoregulation may predispose patients to cerebral hypoperfusion during CPB and resultant stroke or cognitive dysfunction.[84] Cerebral autoregulation is not impaired in the average elderly patient on CPB; however, 20 per cent of all patients do suffer from impaired autoregulation, and the elderly may suffer a greater adverse outcome from the presence of this

impaired autoregulation.[84] Patients with impaired autoregulation are more likely than those with functional autoregulation to have perioperative stroke.[84] Most patients undergoing on-pump cardiac surgery undergo mild hypothermia. It is known that re-warming can disrupt cerebral autoregulation—and in particular, since such a large proportion of the cardiac output passes through the brain, fast re-warming can cause cerebral hyperthermia, which is known to be associated with adverse cognitive outcomes.[87] Cerebral oximetry is a non-invasive method to detect imbalances in the cerebral oxygen supply/demand-ratio and can lead to changes in the intraoperative care to improve the cerebral oxygenation—an important consideration when studies show that a low preoperative and intraoperative cerebral saturation is associated with postoperative delirium after on-pump cardiac surgery in the elderly, and is significantly associated with an increased risk of cognitive decline and prolonged hospital stay after CABG.[99,100] Measurement of cerebral oxygen

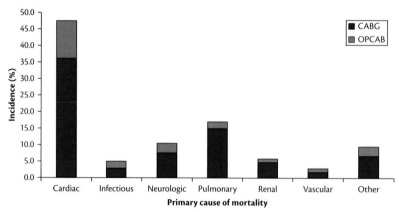

Fig. 21.9 Incidence of primary cause of mortality for decedents after isolated CABG or OPCAB operations. There were several different causes for mortality among those undergoing coronary artery bypass grafting operations. Overall, the most common primary cause of patient mortality was cardiac in origin (47.6%), followed by pulmonary (17.1%) and neurologic (10.5%) etiologies. Renal causes accounted for 5.7% of patient mortality whereas infections were responsible for 4.8% of deaths. *CABG*, Conventional coronary artery bypass grafting; *OPCAB*, off-pump coronary artery bypass grafting. Reprinted from *The Journal of Thoracic and Cardiovascular Surgery*, 141, 1, LaPar DJ, Castigliano M, et al., 'Is off-pump coronary artery bypass grafting superior to conventional bypass in octogenarians?', pp. 81–90, Copyright 2011, with permission from Elsevier, The American Association for Thoracic Surgery, and The Western Thoracic Surgical Association.

saturation has been shown to be an early prediction tool in POCD if desaturation occurs—a feature that may allow for early intervention and therefore prevention (see Fig. 21.10).[99,101,102]

Haematopoietic mechanisms are depressed with ageing, and geriatric tissue fragility and atherosclerosis may cause increased bleeding.[4] Coagulopathy is a common occurrence after any procedure with CPB—as the plasmatic system is affected by haemodilution, hypothermia, rewarming, contact factor activation, and non-physiological flow patterns.[103] In the elderly, blood conservation strategies such as antifibrinolytics, cell saver, and point-of-care tests such as thromboelastography (TEG®) or ROTEM® can be used to guide post-CPB transfusion of fresh frozen plasma, platelets, or other clotting factors if required.[4,80,103] Avoidance of blood or blood product transfusion during or after cardiac surgery is important, as it is associated with increased short-term and long-term mortality.[104] There is no doubt that the physiological reserve of elderly patients is decreased, and excellent/expeditious surgery, meticulous haemostasis, accurate organ perfusion and perfect myocardial protection are absolutely critical for cardiac surgical success.

Postoperative critical care

Depleted physiological reserves and substantial burden of chronic disease place the elderly at greatly increased risk of morbidity and

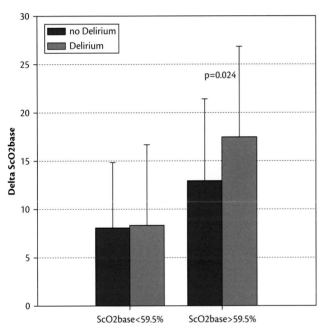

Fig. 21.10 Intraoperative changes in cerebral oximetry (ScO$_2$ox) in patients with or without delirium classified by normal or low preoperative ScO$_2$. Delta ScO$_2$base: difference between preoperative regional cerebral oxygen saturation with oxygen supplementation and minimal intraoperative regional cerebral oxygen saturation; ScO$_2$base: regional cerebral oxygen saturation with supplemental oxygen. In patients who started with low ScO$_2$ox, the groups with and without delirium did not differ in delta ScO$_2$ox. But in patients who started at a normal level of ScO$_2$ox, those patients who developed delirium had larger intraoperative drops in ScO$_2$ox. The positive predictive value for ScO$_2$ox of not more than 59.5% on delirium was 0.56, and the negative predictive value was 0.80. Schoen J, Meyerrose J, et al., 'Preoperative regional cerebral oxygen saturation is a predictor of postoperative delirium in on-pump cardiac surgery patients: a prospective observational trial', *Critical Care*, 15, 5, pp. R218. © 2011 Schoen et al.; licensee BioMed Central Ltd. Reproduced with permission under the Creative Commons Licence 2.0 http://creativecommons.org/licenses/by/2.0/uk/legalcode.

mortality following cardiac surgery. They enter the cardiac theatre with a substantial burden of chronic morbidities, and the stressors of surgery, cardiopulmonary bypass, non-pulsatile circulation, relative hypoperfusion, induced hypothermia, and haemodilution add insult to injury—manifesting as a number of organ dysfunction syndromes. Whilst the surgical procedure is generally similar to younger cohorts, the STS risk calculator demonstrates that the risk incurred with coronary grafting doubles in a 65-year-old versus a 50-year-old—and is increased fivefold in a patient of 80 years.[105] These risks are the result of dysfunction in several organ systems—subclinical in isolation, but significant in combination (see Table 21.2).

Postoperative organ dysfunction begins subclinically in the cardiac theatre. Hence meticulous preprocedural planning and optimal intraoperative management have great relevance to successful outcomes of elderly patients undergoing cardiac surgery.

ICU management

Respiratory

Age-dependant changes are standard in pulmonary function—a progressive decline in FRC and FEV$_1$ occurs from age 65 upwards, with FEV$_1$ change of 50 ml/year.[106] Changes occur at the parenchymal level, as well as the mechanical properties of the lung and chest wall, and decreased oxygen diffusing capacity is associated with survival changes as opposed to FEV$_1$ which is not.[107]

Postoperatively, prolonged ventilation is an independent marker of cost, morbidity and short- and long-term mortality.[108] Early extubation minimizes the need for sedation and therefore potentially reduces vasopressor requirements, optimizes the ability to expectorate, and maximizes chances of early mobilization. Extubation, however, is dependent on adequate and stable cardiac function, minimal bleeding and normal neurological function. Recent data indicates the strong association of positive fluid balance with prolonged ventilation, and all the associated problems.[109] Early diuresis should be encouraged, though not to the detriment of cardiac output or renal dysfunction. High-flow oxygen delivery devices that produce a degree of positive end-expiratory pressure and optimize FRC particularly in patients with a high body mass index, may facilitate early extubation.[110] If early extubation is not safely possible, percutaneous tracheostomy should be considered to allow liberation from the ventilator, optimal toileting of airway and minimization of sedative agents.[111]

Cardiovascular

Protection of perfusion pressure and cardiac output are non-negotiable in post-cardiac surgical patients. Surgical manipulation, cardioplegia, anaesthesia, and CPB all reduce cardiac function in the early postoperative phase, particularly when preoperative cardiac function is impaired. Despite minimal robust data to support its use, it is the authors' opinion that low-dose inotropy may be associated with less adverse effects than copious quantities of fluid given to support the circulation until the heightened inflammatory process diminishes and systolic and diastolic function normalize. Monitoring cardiac function is essential, although data does not support the routine use of a pulmonary artery catheter. Echocardiography in experienced hands provides more direct information on both physiological function as well as mechanical issues including new regional wall motion abnormalities, pericardial collections, and valve function with minimal risk. Whilst

Table 21.2 Physiological comorbidities and changes in the elderly

Physiological system	Age-induced changes	
Cardiovascular	↓ cardiac output ↓ response to inotropes / catecholamines	↑ diastolic dysfunction ↑ atherosclerosis and arterial stiffening ↑ blood pressure ↑ coronary artery disease
Respiratory	↓ vital capacity/DLCO/VO_2 max ↓ elastic recoil of the lung (senile emphysema) ↓ maximum midexpiratory flow rate / FEV_1 ↓ mucociliary function	↑ residual volume/functional residual capacity ↑ A–a gradient ↑ V/Q mismatch ↑ closing volume ↑ kyphosis (decreased chest compliance)
Renal	↓ renal size ↓ glomerular number ↓ creatinine clearance (GFR decrease) ↓ tubular function ↓ Na and K reabsorption	↑ blood urea nitrogen (BUN) ↑ $T_{1/2}$ of renally cleared medications ↑ prostate size ↑ dehydration risk ↑ glomerular and tubulointerstitial fibrosis
Central nervous system	↓ brain size (but no change in intelligence) ↓ motor neuron function ↓ autonomic nervous system adaptability	↑ subclinical cognitive impairment↑ senile dementia ↑ postoperative cognitive dysfunction (POCD)
Haematological	↓ bone marrow response to blood loss ↓ platelet number (thrombocytopenia) ↓ immune function	↑ anaemia ↑ CPB-induced platelet dysfunction
Gastrointestinal	↓ oesophageal function (presbyoesophagus) ↓ intrinsic factor production ↓ colon peristaltic function (chronic constipation) ↓ liver size and synthetic function	↑ atrophic gastritis ↑ achlorhydria ↑ $T_{1/2}$ of hepatic metabolized medications ↑ malnutrition
Endocrine	↓ lean body mass ↓ # and function of pancreatic β cells ↓ glucose homeostasis ↓ vitamin level (vitamin C/folate/thiamine deficiency)	↑ peripheral insulin resistance ↑ adiposity ↑ osteoporosis
Musculoskeletal and Integument	↓ turnover of dermal cells ↓ wound healing ↑ muscle mass/strength/endurance ↑ ability to mobilize and exercise	↑ epidermal atrophy ↑ skin ulcers ↑ degenerative joint disease

optimal imaging with transthoracic echocardiography (TTE) is difficult in the ventilated postoperative cardiac patient, it can be supplemented with TOE. Contrast echocardiography may be utilized to substantially increase the power of TTE, and avoid the sedation and airway support necessitated for TOE.[112,113]

Management of bleeding

Early and immediate management of bleeding minimizes transfusion requirements, reduces hospital stay, and prevents the risk associated with transfusion. Infective risks of transfusion still exist, but are dwarfed by TRALI (transfusion-related acute lung injury) and the mounting data associating perioperative transfusion with increased short- and long-term morbidity and mortality.[104] Determining the cause of bleeding can be difficult, but the perioperative use of point of care technology such as ROTEM* and TEG* may aid in determining the cause of bleeding and is associated with reduced product

requirement.[114] Prolonged blood loss indicates that an early return to theatre may be required to exclude surgical causes of bleeding. Patients who return to theatre in the first 12 hours postoperatively are discharged at the same time as patients who do not require re-opening.[115] Those allowed to bleed for more than 12 hours prior to their return to theatre have a prolonged ICU and hospital stay. There is no randomized controlled study proving blood transfusion is associated with a worse outcome; however data continues to support the association, though more research is needed to guide transfusion requirements in the post cardiac surgical patient.[116]

Renal function

Age-related deterioration in renal function is typical even in a 20-year-old, and the slope of deterioration is increased due to autoregulatory dysfunction typical in the elderly.[117] Non-pulsatile CPB, relative hypoperfusion, inflammation, hypothermia, and relative hypovolaemia all play a part in inducing postoperative renal dysfunction.[118] OPCAB is not associated with a lesser risk of renal dysfunction.[119] Preoperative renal dysfunction has been shown to be an independent predictor of long-term mortality in cardiac surgery patients.[78] It is common, although the majority of patients reach their nadir at the 2nd to 3rd day and begin to recover with optimal fluid management and avoidance of hypoperfusion and nephrotoxins. Drugs such as dopamine and frusemide may induce a diuresis, but do not alter the incidence of renal failure.[120] They may, however, be useful in achieving a negative fluid balance preventing further pulmonary insults or adverse sequelae. If fluid excess cannot be reversed, or metabolic abnormalities are overwhelming, renal replacement should be instituted with the knowledge that post-cardiac surgery patients requiring renal replacement have substantially worse outcomes.[121]

Neurological dysfunction

Neurological dysfunction, common in the standard cardiac surgical population, is much more common in the elderly, and can manifest as delayed wakening post surgery, a confusional state, delirium, or even a dense hemiplegia. Inflammation, hypoperfusion, and embolization in the setting of an abnormal vascular tree all collude to induce alternation in neurological function in up to 70 per cent of patients.[122,123] Excellence in intraoperative management and monitoring of brain perfusion has been shown to reduce both ICU stay and neurological complications.[124] Again, OPCAB has not resulted in improved neurological function.[125]

Nutritional status

Catabolism is normal following any large operation, but may be even more profound in the elderly, who often present to surgery nutritionally deplete. Preoperative assessment and assistance to obtain a nutritionally optimized patient minimizes the risk of postoperative refeeding syndrome and puts the patient in the best position for recovery.[126]

Postoperative pain control

Perioperative pain is poorly assessed and managed, with elderly patients at a higher risk of adverse consequences from under-relieved and under-treated pain.[127] Pre-emptive analgesia has been attempted for cardiac surgery with medications such as gabapentin, although the results have not consistently shown an improvement in postoperative pain scores or decreased opioid usage.[128–130] Oral paracetamol is effective in this patient cohort, and the intravenous form is useful when concerns arise of postoperative gastrointestinal tract stasis. Management of postoperative opioid analgesia in elderly cardiac patients is challenging—effectively treating pain decreases the occurrence of a stress reaction and may even prevent chronic postoperative pain; however, large doses of opioids are associated with sedation and respiratory depression.[131,132] In addition to producing deterioration in physiological, physical, mental and cognitive functions, natural ageing causes changes in the pharmacodynamics and pharmacokinetics of drugs, and sensitivity to the actions of opioids is increased with age while clearance of opioids is reduced.[131] No specific study on the ideal opioid for the elderly has been performed, but it can be concluded that opioids are efficacious in both acute and chronic non-cancer pain in the elderly. Functional impairment of excretory organs is common in the elderly, affecting both the liver and kidneys. For all opioids except buprenorphine, the half-life of the active drug and metabolites is increased in the elderly and in patients with renal dysfunction.[133,134] It is recommended that—except for buprenorphine—doses be reduced, a longer time interval be used between doses, creatinine clearance be monitored, and that buprenorphine may be considered to be the top-line choice for opioid treatment in the elderly once extubated if both hepatic and renal function is affected.[133,134]

One study on postoperative pain control[131] elucidated that after cardiac surgery with inhalation anaesthesia and a fentanyl regimen based on body weight, the fentanyl concentration in plasma was higher in elderly (mean 80 years) than in younger patients (mean 52 years) (see Fig. 21.11).[131]

Additionally, after extubation the plasma levels of intravenously administered standardized doses of oxycodone hydrochloride were similar in the older and the younger patients, but older patients had better pain relief and became more deeply sedated after the 3rd dose of oxycodone hydrochloride (see Fig. 21.12).[131]

Attempting to avoid systemic opioids and utilizing pain control methods such as thoracic epidural anaesthesia or spinal opioids may be better in the elderly,[135,136] because thoracic epidural anaesthesia produces a higher stroke volume index and central venous oxygenation without an increase in heart rate or mean arterial pressure in elderly cardiac surgery patients.[137] However, significant discourse still occurs on this topic,[138] as thoracic epidural anaesthesia does not reduce the time in the ICU or improve the quality of recovery, while unduly putting patients at risk for catastrophic bleeding and neurological complications. Systemic opioids still remain the mainstay of treatment for acute pain post-cardiac surgery in the elderly patient. However, particular attention needs to be paid to the dosing of opioids in elderly surgical patients, who often need a smaller amount for adequate analgesia than younger adults and may require different types of opioids based on organ system dysfunction. There are no clearly superior drugs or regimens, however the appropriate drug should be chosen based on safety and tolerability considerations with an understanding of the differences in pharmacokinetics and pharmacodynamics in the elderly patient.[132,134]

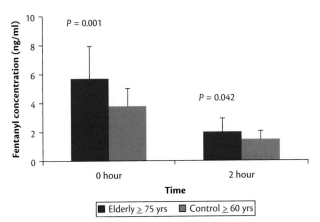

Fig. 21.11 Plasma concentrations of fentanyl after the continuous i.v. infusion at the end of cardiac surgery and 2 h later. At the end of surgery and 2 h later, the mean plasma concentrations of fentanyl were significantly higher in the older patients than in the younger ones (P = 0.042). Reproduced with permission from Pesonen A, Suojaranta-Ylinen R, et al., 'Comparison of effects and plasma concentrations of opioids between elderly and middle-aged patients after cardiac surgery', *Acta Anaesthesiologica Scandinavica*, 53, 1, pp. 101–108, 2009, Wiley © 2008 The Authors. Journal compilation © 2008 The Acta Anaesthesiologica Scandinavica Foundation.

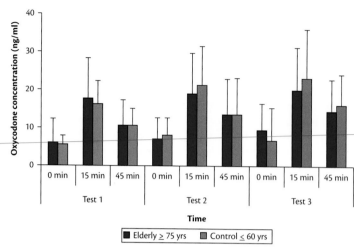

Fig. 21.12 Plasma concentrations of oxycodone during the three tests after extubation in the ICU. The time interval from extubation to the first post-extubation oxycodone hydrochloride dose did not differ between the two groups. At this time, the mean plasma concentration of oxycodone was 6.3 ± 6.2 ng/ml in the older group and 5.7 ± 2.3 ng/ml in the younger group (NS). At the time of the second request of oxycodone, as well as 15 and 45 min later, the mean plasma concentration of oxycodone was slightly higher compared with time 0 of the first oxycodone test, but not to a statistically significant extent, and with no differences between the two age groups. Reproduced with permission from Pesonen A, Suojaranta-Ylinen R, et al., 'Comparison of effects and plasma concentrations of opioids between elderly and middle-aged patients after cardiac surgery', *Acta Anaesthesiologica Scandinavica*, 53, 1, pp. 101–108, 2009, Wiley © 2008 The Authors. Journal compilation © 2008 The Acta Anaesthesiologica Scandinavica Foundation.

Neurocognitive changes after cardiac surgery

The neurological consequences of CABG are well known, but there remains uncertainty about the severity and timing of postoperative cognitive decline and its relationship with any underlying damage to the brain. Adverse cerebral complications after cardiac surgery—including postoperative stroke (CVA), POCD, brain injury (BI), and silent brain injury (SBI)—are associated with prolonged hospitalization, excessive operative mortality, high hospital costs, and altered quality of life.[96] There is a continuum of decline from mild, transient cognitive impairment without evidence of brain insult, to the more devastating occurrence of clinical stroke, and perhaps enhancing the onset of dementia.[139] The American College of Cardiology and the American Heart Association have classified neurological complications after cardiac surgery into two categories, namely type I and type II.[140] Type I neurological deficits include stroke and transient ischaemic attack, coma and fatal cerebral injury; type II neurological deficits are diffuse and not well-defined, and include delirium and POCD, involving deficits of memory, concentration, and psychomotor speed.[140] An understanding of the magnitude, time course, and profile of any cognitive decline following CABG surgery is necessary for risk assessment and possible implementation of neuroprotective strategies.[139] There is a significant divergence in the literature on what the definition of delirium and postoperative cognitive decline after cardiac surgery should encompass, and when patients should be assessed for this cognitive impairment. Murkin and colleagues provided some coherence on the topic in 1995, drafting a consensus statement on the assessment of cognitive function after cardiac surgery.[141] Despite years of study many facets of the incidence, pathogenesis, and consequences of SBI remain to be clarified. It has long been assumed that cerebral embolism associated with CPB, or triggered by intracardiac and intra-aortic manipulation, accounts for both postoperative stroke and POCD.[142] There is a significantly decreased rate of stroke when manipulation of the ascending aorta was avoided during CABG.[143]

No studies isolated the impact of aortic manipulation in the elderly population to determine the true nature of this question, however given that the atherosclerotic burden increases with age it is very likely to be relevant. There are alternative explanations however (e.g. procedure-associated cerebral hypoperfusion or the effects of perioperative drug therapy), with perhaps the most telling observation that POCD can occur in one-third of elderly patients after major non-cardiac surgery.[142] Ageing without any comorbidities is associated with low-grade systemic inflammatory activity which may predispose the elderly individual to a higher likelihood of POCD.[87] Whether focusing on surgery or patient-related causative factors of POCD, a recurring theme is the inflammatory response—and speculation that the systemic inflammation known to be associated with cardiac surgery and to cause dysfunction of several organ systems via inflammatory effects also results in neuronal inflammation and cognitive dysfunction (see Table 21.3).[87]

Two recent meta-analyses demonstrated only very limited differences between on- and off-pump groups.[139,144] OPCAB patients tested better at the Digit Symbol subtest at the earlier time points, while conversely the on-pump group performed better at late follow-up.[139,144] The speculation is that brain vulnerability to transient hypoxia might help explain certain findings in this population—such as the association of early postoperative cognitive decline with intraoperative mean arterial pressure and cerebral oximetry abnormalities—however, simple measures to improve intraoperative brain oxygenation do not improve early cognitive outcome.[100,139] Cardiac surgery may provide the catalyst for a new cognitive deficit in some elderly patients, yet in others it may be an added burden on a neurocognitive system that was already showing decline. In these cases it is important to explore potentially modifiable perioperative risk factors that may be associated with further brain insult. EEG, transcranial Doppler sonography (embolus detection) and cerebral oximetry can indicate acute deficits in brain perfusion and oxygenation during surgery; in fact the simple presence of such neuromonitoring can reduce the incidence of neural injury.[139] SBI is common in healthy elderly people and

Table 21.3 Binary logistic regression with preoperative predictors of delirium in patients undergoing cardiac surgery. Age, MMSE, neurological disease, and ScO_2ox could be identified as independent predictors of delirium

Parameter	P value	Specification	Prevalence delirium, percentage	Odds ratio	95% CI
Age	0.005	<70 years	13.0	Reference	
		≥70 years	40.5	4.30	1.54–12.04
MMSE score	0.018	>27	12.2	Reference	
		24–27	27.4	2.23	0.76–6.52
		≤23	61.3	6.50	1.75–24.13
Additive EuroScore	0.934	0 to 3	12.1	Reference	
		4 to 6	27.2	0.74	0.19–2.83
		7 to 9	37.1	0.98	0.24–3.95
		10 to 20	40.0	0.77	0.17–3.46
Neurological disease	0.001	No	22.0	Reference	
		Yes	55.2	6.22	2.02–19.16
Haemoglobin	0.513	>120 g/L	20.4	Reference	
		≤120 g/L	47.9	0.72	0.27–1.93
NTproBNP	0.447	<1000 pg/ml	17.4	Reference	
		≥1000 pg/ml	41.0	1.43	0.57–3.58
Baseline ScO_2 with O_2	0.027	>59.5%	19.7	Reference	
		≤59.5%	58.3	3.27	1.14–9.37

CI, confidence interval; MMSE, Mini-Mental Status Examination; NTproBNP, N-terminal pro B-type natriuretic peptide; O_2, oxygen; ScO_2ox, cerebral oxygen saturation.

Reproduced with permission from van Harten AE, Scheeren TW, Absalom AR, 'A review of postoperative cognitive dysfunction and neuroinflammation associated with cardiac surgery and anaesthesia', *Anaesthesia*, 67, 3, pp. 280–293, Anaesthesia © 2012 The Association of Anaesthetists of Great Britain and Ireland.

describes a focal ischaemic lesion detected by brain imaging without a history of transient ischaemic attack (TIA) or CVA to explain the imaging findings.[96] The prevalence of postoperative neurological complications in patients with SBI is related to advanced age, renal dysfunction, preoperative cognitive dysfunction, atherosclerosis of the ascending aorta, and intracranial arterial stenosis.[96] Preoperative cognitive impairment is common in patients with SBI and BI, and may reflect diffuse cerebral vascular lesions present preoperatively.[96] MRI examination of the brain both pre- and postoperatively provides a means of identifying and quantifying brain injury even in the absence of clinical signs, and potentially reduces or eliminates the problem of accurate ascertainment of perioperative SBI by neurocognitive testing.[142] However, MRI is contraindicated with certain valve replacements and pacing wires.

Heart transplantation and mechanical assist devices

Data suggests that carefully selected elderly patients have good outcomes and an improved quality of life after cardiac surgery; however, surgical interventions such as heart transplantation and implantation of ventricular assist devices (VADs) are not universally indicated. The lack of biological reserve to withstand such invasive procedures, the severe systemic inflammatory response from VADs, the challenge of extreme immunosuppression for heart transplantation and the higher risk of thromboembolism in the elderly patient top the list of factors that mitigate against their inclusion in such programmes.[145,146] Additionally, the current climate of a worldwide organ shortage and healthcare cost rationing often precludes the very elderly from these life-sustaining procedures.

Individuals being considered for LVAD implantation fall into two general categories: bridge to transplant (BTT) and destination therapy (DT). VADs are approved as DT (permanent use without plans for transplantation) in individuals with advanced heart failure who are not candidates for a cardiac transplant, and as such, they are being increasingly used in older adults. Data from the United States shows that the mean age of individuals undergoing DT from June 2006 to January 2010 was 61.7 (range 23–82), compared with 52.7 (range 19–88) for individuals receiving LVADs for all other indications.[147] Technology is rapidly evolving, and DT is becoming available in many centres, such that an increase in the numbers of older adults considered for this therapy can be expected.[147] Recent studies suggest positive effects of DT on symptom management, quality of life, and functional capacity prompting consideration of mechanical circulatory support as a viable treatment option for individuals with advanced heart failure seeking palliation.[146,148,149] LVAD patients 70 or more years of age in one research analysis[150] had good functional recovery, survival, and quality of life at 2 years, and the authors stated that advanced age should not be used as an independent contraindication when selecting a patient for LVAD therapy at experienced centres. Although LVADs increase quality of life and survival, the associated treatment burdens and complications deserve careful consideration. Clear guidance regarding the use of DT that addresses the risks, burdens and societal costs in older adults is required. In addition, the full inclusion of palliative care and geriatric medicine teams in the care of individuals receiving destination mechanical support is absolutely essential for these devices to be used successfully in this age group.

Weaning from CPB entails the progressive transition from full mechanical support to spontaneous heart activity that provides sufficient blood flow and perfusion to body systems. Elderly patients with numerous comorbidities may require additional pharmacological support, and additionally 1 per cent of patients may need additional mechanical assistance to bridge the gap between CPB and full self-sufficient perfusion.[151] Insertion of IABP should be considered in patients with ongoing instability to reduce LV afterload, improve coronary diastolic blood flow, and increase systemic oxygen delivery.[152] High-risk patients should have the IABP inserted preoperatively or pre-CPB. A recent cohort study of 7440 patients confirms that preoperative IABP is associated with strong trends to reduced mortality despite higher predicted mortality based on risk scoring.[153] Additionally, post-CPB IABP insertion is associated with a higher operative mortality (10 per cent vs 16 per cent).[152,153] Extra-corporeal membrane oxygenation (ECMO) is also a consideration for short-term therapy of cardiorespiratory failure after cardiac surgery—especially for patients with RV failure, severe pulmonary oedema and persistent ventricular dysrhythmias.[152] The advantage or peripherally inserted fem-fem ECMO in comparison to IABP is that it provides not only cardiopulmonary support, but biventricular support, oxygenated blood flow to vital organs, and flow even during periods of severe bradycardia or tachycardia.[151,154] ECMO is a good option for temporary (up to 1 week) support of critically ill patients to gain time for biventricular function to improve and allow for unhurried decisions to be made on the usefulness or futility of further therapy.

Minimally invasive and transcatheter valvular techniques

Emerging techniques are coming to the fore to treat valvular heart disease. Aortic valve stenosis is the most common debilitating valvular heart lesion in adults, and surgical aortic valve replacement is the treatment of choice for the vast majority of affected individuals.[31] Advanced age is a risk factor for mortality after AVR. Hospital mortality after AVR in octogenarians varies from 5–7 per cent; and except for Thourani et al. who reported a mortality of 16.4 per cent in high-risk elderly patients undergoing AVR, there are few studies focusing on mortality in the high-risk elderly group.[34,35,155] In some series, 30–40 per cent of patients are considered too high a risk for surgery and remain untreated—a cohort expected to increase due to the ageing population and improved therapeutic options in patients with multiple comorbidities and advanced medical conditions.[156] Medical management carries a poor prognosis and the effects of percutaneous balloon aortic valvuloplasty are modest and short lived.[157,158] Since AVR in high-risk elderly is associated with higher early morbidity and mortality, and poor 5-year survival, non-conventional methods of AVR are increasingly being offered. Transcatheter aortic valve implantation (TAVI), a minimally invasive technique, minimizes surgical trauma by avoiding sternotomy,

aortotomy, and the use of CPB; and by implanting the prosthesis into a beating heart, avoids cardiac arrest in order to improve postoperative patient outcome. The PARTNER trial compared TAVI to open surgery or medical management with the primary outcome measure to prove non-inferiority to conventional AVR.[159,160] The trial showed TAVI was no worse than surgery at 1 year and better than medical management, albeit with a higher stroke rate—a situation that was maintained at 2-year follow-up.[160] Nevertheless, according to the ACCF/AATS/SCAI/STS expert consensus document TAVI is a complex procedure that requires meticulous attention to detail to avoid complications, and the multi-specialty nature requires a team-based approach at selected high-volume centres.[156] Patient selection should be based on published randomized data. TAVI is recommended in patients with predicted survival more than 12 months, high surgical risk (EuroSCORE ≥20 per cent/STS score ≥10 per cent), and prohibitive surgical risk patients (50 per cent + risk of mortality or morbidity at 30 days) who are judged to have the potential to benefit—although indications are likely to evolve and encompass additional patients in the future.[156,157]

Percutaneous mitral valve procedures are also being performed. Percutaneous edge-to-edge leaflet stitching technique (MitraClip®—Abbott Vascular, Menlo Park, California) for mitral regurgitation is safer than surgery, although less effective.[161] The MitraClip® works on the principle of edge-to-edge (double orifice) repair which involves grasping the free edges of the anterior and posterior leaflets and clipping them together (see Fig. 21.13). Safety and feasibility of this procedure was demonstrated in the EVEREST1 trial.[162,163] EVEREST II trial showed non-inferiority of the MitraClip® to surgery, however MitraClip® was less effective in reducing MR and led to high rates of surgery requiring MVR on potentially repairable valves.[163] The majority of mitral techniques are under development and include: transcatheter leaflet repair, coronary sinus annuloplasty, direct annulus modification, chamber remodelling therapy and transcatheter mitral valve implantation.[161] Currently the mitral procedures are more experimental than practical, and are utilized in trial patients in highly specialized centres (see Table 21.4).[161]

Implantation of both the Edwards SAPIEN and the CoreValve in AS is usually performed via the transfemoral approach, which requires femoral artery access, retrograde crossing of the aortic

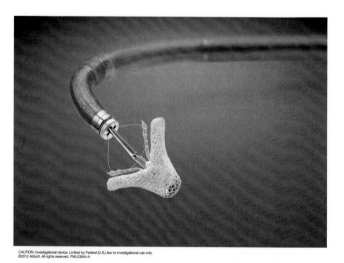

CAUTION: Investigational device. Limited by Federal (U.S.) law to investigational use only.
©2012 Abbott. All rights reserved. PML03944-A

Fig. 21.13 MitraClip device on catheter prior to insertion percutaneously. Reproduced with permission from Abbott Vascular, Santa Clara, California, © Abbott 2012.

Table 21.4 Investigational devices for treating mitral regurgitation

Approach	Devices	Manufacturer	MR types	Vascular access	Current development
Edge-to-edge leaflet repair	MitraClip*	Abbott Vascular Inc.	1, 2	Femoral vein, transseptal	Largest world experience
Coronary sinus annuloplasty (indirect annuloplasty)	MONARC	Edwards Lifesciences	2	Internal jugular vein, coronary sinus	First-in-man study published
	CARILLION™	Cardiac Dimensions	2	Internal jugular vein, coronary sinus	First-in-man study published
	PTMA*	Viacor Inc.	2	Subclavian vein, coronary sinus	First-in-man study published
Direct annulus modification	Percutaneous annuloplasty system (PAS)	Mitralign Guided delivery system	2	Femoral artery, retrograde to LV	First-in-man study performed
	AccuCinch*QuantumCor^a	QuantumCor	2	Femoral artery, retrograde to LV	Preclinical evaluation
Chamber remodelling therapy	PS3	Ample Medical Inc.	2	Transseptal, coronary sinus access	First-in-man study published
Percutaneous mitral valve implantation	EndoValve	EndoValve	1,2	Minithoracotomy and LA purse-string approach, transcatheter approach to follow	Preclinical evaluation

^aQuantumCor access is currently unknown, possibilities are transseptal or femoral artery then retrograde to the left ventricle.

LV: left ventricle; MR: mitral regurgitation; MR type 1: degenerative MR; MR type 2: functional MR; PS3: percutaneous septal sinus shortening system.

Reproduced with permission from Lam YY, Lee PW, et al., 'Investigational devices for mitral regurgitation: state of the art', *Expert Review Medical Devices*, 8, 1, pp. 105–114, © 2011 Expert Reviews Ltd.

valve, and retrograde valve deployment within the native aortic valve (see Figs 21.14–21.16).[164,165]

Deployment may be performed by balloon inflation under rapid ventricular pacing (RVP) or by slowly retracting the outer sheath without RVP.[164] The transfemoral approach may not be feasible in patients with significant aortic or ileo-femoral arterial disease and the transaxillary approach (performed via surgical isolation and direct puncture of the left axillary artery), transapical approach (access to the left ventricular cavity is typically obtained through a small anterolateral thoracotomy), and open surgical access to the retroperitoneal iliac artery and the ascending aorta are other options.[156,157,164] The presence of a patent LIMA graft is a relative contraindication to the use of the transaxillary approach because of the risk of occlusion or dissection, and the transapical approach raises concerns about chest wall discomfort and potential for respiratory compromise and prolonged ventilation in patients with severe respiratory dysfunction.[164,166] A complementary approach using both CE-approved devices and alternative routes tailored to

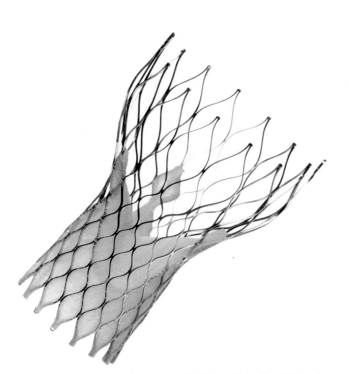

Fig. 21.14 Medtronic CoreValve system. With kind permission from Medtronic.

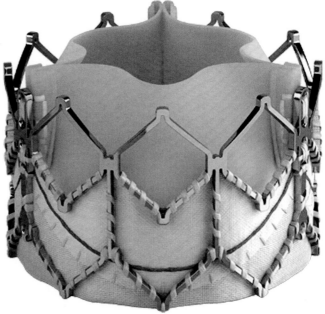

Fig. 21.15 Edwards Sapien valve system. With kind permission from Edwards Lifesciences LLC, Irvine, CA.

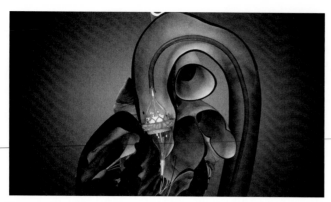

Fig. 21.16 Image of the Sapien valve in deployment phase. With kind permission from Edwards Lifesciences LLC, Irvine, CA.

the anatomy and the comorbidities of the appropriately selected patient is a main component for success.[156,166] The best characterization of risk should be a combination of objective quantitative predictive models (EuroSCORE and the STS) and subjective assessment by experienced surgeons, cardiologists, and anaesthetists.[166] Antiplatelet guidelines for TAVI are not universal, however common practice is administration of aspirin and clopidogrel loading doses before the procedure.[166] To minimize the risk for renal impairment, pre-procedural hydration and N-acetylcysteine can be administered the day before the TAVI.[166,167] Antihypertension drugs, including angiotensin-converting enzyme inhibitors, should be administrated until the day of the procedure; however antiarrhythmic drugs should be discontinued.[165,166]

The anaesthetist must have a participative role in developing monitoring and standards of care in the catheterization laboratory, which must be stocked with additional equipment and drugs that the anaesthetists typically require to manage difficult airways and haemodynamically unstable patients. Ideally, all procedures should be performed in a hybrid operating theatre with an angiography system.[165,168] Patients should be monitored with electrocardiography, pulse oximetry, urinary catheter, temperature, and arterial and central venous lines. External adhesive defibrillator pads should be attached. Pulmonary artery catheterization is reserved for specific situations and is not standard care; however, large-bore peripheral intravenous access is a necessity.[166] Patients suffering from chronic cerebral vasculopathy or those at risk for neurological events may benefit from non-invasive cerebral monitoring.[166] Periprocedural TOE during TAVI may provide useful information beyond X-ray fluoroscopy such as results of balloon valvuloplasty, the position of the prosthetic valve, and identification of procedure-related complications—and may be of particular value when valve calcification is mild and fluoroscopic imaging is difficult.[164,165] However TOE is sometimes limited in its ability to clearly distinguish the prosthesis while mounted on the balloon catheter, may interfere with fluoroscopic imaging necessitating probe withdrawal at the time of implantation, and may increase the operator's preferences for general anaesthesia.[166] Newer modalities, including intracardiac and three-dimensional echocardiography and CT angiography may further assist these procedures.

Anaesthetic management during TAVI has goals of haemodynamic stability typical for any aortic stenosis patient: preload augmentation; low heart rate (50–70 beats/min); sinus rhythm; supraventricular arrhythmia and ventricular ectopy aggressively managed; and hypotension treated early with α-adrenergic agonists.[166,169] During aortic valve ballooning and balloon prosthesis implantation transient partial cardiac standby is induced, usually by RVP, permitting aortic valve deployment and preventing malposition and embolization of the prosthesis.[165,169] RVP is a key feature of the procedure and needs full attention and communication by the anaesthetist as the patient's haemodynamic response to RVP initiation and termination is important. Initial pacing wire testing or valvuloplasty can create severe or prolonged hypotension during and after RVP, and the patient may either require vasopressor before the subsequent pacing period or before initially starting RVP to avoid significant hypotension (see Table 21.5).[170]

Anaesthesia techniques for TAVI vary with the aim of providing less-invasive anaesthesia without compromising the safety of the patient. Local anaesthesia plus sedation is a reliable alternative to general anaesthesia.[171,172] General anaesthesia should provide good haemodynamic stability, cardioprotection, adequate attenuation of stress response, and early awakening. Many centres prefer general anaesthesia with endotracheal intubation because it facilitates valve positioning by maintaining patient immobility; controlling respiratory motion; may be a necessity when the patient is unable to tolerate the operation due to fatigue or difficulty in lying supine; facilitates the potentially complicated introducer sheath placement, removal and eventual surgical repair of arterial access sites; allows the use of TOE; and facilitates management of procedural complications.[166] However, general anaesthesia is associated with potential respiratory complications and haemodynamic instability, and protocols for local anaesthesia plus sedation—sedation accomplished with remifentanil, propofol, local infiltration or preoperative ilioinguinal/iliohypogastric block—are well documented.[166,171,172] With transapical TAVI general anaesthesia is generally considered mandatory; and with transaxillary TAVI, general anaesthesia or local anaesthesia plus sedation can be performed—although superficial cervical plexus block in addition to local infiltration has also been reported.[166] Complications to be vigilant for include: hypotension and myocardial ischaemia secondary to RVP; high-degree A-V block and heart block, especially with the CoreValve*; vascular complications, blood loss and arterial damage at the site of device insertion; aortic regurgitation, malposition and embolization of the device post-deployment; left main coronary artery occlusion; cardiac tamponade; and postoperative renal failure and neurological complications.[165,166] Poor left ventricle function is not a contraindication to extubating the patient immediately post-procedure if the haemodynamic stability is maintained and the procedure went as planned. Postoperative pain is effectively managed with non-steroidal agents/paracetamol and a low dose of opioids if renal function is adequate.[165,169] A brief time in the recovery room and early transfer to an intermediate care unit provided with bedside telemetry is a suitable alternative strategy in selected patients with an uneventful operative course is preferable to ICU admission and remaining intubated (see Table 21.6).[165,170]

There is no doubt that with proper planning, an appropriate hybrid operating theatre set-up, and clear guidelines on patient assessment, TAVI can be done safely and effectively in high-risk patients. Preprocedural multidisciplinary assessment of the patient is essential, and the anaesthetist plays a large role in this process. Bailout strategies, such as intraoperative ECMO, that are clear, planned and individualized to each patient, should be discussed prior to the procedure. It is our practice that ECMO is discontinued prior to moving the patient from the operating theatre.

Table 21.5 Key stages of TAVI procedure and possible complications

TAVI stage	Purpose of TAVI stage	Complications
Vascular access	Placement of guidewires for valve introduction; placement of catheters and guidewires for CPB or ECMO support	Dissection of femoral artery/ascending or descending aorta; vascular perforation and retroperitoneal hematoma; haemorrhage; distal embolic phenomena; distal hypoperfusion; LIMA occlusion if left trans-axillary approach
Trans-apical access	Placement of guidewires for valve introduction; placement of catheters and guidewires for CPB or ECMO support	Lung injury; pneumothorax; haemothorax; chest wall pain; respiratory compromise requiring ventilation; air embolism during LV cannulation; tamponade; stroke; myocardial infarction; atrio-ventricular block;
Placement and testing of RVP wires	Testing temporary pacemaker to achieve ventricular tachycardia (VT) and brief cessation of aortic ejection	Perforation of right atrium or right ventricle with pacing wires; sustained VT; myocardial ischaemia; haemodynamic compromise
Balloon valvuloplasty under RVP	Dilation of the calcified aortic annulus to prepare for valve implantation	Displacement of calcification particles and risk of stroke or myocardial infarction from coronary embolization; acute aortic regurgitation; atrio-ventricular block; aortic root rupture; aortic dissection
Valve positioning	Identification of the position of the transcatheter valve in the native aortic annulus	Displacement of calcification particles and risk of stroke or myocardial infarction from coronary embolization; valve embolization; flow obstruction
Valve deployment	Implantation of the valve in the native aortic annulus	Coronary artery occlusion; myocardial infarction; valve embolization; paravalvular regurgitation (poor adherence of valve to aortic annulus); valvular regurgitation (damaged valve by implantation, patient–prosthesis mismatch); displacement of calcification particles and risk of stroke or myocardial infarction from coronary embolization; atrio-ventricular block; aortic dissection; aortic annular rupture; cardiac perforation and tamponade; mitral valve injury

CPB: cardiopulmonary bypass; ECMO: extracorporeal membrane oxygenation; LIMA: left internal mammary artery; RVP: rapid ventricular pacing; TAVI: transcatheter aortic valve implantation.

Reprinted from *Journal of Cardiothoracic and Vascular Anaesthesia*, 24, 4, Fassl J and Augoustides JGT, 'Transcatheter aortic valve implantation—part 2: anesthesia management', pp. 691–699, Copyright 2012, with permission from European Association of Cardiothoracic Anesthesiologists (EACTA), the Chinese Society of Cardiovascular and Thoracic Anesthesiologists (ICCAF), and Elsevier.

Table 21.6 Comparison of anaesthetic techniques for transfemoral TAVI

Local anaesthesia		General anaesthesia	
Pros	**Cons**	**Pros**	**Cons**
Faster preparation time	Increased patient discomfort for catheter placement	Allows use of procedural TOE	Haemodynamic instability
Allows for neurological assessment at critical stages	Precludes use of TOE	Painless insertion of catheters and guidewires	Possible need for inotropes
May incur more stable haemodynamics during RVP	Movement of patient may occur (making catheter placement, balloon valvuloplasty and valve deployment more concerning stages)	Allows faster interventions if bleeding occurs	Longer preparation time
Shorter implantation time	Haemodynamic instability can occur due to sedation	No patient movement at any stage of procedure	Precludes neurological assessment
Faster recovery time	Time delay if intubation needed	No need to rush into a GA if instability occurs	Increased need for inotropes during and after RVP
Either no need or shorter stay in ICU	Depressed ventilation and hypercapnia due to sedation	No discomfort from a long procedure time	Delayed extubation times
Shorter hospital stay	Limited airway access due to fluoroscopy and TTE access	Better control of respiratory movement (especially during valve positioning and deployment)	Can lead to prolonged ventilation
Early ambulation more likely		Facilitates management of complications	Higher comorbidities
			Alters temperature management
			Longer operation time
			Possibly increased requirement for ICU/ longer hospital stay/increased hospital costs

ICU: intensive care unit; RVP: rapid ventricular pacing; TOE: transoesophageal echocardiography; TTE: transthoracic echocardiography.

Reprinted from *Journal of Cardiothoracic and Vascular Anaesthesia*, 24, 4, Fassl J and Augoustides JGT, 'Transcatheter aortic valve implantation—part 2: anesthesia management', pp. 691–699, Copyright 2012, with permission from European Association of Cardiothoracic Anesthesiologists (EACTA), the Chinese Society of Cardiovascular and Thoracic Anesthesiologists (ICCAF), and Elsevier.

Postoperative standardized monitoring, and patient care pathways and management protocols are required to smooth functioning of the process and patient safety.[169]

Conclusion

The procedures that are being developed and are available for younger patients are also of great value to the elderly patient with cardiovascular disease. Outcomes both functional and symptomatic are good and there is no longer any age limit to the provision of cardiac surgical intervention. Relatively non-invasive interventional techniques offer clear advantages to the elderly who are more prone to cognitive dysfunction following operations based on CPB provided that full rescue facilities are available in the event of procedural complications. The improvement in functional ability achieved by these cardiac surgical procedures can make all the difference between maintaining an independent life and one of increasing dependency and isolation but this depends on meticulous assessment and planning throughout the patient's perioperative journey.

References

1. Available from: <http://epp.eurostat.ec.europa/cache/ITY_OFFPUB/KS-SF-08-072/EN/KS-SF-08-072-EN.PDF>.
2. Shirani J, Yousefi J, Roberts WC. Major cardiac findings at necropsy in 366 American octogenarians. *Am J Cardiol*. 1995;75(2):151–156.
3. Ghanta RK, Shekar PS, McGurk S, Rosborough DM, Aranki SF. Long-term survival and quality of life justify cardiac surgery in the very elderly patient. *Ann Thorac Surg*. 2011;92(3):851–857.
4. Silvay G, Castillo JG, Chikwe J, Flynn B, Filsoufi F. Cardiac anesthesia and surgery in geriatric patients. *Semin Cardiothorac Vasc Anesth*. 2008;12(1):18–28.
5. Freitas WM, Carvalho LS, Moura FA, Sposito AC. Atherosclerotic disease in octogenarians: a challenge for science and clinical practice. *Atherosclerosis*. 2012;225(2):281–289.
6. Fleg JL, Strait J. Age-associated changes in cardiovascular structure and function: a fertile milieu for future disease. *Heart Fail Rev*. 2012;17(4–5):545–554.
7. Wadley AJ, Veldhuijzen van Zanten JJ, Aldred S. The interactions of oxidative stress and inflammation with vascular dysfunction in ageing: the vascular health triad. *Age (Dordr)*. 2013;35(3):705–718.
8. Dyer C. The interaction of ageing and lung disease. *Chron Respir Dis*. 2012;9(1):63–67.
9. Vaz Fragoso CA, Gill TM. Respiratory impairment and the aging lung: a novel paradigm for assessing pulmonary function. *J Gerontol A Biol Sci Med Sci*. 2012;67(3):264–275.
10. Esposito C, Dal Canton A. Functional changes in the aging kidney. *J Nephrol*. 2010;23(Suppl 15):S41–S45.
11. Gunasekaran U, Gannon M. Type 2 diabetes and the aging pancreatic beta cell. *Aging (Albany NY)*. 2011;3(6):565–575.
12. Trifiro G, Spina E. Age-related changes in pharmacodynamics: focus on drugs acting on central nervous and cardiovascular systems. *Curr Drug Metab*. 2011;12(7):611–620.
13. Price EA, Mehra R, Holmes TH, Schrier SL. Anemia in older persons: etiology and evaluation. *Blood Cells Mol Dis*. 2011;46(2):159–165.
14. Doherty TM, Fitzpatrick LA, Inoue D, et al. Molecular, endocrine, and genetic mechanisms of arterial calcification. *Endocr Rev*. 2004;25(4):629–672.
15. Witteman JC, Kannel WB, Wolf PA, et al. Aortic calcified plaques and cardiovascular disease (the Framingham Study). *Am J Cardiol*. 1990;66(15):1060–1064.
16. Naylor AR, Mehta Z, Rothwell PM, Bell PR. Carotid artery disease and stroke during coronary artery bypass: a critical review of the literature. *Eur J Vasc Endovasc Surg*. 2002;23(4):283–294.

17. Wanamaker KM, Moraca RJ, Nitzberg D, Magovern GJ Jr. Contemporary incidence and risk factors for carotid artery disease in patients referred for coronary artery bypass surgery. *J Cardiothorac Surg*. 2012;7:78–78.
18. Mahmoudi M, Hill PC, Xue Z, et al. Patients with severe asymptomatic carotid artery stenosis do not have a higher risk of stroke and mortality after coronary artery bypass surgery. *Stroke*. 2011;42(10):2801–2805.
19. Salasidis GC, Latter DA, Steinmetz OK, Blair JF, Graham AM. Carotid artery duplex scanning in preoperative assessment for coronary artery revascularization: the association between peripheral vascular disease, carotid artery stenosis, and stroke. *J Vasc Surg*. 1995;21(1):154–160; discussion 61-2.
20. Fukuda I, Gomi S, Watanabe K, Seita J. Carotid and aortic screening for coronary artery bypass grafting. *Ann Thorac Surg*. 2000;70(6):2034–2039.
21. Stamou SC, Hill PC, Dangas G, et al. Stroke after coronary artery bypass: incidence, predictors, and clinical outcome. *Stroke*. 2001;32(7):1508–1513.
22. Berens ES, Kouchoukos NT, Murphy SF, Wareing TH. Preoperative carotid artery screening in elderly patients undergoing cardiac surgery. *J Vasc Surg*. 1992;15(2):313–321; discussion 22-3.
23. Ederle J, Dobson J, Featherstone RL, et al. Carotid artery stenting compared with endarterectomy in patients with symptomatic carotid stenosis (International Carotid Stenting Study): an interim analysis of a randomised controlled trial. *Lancet*. 2010;375(9719):985–997.
24. Lytle BW, Loop FD, Cosgrove DM, Ratliff NB, Easley K, Taylor PC. Long-term (5 to 12 years) serial studies of internal mammary artery and saphenous vein coronary bypass grafts. *J Thorac Cardiovasc Surg*. 1985;89(2):248–258.
25. FitzGibbon GM, Leach AJ, Kafka HP, Keon WJ. Coronary bypass graft fate: long-term angiographic study. *J Am Coll Cardiol*. 1991;17(5):1075–1080.
26. Ottino G, De Paulis R, Pansini S, et al. Major sternal wound infection after open-heart surgery: a multivariate analysis of risk factors in 2,579 consecutive operative procedures. *Ann Thorac Surg*. 1987;44(2):173–179.
27. Wouters R, Wellens F, Vanermen H, De Geest R, Degrieck I, De Meerleer F. Sternitis and mediastinitis after coronary artery bypass grafting. Analysis of risk factors. *Tex Heart Inst J*. 1994;21(3):183–188.
28. Turrentine FE, Wang H, Simpson VB, Jones RS. Surgical risk factors, morbidity, and mortality in elderly patients. *J Am Coll Surg*. 2006;203(6):865–877.
29. Williams DB, Carrillo RG, Traad EA, et al. Determinants of operative mortality in octogenarians undergoing coronary bypass. *Ann Thorac Surg*. 1995;60(4):1038–1043.
30. Ko W, Krieger KH, Lazenby WD, et al. Isolated coronary artery bypass grafting in one hundred consecutive octogenarian patients. A multivariate analysis. *J Thorac Cardiovasc Surg*. 1991;102(4):532–538.
31. Lindroos M, Kupari M, Heikkila J, Tilvis R. Prevalence of aortic valve abnormalities in the elderly: an echocardiographic study of a random population sample. *J Am Coll Cardiol*. 1993;21(5):1220–1225.
32. Ross J Jr, Braunwald E. Aortic stenosis. *Circulation*. 1968;38(1 Suppl):61–67.
33. Nowicki ER, Birkmeyer NJ, Weintraub RW, et al. Multivariable prediction of in-hospital mortality associated with aortic and mitral valve surgery in Northern New England. *Ann Thorac Surg*. 2004;77(6):1966–1977.
34. Cerillo AG, Assal Al, Kodami A, et al. Aortic valve surgery in the elderly patient: a retrospective review. *Interact Cardiovasc Thorac Surg*. 2007;6(3):308–313.
35. Litmathe J, Feindt P, Kurt M, Gams E, Boeken U. Aortic valve replacement in octogenarians: outcome and predictors of complications. *Hellenic J Cardiol*. 2011;52(3):211–215.
36. Varadarajan P, Kapoor N, Bansal RC, Pai RG. Survival in elderly patients with severe aortic stenosis is dramatically improved by aortic valve replacement: Results from a cohort of 277 patients aged ≥80 years. *Eur J Cardiothorac Surg*. 2006;30(5):722–727.
37. Bonow RO, Carabello BA, Kanu C, et al. ACC/AHA 2006 guidelines for the management of patients with valvular heart disease: a report of the American College of Cardiology/American Heart Association

Task Force on Practice Guidelines (writing Committee to revise the 1998 guidelines for the management of patients with valvular heart disease): developed in collaboration with the Society of Cardiovascular Anesthesiologists: endorsed by the Society for Cardiovascular Angiography and Interventions and the Society of Thoracic Surgeons. *Circulation.* 2006;114(5):e84–e231.

38. Vahanian A, Baumgartner H, Bax J, et al. Guidelines on the management of valvular heart disease: The Task Force on the Management of Valvular Heart Disease of the European Society of Cardiology. *Eur Heart J.* 2007;28(2):230–268.

39. Hannan EL, Samadashvili Z, Lahey SJ, et al. Aortic valve replacement for patients with severe aortic stenosis: risk factors and their impact on 30-month mortality. *Ann Thorac Surg.* 2009;87(6):1741–1749.

40. Florath I, Albert A, Rosendahl U, Alexander T, Ennker IC, Ennker J. Mid term outcome and quality of life after aortic valve replacement in elderly people: mechanical versus stentless biological valves. *Heart.* 2005;91(8):1023–1029.

41. Kirsch M, Nakashima K, Kubota S, Houel R, Hillion ML, Loisance D. The risk of reoperative heart valve procedures in octogenarian patients. *J Heart Valve Dis.* 2004;13(6):991–996; discussion 6.

42. Odell JA, Mullany CJ, Schaff HV, Orszulak TA, Daly RC, Morris JJ. Aortic valve replacement after previous coronary artery bypass grafting. *Ann Thorac Surg.* 1996;62(5):1424–1430.

43. Khaladj N, Shrestha M, Peterss S, et al. Isolated surgical aortic valve replacement after previous coronary artery bypass grafting with patent grafts: is this old-fashioned technique obsolete? *Eur J Cardiothorac Surg.* 2009;35(2):260–264.

44. Brunvand H, Offstad J, Nitter-Hauge S, Svennevig JL. Coronary artery bypass grafting combined with aortic valve replacement in healthy octogenarians does not increase postoperative risk. *Scand Cardiovasc J.* 2002;36(5):297–301.

45. Vasques F, Lucenteforte E, Paone R, Mugelli A, Biancari F. Outcome of patients aged ≥80 years undergoing combined aortic valve replacement and coronary artery bypass grafting: a systematic review and meta-analysis of 40 studies. *Am Heart J.* 2012;164(3):410–418 e1.

46. Vasques F, Messori A, Lucenteforte E, Biancari F. Immediate and late outcome of patients aged 80 years and older undergoing isolated aortic valve replacement: a systematic review and meta-analysis of 48 studies. *Am Heart J.* 2012;163(3):477–485.

47. Barreiro CJ, Patel ND, Fitton TP, et al. Aortic valve replacement and concomitant mitral valve regurgitation in the elderly: impact on survival and functional outcome. *Circulation.* 2005;112(9 Suppl):I443–I447.

48. Gill M, Dunning J. Is reduction aortoplasty (with or without external wrap) an acceptable alternative to replacement of the dilated ascending aorta? *Interact Cardiovasc Thorac Surg.* 2009;9(4):693–697.

49. Bauer M, Pasic M, Schaffarzyk R, et al. Reduction aortoplasty for dilatation of the ascending aorta in patients with bicuspid aortic valve. *Ann Thorac Surg.* 2002;73(3):720–723.

50. Szabo TA, Toole JM, Payne KJ, Giblin EM, Jacks SP, Warters RD. Management of aortic valve bypass surgery. *Semin Cardiothorac Vasc Anesth.* 2012;16(1):52–58.

51. Glower DD, Lee T, Desai B. Aortic valve replacement through right minithoracotomy in 306 consecutive patients. *Innovations (Phila).* 2010;5(5):326–330.

52. Nkomo VT, Gardin JM, Skelton TN, Gottdiener JS, Scott CG, Enriquez-Sarano M. Burden of valvular heart diseases: a population-based study. *Lancet.* 2006;368(9540):1005–1011.

53. Mehta RH, Eagle KA, Coombs LP, et al. Influence of age on outcomes in patients undergoing mitral valve replacement. *Ann Thorac Surg.* 2002;74(5):1459–1467.

54. Chikwe J, Goldstone AB, Passage J, et al. A propensity score-adjusted retrospective comparison of early and mid-term results of mitral valve repair versus replacement in octogenarians. *Eur Heart J.* 2011;32(5):618–626.

55. Savage EB, Ferguson TB, Jr., DiSesa VJ. Use of mitral valve repair: analysis of contemporary United States experience reported to the Society of Thoracic Surgeons National Cardiac Database. *Ann Thorac Surg.* 2003;75(3):820–825.

56. Gillinov AM, Blackstone EH, Rajeswaran J, et al. Ischemic versus degenerative mitral regurgitation: does etiology affect survival? *Ann Thorac Surg.* 2005;80(3):811–819.

57. Boon A, Cheriex E, Lodder J, Kessels F. Cardiac valve calcification: characteristics of patients with calcification of the mitral annulus or aortic valve. *Heart.* 1997;78(5):472–474.

58. Iribarne A, Easterwood R, Russo MJ, Chan EY, Smith CR, Argenziano M. Comparative effectiveness of minimally invasive versus traditional sternotomy mitral valve surgery in elderly patients. *J Thorac Cardiovasc Surg.* 2012;143(4 Suppl):S86–S90.

59. Vollroth M, Seeburger J, Garbade J, et al. Minimally invasive mitral valve surgery is a very safe procedure with very low rates of conversion to full sternotomy. *Eur J Cardiothorac Surg.* 2012;42(1):e13–e15.

60. Holzhey DM, Shi W, Borger MA, et al. Minimally invasive versus sternotomy approach for mitral valve surgery in patients greater than 70 years old: a propensity-matched comparison. *Ann Thorac Surg.* 2011;91(2):401–405.

61. Bickerstaff LK, Pairolero PC, Hollier LH, et al. Thoracic aortic aneurysms: a population-based study. *Surgery.* 1982;92(6):1103–1108.

62. Shah PJ, Estrera AL, Miller CC 3rd, et al. Analysis of ascending and transverse aortic arch repair in octogenarians. *Ann Thorac Surg.* 2008;86(3):774–779.

63. Anagnostopoulos CE, Prabhakar MJ, Kittle CF. Aortic dissections and dissecting aneurysms. *Am J Cardiol.* 1972;30(3):263–273.

64. Hagan PG, Nienaber CA, Isselbacher EM, et al. The International Registry of Acute Aortic Dissection (IRAD): new insights into an old disease. *JAMA.* 2000;283(7):897–903.

65. Tsai TT, Evangelista A, Nienaber CA, et al. Long-term survival in patients presenting with type A acute aortic dissection: insights from the International Registry of Acute Aortic Dissection (IRAD). *Circulation.* 2006;114(1 Suppl):I350–I356.

66. Piccardo A, Regesta T, Zannis K, et al. Outcomes after surgical treatment for type A acute aortic dissection in octogenarians: a multicenter study. *Ann Thorac Surg.* 2009;88(2):491–497.

67. Mehta RH, O'Gara PT, Bossone E, et al. Acute type A aortic dissection in the elderly: clinical characteristics, management, and outcomes in the current era. *J Am Coll Cardiol.* 2002;40(4):685–692.

68. Caus T, Frapier JM, Giorgi R, et al. Clinical outcome after repair of acute type A dissection in patients over 70 years-old. *Eur J Cardiothorac Surg.* 2002;22(2):211–217.

69. Geirsson A, Szeto WY, Pochettino A, et al. Significance of malperfusion syndromes prior to contemporary surgical repair for acute type A dissection: outcomes and need for additional revascularizations. *Eur J Cardiothorac Surg.* 2007;32(2):255–262.

70. Neri E, Toscano T, Massetti M, et al. Operation for acute type A aortic dissection in octogenarians: is it justified? *J Thorac Cardiovasc Surg.* 2001;121(2):259–267.

71. Sundermann S, Dademasch A, Praetorius J, et al. Comprehensive assessment of frailty for elderly high-risk patients undergoing cardiac surgery. *Eur J Cardiothorac Surg.* 2011;39(1):33–37.

72. Afilalo J, Mottillo S, Eisenberg MJ, et al. Addition of frailty and disability to cardiac surgery risk scores identifies elderly patients at high risk of mortality or major morbidity. *Circ Cardiovasc Qual Outcomes.* 2012;5(2):222–228.

73. Katz S, Ford AB, Moskowitz RW, Jackson BA, Jaffe MW. Studies of Illness in the Aged. The Index of Adl: a standardized measure of biological and psychosocial function. *JAMA.* 1963;185:914–919.

74. Lee DH, Buth KJ, Martin BJ, Yip AM, Hirsch GM. Frail patients are at increased risk for mortality and prolonged institutional care after cardiac surgery. *Circulation.* 2010;121(8):973–978.

75. Chow WB, Rosenthal RA, Merkow RP, Ko CY, Esnaola NF. Optimal preoperative assessment of the geriatric surgical patient: a best practices guideline from the American College of Surgeons National Surgical Quality Improvement Program and the American Geriatrics Society. *J Am Coll Surg.* 2012;215(4):453–466.

76. Contrada RJ, Boulifard DA, Hekler EB, *et al.* Psychosocial factors in heart surgery: presurgical vulnerability and postsurgical recovery. *Health Psychol.* 2008;27(3):309–319.

77. Sieber FE, Barnett SR. Preventing postoperative complications in the elderly. *Anesthesiol Clin.* 2011;29(1):83–97.

78. Dhanani J, Mullany DV, Fraser JF. Effect of preoperative renal function on long-term survival after cardiac surgery. *J Thorac Cardiovasc Surg.* 2013;146(1):90–95.

79. Biancari F, Rimpilainen R. Meta-analysis of randomised trials comparing the effectiveness of miniaturised versus conventional cardiopulmonary bypass in adult cardiac surgery. *Heart.* 2009;95(12):964–969.

80. Rozental T, Shore-Lesserson L. Pharmacologic management of coagulopathy in cardiac surgery: an update. *J Cardiothorac Vasc Anesth.* 2012;26(4):669–679.

81. Ng CS, Wan S. Limiting inflammatory response to cardiopulmonary bypass: pharmaceutical strategies. *Curr Opin Pharmacol.* 2012;12(2):155–159.

82. Vohra HA, Whistance R, Modi A, Ohri SK. The inflammatory response to miniaturised extracorporeal circulation: a review of the literature. *Mediators Inflamm.* 2009;2009:707042.

83. Black KM, Barnett RJ, Bhasin MK, *et al.* Microarray and proteomic analysis of the cardioprotective effects of cold blood cardioplegia in the mature and aged male and female. *Physiol Genomics.* 2012;44(21):1027–1041.

84. Ono M, Joshi B, Brady K, *et al.* Risks for impaired cerebral autoregulation during cardiopulmonary bypass and postoperative stroke. *Br J Anaesth.* 2012;109(3):391–398.

85. Newman MF, Croughwell ND, Blumenthal JA, *et al.* Effect of aging on cerebral autoregulation during cardiopulmonary bypass. Association with postoperative cognitive dysfunction. *Circulation.* 1994;90(5 Pt 2):II243–II249.

86. Bellapart J, Geng S, Dunster K, *et al.* Intraaortic balloon pump counterpulsation and cerebral autoregulation: an observational study. *BMC Anesthesiol.* 2010;10:3–3.

87. van Harten AE, Scheeren TW, Absalom AR. A review of postoperative cognitive dysfunction and neuroinflammation associated with cardiac surgery and anaesthesia. *Anaesthesia.* 2012;67(3):280–293.

88. Cooper EA, Edelman JJ, Wilson MK, Bannon PG, Vallely MP. Off-pump coronary artery bypass grafting in elderly and high-risk patients—a review. *Heart Lung Circ.* 2011;20(11):694–703.

89. Demaria RG, Carrier M, Fortier S, *et al.* Reduced mortality and strokes with off-pump coronary artery bypass grafting surgery in octogenarians. *Circulation.* 2002;106(12 Suppl 1):I5–I10.

90. Ricci M, Karamanoukian HL, Abraham R, *et al.* Stroke in octogenarians undergoing coronary artery surgery with and without cardiopulmonary bypass. *Ann Thorac Surg.* 2000;69(5):1471–1475.

91. LaPar DJ, Bhamidipati CM, Reece TB, Cleveland JC, Kron IL, Ailawadi G. Is off-pump coronary artery bypass grafting superior to conventional bypass in octogenarians? *J Thorac Cardiovasc Surg.* 2011;141(1):81–90.

92. Moller CH, Penninga L, Wetterslev J, Steinbruchel DA, Gluud C. Off-pump versus on-pump coronary artery bypass grafting for ischaemic heart disease. *Cochrane Database Syst Rev.* 2012;3:CD007224.

93. Evered LA, Silbert BS, Scott DA. Postoperative cognitive dysfunction and aortic atheroma. *Ann Thorac Surg.* 2010;89(4):1091–1097.

94. Schachner T, Nagele G, Kacani A, Laufer G, Bonatti J. Factors associated with presence of ascending aortic atherosclerosis in CABG patients. *Ann Thorac Surg.* 2004;78(6):2028–2032; discussion 32.

95. Yamaguchi A, Adachi H, Tanaka M, Ino T. Efficacy of intraoperative epiaortic ultrasound scanning for preventing stroke after coronary artery bypass surgery. *Ann Thorac Cardiovasc Surg.* 2009;15(2):98–104.

96. Ito A, Goto T, Maekawa K, Baba T, Mishima Y, Ushijima K. Postoperative neurological complications and risk factors for pre-existing silent brain infarction in elderly patients undergoing coronary artery bypass grafting. *J Anesth.* 2012;26(3):405–411.

97. Rosenberger P, Shernan SK, Loffler M, *et al.* The influence of epiaortic ultrasonography on intraoperative surgical management in 6051 cardiac surgical patients. *Ann Thorac Surg.* 2008;85(2):548–553.

98. Sylivris S, Calafiore P, Matalanis G, *et al.* The intraoperative assessment of ascending aortic atheroma: epiaortic imaging is superior to both transesophageal echocardiography and direct palpation. *J Cardiothorac Vasc Anesth.* 1997;11(6):704–707.

99. Schoen J, Meyerrose J, Paarmann H, Heringlake M, Hueppe M, Berger KU. Preoperative regional cerebral oxygen saturation is a predictor of postoperative delirium in on-pump cardiac surgery patients: a prospective observational trial. *Crit Care.* 2011;15(5):R218.

100. Slater JP, Guarino T, Stack J, *et al.* Cerebral oxygen desaturation predicts cognitive decline and longer hospital stay after cardiac surgery. *Ann Thorac Surg.* 2009;87(1):36–44; discussion -5.

101. de Tournay-Jette E, Dupuis G, Bherer L, Deschamps A, Cartier R, Denault A. The relationship between cerebral oxygen saturation changes and postoperative cognitive dysfunction in elderly patients after coronary artery bypass graft surgery. *J Cardiothorac Vasc Anesth.* 2011;25(1):95–104.

102. Fedorow C, Grocott HP. Cerebral monitoring to optimize outcomes after cardiac surgery. *Curr Opin Anaesthesiol.* 2010;23(1):89–94.

103. Besser MW, Klein AA. The coagulopathy of cardiopulmonary bypass. *Crit Rev Clin Lab Sci.* 2010;47(5-6):197–212.

104. Bhaskar B, Dulhunty J, Mullany DV, Fraser JF. Impact of blood product transfusion on short and long-term survival after cardiac surgery: more evidence. *Ann Thorac Surg.* 2012;94(2):460–467.

105. Surgery S-SoT risk calculator. <http://riskcalc.sts.org/STSWebRiskCalc273/de.aspx> (accessed 21 March 2013).

106. Griffith KA, Sherrill DL, Siegel EM, Manolio TA, Bonekat HW, Enright PL. Predictors of loss of lung function in the elderly: the Cardiovascular Health Study. *Am J Respir Crit Care Med.* 2001;163(1):61–68.

107. Liptay MJ, Basu S, Hoaglin MC, *et al.* Diffusion lung capacity for carbon monoxide (DLCO) is an independent prognostic factor for long-term survival after curative lung resection for cancer. *J Surg Oncol.* 2009;100(8):703–707.

108. Bailey ML, Richter SM, Mullany DV, Tesar PJ, Fraser JF. Risk factors and survival in patients with respiratory failure after cardiac operations. *Ann Thorac Surg.* 2011;92(5):1573–1579.

109. Pearse B, Cole C, Barnett A, Pohlner P, Fraser J. A positive fluid balance post cardiac surgery results in prolonged ventilation, intensive care unit and hospital length of stay. *Aust Crit Care.* 2012;25(2):137.

110. Corley A, Caruana LR, Barnett AG, Tronstad O, Fraser JF. Oxygen delivery through high-flow nasal cannulae increase end-expiratory lung volume and reduce respiratory rate in post-cardiac surgical patients. *Br J Anaesth.* 2011;107(6):998–1004.

111. Yavas S, Yagar S, Mavioglu L, *et al.* Tracheostomy: how and when should it be done in cardiovascular surgery ICU? *J Card Surg.* 2009;24(1):11–18.

112. Platts DG, Fraser JF. Contrast echocardiography in critical care: echoes of the future? A review of the role of microsphere contrast echocardiography. *Crit Care Resusc.* 2011;13(1):44–55.

113. Platts DG, Fraser JF. Microsphere contrast echocardiography in the critical care complex. *Crit Care.* 2011;15(2):417–417.

114. Weber CF, Gorlinger K, Meininger D, *et al.* Point-of-care testing: a prospective, randomized clinical trial of efficacy in coagulopathic cardiac surgery patients. *Anesthesiology.* 2012;117(3):531–547.

115. Karthik S, Grayson AD, McCarron EE, Pullan DM, Desmond MJ. Reexploration for bleeding after coronary artery bypass surgery: risk factors, outcomes, and the effect of time delay. *The Annals of Thoracic Surgery.* 2004;78(2):527–534.

116. Bhaskar B, Bidstrup BP, Fung YL, Fraser JF. To transfuse, or not to transfuse: that is the question. *Crit Care Resusc.* 2009;11(1):71–77.

117. Fliser D, Ritz E, Franek E. Renal reserve in the elderly. *Semin Nephrol.* 1995;15(5):463–467.

118. Suen WS, Mok CK, Chiu SW, *et al.* Risk factors for development of acute renal failure (ARF) requiring dialysis in patients undergoing cardiac surgery. *Angiology.* 1998;49(10):789–800.

119. Chukwuemeka A, Weisel A, Maganti M, *et al.* Renal dysfunction in high-risk patients after on-pump and off-pump coronary artery bypass surgery: a propensity score analysis. *Ann Thorac Surg.* 2005;80(6):2148–2153.

120. Bellomo R, Chapman M, Finfer S, Hickling K, Myburgh J. Low-dose dopamine in patients with early renal dysfunction: a placebo-controlled randomised trial. Australian and New Zealand Intensive Care Society (ANZICS) Clinical Trials Group. *Lancet.* 2000;356(9248):2139–2143.

121. Wijeysundera DN, Karkouti K, Dupuis JY, et al. Derivation and validation of a simplified predictive index for renal replacement therapy after cardiac surgery. *JAMA.* 2007;297(16):1801–1809.

122. Redmond JM, Greene PS, Goldsborough MA, et al. Neurologic injury in cardiac surgical patients with a history of stroke. *Ann Thorac Surg.* 1996;61(1):42–47.

123. Hogue CW, Jr., Murphy SF, Schechtman KB, Davila-Roman VG. Risk factors for early or delayed stroke after cardiac surgery. *Circulation.* 1999;100(6):642–647.

124. Selnes OA, Grega MA, Borowicz LM, Jr., Royall RM, McKhann GM, Baumgartner WA. Cognitive changes with coronary artery disease: a prospective study of coronary artery bypass graft patients and nonsurgical controls. *Ann Thorac Surg.* 2003;75(5):1377–1384.

125. Breuer AC, Furlan AJ, Hanson MR, et al. Central nervous system complications of coronary artery bypass graft surgery: prospective analysis of 421 patients. *Stroke.* 1983;14(5):682–687.

126. Chermesh I, Hajos J, Mashiach T, et al. Malnutrition in cardiac surgery: food for thought. *Eur J Prev Cardiol.* 2012;Jun 27. Epub ahead of print.

127. Aubrun F, Gazon M, Schoeffler M, Benyoub K. Evaluation of perioperative risk in elderly patients. *Minerva Anestesiol.* 2012;78(5):605–618.

128. Ucak A, Onan B, Sen H, Selcuk I, Turan A, Yilmaz AT. The effects of gabapentin on acute and chronic postoperative pain after coronary artery bypass graft surgery. *J Cardiothorac Vasc Anesth.* 2011;25(5):824–829.

129. Rapchuk IL, O'Connell L, Liessmann CD, Cornelissen HR, Fraser JF. Effect of gabapentin on pain after cardiac surgery: a randomised, double-blind, placebo-controlled trial. *Anaesth Intensive Care.* 2010;38(3):445–451.

130. Menda F, Koner O, Sayin M, Ergenoglu M, Kucukaksu S, Aykac B. Effects of single-dose gabapentin on postoperative pain and morphine consumption after cardiac surgery. *J Cardiothorac Vasc Anesth.* 2010;24(5):808–813.

131. Pesonen A, Suojaranta-Ylinen R, Hammaren E, Tarkkila P, Seppala T, Rosenberg PH. Comparison of effects and plasma concentrations of opioids between elderly and middle-aged patients after cardiac surgery. *Acta Anaesthesiol Scand.* 2009;53(1):101–108.

132. van Ojik AL, Jansen PA, Brouwers JR, van Roon EN. Treatment of chronic pain in older people: evidence-based choice of strong-acting opioids. *Drugs Aging.* 2012;29(8):615–625.

133. Pergolizzi J, Boger RH, Budd K, et al. Opioids and the management of chronic severe pain in the elderly: consensus statement of an International Expert Panel with focus on the six clinically most often used World Health Organization Step III opioids (buprenorphine, fentanyl, hydromorphone, methadone, morphine, oxycodone). *Pain Pract.* 2008;8(4):287–313.

134. Huang AR, Mallet L. Prescribing opioids in older people. *Maturitas.* 2013;74(2):123–129.

135. Monaco F, Biselli C, De Luca M, Landoni G, Lembo R, Zangrillo A. Thoracic epidural anesthesia in elderly patients undergoing cardiac surgery for mitral regurgitation feasibility study. *Ann Card Anaesth.* 2012;15(2):164–165.

136. Mukherjee C, Koch E, Banusch J, Scholz M, Kaisers UX, Ender J. Intrathecal morphine is superior to intravenous PCA in patients undergoing minimally invasive cardiac surgery. *Ann Card Anaesth.* 2012;15(2):122–127.

137. Jakobsen CJ, Bhavsar R, Nielsen DV, Ryhammer PK, Sloth E, Greisen J. High thoracic epidural analgesia in cardiac surgery: part 1-high thoracic epidural analgesia improves cardiac performance in cardiac surgery patients. *J Cardiothorac Vasc Anesth.* 2012;26(6):1039–1047.

138. Nielsen DV, Bhavsar R, Greisen J, Ryhammer PK, Sloth E, Jakobsen CJ. High thoracic epidural analgesia in cardiac surgery: part 2-high thoracic epidural analgesia does not reduce time in or improve quality of recovery in the intensive care unit. *J Cardiothorac Vasc Anesth.* 2012;26(6):1048–1054.

139. Cormack F, Shipolini A, Awad WI, et al. A meta-analysis of cognitive outcome following coronary artery bypass graft surgery. *Neurosci Biobehav Rev.* 2012;36(9):2118–2129.

140. Eagle KA, Guyton RA, Davidoff R, et al. ACC/AHA guidelines for coronary artery bypass graft surgery: executive summary and recommendations: A report of the American College of Cardiology/American Heart Association Task Force on Practice Guidelines (Committee to revise the 1991 guidelines for coronary artery bypass graft surgery). *Circulation.* 1999;100(13):1464–1480.

141. Murkin JM, Newman SP, Stump DA, Blumenthal JA. Statement of consensus on assessment of neurobehavioral outcomes after cardiac surgery. *Ann Thorac Surg.* 1995;59(5):1289–1295.

142. Sun X, Lindsay J, Monsein LH, Hill PC, Corso PJ. Silent brain injury after cardiac surgery: a review: cognitive dysfunction and magnetic resonance imaging diffusion-weighted imaging findings. *J Am Coll Cardiol.* 2012;60(9):791–797.

143. Edelman JJ, Yan TD, Padang R, Bannon PG, Vallely MP. Off-pump coronary artery bypass surgery versus percutaneous coronary intervention: a meta-analysis of randomized and nonrandomized studies. *Ann Thorac Surg.* 2010;90(4):1384–1390.

144. Marasco SF, Sharwood LN, Abramson MJ. No improvement in neurocognitive outcomes after off-pump versus on-pump coronary revascularisation: a meta-analysis. *Eur J Cardiothorac Surg.* 2008;33(6):961–970.

145. Wiedemann D, Bernhard D, Laufer G, Kocher A. The elderly patient and cardiac surgery—a mini-review. *Gerontology.* 2010;56(3):241–249.

146. Butler CR, Jugdutt BI. Mechanical circulatory support for elderly heart failure patients. *Heart Fail Rev.* 2012;17(4-5):663–669.

147. Kirklin JK, Naftel DC, Kormos RL, et al. Third INTERMACS Annual Report: the evolution of destination therapy in the United States. *J Heart Lung Transplant.* 2011;30(2):115–123.

148. Flint KM, Matlock DD, Lindenfeld J, Allen LA. Frailty and the selection of patients for destination therapy left ventricular assist device. *Circ Heart Fail.* 2012;5(2):286–293.

149. Brouwers C, Denollet J, de Jonge N, Caliskan K, Kealy J, Pedersen SS. Patient-reported outcomes in left ventricular assist device therapy: a systematic review and recommendations for clinical research and practice. *Circ Heart Fail.* 2011;4(6):714–723.

150. Adamson RM, Stahovich M, Chillcott S, et al. Clinical strategies and outcomes in advanced heart failure patients older than 70 years of age receiving the HeartMate II left ventricular assist device: a community hospital experience. *J Am Coll Cardiol.* 2011;57(25):2487–2495.

151. Sansone F, Campanella A, Rinaldi M. Extracorporeal membrane oxygenation as a 'bridge to recovery' in a case of myotomy for myocardial bridge complicated by biventricular dysfunction. *J Artif Organs.* 2010;13(2):97–100.

152. Licker M, Diaper J, Cartier V, et al. Clinical review: management of weaning from cardiopulmonary bypass after cardiac surgery. *Ann Card Anaesth.* 2012;15(3):206–223.

153. Zaky SS, Hanna AH, Sakr Esa WA, et al. An 11-year, single-institution analysis of intra-aortic balloon pump use in cardiac surgery. *J Cardiothorac Vasc Anesth.* 2009;23(4):479–483.

154. Dardas P, Mezilis N, Ninios V, et al. ECMO as a bridge to high-risk rotablation of heavily calcified coronary arteries. *Herz.* 2012;37(2):225–230.

155. Thourani VH, Ailawadi G, Szeto WY, et al. Outcomes of surgical aortic valve replacement in high-risk patients: a multiinstitutional study. *Ann Thorac Surg.* 2011;91(1):49–55.

156. Agnihotri A. 2012 ACCF/AATS/SCAI/STS expert consensus document on transcatheter aortic valve replacement: executive summary. *J Thorac Cardiovasc Surg.* 2012;144(3):534–537.

157. Boothroyd LJ, Spaziano M, Guertin JR, et al. Transcatheter aortic valve implantation: recommendations for practice based on a multidisciplinary review including cost-effectiveness and ethical and organizational issues. *Can J Cardiol.* 2013;29(6):718–726.

158. Sinning JM, Werner N, Nickenig G, Grube E. Transcatheter aortic valve implantation: the evidence. *Heart.* 2012;98 Suppl 4:iv65–iv72.

159. Leon MB, Smith CR, Mack M, et al. Transcatheter aortic-valve implantation for aortic stenosis in patients who cannot undergo surgery. *N Engl J Med.* 2010;363(17):1597–1607.

160. Kodali SK, Williams MR, Smith CR, *et al*. Two-year outcomes after transcatheter or surgical aortic-valve replacement. *N Engl J Med*. 2012;366(18):1686–1695.

161. Lam YY, Lee PW, Yong G, Yan BP. Investigational devices for mitral regurgitation: state of the art. *Expert Rev Med Devices*. 2011;8(1):105–114.

162. Feldman T, Kar S, Rinaldi M, *et al*. Percutaneous mitral repair with the MitraClip system: safety and midterm durability in the initial EVEREST (Endovascular Valve Edge-to-Edge REpair Study) cohort. *J Am Coll Cardiol*. 2009;54(8):686–694.

163. Glower D, Ailawadi G, Argenziano M, *et al*. EVEREST II randomized clinical trial: predictors of mitral valve replacement in de novo surgery or after the MitraClip procedure. *J Thorac Cardiovasc Surg*. 2012;143(4 Suppl):S60–S63.

164. Bapat V, Attia R. Transaortic transcatheter aortic valve implantation: step-by-step guide. *Semin Thorac Cardiovasc Surg*. 2012;24(3):206–211.

165. Huffmyer J, Tashjian J, Raphael J, Jaeger JM. Management of the patient for transcatheter aortic valve implantation in the perioperative period. *Semin Cardiothorac Vasc Anesth*. 2012;16(1):25–40.

166. Franco A, Gerli C, Ruggeri L, Monaco F. Anaesthetic management of transcatheter aortic valve implantation. *Ann Card Anaesth*. 2012;15(1):54–63.

167. Barbash IM, Ben-Dor I, Dvir D, *et al*. Incidence and predictors of acute kidney injury after transcatheter aortic valve replacement. *Am Heart J*. 2012;163(6):1031–1036.

168. Fusari M, Bona V, Muratori M, *et al*. Transcatheter vs. surgical aortic valve replacement: a retrospective analysis assessing clinical effectiveness and safety. *J Cardiovasc Med (Hagerstown)*. 2012;13(4):229–241.

169. Covello RD, Landoni G, Zangrillo A. Anesthetic management of transcatheter aortic valve implantation. *Curr Opin Anaesthesiol*. 2011;24(4):417–425.

170. Fassl J, Augoustides JG. Transcatheter aortic valve implantation—part 2: anesthesia management. *J Cardiothorac Vasc Anesth*. 2010;24(4):691–699.

171. Yamamoto M, Meguro K, Mouillet G, *et al*. Effect of local anesthetic management with conscious sedation in patients undergoing transcatheter aortic valve implantation. *Am J Cardiol*. 2013;111(1):94–99.

172. Ben-Dor I, Looser PM, Maluenda G, *et al*. Transcatheter aortic valve replacement under monitored anesthesia care versus general anesthesia with intubation. *Cardiovasc Revasc Med*. 2012;13(4):207–210.

CHAPTER 22

Neuroanaesthesia in the elderly

Bernard Graf and Chris Dodds

Introduction

The administration of anaesthesia to aged neurosurgical patients is increasingly common and requires not only an understanding of the basic principles of neurophysiology and the effects of anaesthetic agents on intracranial dynamics but also an understanding of the anatomy and physiology of the central nervous system in elderly patients. The practice of neuroanaesthesia is unique in that the target organ of both the surgeon and the anaesthetist is the same. The impact of the surgery has a profound influence on the anaesthetic management of the elderly patient especially as often the only aspect of the elderly patient that does not suffer from loss of reserve appears to be their personality.

General preoperative evaluation

Neurosurgical procedures generally differ from other surgical procedures by their length of operating time, the positioning of the patient, and the need for techniques such as hyperventilation, cerebral dehydration, and deliberate hypotension. When assessing the elderly patient for these procedures their comorbid status and medication must be incorporated into the anaesthetic plan. Not all elderly patients will be able to tolerate either the duration of surgery, positioning, or use of means to reduce intracranial volume.

The common comorbidities in the elderly of cardiac, pulmonary, and renal diseases have to be evaluated in the context, for instance, of the risk of administering osmotically active agents such as mannitol with sudden changes in intravascular volume or using hyperventilation to reduce intracranial volume. When the duration of surgery is likely to be long optimization of cardiac, respiratory, or renal dysfunction is important and unless surgery is urgent should be instituted before operation.

The preoperative evaluation in these patients must also include a complete and written neurological examination with special attention to the patient's level of consciousness, presence or absence of increased ICP, and extent of focal neurological deficits. This evaluation is important for the postoperative judgement of the neurological status as well as the postoperative detection of cognitive dysfunctions. Preoperative activity levels and cognitive function have to be screened and documented accurately, because these parameters will determine postoperative outcome and therefore the choice of the surgical and anaesthetic techniques.[1]

The elderly have a greater tolerance of a rising intracranial pressure (ICP) (see later) and exhibit the typical signs of intracranial hypertension relatively late compared to younger patients. The presence of a headache, nausea, papilloedema, unilateral pupillary dilation, and oculomotor or abducens palsy indicate the need for urgent action to reduce ICP whereas a depressed level of consciousness and irregular respiration is a life threatening neurosurgical emergency. Clinical signs do not reliably indicate the level of the ICP. Only directly cerebrospinal pressure measurement can be used to quantitate this; however, indirect evidence of elevated ICP can be determined by evaluating the computed tomography (CT) or more commonly the magnetic resonance imaging (MRI) scan for a mass lesion that is accompanied by a midline shift of 0.5 cm or greater and/or an encroachment of expanding brain on cerebrospinal fluid (CSF) cisterns.

Fluid and electrolyte abnormalities are very common in patients with reduced levels of consciousness. Elderly patients are usually dehydrated and develop electrolyte abnormalities because of age-related decreased fluid intake, iatrogenic water restriction, neuroendocrine abnormalities, and diuresis from diuretics. Fluid and electrolyte abnormalities should be corrected before the induction of anaesthesia in order to prevent cardiovascular instability. Normally, except for acute neurosurgical emergencies (e.g. head trauma, impending herniation, and spinal cord compression with paraplegia), most neurosurgical procedures can be delayed in order to optimize patients with medically unstable conditions.

General intraoperative management

In common with the anaesthetic management of elderly patients for other forms of surgery a balanced technique with a smooth induction and recovery is important. This is especially true to maintain an appropriate cerebral perfusion pressure (CPP). In particular, intracranial hypertension or hypotension should be avoided to provide optimal surgical conditions but also to ensure perfusion to vascular watershed areas of the brain. At the moment there are few indications for regional anaesthesia during neurosurgery (see 'Awake craniotomy' section).

Invasive monitoring is required for all but the most minor procedures. It is especially indicated in prolonged procedures in frail elderly patients. Full haemodynamic monitoring allows for the provision of a stable ICP and an adequate CPP. Beat to beat haemodynamic monitoring allows rapid identification of changes and opportunities to restore CPP.

Most anaesthetic agents reduce neuronal activity and in parallel reduce the cerebral metabolic requirement for oxygen ($CMRO_2$). They therefore provide a protective mechanism when oxygen demand may outweigh supply.

Unfortunately, many anaesthetic agents also reduce the mean arterial blood pressure by causing arterial vasodilatation. This induced hypotension directly reduces the CPP.

Anaesthetic drugs with minimal effects on arterial blood pressure should be used in the critically ill aged patients. However, if hypotension does occur the use of directly acting vasoconstrictors can restore perfusion pressure and may provide a stable CPP during induction and maintenance of anaesthesia provided that the patient does not have incipient cardiac failure.

Intraoperative positioning, especially if marked head up or sitting, can lead to postural hypotension which can be difficult to treat. Recovery after surgery should be swift to allow neurological assessment postoperatively. The modern anaesthetic agents and opioids provide both intraoperative control and a fast return of consciousness. As the surgical procedures may last many hours, drugs with prolonged context sensitive half-times are best avoided if early neurological assessment in necessary.

Principle of neuroanaesthesia

The cornerstone of neuroanaesthesia is the maintenance of a stable CPP. One of the major determinants of the CPP is the pressure/volume relationship within the cranial vault. The CPP is the calculated difference between the mean arterial pressure (MAP) and the sum of the intracranial pressure (ICP) and the central venous pressure (CVP):

$$CPP = MAP - (ICP + CVP)$$

Under normal physiological conditions, the ICP remains at 1–2 kPa (5–12 mmHg). The venous pressure is physiologically zero in younger subjects but is normally increased in the elderly because of an age-dependent rise in venous pressure due to diastolic dysfunction and tricuspid insufficiency. MAP is the main factor for determining the CPP. In the presence of a raised ICP, a raised venous pressure or a low MAP, the CPP is explicitly reduced. As the therapeutic aim is to maintain an optimal CPP, this can be achieved by lowering ICP with the use of drugs, hyperventilation, or decompression, by increasing the MAP moderately using drugs or volume, and by avoiding obstruction of venous backflow and venous volume overload.

Physiological stability of cerebral blood flow (CBF) during changes in MAP and CPP cerebral vessels is maintained by alterations in cerebrovascular resistance as a process of cerebral autoregulation. If the perfusion pressure falls or metabolic activity increases the cerebral vessels dilate to keep the CBF constant or vice versa they constrict if MAP increases or metabolism decreases. This autoregulation is active between 50 and 150 mmHg, but it can be disturbed by anaesthetics,[2] other drugs, metabolic disorders, and intracranial bleeds (either from strokes[3] or aneurysmal bleeds). Although cerebral autoregulation is normally maintained throughout life, the CBF by itself is decreases with age probably caused by diminished metabolic activity and fewer neurons.

In the presence of a space-occupying pathological lesion, e.g. blood, tumour, or oedema, the brain has only limited compensatory mechanisms before ICP increases significantly. The geriatric brain itself has more space within the cranium for compensation than the younger because the cerebral ventricle system as well as the epidural space is relatively increased because of the decreased amount of cerebral tissue. Daily nearly 50 000 neurons die and most of them are not replaced by neuronal connective tissue, so

that more space is available for compensating intracerebral pressure undulations. As the compensating mechanisms are exhausted there is a rapid increase of ICP. The increase of ICP is a late sign in elderly patients but the rapidity of rise once compensation is lost is much worse.

To avoid displacement of brain tissue and cerebellar tonsillar herniation through the foramen magnum caused by increasing ICP moderate hyperventilation to reduce carbon dioxide tensions and ensure adequate oxygen tension and achieve vasoconstriction as well as intracellular liquid mobilization by hyperoncotic mannitol or sodium chloride infusions have to be initiated. If these manoeuvres fail to reduce ICP then emergency decompressive craniectomy may be necessary. The symptoms of a slowly increasing ICP are headache and nausea, whereas a sudden catastrophic increase in ICP by intracerebral haemorrhage causes widespread ischaemia and infarction. This ischaemia in turn initiates a vicious circle of swelling around the infarcted tissue and a further increase in ICP.

If signs of raised ICP are identified, attempts to temporarily reduce the ICP until more definitive management can be instituted include:

- Hyperventilation reduces brain volume by decreasing the CBF through cerebral vasoconstriction. This effect may be effective for 4–6 hours depending on the pH of the CSF. For every 1 kPa change in $PaCO_2$, CBF changes by 7–14 ml/100 g/min. Hyperventilation is only effective as long as the CO_2 reactivity of the cerebro-vasculature is intact, which can be affected by ischaemia, trauma, tumour, and infection. Anaesthetic agents do not appear to have an impact on the efficacy of hyperventilation.[4] Whilst in humans hyperventilation-dependent vasoconstriction is preserved lifelong, the aged brain (as in neonates) is more vulnerable to ischaemia with profound cerebral vasoconstriction, and special care has to be taken to avoid excessive cerebral $PaCO_2$-lowering. The typical target $PaCO_2$ is 4–4.5 kPa (30–35 mmHg), whereby a $PaCO_2$ less than 4 kPa (30 mmHg) may be associated with ischaemia caused by extreme cerebral vasoconstriction in elderly patients.[5,6]

- For most neurosurgical patients, a neutral head position, elevated 15–30°, is recommended which decreases ICP by improving venous drainage. Conversely, flexing or turning of the head may obstruct cerebral venous outflow causing a dramatic ICP elevation that resolves with resumption of a neutral head position. Lowering the head impairs cerebral venous drainage, which can quickly result in an increase in brain bulk and ICP. The application of positive end-expiratory pressure (PEEP) to mechanically ventilated patients can potentially increase ICP, however a compromise between effects on ICP and optimizing ventilation is normally agreed.

- The administration of pharmacological agents that increase cerebral vascular resistance can acutely reduce ICP. Thiopentone and propofol are used for this purpose as they lower CBF by reducing cerebral metabolism. Hypertonic saline (HTS) and hyperoncotic mannitol are also used to treat intracranial hypertension. The principal mechanism underlying these effects is the induction of a water shift from brain tissues to the intravascular space by the hyperosmolarity of HTS and mannitol because the blood-brain barrier is impermeable to sodium and mannitol. Mannitol is also an osmotic diuretic and can have significant beneficial effects on ICP, CBF, and brain metabolism. Immediately after bolus administration they expand circulating volume, decrease blood viscosity and therefore increase CBF and cerebral oxygen delivery. Their hyperoncotic properties set up an osmotic gradient and draw water out of neurons. This is however a short term effect, since a continuous infusion or repeated boluses of mannitol do penetrate the blood-brain-barrier and thereby may exacerbate cerebral oedema. Therefore mannitol is best used by bolus administration for acute reduction in ICP. In elderly patients careful consideration should be given before either mannitol or hypertonic sodium chloride are administered, since they are wholly excreted in the urine and cause a rise in serum urine and osmolality. As the elderly are more prone to renal dysfunction, they are at risk from developing acute tubular necrosis, particularly in connection with hypovolaemia.

◆ Fluid restriction is option in less acute situations to reduce ICP but in elderly patients especially with compromised renal function this is relatively contraindicated. This is because it is frequently necessary to induce general anaesthesia for surgical management and maintained normovolaemia is important to limit the potential hypotension in response to anaesthetic agents and positive-pressure ventilation.

Anaesthesia for craniotomy for tumour or intracranial bleeding

Craniotomy in geriatric patients is usually for the removal of intracerebral tumours or more often decompression of intracerebral bleeding. In both groups the patient's history and examination are important to detect signs and symptoms of convulsions, nerve palsies and reduced levels of consciousness. Depending on the location of the tumour neuronal lesions, bulbar palsies and lower cranial nerve paralysis can be seen, whereby lesions of cranial nerves increase the risk of laryngeal incompetence and lead to chronic or acute aspiration of gastric contents and hypoxia.

Intracerebral bleeds are far more common in the elderly, and both acute subarachnoid haemorrhage (SAH) and chronic subdural haematoma (SDH) are seen. SAH usually presents as an emergency and can cause massive release of catecholamines leading to acute heart failure and malignant arrhythmias with no-specific electrocardiogram (ECG) changes. SDH shows a clear male predominance in older patients, and in most cases follows, often long forgotten minor trauma, or chronic anticoagulation by antiplatelet drugs.

Intracerebral tumours

Tumours (meningiomas, gliomas, and metastatic lesions) are initially small and slowly expanding. Particularly in aged patients with their increased ventricles and sulci it takes longer for identifiable increases in ICP because volume-spatial compensation occurs by compression of the CSF compartment and cerebral veins. Because of this increased ability of the elderly intracranial compartment to compensate, patients may exhibit minimal neurological dysfunction despite the presence of a large mass, an elevated ICP, and shifts in the position of brain structures. But as soon as the compensatory mechanisms become exhausted any further increase in tumour mass will cause progressively greater increases in ICP. In addition ICP is increased by the brain oedema surrounding the tumour. Cerebral autoregulation is compromised in the area around the tumour. Inadvertent increases in arterial pressure, hypercarbia, hypoxia, vasodilating agents, and jugular venous obstruction can produce significant increases in CBF, which can increase intracranial volume and ICP causing potentially life-threatening cerebral ischaemia and herniation.

If the tumour is located in the posterior fossa, which is a relatively confined space because it contains the medulla, pons, cerebellum, major motor and sensory pathways, primary respiratory and cardiovascular centres, and lower cranial nerve nuclei, decompensation occurs early. This is true even in the elderly with relatively more available space within the skull, where a small, localized tumour can compromise vital structures, causing profound neurological damage at an early stage and without increased ICP compared to tumours in the cerebrum.

Anaesthesia for cerebral tumours

Premedication should be prescribed with special care, particularly if there is any doubt about the patient's level of consciousness. A gross neurological examination should anyways be repeated and documented before induction of anaesthesia to have a documented neurological status quo. Preoperative medications, especially anticonvulsants, steroids, and cardiac drugs, should be continued until and including the day of surgery if possible. In addition to the routine monitoring, direct measurement of arterial blood pressure, arterial blood gases, central venous pressure, and urine output is recommended for all major neurosurgical procedures. In elderly patients invasive haemodynamic monitoring should be placed before induction of anaesthesia because they are at high risk for severe hypotension during induction of narcosis. In addition the arterial cannula allows measurement of the $paCO_2$ and an estimate of the ventilation–perfusion mismatch that is more evident in the elderly and means that the end-tidal CO_2 may correlate poorly with the $PaCO_2$. ICP is normally not available for induction of anaesthesia. In more patients where aggressive ICP management has been instituted before surgery ICP monitors may have been placed but this is a relatively painful procedure that itself may cause bleeding or infection.

It is most important to maintain blood pressure near the preoperative values to preserve CBF during induction of anaesthesia. The prolonged circulation time in the elderly can make this difficult if induction doses of anaesthetic agents are not titrated carefully. The same is true for non-depolarizing muscle relaxants as their onset time will be prolonged by several minutes to full relaxation. The stress response to intubation may be ameliorated by opioids, or a small bolus of propofol or lignocaine. If a rapid sequence technique is necessary, for instance because of known oesophageal reflux, high-dose rocuronium may be preferable to suxamethonium to avoid the potential spike in ICP which can occur with depolarizing relaxants. If there is concern about any difficulty in achieving tracheal intubation a planned approach is necessary because prolonged attempts at laryngoscopy are extremely stimulating and increase cerebral oxygen demand and ICP.

A major challenge of neurosurgical procedures is related to the positioning of the patient for difficult to access tumours, for example, those with an infratentorial location. Positioning can have direct problems from the actual position itself, from postural hypotension, from venous air embolism, or from direct pressure damage. Exploration of the posterior fossa has been traditionally performed in the sitting position because it provides excellent surgical exposure and facilitates venous and CSF drainage. From the anaesthetic perspective the sitting position compared to the Concorde or modified park bench positions provides better ventilation and easier access to the chest, airway, endotracheal tube, and extremities and reduces facial and conjunctival oedema. However, the sitting position is associated with significant risks for older patients, since it can produce intractable cardiovascular instability. The main risk of this position is that of venous air emboli, which can be lethal. In many centres worldwide the sitting position is no longer used in elderly or frail patients as there is no evidence of long-term differences in outcome dependent on the surgical positioning alone.

Independent of the decision for sitting or semi-reclined positions in elderly patients any flexion of the head on the cervical spine may be hazardous. This may occur on any occasion when pin fixation of the head is necessary. A preoperative examination of the mobility of the cervical spine, including a review of radiological studies to determine the width of the cervical canal, should be performed and recorded in geriatric patients.

Recovery has to be actively managed following neurosurgery, especially if this involves removal of a tumour or evacuation of haematoma when bleeding or rebleeding can be catastrophic. As with all such procedures the conduct of the anaesthetic is aimed at awakening and extubating the patient to permit an early assessment of surgical results and postoperative neurological status.

When the patient is completely stable, the risk of rebleeding is minimal and the reflexes of the patients are fully reversed, the choice of an early versus a delayed recovery in aged neurosurgical patients can be made.[7] In our institution an intravenous lidocaine bolus (1.5 mg/kg) is routinely administered 90 seconds before suctioning and extubation to minimize coughing, straining, and hypertension. Close monitoring and frequent neurological examinations are continued in the recovery room and for elderly patients this may be extended into overnight observation in the neurosurgical intensive care unit.

Awake craniotomy

Awake craniotomy is increasingly being used for neurosurgical procedures for removal of tumours involving the eloquent cortex. A neuropsychologist performs neurocognitive testing and/or monitors motor responses during tumour resection, which allows maximal tumour resection with minimal postoperative neurological deficits from retraction, oedema and/or resection of eloquent tissue. In our institution we perform awake craniotomy without any sedation, using only cranial blocks with long-acting local anaesthetics. The preoperative evaluation and preparation of these patients for awake craniotomy is rather different than for general anaesthesia. The main requirements for these patients are that they are cooperative, able to participate in neurocognitive testing, and stoical enough to cope with the stress of an awake craniotomy. At the moment the use of awake craniotomy is very restricted in the elderly and not routinely used in our institute.

Intracranial bleeding

Intracranial bleeding can be caused by direct traumatic brain injury (TBI) or by the rupture of an intracranial vessel or aneurysm. Both are devastating diseases and despite considerable advances in their management the outcome remains poor, particularly for geriatric patients. Intracranial bleeding may be from the rupture of a superficial arterial aneurysm causes in subarachnoid haemorrhage or hypertensive leaking from an intracerebral vessel leading to a deep intracerebral haematoma. Whilst SAH has an overall incidence of 8–10 per 100 000 people and a peak incidence for rupture in the fifth and sixth decades, the incidence of stroke continues to increase after 55 years of age. Approximately 15 per cent of strokes are haemorrhagic and rapid assessment and differentiation between thrombotic or haemorrhagic causes allows the choice of appropriate early treatment.

In subarachnoid bleeds, as soon as blood enters the subarachnoid space an abrupt, marked rise in ICP occurs, which causes an acute onset of severe headache with a stiff neck, photophobia, nausea and vomiting, systemic hypertension, and dysrhythmias. Frequently this is seen in parallel with a transient loss of consciousness. Warning symptoms and signs tend to be mild and no-specific (headache, dizziness, orbital pain, slight motor or sensory disturbance), so that they are generally ignored or misdiagnosed particularly by older patients and their physicians. The diagnosis of SAH is routinely made by the combination of clinical signs and a non-contrast CT scan of the head, where high density blood clot can be seen in the basal subarachnoid cisterns. Recently, sensitive spiral CT angiography as well as MRI scans have been used for detection and evaluation of intracranial aneurysms, which have high specificity, sensitivity, and diagnostic accuracy in detecting intracranial aneurysms. Increasingly, the choice of management of for acute and multiple aneurysms in by interventional neuroradiology aimed at embolizing the aneurysmal sac.[8] The care of unruptured aneurysms may be either by surgical clipping and occlusion or by interventional neuroradiology as for acute bleeds. The 2003 the International Study of Unruptured Intracranial Aneurysms (ISUIA)[9] demonstrated that no significant differences were observed in outcome between open surgical or endovascular procedures. In this study the strongest predictors of surgical outcome were the patient's age, size, and the location of the aneurysm.

Surgical decompression of an intracranial bleed from a stroke is becoming increasingly common, as the management of strokes is more active and interventional. A bleed volume of 30 ml or more with signs of raised ICP is the usual trigger for intervention. The procedure may vary from simple aspiration of the haematoma to decompressive hemicraniectomy.[10] The risk of further neurological damage associated with an acute intervention in these critically ill elderly patients is high but lacks the detailed evidence available for aneurysmal bleeds.

Conduct of anaesthesia for intracranial bleeding

Aneurysmal SAH is usually classified according to either the Hunt and Hess[11] (see Table 22.1) or the World Federation of Neurosurgical Societies (WFNS)[12] classifications. The outcome of these patients is also strongly influenced by the presence of cerebral vasospasm and intracranial hypertension, although the patient's age, the size, and location of the aneurysm are the main predictors of surgical mortality and outcome.

Severity, acuteness, and the stage of the SAH as well as the presence of complications determine the time of surgery. The debate over 'early versus late' surgery has still not been resolved.[13–15] The outcomes appear to show a benefit from early surgery in high grade

Table 22.1 Hunt and Hess classification of patients with subarachnoid haemorrhage

Grade	Criteria
0	Unruptured aneurysm
I	Asymptomatic, or minimal, headache and slight nuchal rigidity
II	Moderate to severe headache, nuchal rigidity, no neurological deficit other than cranial nerve palsy
III	Drowsiness, confusion, or mild focal deficit
IV	Stupor, moderate to severe hemiparesis, early decerebration, vegetative disturbance
V	Deep coma, decerebrate rigidity, moribund

Reproduced from Hunt WE, Hess RM, 'Surgical risk as related to time of intervention in the repair of intracranial aneurysms', *Journal of Neurosurgery*, 28, 1, pp. 14–20, copyright 1968, with permission from American Association of Neurological Surgeons.

(1 or 2) patients, although there is no difference in the incidence of intra-operative rupture between early and late surgery. The primary reason for early surgery is to reduce the incidence of rebleeding that occurs with conservative management of SAH. Rebleeding occurs most commonly during the first 24 hours following the initial SAH. The chance of rebleeding is about 4 per cent within the first day; after 48 hours, it is 1.5 per cent per day, with a cumulative rebleeding rate of 19 per cent by the end of 2 weeks.[16]

Acute SAH can be accompanied by ECG changes (ST-segment depression or elevation, T-wave inversion or flattening, U waves, prolonged QT intervals) dysrhythmia, temperature instability, various changes in endocrine functions, various electrolyte disturbances, particularly hyponatraemia, volume shifts, sympathetic overactivity. These are usually attributed to the effect of the bleed from the circle of Willis and the proximity of the hypothalamus. This triggers hypothalamic dysfunctional responses that can include an overstimulation of both the adrenal cortex and medulla, which can also contribute to hypertension and diabetes.

Elderly patients with poorly compensated organ function are at risk for decompensation for elective surgery, and this is even more so when hypertension and dysrhythmias are present after a bleed. Treating the hypertension before surgery, usually with β-blockers such as esmolol or labetalol, without causing major changes in intracranial blood volume of ICP can be difficult. Frequent neurological assessments are necessary to identify any new events that could be due to ischaemia caused by lowering the blood pressure below the perfusion threshold for cerebral circulations vulnerable to vasospasm.

Aneurysm surgery can be performed as open or endovascular interventional neuroradiology (INR) procedure. Endovascular embolization is a therapeutic option to surgical clipping of the cerebral aneurysm. Patients with high-risk, inaccessible aneurysms and/or comorbid medical conditions are candidates for INR procedures. Increasingly, this is the procedure recommended for older patients, if the condition, location, and size of the intracranial aneurysms allow it.[8] Endovascular techniques are rapidly evolving and new techniques and investigational devices are being developed and investigated continually. An anaesthetist or intensivist should be present for all of these procedures to monitor the patient, to provide appropriate anaesthesia or analgo-sedation for the procedure and to manage fulminating complications. During embolization procedures it is important to maintain a stable cerebral circulation to enable the neuroradiologist to enter the vessel and safely embolize the aneurysm. If the flow changes this may flush the embolizing material into normal vessels with clear adverse effects.

For intracranial aneurysm surgery the primary aim of anaesthesia is to prevent rupture of the aneurysm by maintaining a stable transmural pressure within the affected vessel and sac and keeping the CPP above the ischaemic threshold. Once the craniectomy is complete and the dissection is about to start most surgeons prefer a 'slack' brain to limit traction damage to the underlying brain tissue.

Standard monitoring, including placement of an arterial line and if necessary advanced haemodynamic monitoring as well as electrophysiological monitoring to assess the adequacy of cerebral perfusion, is recommended before induction.

Induction drugs should maintain mean arterial pressure und ICP, so that CPP is constant, since this keeps the transmural pressure also stable, while an increase in mean arterial pressure or fall in ICP will increase transmural pressure and consequently the risk of the life-threatening aneurysm rupture. Intravenous lidocaine and the short-acting β-adrenergic antagonists are recommended to avoid hypertension during laryngoscopy and intubation.

If ICP following induction is normal, then the anaesthetist should maintain normoxyia, normocarbia, normothermia, normovolaemia, normotension, and normoglycaemia. If intracranial hypertension is present, the $PaCO_2$ can be moderately lowered to 4–4.5kPa (30–35 mmHg). General anaesthesia should be deep enough to avoid a hypertensive response to insertion of head pins, the scalp incision, turning the bone flap, and opening the dura. The drugs most frequently used to maintain anaesthesia during aneurysm surgery are intravenous opioids such as fentanyl or remifentanil and propofol infusions with or without 0.5 minimum alveolar concentration (MAC) of a potent inhalation agent such as sevoflurane or desflurane in oxygen and a non-depolarizing muscle relaxant. Where there is very poor intracranial compliance, a continuous infusion of thiopental (1–3 mg/kg/hour following a bolus dose of 5 mg/kg) may be substituted for propofol as the primary anaesthetic although this may be more hazardous in elderly patients because of the blood pressure instability and prolonged recovery from anaesthesia.

If further reduction in intracranial volume is necessary osmotic diuretics, CSF drainage or further hyperventilation may be effective but are more risky in the elderly because of the risk of sudden transmural pressure changes.

For the definitive aneurysm clipping either induced hypotension or temporary occlusion of a major intracranial vessel may be necessary to allow safe placement of the permanent clip. When considering the use of controlled hypotension during aneurysm dissection, the risk/benefit ratio must be assessed for the older patients. Older patients with their higher incidence of cardiovascular diseases, of occlusive cerebrovascular diseases, anaemia, and renal diseases are at high risk during controlled hypotension. The first choice in elderly patients should be temporary occlusion with normotension in order to maintain maximal collateral perfusion. Only if this fails can a moderate reduction in systemic blood pressure (20–30 mmHg) be accepted. This may be achieved with short-acting drugs like sodium nitroprusside, inhalational anaesthetics, and esmolol. Mild intraoperative hypothermia (32 to 34°C) during aneurysm surgery to enhance the brain's ability to tolerate ischaemia is not indicated and doesn`t improve outcome in geriatric neurosurgical patients.[17–19] When the aneurysm is secured, any intraoperative fluid deficits are replaced and additional volume is moderately administered.

When an aneurysm ruptures intraoperatively, there is a high risk of major ischaemic damage or haemorrhagic death if the surgeon can`t gain control with suction and apply either a temporary or the permanent clip to the neck of the aneurysm. When bleeding is excessive and the surgeon loses control of the blood loss, aggressive fluid resuscitation and blood transfusion must commence immediately. Immediate, high-dose administration of cerebroprotective agents is questionable because of associated negative haemodynamic effects.

Cerebral vasospasm

Cerebral vasospasm is a severe and frequent complication in SAH patients and as dangerous as rebleeding, intracranial hypertension, and hydrocephalus. The clinical syndrome of vasospasm is often heralded by a worsening headache and increasing blood pressure; characterized by progressive symptoms of confusion and lethargy, followed by focal motor and speech impairments depending on the arterial territory involved. The syndrome may resolve gradually or progress to coma and death within a period of hours to days. The diagnosis of vasospasm was confirmed by angiography but is increasingly being assessed with transcranial Doppler (TCD). This is a safe, repeatable, non-invasive method to identify and quantify vasospasm and to guide therapeutic interventions. Although the mechanism responsible for vasospasm is still unknown, there is evidence that vasospasm after SAH correlates with the amount of blood in the subarachnoid space, and is possibly caused by oxyhaemoglobin. Another theory is that spreading depolarization from the bleeding spot causes the vasoconstriction.[20] The oral calcium channel blocker nimodipine has become standard prophylactic therapy, although meta-analysis could not proof significant outcome improvements with nimodipine prophylaxis.[21] At present the 'triple-H' therapy—hypervolaemia, hypertension, and haemodilution—is the treatment of first choice for ischaemic neurological deficits caused by cerebral vasospasm.[22] However in elderly patients with compromised cardiac reserve hypervolaemia and haemodilution are restricted to prevent cardiac decompensating. Therefore advanced haemodynamic monitoring is required to avoid cardiac failure and pulmonary oedema. Caution is also necessary because hypervolaemia and hypertension can worsen cerebral oedema, increase ICP, and cause haemorrhagic infarction. In the geriatric population the preferred therapeutic interventions for treating symptomatic vasospasm are controlled moderate hypervolemia supported by inotropic drugs where necessary, and cerebral transluminal angioplasty under general anaesthesia and continuous superselective intra-arterial infusion of papaverine, nimodipine or verapamil, which can dilate distal vessels not easily accessible to angioplasty.[23,24]

Traumatic brain injury

TBI is typically a disease of younger people and a frequent cause of death in them, but it is becoming more and more a global disease burden in elderly patients. The main causes in geriatric patients are falls, followed by motor vehicle accidents as pedestrians. The injuries are unfortunately aggravated by their comorbidities and the common use of antiplatelet and anticoagulant medications in the elderly.

TBI is dependent not only on the extent of the direct irreversible neuronal damage at the time of injury, but also on the occurrence of any secondary insults. These additional insults include:

♦ Systemic factors such as hypoxaemia, hypercapnia, or hypotension.

♦ Formation and expansion of an epidural, subdural, or intracerebral haematoma.

♦ Sustained intracranial hypertension.

Post-traumatic surgical and anaesthetic management is focused on preventing these secondary insults. The Glasgow Coma Scale (GCS) score[25,26] (see Table 22.2) generally correlates well with the severity of injury and outcome.

Depending on the mechanism of injury cerebral contusions in elderly patients may be limited to the surface of the brain or may involve haemorrhage in deeper hemispheric structures or the brain stem, and each will present with different clinical symptoms. The operative treatment in this population group is usually for depressed skull fractures, evacuation of displacing epidural, subdural, and some intracerebral haematomas, and debridement of penetrating injuries. Developing intracranial hypertension (ICP) can be treated with moderate hyperventilation, mannitol or hyperosmolar sodium chloride infusions and boluses of barbiturates or propofol. Placing an intracerebral pressure sensor appears to be reasonable, since during increases in ICP the CPP should be maintained constantly. An ICP greater than 60 mmHg results in irreversible brain oedema in geriatric patients.

Conduct of anaesthesia for traumatic brain injury

The anaesthetic care of patients with severe head trauma begins in the emergency department. Elderly patients are at risk for hypoxaemia, hypoventilation, and hypotension from other injuries. Therefore supplemental oxygen should be given to all geriatric trauma patients. All trauma patients must be assumed to have a cervical spine injury until proven otherwise. Patients with obvious hypoventilation, an absent gag reflex, and/or a persistent score below 8 on the GCS require immediate tracheal intubation and moderate hyperventilation.

For emergency intubation all patients should be regarded as having a full stomach. Consequently a rapid sequence induction with

Table 22.2 Glasgow Coma Scale (GCS) score[25]

Eye opening	Best verbal response	Best motor response
Spontaneously 4	Oriented, conversing 5	Obeys verbal commands 6
To verbal command 3	Disoriented, conversing 4	Localizes to pain 5
To pain 2	Inappropriate words 3	Flexion/withdrawal 4
None 1	Incomprehensible sounds 2	Abnormal flexion (decorticate) 3
	No verbal response 1	Extension (decerebrate) 2

Mild head injury = 13–15; moderate = 9–12; severe = ≤8. Reprinted from *The Lancet*, 304, 7872, Teasdale G and Jennett B, 'Assessment of coma and impaired consciousness: A practical scale', pp. 81–84, Copyright 1974, with permission from Elsevier.

manual in-line axial stabilization of the cervical spine is necessary. Administration of thiopental, 1–2 mg/kg, or propofol, 1.0 mg/kg, opioids and suxamethonium or rocuronium as relaxant is indicated. The lower doses of induction agents is important in elderly patients and even more so if they are haemodynamically unstable or hypotensive.

If a difficult intubation is anticipated, consideration of the need for awake fibreoptic intubation or even tracheostomy is necessary, since the head should be immobilized for intubation because of the potential unstable cervical spine. Blind nasal intubation is absolutely contraindicated in the presence of a basilar skull fracture, which is suggested by CSF rhinorrhoea or otorrhoea or haemotympanum. Once the patient is stable the decision between operative and medical management of head trauma is made based on radiographic as well as clinical features; not all TBI patients have to be operated upon. In the event of neurological deterioration and increased ICP, administration of intravenous mannitol and thiopental could be considered, followed by moderate hyperventilation.

If surgical intervention is planned the anaesthetic management is no different to that for other mass lesions associated with intracranial hypertension. Invasive arterial blood pressure and central venous pressure monitoring should be established if not already present. However, in an emergency procedure arterial or venous cannulation should not delay surgical decompression in a rapidly deteriorating patient. An intravenous technique is commonly used, while nitrous oxide is contraindicated since air could be entrapped within the cranium.

For hypertension additional doses of the induction agent can be administered, but also increased concentrations of inhalational anaesthetics or antihypertensives may be used. CPP should be maintained between 70 and 110 mmHg. Disseminated intravascular coagulation may be seen with severe head injuries and is in addition to the bleeding caused by the routine use of antiplatelet and anticoagulant drugs in this age group. The decision whether to extubate the trachea at the end of the surgical procedure depends on the severity of the injury, the presence of concomitant abdominal or thoracic injuries, comorbidities, and the preoperative level of consciousness.

Chronic SDH represents one of the most frequent clinical entities encountered in daily neurosurgical practice for older patients with other associated serious systemic problems. Minor trauma, often long forgotten by the time of presentation, is postulated to be the initial cause in most cases. Pathophysiologically, cerebral atrophy and the concomitant stretching of the bridging veins are the main reasons for SDH. These veins rupture following even minor insult such as a fall, particularly when the patient is on antiplatelet or anticoagulant medication. Because of the cerebral atrophy in ageing patients significant blood collection can occur in the subdural space before a rise in ICP is seen, which is probably the reason for the late presentation. Clinical signs are seizures, focal neurological signs, subtle cognitive deficits such as confusion, memory loss, etc. which mimic many neurological and psychiatric illnesses. The diagnosis of SDH is usually confirmed by CT scan. Surgical intervention and evacuation of the haematoma by burr holes or the wait-and-see attitude depends on the progression or otherwise of symptoms and signs of spreading. For surgical intervention coexisting systemic diseases usually pose a problem for general anaesthesia in this particular patient group, so that an alternative method to general anaesthesia, local anaesthesia, has to be discussed. As this is a relatively superficial procedure many units use a local anaesthetic technique, usually without any sedation.

Novel neurosurgical procedures

Stem cell implantation for neurodegenerative disorders or following trauma/stroke has been suggested for many years. Early trials, which did show some effects, used mesodermal rather than ectodermal cell lines and thus were unlikely to provide new neurological tissue. Recent use of ectodermal progenitor cell lines has been reported to improve outcome following stroke. Conditions such as Parkinson's disease or Alzheimer's disease where a more progressive cell loss occurs may also benefit from such therapy. The surgical procedures would be stereotactic in nature and may be prolonged. As the majority will be provided for elderly patients anaesthetists will have to develop appropriate techniques to provide optimal surgical operating conditions whilst developing an understanding of the impact that anaesthetic agents may have on such vulnerable cell lines.

Anaesthesia for surgery on the spine

Spinal surgery is most often performed for symptomatic nerve root or cord compression secondary to degenerative diseases or trauma. The compression of the spinal cord may occur, on the one hand, by the severe forces caused by blunt trauma, falls, motor vehicle collisions, etc. The spinal cord can also be scrunched or totally severed by disrupted intervertebral bands or dislocated vertebral bodies. On the other hand, age-depending osteophytic bones, osteoporosis, or protrusion of an intervertebral disc into the spinal canal can severely damage the spinal cord or nerve roots. Spondylitis, a common feature of rheumatoid arthritis, tends to affect the lower cervical spine more than the lumbar spine and typically affects older patients. Operations on the spinal column can decompress the cord, and fuse the spine if disrupted by blunt trauma. Spinal surgery may also be performed to resect a tumour or vascular malformation or to drain an epidural abscess or haematoma in elderly patients. Spinal decompression, discectomy as well as vertebroplasty are also performed in geriatric patients, since the outcome in terms of restored/retained function nearly match those of younger patients.

The blood flow to the spinal cord is dependent on relatively few arteries and these can be compromised by the same medium vessel diseases as coronary or peripheral vessels. As the vertebral column is progressively subject to stresses from posture and minor injuries throughout life, the elderly are more prone to compression from osteophytes, ligamental calcification, and rigidity. The combination of these two processes means that the spinal cord perfusion pressure must be maintained to preserve cord perfusion. The same care that is necessary to maintain the CPP has to be delivered in spinal surgery in the elderly.

Conduct of anaesthesia for spine surgery

As the majority of spinal surgery is performed in the prone position the preoperative evaluation of these older patients should particularly focus on their ability to compensate for the changes in physiology in that position and the magnitude of the surgical procedure and its associated stress response. Anterior cervical procedures are less demanding of the patient but do have their own risk of serious complications. In common with cranial surgery it is important to document accurately all existing neurological deficits for legal reasons and this is best performed by an independent specialist or neurologist.

The movement of the patient into the prone position means that a thorough examination of the patient's musculoskeletal system should be performed to assess limitations to movement and especially flexion/extension of the neck in case of vertebro-basilar compromise. Osteoporosis and cervical spondylosis may be asymptomatic but close to critically compressing the nerve root canals and cord. Increasingly, obesity is more common in the elderly and this can have a marked influence on the abdominal pressures generated once prone.

Many elderly patients with severe arthritis or degenerative spinal diseases will be on analgesic and non-steroidal anti-inflammatory drugs (NSAIDs). Some will also be on potent opiates. The perioperative management of these patients is complex and may require support from an acute pain management team. Stopping the drugs will immobilize the patient and manipulation of tender joints under anaesthesia will cause extreme, widespread pain on recovery that is unrelated to the spinal surgery itself. The risk of renal dysfunction caused by dehydration and the NSAIDs in the elderly is very real. Premedication should be used sparingly especially in patients with difficult airways or ventilatory impairment. The risk of airway compromise or hypoxia from obstructive sleep apnoea means that these patients should be very closely monitored if premedication is prescribed, whether opioid or sedative.

Monitoring and induction should be as precisely controlled as for craniotomy because the spinal perfusion pressure is just as precarious as the CPP. As mentioned earlier, the anaesthetic management is complicated by the prone position, which is preferred for most surgical procedures on the spine. Following induction of anaesthesia and tracheal intubation in the supine position, the patient is normally turned prone. Special care must be taken to maintain the neck in a neutral position to secure spinal cord perfusion. Once in the prone position, the head can be turned to the side or can remain face down on a special soft holder. Extreme caution is also necessary to avoid positional and pressure damages to the eyes, nose, breasts, and genitals as well as to nerve and muscle. Corneal abrasions or retinal ischaemia from pressure occur, albeit infrequently. The prone position also needs appropriate positioning supports to aid ventilation and maintain cardiac function. The chest should rest on rolls or special supports whilst the arms may be at the sides in a comfortable position or extended with the elbows flexed as far this is possible in elderly patients. Turning the geriatric patient prone is a critical manoeuvre for the patient and the anaesthetist. There is a risk of hypotension resulting from abdominal compression, particularly in obese patients, where venous return is impeded because of caval compression and cardiac filling is diminished. The caval compression also leads to the engorgement of epidural veins, which makes the operative field hazardous and if the epidural veins are damages contributes to massive intraoperative blood loss. For this reason the abdomen should be dependent and free of direct compression. One occult cause of massive bleeding is damage to the aorta if the anterior longitudinal ligament is damaged during dissection for complex disc or vertebral surgery. This blood loss may catastrophic but into the retroperitoneal space.

The supine position is used for an anterior approach to the cervical spine. This approach may indeed facilitate the anaesthetic management of spine surgery in the cervical and upper thoracic areal, but increase the risk of surgical complications involving the trachea, oesophagus, recurrent laryngeal nerve, sympathetic chain, carotid artery, or jugular vein. Cervical traction through a two-pin system may be used to improve the operative access but is more hazardous in the elderly patient who may not tolerate the distraction. The transoral approach is necessary for anterior surgery on the first three cervical discs and odontoid process. The postoperative oedema from these anterior approaches may compromise the airway in recovery, especially if there is also poor haemostasis and a haematoma forms. This may cause a life-threatening loss of airway.

Anterior surgery on the thoracic spine, for instance, for decompression of vertebral collapse may require a transthoracic approach and the need for one-lung ventilation. This may be poorly tolerated in the elderly and modification of the surgical approach may be necessary. A sitting or lateral decubitus position may occasionally be used but is the exception for these procedures.

Spinal surgery may have as massive and acute blood loss as major vascular surgery. This is more likely if there is caval and abdominal compression. In the elderly with reduced cardiovascular reserve identical monitoring and provision for rapid, warmed blood transfusion and red cell salvage should be available as for major vascular cases. Elective hypotension carries a much greater risk of critically reducing cord perfusion and should be avoided.

Some forms of spinal surgery require intraoperative assessment of function and techniques for 'wake-up' are well developed. It is rare for this to be necessary in the elderly and the increasing use of somatosensory and motor evoked potentials are more likely to be utilized. There is, however, still a need for the rapid neurological assessment of function after surgery and therefore a need for a rapid and full return to consciousness. Close haemodynamic monitoring should continue until postoperative variables confirm that insidious blood loss is absent. Pain control and rapid mobilization are important to recovery and may need support from the acute pain team if there is a degree of cognitive impairment. The inhumane restriction of appropriate analgesia to the elderly neurosurgical patient is more likely to trigger delirium than cause respiratory complications.

Rehabilitation and convalescence of the elderly neurosurgical patient may be slow and take some months to achieve the maximum outcome following surgery. This is partly due to the elderly's limited physiological reserve and partly to the reduced resilience of their neuronal pathways. There is little scientific evidence on the impact of ageing on recovery but major surgery does appear to take at least 6 months to return to their pre-surgical fitness.

Conclusion

The elderly patient is just as likely to benefit from neurosurgery as their younger cohorts. Increasingly, the acute management of intracranial bleeds by decompression has improved outcome from stroke in terms of both mortality and morbidity. Reconstructive and decompressive spinal surgery for trauma and tumour relieve pain and increase mobility that in turn maintain independence of individual patients. The challenges for the future when stem cell implantation becomes feasible and modification of degenerative diseases realistic will change neurosurgical demands and the anaesthetic care that allows these novel procedures to be performed safely.

References

1. Dodds C, Kumar CM, Servin F (eds) *Anaesthesia for the elderly patient.* Oxford: Oxford University Press, 2007.

2. Dagal A, Lam AM. Cerebral autoregulation and anesthesia. *Curr Opin Anaesthesiol.* 2009;22(5):547–552.

3. Aries MJ, Elting JW, De Keyser J, Kremer BP, Vroomen PC. Cerebral autoregulation in stroke: a review of transcranial Doppler studies. *Stroke.* 2010;41(11):2697–2704.

4. Citerio G, Pesenti A, Latini R, *et al.* A multicentre, randomised, open-label, controlled trial evaluating equivalence of inhalational and intravenous anaesthesia during elective craniotomy. *Eur J Anaesthesiol.* 2012;29(8):371–379.

5. Obrist WD, Langfitt TW, Jaggi JL, *et al.* Cerebral blood flow and metabolism in comatose patients with acute head injury. Relationship to intracranial hypertension. *J Neurosurg.* 1984;61(2):241–253.

6. Coles JP, Minhas PS, Fryer TD, *et al.* Effect of hyperventilation on cerebral blood flow in traumatic head injury: clinical relevance and monitoring correlates. *Crit Care Med.* 2002;30:1950–1959.

7. Bruder N, Ravassin P. Recovery from anesthesia and postoperative extubation of neurosurgical patients: a review. *J Neurosurg Anesthesiol.* 1999;11:282–293.

8. Wilson TJ, Davis MC, Stetler WR, *et al.* Endovascular treatment for aneurysmal subarachnoid hemorrhage in the ninth decade of life and beyond. *J Neurointerv Surg.* 2013;Mar 27. [Epub ahead of print]

9. The International Study of Unruptured Intracranial Aneurysms Investigators. Unruptured intracranial aneurysms: natural history, clinical outcome, and risks of surgical and endovascular treatment. *Lancet.* 2003;362:103–11.

10. Inamasu J, Kaito T, Watabe T, *et al.* Decompressive hemicraniectomy for malignant hemispheric stroke in the elderly: comparison of outcomes between individuals 61-70 and >70 years of age. *J Stroke Cerebrovascular Dis.* 2013;Mar 10. [Epub ahead of print]

11. Hunt WE, Hess RM. Surgical risk as related to time of intervention in the repair of intracranial aneurysms. *J Neurosurg.* 1968;28:14–20.

12. Teasdale GM, Drake CG, Hunt W, *et al.* A universal subarachnoid hemorrhage scale: report of a committee of the World Federation of Neurosurgical Societies. *J Neurol Neurosurg Psychiatry.* 1988;51(11):1457.

13. Kassell NF, Torner JC, Haley EC Jr, *et al.* The International Cooperative Study on the Timing of Aneurysm Surgery. Part I: overall management results. *J Neurosurg.* 1990;73:18–36.

14. Golchin N, Ramak Hashem SM, Abbas Nejad E, Noormohamadi S. Timing of surgery for aneurysmal subarachnoid hemorrhage. *Acta Medica Iranica.* 2012;50(5):300–304.

15. Siddiq F, Chaudhry SA, Tummala RP, Suri MF, Qureshi AI. Factors and outcomes associated with early and delayed aneurysm treatment in subarachnoid hemorrhage patients in the United States. *Neurosurgery.* 2012;71(3):670–677.

16. Dorhout Mees SM, Molyneux AJ, Kerr RS, Algra A, Rinkel GJ. Timing of aneurysm treatment after subarachnoid hemorrhage: relationship with delayed cerebral ischemia and poor outcome. *Stroke.* 2012;43(8):2126–2129.

17. Kassell NF, Torner JC. Aneurysmal rebleeding: a preliminary report from the Cooperative Aneurysm Study. *J Neurosurg.* 1983;13:479–481.

18. Todd MM, Hindman BJ, Clark WR, *et al.* Mild inoperative hypothermia during surgery for intracranial aneursym. *N Engl J Med.* 2005;352(2):135–145.

19. Moore L, Berkow L, Zickmann J, *et al.* A survey of SNACC members' clinical practice of neuroanesthesia. *J Neurosurg Anesthesiol.* 2002;14(4):A1100.

20. Dreier JP. The role of spreading depression, spreading depolarization and spreading ischemia in neurological disease. *Nat Med.* 2011;17(4):439–447.

21. Barker FG, Ogilvy CS. Efficacy of prophylactic nimodipine for delayed ischemic deficit after subarachnoid hemorrhage: a meta-analysis. *J Neurosurg.* 1996;84:405.

22. Sen J, Belli A, Alban H, *et al.* Triple-H therapy in the management of aneurysmal subarachnoid hemorrhage. *Lancet Neurol.* 2003;2(10):614–621.

23. Bendo AA, Kass IS, Hartung J, *et al.* Anesthesia for neurosurgery. In Barash PG, Cullen BF, Stoelting RK (eds) *Clinical anesthesia,* 4th edn (pp. 743–790). Philadelphia, PA: Lippincott Williams & Wilkins, 2001.

24. Feng L, Fitzsimmons B-F, Young WL, *et al.* Intraarterially administered verapamil as adjunct therapy for cerebral vasospasm: safety and 2-year experience. *AJNR.* 2002;23:1284–1290.

25. Teasdale G, Jennett B. Assessment of coma and impaired consciousness: a practical scale. *Lancet.* 1974;2:81–84.

26. Jennett B. Assessment of the severity of head injury. *J Neurol Neurosurg Psychiatry.* 1976;39:647–655.

CHAPTER 23

Major abdominal surgery in the elderly

Dave Murray

Introduction

The elderly population represents a considerable consumer of healthcare resources. Approximately 25 per cent of surgical patients in Western countries are over 65 years old, a figure that is set to increase.[1] Data from UK Office of National Statistics estimates that the number of people over the age of 85 will double by 2030.[2] In addition, the number of elderly patients undergoing surgery is also increasing independently of this rise.[3] This chapter will consider management of the elderly patient undergoing major intra-abdominal surgery. It begins with an overview of general anaesthetic management, and then continues with a more in-depth discussion of specific clinical issues.

Preoperative assessment

See also Chapter 15.

Patients aged 80 and above have a high incidence of chronic medical illness when compared to younger patients. In particular, cardiorespiratory and cerebrovascular disease, diabetes, and renal impairment are all common place. The impact of this is compounded by the loss of physiological reserve brought about by the ageing process, and it can sometimes be difficult to distinguish between the two. The challenge of preoperative assessment for major intra-abdominal surgery is to:

- Accurately define the extent of existing disease states.

- Identify areas where the patient might benefit from optimization of their medical condition, taking into account the time constraints imposed by the surgical pathology. The surgical window may also be constrained by preoperative chemo- and radiotherapy.

- Ensure the patient is fully informed of the risk and benefit of the proposed surgery

Preoperative investigations for major abdominal surgery

There are various guidelines published that provide evidence based approaches to preoperative tests.[4,5] National Institute for Health and Clinical Excellence (NICE) guidelines include specific recommendations for patients aged over 80 years. Patients undergoing major surgery aged 80 and over, should have a full blood count and renal function performed, regardless of American Society of Anesthesiologists (ASA) grade. An electrocardiogram should also be performed. Tests of clotting function are unlikely to be abnormal without significant liver disease or anticoagulant therapy, and the NICE guidelines state that the clinician should consider tests of coagulation on an individual patient basis.

Anaemia is relatively common in the elderly due to poor nutrition and chronic diseases states. Patients may not have sufficient haematinic stores to restore their haemoglobin levels themselves in the postoperative period. In addition, haemoglobin levels may be low due to gastrointestinal losses from a tumour site.

Major surgery is associated with significant fluid shifts in the perioperative period, and hence estimation of renal function is important. Abnormal serum urea and electrolyte values are relatively common. However, reduced dietary intake and muscle mass mean that the respective values of urea and creatinine are lower in the elderly, and hence normal values may still be seen despite a reduction in renal function. Estimation of glomerular filtration rate may be useful in these cases.

Assessing risk and benefit in major intra-abdominal surgery

Whilst 30-day mortality rates for patients of all ages undergoing major surgery may be in the region of 5 per cent, major surgery clearly holds a higher risk for the elderly patient. One of the challenges facing the anaesthetist is accurately assessing that risk for an individual patient. Without it, it can be difficult to have an informed discussion with the patient about the consequences of proceeding to surgery. Age and ASA classification have clearly been identified as predictors of mortality in several scoring systems. However there are limitations to many of these. POSSUM (Physiological and Operative Severity Score for Enumeration of Mortality and Morbidity) is well validated, but is designed to compare risk on a population basis rather than an individual patient basis.[6] Disease-specific models, such as that available for colorectal surgery (CR-POSSUM), and the model developed by the Association of Coloproctology of Great Britain and Ireland generally outperform generic models in estimating operative mortality.[7–10]

Given these difficulties in accurately predicting individual patient risk, it is of vital importance that the anaesthetist has a full and frank discussion with the patient in advance of surgery. This will allow the anaesthetist to discuss with the patient their expectations and desires for the forthcoming surgery. It is not uncommon for patients with cancer to still opt for surgery, despite being quoted an estimated 30-day mortality of 15–20 per cent. There is still a stigma associated with a cancer diagnosis, especially in this age group of patients, and patients will often express a strong desire for surgery in order for the cancer to be removed. Quality of life also features highly for elderly patients. Symptoms may be a limiting factor, particularly if the surgical diagnosis (such as colorectal cancer) is associated with symptoms of faecal frequency and incontinence. Similar issues arise in patients with entero-vaginal fistulae from severe diverticular disease. These may be of such severity that the patient does not venture outside their home. Hence surgery is perceived as being associated with an immediate improvement in their quality of life, even if the disease process is not life threatening.

Another important factor that needs to be considered is the length of time that it will take for the patient to resume their normal daily activities. Whilst the patient might be discharged from hospital within a week or so, full return to the same preoperative level of functioning may take much longer. For major surgery, this may be up to a year. For an elderly patient who is just coping to live independently in their own home, this protracted recovery period may mean that they cannot return to their own home in the immediate postoperative period without additional help. Failing to recognize this in the preoperative period will lead to delays in discharge whilst this additional support is put in place. In some cases, major surgery may mean that a patient is unable to return to their current home at all. It is also not uncommon for the patient undergoing surgery to be the main carer for a spouse whose needs will also need to be considered. The availability of family support can be vital in reaching a decision.

It can be helpful to have a patient's relatives present at the preoperative assessment visit. Deafness and cognitive impairment may severely restrict the ability to obtain an accurate history, and relatives may be able to corroborate the history. Patients will often require time to consider the implications of any discussion, and it is helpful if relatives have been present at that discussion. Prehabilitation and comprehensive geriatric assessment may also be important in improving patient outcomes.[11] The risk/benefit assessment is particularly difficult when considering emergency surgery. There is debate about the appropriateness of surgery when faced with an elderly patient with acute abdominal pathology and significant comorbidities.[12] On one hand, a small study demonstrated that 66 per cent of elderly ASA 5 patients survived 30 days and 33 per cent were discharged from hospital.[13] On the other hand, the Scottish Audit of Surgical Mortality found that the most common 'adverse event' was an assessment that, in retrospect, the operation should not have been carried out.[14] This emphasizes the difficulty in deciding on the most appropriate course of action given the lack of a robust risk assessment method for predicting outcomes.

It is good practice for the anaesthetist to be present at any multidisciplinary meetings where options for surgery can be discussed. Less invasive techniques or a palliative procedure may be appropriate. Malignant polyps might be amenable to a per-anal approach, rather than full resection. The greater chance of surgical cure following resection needs to be balanced against the benefits of less invasive surgery. A transverse rather than a longitudinal abdominal incision may be used, although this is becoming less of an issue with the rise in minimally invasive approaches and enhanced recovery programmes. In the emergency situation, obstructive symptoms may be relieved by a loop ileostomy or colostomy without the need to undergo a full laparotomy. Endoscopic stents may relieve an obstructing tumour, allowing the patient to receive surgery as a non-urgent case, and may even mean that surgery can be avoided altogether in a patient with significant comorbidity.

Ultimately a final decision should be made taking into account various issues. These include the patient's wishes, quality of life, and opinions from surgeons, anaesthetists, and intensive care specialists, guided by preoperative evaluation and based on clinical experience.

Perioperative care

Anaesthetic technique

Virtually any anaesthetic technique may be used when anaesthetizing the elderly patient for major intra-abdominal surgery. There is little evidence that any one anaesthetic technique offers specific advantages over an alternative. Clearly the effects of age related changes to normal physiology and the effects of any active disease process need to be borne in mind, and some modification to technique is likely to be required in order to provide safe anaesthesia. The majority of major abdominal surgery will require a general anaesthetic technique due to the requirements for adequate surgical access, especially if laparoscopic surgery is planned. In addition, major surgery can be prolonged; whilst an open hemicolectomy is frequently performed within 2 hours, an abdomino-perineal resection may take over 4 hours. Laparoscopic surgery may take longer still. Hence whilst a regional technique might be feasible, it may be difficult for patients to tolerate regional anaesthesia for this duration. Despite this, there are several series published that have successfully used continuous regional techniques for open surgery particularly in patients considered high risk for general anaesthesia due to respiratory comorbidity.[15]

Minor rectal surgery, such as rectal prolapse repair, is more amenable to a regional technique, especially as these procedures are shorter and therefore better tolerated. The anaesthetist needs to be aware of the risks of haemodynamic instability in an elderly patient with reduced cardiovascular reserve, and ensure that any treatment is provided promptly. Major surgery is not infrequently preceded by more minor surgery such as examination under anaesthesia and per-anal resection of polyp in order to gain a tissue diagnosis. This provides the anaesthetist with the opportunity to assess the patient's response to anaesthesia prior to more definitive surgery.

The usual technique for major abdominal surgery is endotracheal intubation, facilitated by appropriate muscle relaxants, and intermittent positive pressure ventilation. The use of pressure controlled modes of ventilation may have benefits in terms of reduction in volutrauma. Small amounts of positive end-expiratory pressure (e.g. 5 cmH$_2$O) may be beneficial in reducing basal atelectasis.

Maintenance is usually with a volatile anaesthetic agent, although total intravenous techniques may also be used. Analgesia may be provided by a variety of techniques and is covered later in the chapter.

Fluid management

Patients undergoing major abdominal surgery require careful attention to fluid management. Large-bore intravenous access is generally required, and due to skin fragility, care is required when securing intravenous cannulae with adhesive tape and dressings.

The National Enquiry into Perioperative Deaths highlighted hypovolaemia as a major contributor to hypotension during the peri- and postoperative period, particularly after emergency abdominal surgery.[16] In the past, preoperative fluid depletion was a common occurrence due to prolonged starvation periods and the use of purgative bowel preparation. However with the adoption of enhanced recovery programmes, purgative bowel preparation is now used less, and patients are actively given oral fluids as part of preoperative carbohydrate loading.

Fluid replacement may be guided by various means. Traditionally, central venous pressure monitoring was the mainstay of monitoring, particularly if extensive fluid loss was anticipated. A worsening base deficit on arterial blood gas analysis may suggest inadequate fluid replacement. A urinary catheter allows urine output to be monitored throughout the perioperative period.

More recently, goal-directed fluid therapy, particularly using the oesophageal Doppler, has been seen as offering advantages over conventional invasive monitoring, and many of these trials have included elderly patients.[17] Its use is associated with the administration of increased volumes of fluid earlier on during surgery, with quicker recovery of bowel function and shorter postoperative stay.[18] However it may be difficult to isolate the benefits of cardiac output monitoring from the benefits of enhanced recovery programmes.

Furthermore, there is controversy surrounding which fluid is best for goal directed fluid therapy, and whether liberal or restrictive regimes should be utilized.[19–22]

Blood loss

Blood loss may be variable depending on the extent of surgery. Whilst straightforward surgery may result in minimal blood loss of less than 300 ml, losses in excess of 3000 ml may occur especially if extensive pelvic dissection is required, or if there has been previous intra-abdominal surgery or radiotherapy. Blood loss may be insidious, with the majority of it collected in swabs rather than in suction containers. The use of laparoscopic surgery means that blood loss may not be immediately apparent until it is suctioned from the abdomen, and will be diluted with irrigation fluid. All irrigation fluid should be measured to aid accurate blood loss estimation, and swabs should also be weighed. For operations where large blood losses are expected, cell salvage may also be used and is associated in a reduction in the need for allogeneic blood transfusion.[23] The need for blood transfusion should be guided by transfusion triggers based on near patient testing of haemoglobin or haematocrit. The actual transfusion trigger should reflect patient pathology, particularly cardiac disease, and also account for anticipated ongoing blood loss in the postoperative period.

Monitoring

Minimum standards of patient monitoring should be commenced upon entering the anaesthetic room and should continue until the patient is ready to leave the recovery area.[24] The use of invasive monitoring should be guided by both the patient's clinical status and planned surgery. An invasive arterial cannula allows real time beat to beat monitoring of arterial blood pressure. This may be advantageous in the elderly, not only because of the presence of cardiac disease, but also because of the high incidence of atrial fibrillation. The latter may render automated non-invasive blood pressure monitoring inaccurate and prone to delay due to the beat-to-beat variation in pulse pressure. Arterial access also allows the clinician to more easily monitor haemoglobin concentration and acid–base status due to the ease of blood sampling for near-patient testing. In addition, there are several cardiac output monitors that utilize waveform analysis from an invasive arterial line in order to derive values for cardiac output. The introduction of newer monitors now allows for real time continuous measurement of haemoglobin concentration without the need for patient sampling. A central venous catheter allows the clinician to monitor central pressures, provides appropriate venous access should vasopressors be required, and also facilitates blood sampling. Access is most easily achieved via the internal jugular vein, whilst the use of a long-line sited in the antecubital fossa offers a less invasive alternative. Core body temperature should be monitored in all but the shortest surgery.

Temperature management

See also Chapter 34.

Maintenance of body temperature is an important part of perioperative care and should start before the patient enters the theatre environment. Major intra-abdominal surgery is usually lengthy and therefore the elderly patient is at high risk of hypothermia. There is evidence that failing to maintain normothermia may increase complications such as cardiac morbidity, wound infection rates and blood loss, all of which may results in increased length of hospital stay.[25] The elderly are more prone to developing hypothermia during surgery than younger patients. This is predominantly due to the effects of ageing which cause both an increase in heat loss, and a reduction in the ability to restore body temperature via the usual metabolic processes. Whilst the elderly have an increased body fat content compared to younger patients, they are more likely to have a reduced body mass index (BMI) due to poor nutrition, the effects of ageing, and the disease process, and hence will lose heat at a greater rate than patients with a higher BMI. There is also a reduction in metabolic and muscular reserve such that the elderly may be unable to restore their body temperature back to normal levels. Despite this reduced muscle bulk, the oxygen demand created by shivering may still impose a requirement that exceeds respiratory and cardiac reserve.

It is not unusual for an elderly patient to arrive in the theatre complex from the ward environment with a degree of hypothermia. Preparation for surgery involves the patient changing into hospital gowns that do not provide the same heat conservation as normal clothing. Hence attempts to preserve normal body temperature are required throughout all stages of the perioperative process and should ideally start before the patient enters the theatre environment. Active warming with hot air blankets have been successfully used on the ward prior to transfer to theatre.[26] The patient is at additional risk of increased hypothermia in the anaesthetic room if there is a need to perform regional anaesthesia and site invasive monitoring. Once in theatre, additional evaporative heat losses occur from the exposed surgical site, although this is reduced in laparoscopic surgery. Because of these factors, steps should be taken to preserve normothermia in all elderly patients. It may be difficult to restore normothermia in patients undergoing anything but the shortest surgery, unless all available measures are used. Reflective drapes and warmed intravenous fluids are passive measures that can only help to prevent heat loss. Heat loss from the lower extremities is magnified through the use of epidural anaesthesia due to sympathetically mediated vasodilatation. Active warming with forced warm air systems and warming mattresses will be required to restore a hypothermic patient to normothermia, particularly if placed on the lower extremities. However patient positioning may make it difficult to effectively use all these techniques, especially the Lloyd-Davis position where the legs are held in an adducted position in order to provide surgical access. In this case the author's preference is to use reflective drapes on the legs and head, and forced air warming on the torso. It may be necessary to continue active warming in the recovery area, and core temperature should be within normal limits before the patient leaves the recovery area.

Core temperature is easily monitored in the awake patient by tympanic measurement, and with a naso-pharyngeal temperature probe in the asleep patient.

Patient positioning

Colorectal surgery often takes place in the Lloyd-Davies position where the legs are elevated and adducted in stirrups. The left lateral position is often used for peri-anal procedures, and the prone jack-knife position is increasingly used to perform the peri-anal part of an abdomino-peroneal resection. Patient positioning may be challenging in the elderly because of several factors. Ageing itself is associated with a loss of joint mobility. This is compounded by the high incidence of arthritis in the elderly. In addition, these patients frequently have a prosthetic joint replacement which both reduces range of movement, and requires care in positioning in order to avoid dislocation. Even in the supine position this can cause problems as it is not always possible to place patient's arms flat by their sides, or out on arm boards due to a reduction in elbow extension. It is important to assess the patient for vertebro-basilar insufficiency as prolonged neck extension in the prone position may lead to arterial occlusion, and alternative positions should be considered.

It is vital that care is taken to ensure that pressure areas are well padded in order to avoid nerve injury. Appropriate mattresses should be used in order to prevent pressure sores which may be particularly debilitating and entail a hospital stay longer than that for the original surgery.

Perioperative and postoperative analgesia

Simple oral analgesia may be sufficient for less invasive procedures. Single shot caudal injections are useful in surgery such as repair of rectal prolapse. For major intra-abdominal procedures, patients will require significant levels of peri- and postoperative analgesia. Inadequate postoperative analgesia may increase the risk of adverse outcomes in addition to be inhumane.[27,28] Perioperative analgesia is usually provided by long-acting opiates such as morphine, or short-acting opiates, such as remifentanil infusions or alfentanil, supplemented by regional anaesthesia. Intravenous paracetamol is a useful adjunct to more invasive analgesia techniques.

Postoperative analgesia traditionally involved either patient-controlled analgesia (PCA) using morphine, or patient-controlled epidural analgesia (PCEA).[29] With the increased use of laparoscopic techniques for intra-abdominal surgery, the need for epidural analgesia has been questioned as being unnecessary due to the less invasive nature of surgery. The same applies for laparoscopically assisted surgery where the patient will have a lower midline or Pfannenstiel incision rather than a traditional full midline incision.

Transversus abdominis plane (TAP) blocks may be used to provide postoperative analgesia, and may reduce postoperative analgesic requirements. Spinal analgesia may be used for laparoscopic surgery, and may be associated with improved outcomes compared to epidural analgesia. However, specific studies of the efficacy of TAP blocks and spinal analgesia in the elderly are lacking. Local anaesthetic wound infusions may also be used, but again further studies are required.[30–34]

Non-steroidal anti-inflammatory drugs (NSAIDS) can provide useful benefits in the treatment of postoperative pain, but their use needs to be carefully considered in the elderly patient undergoing major abdominal surgery. There is a real risk of renal complications when using these drugs in patients due to pre-existing age-related renal dysfunction and impaired fluid handling, coupled with the fluid shifts that accompany major surgery. Whilst COX-2 inhibitors may provide some protection against further renal dysfunction, there have been concerns over increased cardiac morbidity.[35,36]

The choice of analgesic technique is dependent on the risks and benefits of each option, and should take into account facilities available for postoperative care. Patient preference also needs to be considered. In addition, confusion and cognitive dysfunction may make assessment of pain problematic, and patients may not necessarily have the ability to understand how to use patient-controlled techniques effectively.

For major abdominal surgery, the choice of postoperative analgesia is usually between epidural analgesia and patient-controlled intravenous analgesia. Either option offers advantages and disadvantages. The evidence that epidural analgesia is associated with improved outcomes is not overwhelming.[27] Whilst a reduction is respiratory and thrombotic complications have been demonstrated, this has not translated into improvements in long-term outcome.[37] This may be in part due to the high levels of care that patients receive regardless of analgesic regimen, particularly with the introduction of enhanced recovery programmes that emphasize the importance of each element of care. In addition, whilst epidural analgesia may offer better quality postoperative analgesia than other regimens, there is little evidence from trials carried out exclusively in the elderly. Epidural analgesia may also be associated with a significant failure rate unless intensive and active follow-up is implemented.[28,38,39] PCA analgesia is an acceptable form of analgesia in the elderly and is associated with good quality pain relief.[40]

Postoperative care

The elderly are at highest risk of postoperative complications following major abdominal surgery when compared to all other surgical populations and therefore should receive postoperative care in an environment that reflects this increased risk.[28,41] The use of high dependency care, and even intensive care, may be advantageous in reducing postoperative complications. Whilst age is an un-modifiable risk factor for higher morbidity and mortality, there is evidence that attention to treating postoperative complications in a prompt and timely fashion can reduce early mortality after major surgery.[42] Patients who are electively admitted to a critical care environment following high-risk surgery also show an improved outcome compared to patients who require subsequent admission from a ward due to deterioration in their condition.[43]

High dependency care allows invasive monitoring to be continued such that closer attention may be paid to oxygenation, fluid balance, acid–base status and analgesia. The patient should receive continuous humidified oxygen particularly if epidural or PCA opiates are being used. Chest physiotherapy and incentive spirometry may be required. The success of enhanced recovery programmes have emphasized the importance of early mobilization, prompt resumption of enteral feeding, and minimal use of intravenous fluids. Some of these aims are clearly in conflict with some of the care provided within a high dependency environment where invasive monitoring effectively confines a patient to the bed. It is therefore important that care is individualized as appropriate. Epidural and intravenous PCA is usually continued for 1–4 days (the shorter durations being used in enhanced recovery), supplemented by simple analgesics such as paracetamol. Oral analgesia is then usually provided as step-down analgesia.

Gastric surgery

The majority of gastric surgery is for either gastric carcinoma or gastric haemorrhage. Gastric cancer is the third most common cause of cancer death in men in the United Kingdom, with a peak age of 60 years of age.[44]

Whilst the elderly are underrepresented in clinical trials the outcome following surgery is such that it is a viable option for treatment of gastric cancer in the elderly.[45] However it is associated with longer length of stay, higher risk of complications and a higher mortality compared to younger patients.[46]

The surgical approach is dictated by the tumour site and usually results in either a subtotal or total gastrectomy. Morbidity and mortality is higher with more extensive surgery, and this is exacerbated by increasing age. Hence the elderly may be offered a more limited gastric resection due to concerns over limited physiological reserve, in an attempt to reduce perioperative comorbidity.

Distal and antral tumours can cause gastric outflow obstruction and these patients are at risk of regurgitation and aspiration on induction of anaesthesia. Hence a 'rapid sequence induction' which protects the airway during induction may be appropriate. There is also a predisposition to oesophageal reflux. This, coupled with a fall in sensitivity of the cough reflexes in the elderly, may mean that the patient's lung function is reduced preoperatively due to silent aspiration. The anaesthetist needs to be aware of this possibility as there may be potential to improve lung function with appropriate treatment.

Gastric haemorrhage due to peptic ulcer disease is usually treated in the first instance by endoscopic techniques. If this is unsuccessful then surgical intervention is required as an emergency procedure. In this case, the patient is likely to be in a moribund state due to blood loss and hypovolaemia. Their poor preoperative status may be compounded due to the effects of any sedation given for the initial endoscopy. These patients require careful attention in order to ensure safe conduct of anaesthesia. It may not be possible to fully resuscitate the patient prior to induction of anaesthesia due to ongoing haemorrhage, as the surgical procedure in fact constitutes part of the resuscitation technique.

Hepatobiliary surgery

Hepatic surgery is carried out for resection of primary hepatocellular carcinoma, or for resection of colorectal metastases following colorectal resection. There is a lack of clinical trials that include elderly patients. However retrospective reviews suggest that such surgery is a feasible option for the elderly as it offers a reasonable outcome.[47] For instance, one review of over 900 patients found that patients over 70 years of age had similar mortality and morbidity rates to younger patients. Although age was found to be associated with poorer outcome, 5-year survival in the over 70s was 31.8 per cent compared to 37.5 per cent in younger patients.[48] A similar situation is found in patients undergoing surgery for hepatocellular carcinoma.[49]

Conversely, pancreatic surgery is not often performed in elderly patients. Whilst the incidence of pancreatic cancer increases with increasing age, the only viable surgical option is a pancreaticoduodenectomy (Whipple's procedure). It is only of value if the primary tumour is small, free of major blood vessels with no metastatic spread. Few patients meet these criteria, and the magnitude of surgery is such that it is only contemplated in the fittest of patients.[44]

Colorectal surgery

The elderly patient may undergo colorectal surgery for a variety of different pathologies, including diverticular disease, cancer, and inflammatory bowel disease.

Diverticular disease is very common in the elderly, affecting around half those aged over 80 years of age. A proportion of these patients will require surgical resection for the treatment of diverticular abscess, bowel obstruction, perforation, or fistulae.[50]

The incidence of inflammatory bowel disease (ulcerative colitis and Crohn's disease) has a secondary peak in the 70s. Elective surgery takes place to relieve chronic debilitating symptoms, or if there is a high risk of cancer. For ulcerative colitis, a panproctocolectomy with formation of an ileo-anal pouch is the procedure of choice in the elderly, assuming there is adequate sphincter function. In Crohn's disease, the options for surgery will depend on whether additional parts of the bowel are affected. Emergency surgery may be performed if there has been failed medical treatment of an acute flare-up of colitis, and toxic dilatation of the colon may develop. Patients with inflammatory bowel disease are often very debilitated due to chronic disease and long-term steroid use.[51]

Colorectal cancer is the fourth most common form of cancer worldwide, and is also increasing.[52] It is approximately four times more common amongst 80-year-olds compared to 60-year-olds, and in Great Britain and Ireland over 70 per cent of patients undergoing surgery for colorectal cancer are older than 65 years.[8] Resection depends on the cancer site. For colonic cancers, this will involve either a hemicolectomy, sigmoid colectomy, or a total colectomy if there are multiple malignant polyps. An anterior resection is performed for high rectal tumours, and an abdomino-perineal resection for low rectal tumours.

A loop ileostomy is often performed to defunction the distal bowel and allow the anastomosis to heal. The patient will require this to be reversed, usually 9–12 months following the initial resection. The impact of repeat surgery needs to be borne in mind when the elderly patient is being offered their initial surgery.

Enhanced recovery

Enhanced recovery programmes have received considerable attention in the last few years. They have been successful in reducing not only length of stay, but there is also evidence of improved long-term outcome. The main elements of enhanced recovery consist of:

♦ Preoperative assessment, planning, and preparation prior to admission.

♦ Reducing the stress response to surgery.

♦ A structured approach to perioperative and immediate postoperative management, including pain relief.

♦ Early mobilization.

This is achieved with measures such as:

♦ Minimal bowel preparation, preoperative carbohydrate loading, and goal-directed fluid therapy.

♦ Minimally invasive surgical techniques.

♦ Early postoperative oral nutrition and avoidance of naso-gastric tubes.

♦ Minimal use of drains, postoperative intravenous fluids, and urinary catheters.

The initial enhanced recovery programmes were set up within colorectal surgery, and have more recently been extended to other forms of surgery such as urological, gynaecological, and orthopaedic surgery. Prior to these programmes, length of stay following major colorectal resection was in the order of 12–14 days, but this has fallen steadily to around 3–4 days.

Whist the recovery of mobility and the length of stay is more prolonged than in younger patients, elderly patients do not have a worse outcome, and still benefit from an enhanced recovery programme when compared to more traditional perioperative car.[53,54]

Laparoscopic surgery in the elderly

Minimally invasive laparoscopic surgery has received considerable attention with advantages in short-term outcome and length of stay. These benefits are just as applicable to the elderly patient. There is evidence for improved early mortality and shorter length of stay compared to open surgery, and hence age should not be considered a barrier to laparoscopic surgery.[55-58] However, recent reviews have stated that whilst there are short-term advantages to laparoscopic surgery compared to open surgery, there is less evidence demonstrating improved long-term outcomes. It may be difficult to tease out the benefits of laparoscopic surgery as this technique is frequently performed as part of an enhanced recovery programme.[59,60]

Emergency intra-abdominal surgery in the elderly

Emergency laparotomy is one of the commonly performed surgical procedures in the NHS. The majority of the procedures are performed for bowel related pathologies, usually obstruction or perforation, with associated intra-abdominal sepsis. It accounts for the largest number of emergency general surgical deaths in the United Kingdom.[61] Approximately 40 per cent of these patients get admitted to critical care, making it the commonest surgical admission to critical care unit in a district general hospital without vascular or neurosurgical services.[62] Emergency surgery in the elderly is potentially a catastrophic event. Outcomes are poor when compared to both elective surgery in the elderly, and emergency surgery in younger patients.[12,63-65]

Pearse[43] reviewed mortality rates following high risk surgery according to UK Healthcare Resource Groups, and found that major emergency intra-abdominal surgery in patients over 69 years of age had the third highest mortality of 15 per cent. Several other retrospective studies have also found that patients older than 80 years of age undergoing emergency colectomy have far worse outcome, with a greater incidence of complications and less likely to return home when compared to similarly aged elective patients. Louis reports a 32 per cent mortality rate for emergency colorectal surgery in the elderly, and Ford reports a 42 per cent mortality rate for emergency general surgery.[66,67]

A prospective audit by the UK Emergency Laparotomy Network of almost 1900 patients undergoing emergency laparotomy found a mortality rate of 15 per cent. However this increased to 22 per cent in patients aged 71 to 90, and was found to be 32 per cent in patients over 90 years of age.[68] Elderly patients are also more likely to undergo emergency intra-abdominal surgery than elective surgery.

Several factors have been identified that are associated with poorer outcome. These include age, septic shock at presentation, large estimated intraoperative blood loss, delay to operation, and development of a postoperative complication.[66,69] One study found that mortality increased fivefold in patients whose surgery was delayed greater than 24 hours.[70] This supports evidence back as far as 1990 that found that death rates amongst the elderly undergoing laparotomy increased from 6 per cent to 45 per cent when surgery took place more than 24 hours after admission.[71] Given the role that sepsis plays in the pathophysiology of the patient requiring an emergency laparotomy, prompt antibiotic administration is associated with improved outcome.[72]

The Royal College of Surgeons of England has published guidance on standards of care that should apply to the patient undergoing emergency laparotomy. These include standards in the use of pre- and postoperative risk prediction in order to identify higher risk patients who require postoperative critical care, grade of clinical staff, the use of goal-directed fluid therapy, and prompt antibiotic administration.[73]

Conclusion

Elderly patients undergoing major intra-abdominal surgery represent an extremely heterogenous group. On one hand, the elderly have been successfully included in accelerated recovery programmes. On the other, they have the highest incidence of postoperative complications, especially after emergency surgery. There is a range of pathophysiological disease and ageing processes that need to be considered during the perioperative period. In addition, risk prediction is an inexact science that is not well suited to providing patient-specific risk. When providing anaesthesia for major intra-abdominal surgery, the anaesthetist needs to consider tailor perioperative care to ensure that patients' needs are met on an individual patient basis.

References

1. Priebe HJ. The aged cardiovascular risk patient. *Br J Anaesth.* 2000;85(5):763–778.
2. Office for National Statistics. *2010-based National Population Projections.* <http://www.ons.gov.uk> (accessed 8 October 2011).
3. Klopfenstein CE, Herrmann FR, Michel JP, Clergue F, Forster A. The influence of an aging surgical population on the anesthesia workload: a ten-year survey. *Anesth Analg.* 1998;86(6):1165–1170.
4. Practice advisory for preanesthesia evaluation: a report by the American Society of Anesthesiologists Task Force on Preanesthesia Evaluation. *Anesthesiology.* 2002;96(2):485–496.
5. National Institute for Health and Clinical Excellence. *Preoperative Tests. The use of routine preoperative tests for elective surgery.* CG3. London: NICE, 2003. <http://www.nice.org.uk> (accessed 21 November 2011).
6. Copeland GP, Jones D, Walters M. POSSUM: a scoring system for surgical audit. *Br J Surg.* 1991;78(3):355–360.
7. Horzic M, Kopljar M, Cupurdija K, Bielen DV, Vergles D, Lackovic Z. Comparison of P-POSSUM and Cr-POSSUM scores in patients undergoing colorectal cancer resection. *Arch Surg.* 2007;142(11):1043–1048.
8. Tekkis PP, Poloniecki JD, Thompson MR, Stamatakis JD. Operative mortality in colorectal cancer: prospective national study. *BMJ.* 2003;327(7425):1196–1201.
9. Tez M, Yoldas O, Gocmen E, Kulah B, Koc M. Evaluation of P-POSSUM and CR-POSSUM scores in patients with colorectal cancer undergoing resection. *World J Surg.* 2006;30(12):2266–2269.
10. Yan J, Wang YX, Li ZP. Predictive value of the POSSUM, p-POSSUM, cr-POSSUM, APACHE II and ACPGBI scoring systems in colorectal cancer resection. *J Int Med Res.* 2011;39(4):1464–1473.
11. Cheema FN, Abraham NS, Berger DH, Albo D, Taffet GE, Naik AD. (2011). Novel approaches to perioperative assessment and intervention may improve long-term outcomes after colorectal cancer resection in older adults. *Ann Surg.* 2011;253(5):867–874.
12. Cook TM, Day CJ. Hospital mortality after urgent and emergency laparotomy in patients aged 65 yr and over. Risk and prediction of risk using multiple logistic regression analysis. *Br J Anaesth.* 1998;80(6):776–781.
13. Church JM. Laparotomy for acute colorectal conditions in moribund patients: is it worthwhile? *Dis Colon Rectum.* 2005;48(6)1147–1152.
14. Scottish Audit of Surgical Mortality. *Scottish Audit of Surgical Mortality Annual Report 2010.* <http://www.sasm.org.uk> (accessed 23 June 2011).
15. Kumar CM, Corbett WA, Wilson RG. Spinal anaesthesia with a micro-catheter in high-risk patients undergoing colorectal cancer and other major abdominal surgery. *Surg Oncol.* 2008;17(2):73–79.
16. National Confidential Enquiry into Perioperative Deaths, London. *Extremes of Age 1999.* <http://www.ncepod.org.uk/> (accessed 10 August 2011).
17. Conway DH, Mayall R, bdul-Latif MS, Gilligan S, Tackaberry C. Randomised controlled trial investigating the influence of intravenous fluid titration using oesophageal Doppler monitoring during bowel surgery. *Anaesthesia.* 2002;57(9):845–849.
18. Gan TJ, Soppitt A, Maroof M, *et al.* Goal-directed intraoperative fluid administration reduces length of hospital stay after major surgery. *Anesthesiology.* 2002;97(4):820–826.
19. Brandstrup B, Tonnesen H, Beier-Holgersen R, *et al.* Effects of intravenous fluid restriction on postoperative complications: comparison of two perioperative fluid regimens: a randomized assessor-blinded multicenter trial. *Ann Surg.* 2003;238(5):641–648.
20. Morris C, Rogerson D. What is the optimal type of fluid to be used for peri-operative fluid optimisation directed by oesophageal Doppler monitoring? *Anaesthesia.* 2011;6(9):819–827.
21. Nisanevich V, Felsenstein I, Almogy G, Weissman C, Einav S, Matot I. Effect of intraoperative fluid management on outcome after intraabdominal surgery. *Anesthesiology.* 2005;103(1):25–32.
22. Rahbari NN, Zimmermann JB, Schmidt T, Koch M, Weigand MA, Weitz J. Meta-analysis of standard, restrictive and supplemental fluid administration in colorectal surgery. *Br J Surg.* 2009;96(4):331–341.
23. Ashworth A, Klein AA. Cell salvage as part of a blood conservation strategy in anaesthesia. *Br J Anaesth.* 2010;105(4):401–416.
24. The Association of Anaesthetists of Great Britain and Ireland. *Recommendations For Standards Of Monitoring During Anaesthesia And Recovery.* <http://www.aagbi.org> (accessed 7 November 2011).
25. Harper CM, McNicholas T, Gowrie-Mohan S. Maintaining perioperative normothermia. *BMJ.* 2003;326(7392):721–722.
26. National Institute for Health and Clinical Excellence. *The management of inadvertent perioperative hypothermia in adults.* CG65. London: NICE, 2008. <http://www.nice.org.uk> (accessed 21 August 2011).
27. Ballantyne JC. (2004). Does epidural analgesia improve surgical outcome? *Br J Anaesth.* 2004;92(1):4–6.
28. Jin F, Chung F. Minimizing perioperative adverse events in the elderly. *Br J Anaesth.* 2001;87(4):608–624.
29. Gagliese L, Jackson M, Ritvo P, Wowk A, Katz J. Age is not an impediment to effective use of patient-controlled analgesia by surgical patients. *Anesthesiology.* 2000;93(3):601–610.
30. Conaghan P, Maxwell-Armstrong C, Bedforth N, *et al.* Efficacy of transversus abdominis plane blocks in laparoscopic colorectal resections. *Surg Endosc.* 2010;24(10):2480–2484.
31. Levy BF, Scott MJ, Fawcett W, Fry C, Rockall TA. Randomized clinical trial of epidural, spinal or patient-controlled analgesia for patients undergoing laparoscopic colorectal surgery. *Br J Surg.* 2011;98(8):1068–1078.
32. McDonnell JG, O'Donnell B, Curley G, Heffernan A, Power C, Laffey JG. The analgesic efficacy of transversus abdominis plane block after abdominal surgery: a prospective randomized controlled trial. *Anesth Analg.* 2007;104(1):193–197.
33. Thornton PC, Buggy DJ. Local anaesthetic wound infusion for acute postoperative pain: a viable option? *Br J Anaesth.* 2011;107(5):656–658.
34. Zafar N, Davies R, Greenslade GL, Dixon AR. The evolution of analgesia in an 'accelerated' recovery programme for resectional laparoscopic colorectal surgery with anastomosis. *Colorectal Dis.* 2010;12(2):119–124.
35. Jones R. Efficacy and safety of COX 2 inhibitors. *BMJ.* 2002;325(7365):607–608.
36. Juni P, Reichenbach S, Egger M. COX 2 inhibitors, traditional NSAIDs, and the heart. *BMJ.* 2005;330(7504):1342–1343.
37. Kehlet H, Holte K. Effect of postoperative analgesia on surgical outcome. *Br J Anaesth.* 2001;87(1):62–72.
38. Block BM, Liu SS, Rowlingson AJ, Cowan AR, Cowan JA Jr, Wu CL. Efficacy of postoperative epidural analgesia: a meta-analysis. *JAMA.* 2003;290(18):2455–2463.
39. Rigg JR, Jamrozik K, Myles PS, *et al.* Epidural anaesthesia and analgesia and outcome of major surgery: a randomised trial. *Lancet.* 2002;359(9314):1276–1282.
40. Mann C, Pouzeratte Y, Boccara G, *et al.* Comparison of intravenous or epidural patient-controlled analgesia in the elderly after major abdominal surgery. *Anesthesiology.* 2000;92(2):433–441.
41. Khuri SF, Henderson WG, DePalma RG, Mosca C, Healey NA, Kumbhani DJ. Determinants of long-term survival after major surgery and the adverse effect of postoperative complications. *Ann Surg.* 2005;242(3):326–341.
42. Ghaferi AA, Birkmeyer JD, Dimick JB. Variation in hospital mortality associated with inpatient surgery. *N Engl J Med.* 2009;361(14):1368–1375.
43. Pearse RM, Harrison DA, James P, *et al.* Identification and characterisation of the high-risk surgical population in the United Kingdom. *Crit Care.* 2006;10(3):R81.
44. Bowles MJ, Benjamin IS. ABC of the upper gastrointestinal tract: cancer of the stomach and pancreas. *BMJ.* 2001;323(7326):1413–1416.
45. Saif MW, Makrilia N, Zalonis A, Merikas M, Syrigos K. Gastric cancer in the elderly: an overview. *Eur J Surg Oncol.* 2010;36(8):709–717.
46. Hager ES, Abdollahi H, Crawford AG, *et al.* Is gastrectomy safe in the elderly? A single institution review. *Am Surg.* 2011;77(4):488–492.

47. Cannon RM, Martin RC, Callender GG, McMasters KM, Scoggins CR. Safety and efficacy of hepatectomy for colorectal metastases in the elderly. *J Surg Oncol.* 2011;104(7):804–808.

48. Kulik U, Framke T, Grosshennig A. Liver resection of colorectal liver metastases in elderly patients. *World J Surg.* 2011;35(9):2063–2072.

49. Nanashima A, Abo T, Nonaka T, *et al.* Prognosis of patients with hepatocellular carcinoma after hepatic resection: are elderly patients suitable for surgery? *J Surg Oncol.* 2011;104(3):284–291.

50. Jones DJ. ABC of colorectal diseases. Diverticular disease. *BMJ.* 1992;304(6839):1435–1437.

51. Pettit S, Irving MH. ABC of colorectal diseases. Non-specific inflammatory bowel disease. *BMJ.* 1992;304(6838):1367–1371.

52. Boyle P, Langman JS. ABC of colorectal cancer: epidemiology. *BMJ.* 2000;321(7264):805–808.

53. Basse L, Thorbol JE, Lossl K, Kehlet H. Colonic surgery with accelerated rehabilitation or conventional care. *Dis Colon Rectum.* 2004;47(3):271–277.

54. Hendry PO, Hausel J, Nygren J, *et al.* Determinants of outcome after colorectal resection within an enhanced recovery programme. *Br J Surg.* 2009;96(2):197–205.

55. Bardram L, Funch-Jensen P, Kehlet H. Rapid rehabilitation in elderly patients after laparoscopic colonic resection. *Br J Surg.* 2000;87(11):1540–1545.

56. Kurian AA, Suryadevara S, Vaughn D, *et al.* Laparoscopic colectomy in octogenarians and nonagenarians: a preferable option to open surgery? *J Surg Educ.* 2010;67(3):161–166.

57. Lian L, Kalady M, Geisler D, Kiran RP. Laparoscopic colectomy is safe and leads to a significantly shorter hospital stay for octogenarians. *Surg Endosc.* 2010;24(8):2039–2043.

58. Mutch MG. Laparoscopic colectomy in the elderly: when is too old? *Clin Colon Rectal Surg.* 2006;19(1):33–39.

59. Bartels SA, Vlug MS, Ubbink DT, Bemelman WA. Quality of life after laparoscopic and open colorectal surgery: a systematic review. *World J Gastroenterol.* 2010;16(40):5035–5041.

60. Kunzli BM, Friess H, Shrikhande SV. Is laparoscopic colorectal cancer surgery equal to open surgery? An evidence based perspective. *World J Gastrointest Surg.* 2010;2(4):101–108.

61. Association of Surgeons of Great Britain and Ireland, London. *Emergency general surgery: the future. A consensus statement June 2007.* <http://www.asgbi.org.uk> (accessed November 2011).

62. Jhanji S, Thomas B, Ely A, Watson D, Hinds CJ, Pearse RM. Mortality and utilisation of critical care resources amongst high-risk surgical patients in a large NHS trust. *Anaesthesia.* 2008;63(7):695–700.

63. Clarke A, Murdoch H, Thomas MJ, Cook TM, Peden CJ. Mortality and postoperative care after emergency laparotomy. *Eur J Anaesthesiol.* 2011;28(1):16–19.

64. Kurian A, Suryadevara S, Ramaraju D, *et al.* In-hospital and 6-month mortality rates after open elective vs open emergent colectomy in patients older than 80 years. *Dis Colon Rectum.* 2011;54(4):467–471.

65. Morse BC, Cobb WS, Valentine JD, Cass AL, Roettger RH. Emergent and elective colon surgery in the extreme elderly: do the results warrant the operation? *Am Surg.* 2008;74(7):614–618.

66. Ford PN, Thomas I, Cook TM, Whitley E, Peden CJ. (2007). Determinants of outcome in critically ill octogenarians after surgery: an observational study. *Br J Anaesth.* 2007;99(6):824–829.

67. Louis DJ, Hsu A, Brand MI, Saclarides TJ. Morbidity and mortality in octogenarians and older undergoing major intestinal surgery. *Dis Colon Rectum.* 2009;52(1):59–63.

68. Saunders D, Pichel A, Varley S, Peden C, Murray D. Variations in mortality following emergency laparotomy; the first report of the United Kingdom Emergency Laparotomy Network. *Br J Anaesth.* 2012;109(3):368–375.

69. McGillicuddy EA, Schuster KM, Davis KA, Longo WE. Factors predicting morbidity and mortality in emergency colorectal procedures in elderly patients. *Arch Surg.* 2009;144(12):1157–1162.

70. Su YH, Yeh CC, Lee CY. Acute surgical treatment of perforated peptic ulcer in the elderly patients. *Hepatogastroenterology.* 2010;57(104):1608–1613.

71. Monod-Broca P. [Mortality in emergency abdominal surgery. 304 cases. A plea for better clinical practice]. *Ann Gastroenterol Hepatol (Paris).* 1990;26(4):184–186. [Article in French.]

72. Kumar A, Roberts D, Wood KE, *et al.* Duration of hypotension before initiation of effective antimicrobial therapy is the critical determinant of survival in human septic shock. *Crit Care Med.* 2006;34(6):1589–1596.

73. Report of the Royal College of Surgeons of England/Department of Health Working Group on Peri-Operative Care of the Higher-Risk General Surgical Patient. *The higher risk general surgical patient: towards improved care for a forgotten group.* <http://www.rcseng.ac.uk> (accessed 17 November 2011).

CHAPTER 24

Gynaecological surgery in the elderly

Onyi Onuoha and Ashish C. Sinha

Introduction

Individuals over 65 years of age are estimated to constitute 20 per cent of the population by the year 2030.[1] More notably, the most recent 2010 Census data indicates that women comprise 50.8 per cent of the current 308.7 million people in the United States. With the projected increase in women aged 65 and older in the next few decades, the number of women seeking routine and acute gynaecological surgical interventions is expected to increase dramatically.

A basic understanding of the elderly population and the common surgical procedures that are expected to increase as the population ages is therefore critical. The goal of this chapter is to discuss some of the common gynaecological surgical procedures as well as the anesthetic implications involved in caring for the elderly. The elderly woman will remain a significant part of our society in the future and will continue to require an extensive array of medical services including gynaecological surgeries well into their advanced age.

Common gynaecological surgical procedures in the elderly

Mains et al. (2007) reported an increased risk of perioperative morbidity and mortality in elderly women (mean age 83.1 years) undergoing major gynaecologic surgery[2]. In their retrospective chart review, results showed a postoperative complication in approximately 45 per cent of the patients with 8.1 per cent experiencing a major complication. Although advanced age (85+ years) was not associated with any of the outcomes of interest in this study, the increased perioperative morbidity in the elderly should be considered when performing surgery on women in this age group. Most studies have limited power and are susceptible to bias given the study design. Larger and better-designed prospective studies are definitely needed to confirm these results.

Some of the major gynaecological surgeries in this population include procedures performed for cancer or a mass, for pelvic organ prolapse (POP) or urinary incontinence. These procedures can be performed abdominally, vaginally, or laparoscopically.[2]

Urinary incontinence surgery

Urinary incontinence is a significant health problem among elderly women worldwide with considerable social and economic impact.[3,4] The magnitude varies by geography, culture, and definition, hence

the reason for the wide variation in actual statistics. Luber describes an observed prevalence of stress urinary incontinence (SUI) ranging from 4 per cent to 35 per cent.[4] Elderly women are twice as likely as men to experience incontinence.[5] POP is another ailment affecting millions of women worldwide with a woman possessing an estimated lifetime risk of 11 per cent to undergo surgery for either prolapse or incontinence.[6] Despite the high prevalence of this disease, there is a paucity of high-quality epidemiological studies to accurately estimate its prevalence.[6]

According to Whiteside and Walters, the current consensus on the pathophysiology of SUI is that multiple physiological factors contribute to the presence and severity of this condition in women.[1] Some theories include maternal characteristics like age and anatomical or neurological injury during childbirth. These can subsequently unmask a genetic susceptibility to SUI and can be exacerbated by environmental factors such as nutrition, smoking, and exercise. 'Optimal therapy for urinary incontinence depends on several factors, including the type and severity of the incontinence, the presence of associated conditions such as prolapse or other abdominal pathology, prior surgical or nonsurgical therapy, the patient's medical status, and her ability or willingness to cooperate with treatment'.[1] Recent advances in non-surgical treatments for SUI and POP have made this mode of treatment a reasonable choice especially in the elderly. Non-surgical therapy include behavioural intervention (pelvic floor muscle training and exercise, bladder training, and the use of a bladder diary), electrical stimulation, weight loss, pharmacological agents like oestrogen replacement therapy and other non-Food and Drug Administration (FDA) approved agents like adrenergic agonists (midodrine), beta adrenergic receptor antagonists and agonists, tricyclic antidepressants, and serotonergic and noradrenergic reuptake inhibitors (duloxetine).[1,7,8] Urethral devices including inserts and occlusive devices also exist and may be options in selected patients.[9]

Nevertheless for patients who fail with non-surgical interventions, surgical procedures exist. Marshall et al. first described retropubic urethrovesical suspension for the treatment of SUI in 1949.[1] All the different variants of retropubic procedures aim at suspending and stabilizing the anterior vaginal wall and consequently, the bladder neck and proximal urethra, in a retropubic position to prevent descent and allow urethral compression against a stable suburethral layer. The Burch colposuspension is often preferred for urodynamic stress incontinence with bladder neck hypermobility and adequate resting urethral sphincter function and is combined with a paravaginal defect repair when the patient has a stage 2 or 3 anterior vaginal prolapse.[1,10,11] Retropubic urethrovesical suspension procedures are therefore indicated for the diagnosis of urodynamic SUI with a hypermobile proximal urethra and bladder neck. Although these procedures can be used for intrinsic sphincter deficiency with urethral hypermobility, other more obstruction procedures like a sling most likely yield better long-term results.[1] The postoperative complications of wound and urinary infections are the most common surgical complications.[1] Other rare complications include bladder lacerations, sutures through the bladder and urethra resulting in vesical stone formation, painful voiding, recurrent cystitis, or fistula. Ureteral obstruction, although rare, can also be seen. This results from ureteral stretching or kinking after elevation of the vagina and bladder base.[1]

Postoperative voiding difficulties vary widely among patients after colposuspension.[1] Other well recognized postoperative complications include overactive bladder, osteitis pubis, and enterocoele/rectocoele formation.[1]

The use of laparoscopy and mini-incision laparotomy to perform similar procedures in the retropubic space is now expanding. Both the Burch colposuspension and paravaginal defect repair can be performed laparoscopically. Nevertheless, most laparoscopic colposuspensions have been done only for primary SUI due to the difficulty with dissection with the presence of prior retropubic adhesions.[1] Advantages to laparoscopic surgery in this population include improved visualization of the peritoneal cavity due to magnification, improved haemostasis, shortened length of hospital stay resulting in a potential cost reduction, decreased postoperative pain, rapid recovery and return back to work (if necessary), and better cosmetic appearance due to smaller incisions.[1,11] The existing disadvantages have however, limited the widespread use of this technique for the treatment of SUI and POP. These include inadequate experience and technical skills of the operator, increased operating time early in the surgeon's career, which could lead to increased hospital costs.[1] Of note however is that outcomes (e.g. cure rate) of the laparoscopic approach appear to be subjectively comparable to open techniques.[11,12] A meta-analysis of four randomized clinical trials (RCTs) demonstrated no difference in the subjective perception of cure between the laparoscopic group and the open group after 6–18 months of follow-up.[13] Urodynamic studies, however, showed a significantly lower success rate for laparoscopic compared to open colposuspension techniques. With the exclusion of one of the poor quality RCT, cure rates remained lower for the laparoscopic approach but not statistically significant.[13] The choice between laparoscopic versus open retropubic colposuspension depends on several factors: age, weight, the ability to undergo general anaesthesia, history of previous pelvic or anti-incontinence surgery, presence or history of severe abdominopelvic infection or adhesions, patient preference, operator experience, and ability.[1]

Suburethral sling procedures, including proximal urethral and midurethral tension-free slings, are the most commonly used procedures for the surgical correction of urodynamic SUI. These vaginal procedures have been reserved for patients with severe SUI, previous surgical failures, and patients with intrinsic sphincter deficiency.[1] It was first described in 1907 and has evolved since with many variations of muscular and fascial slings. The procedure involves the use of two strips of rectus fascia sutures in the midline below the urethra through a separate incision. These fascial strips are brought down through the rectus muscle, behind the symphysis pubis and united as a sling behind the urethra.[1] Synthetic grafts can also be used as a replacement of the autologous sling material. These have been demonstrated to be comparable.[1] Complications include injury to the bladder or urethra, voiding dysfunction and retention, detrusor overactivity, and irritative voiding symptoms (frequency, urge incontinence, dysuria, urgency), recurrent or persistent incontinence, haemorrhage, infection and erosion, nerve damage (most commonly, the common peroneal nerve due to lithotomy positioning, ilioinguinal nerve damage).[1,14,15] Long-term data suggest comparable objective cure rates of about 80 per cent and additional improvement in about 10 per cent of patients for the Burch colposuspension and the sling procedures.[1]

Gynaecological cancer surgery

Procedures performed for cancer or the removal of a mass remain quite prevalent among the elderly population. Endometrial cancer is the most common gynaecological malignancy in the United States, with advanced age as an independent predictor for survival and poor outcomes.[16] With the increasing ageing population, gynaecological oncologists are also faced with an increasing prevalence of geriatric ovarian cancer.[17] The appropriate and aggressiveness of the treatment for such patients given age and a higher incidence of pre-existing comorbidities still remains a topic of debate. Many studies indicate feasibility and acceptable complication rates for debulking or cytoreductive surgery in women over 70 years of age with improved survival among optimally debulked patients.[18] This early management of ovarian cancer however, demands a critical clinical assessment for appropriate patient selection. Limited data exists on patients over 80 years of age. For these oldest patients (over 80 years of age) however, the decision is often a less aggressive treatment regimen.[18] A disparity of surgical operations performed in older patients compared to younger patients exists with optimal cytoreduction decreasing with age. This disparity is often not due to older patients being less willing to undergo surgery but the presence of severe medical comorbidities and a concern for higher surgical mortality and morbidity in these patients.[19,20] Higher rates of serious morbidity, postoperative mortality, and intensive care monitoring have been reported with cytoreductive surgeries in this patient population.[19,20] However, with improvements in surgical techniques and postoperative care, surgical morbidity in the elderly has improved over the past decades with women older than 70 having significantly shorter hospital stays, lower transfusion rates, morbidity, and perioperative mortality when compared to similar patients at the same hospital a decade earlier.[21] Of note, the mean age in this study was 73 and most of these studies have been retrospective reviews hence, the susceptibility for bias. Prospective trials in higher-risk populations such as patients 80 years and above are still lacking. Unfortunately, a bias against performing surgery in the elderly still exists with misconceptions of age as a surgical risk. There is no ethical or moral basis for denying appropriate care based on age alone if the proposed surgery can improve the quality of the remaining years.[22] Delaying or refusing surgery based on age alone is still not supported by existing literature.[23,24]

Quality of life (QOL) is positively altered by surgery in elderly women with ovarian cancer especially in the physical and functional domains.[25,26] Most studies, however, follow women who had a combination of surgery and adjuvant chemotherapy. Others are quite varied with no controls or different definitions for elderly.

Palliative surgery, especially for ovarian cancer, can be non-curative but is done to alleviate symptoms of tumour or complications that can arise from medical treatment.[27] At this point, optimizing QOL becomes the goal of medical care.

Anaesthetic considerations in the elderly

The anaesthetic management of elderly patients presents special challenges due to multiple factors including, physiological processes of ageing, numerous coexisting age-related diseases, and a variety of pharmacological agents often prescribed for chronic diseases.[28] The anaesthetic technique of choice (sedation, regional, or general) would therefore depend on the patient's medical condition including her comorbidities and current medications, the procedure to be performed (its invasiveness and expected complications), the urgent/emergent nature of the procedure, history of tolerance to prior surgery, and most importantly, the patient's wishes. In the elderly, the optimal anaesthetic technique is designed on an individual-to-individual basis.

Preoperative evaluation and preparation

See also Chapter 15.

Detailed medical history and physical examination

The care of the elderly female begins with eliciting a detailed medical history investigating the presence or absence of comorbidities prevalent in older adults, determining the functional status of all vital organs, performing a physical exam, and obtaining a complete medication list. Functional capacity provides an excellent estimate of reserve.[23] This may involve obtaining medical information from family members or a caregiver. A thorough pre-op evaluation cannot be overemphasized in this population. The adequacy of the optimal medical management of pre-existing comorbidities is determined at this stage and recommendations are made for further management if necessary.

Preoperative tests

Based on the elicited history and physical exam, pre-op tests are obtained as needed. Routine pre-op testing in geriatric surgical patients without any clinical indications yields a small percentage of abnormal results.[29,30] For intermediate risk surgery, pre-op testing should be obtained only if the functional status of the patient is questionable. No invasive testing is required for patients with moderate functional capacity (4–7 metabolic equivalents (METs)) and intermediate clinical predictors (mild stable angina, prior myocardial infarction, diabetes mellitus, compensated or prior congestive heart failure).[31] Most gynaecological procedures are low or intermediate risk procedures. Tests should be ordered when the history or physical examination would have indicated the need for testing even if surgery had not been planned.[29,32]

Education/informed consent

The patient, caregiver, and family are educated about the procedure including the efficacy, complications, and expectations. A thorough and well-documented consent form delineating details, possible outcomes, and risk both of the surgery and anaesthesia should be completed to ensure that the patient's expectations of surgery, recovery, and final outcomes are realistic and appropriate.[33] The patient should be aware of her right to refuse surgical therapy. Her wishes through living wills, healthcare proxies, and healthcare directives should be evaluated to ensure that both parties understand what will or will not be performed in the case of an event.[29]

Premedication

Maintain home medications unless discontinuation is absolutely indicated. Data suggests that withholding beta-blockers in patients on chronic beta blockade increases the risk of perioperative ischemia.[34]

Support

For the elderly female, issues like adequate living conditions post surgery to provide support for a successful recovery should be addressed.[29]

Intraoperative management

Induction

A reduction in induction doses of intravenous anaesthetic agents remains key. Almost any standard technique is safe if performed carefully.[29] Regional anaesthesia (RA) has been shown to possess some advantages over general anaesthesia (GA) especially in the elderly including decreased incidence of postoperative thromboembolic events, decreased stress response to surgery, decreased blood loss and decreased incidence of postoperative cognitive delirium.[35] There is however no superiority of RA over GA when considering outcome measures like mortality and morbidity in this patient population.[35] Regardless of technique, caution should be taken to consider physiological implications associated with the elderly during induction.

Maintenance

Intravascular volume status in the elderly is critical because of the greater dependence of cardiac output on preload.[31,36] Invasive monitoring should be considered in patients with significant cardiovascular/pulmonary disease or where volume status is unknown.[23] Other pertinent issues like correct positioning, adequate padding and sufficient warming to prevent hypothermia should be optimized during this phase. Hypothermia is more pronounced and prolonged in the elderly due to several factors including a low basal metabolic rate, hypothyroidism, high ratio of surface area to body mass, impairment of autonomic mechanisms for thermoregulation, less effective cold-induced vasoconstriction and delayed shivering.[24,29] Shivering is delayed in persons over 80 years old until core temperature falls much lower than that in younger adults. Consequently, a reduction in skeletal muscle mass decreases in post-op shivering and inhibition of thermoregulatory responses by anaesthetics limits the rate at which temperature homeostasis is re-instituted in the elderly.[24,29] One suggestion for this is to keep the operating room warm, at about 80° Fahrenheit.

Emergence

The older patient often exhibit slower emergence from general anaesthesia than their younger counterparts due to a longer duration of action for drugs, synergistic drug interactions, relative drug overdoses, and a higher propensity for hypothermia which further prolongs the duration of drug action.[37]

Postoperative management

Supplemental oxygen is often required during transport to the post-anaesthesia care unit (PACU) due to a blunted response to hypoxia and hypercapnia in the elderly.[29,36]

Postoperative analgesia

Adequate pain control is a major goal with cautious titration of opioid to desired effect due to increased sensitivity. Optimal analgesia is needed to prevent associated adverse outcomes of sleep deprivation, respiratory impairment, ileus, suboptimal mobilization, tachycardia, hypertension, and insulin resistance which all result in subsequent longer hospitalization and delirium.[38,39] Patients should be frequently monitored for sedation and respiratory depression. Epidural analgesia has been shown to be superior to intravenous therapy even in the elderly.[29,40]

Triage

It is important to safely triage the elderly to the appropriate area for immediate acute recovery (PACU vs ICU).

Conclusion

An ageing population increases the number of patients who would require surgical treatment for urological and gynaecological diseases in the future. The outcome from these interventions depends on careful assessment of the patient's ability to withstand the demands of surgery. This chapter addresses specific problems encountered by the elderly during gynaecologic surgery and offers suggestions for their safe management.

References

1. Walters MD, Karram MM. *Urogynecology and reconstructive pelvic surgery*, 3rd edn. St. Louis, MO: Mosby-Elsevier.
2. Mains LM, Magnus M, Finan M. Perioperative morbidity and mortality from major gynecologic surgery in the elderly woman. *J Reprod Med.* 2007;52(8):677–684.
3. Milsom I. Epidemiology of stress, urgency, and mixed incontinence: where do the boundaries cross? *Eur Urol Suppl.* 2006;5(16):835–870.
4. Luber KM. The definition, prevalence, and risk factors for stress urinary incontinence. *Rev Urol.* 2004;6(suppl 3):S3–S9.
5. Hannestad YS, Rortveit G, Sandvik H, Hunskaar S. A community-based epidemiological survey of female urinary incontinence: the Norwegian EPINCONT Study. *J Clin Epidemiol.* 2000;53:1150–1157.
6. Schorge JO, Schaffer JI, Halvorson LM, et al. *Williams gynecology*, 6th edn. New York: McGraw-Hill Medical, 2008.
7. Al-Badr A, Ross S, Soroka D, Drutz HP. What is the available evidence for hormone replacement therapy in women with stress urinary incontinence? *J Obstet Gynaecol Can.* 2003;25:567–574.
8. Alhassso A, Glazener CM, Pickard R, et al. Adrenergic drugs for urinary incontinence in adults. *Cochrane Database Syst Rev.* 2005;3:CD001842.
9. Bachmann G, Wiita B. External occlusive devices for management of female urinary incontinence. *J Womens Health.* 2002;11:793–800.
10. Korda A, Ferry J, Hunter P. Colposuspension for the treatment of female urinary incontinence. *Aust N Z J Obstet Gynaecol.* 1989;29:146–149.
11. Carey MP, Goh JT, Rosamilia A, et al. Laparoscopic versus open Burch colposuspension: a randomized controlled trial. *Br J Obstet Gynaecol.* 2006;113(9):999–1006.
12. Reid F, Smith AR. Laparoscopic versus open colposuspension: which one should we choose? *Curr Opin Obstet Gynecol.* 2007;19(4):345–349.
13. Moehrer B, Carey M, Wilson D. Laparoscopic colposuspension: a systematic review. *Br J Obstet Gynaecol.* 2003;110:230–235.
14. Klutke C, Siegel S, Carlin B, Paszkiewicz E, Kirkemo A, Klutke J. Urinary retention after tension free vaginal tape procedure: incidence and treatment. *Urology.* 2001;58:697–701.
15. Miyazaki F, Shook G. Ilioinguinal nerve entrapment during needle suspension for stress incontinence. *Obstet Gynecol.* 1992;80:246–248.
16. Jemal A, Siegel R, Ward E, et al. Cancer statistics. 2008. *CA Cancer J Clin.* 2008;58:71–96.
17. Susini T, Amunni G, Busi E, et al. Ovarian cancer in the elderly: feasibility of surgery and chemotherapy in 89 geriatric patients. *Int J Gynecol Cancer.* 2007;17(3):581–588.
18. Gardner GJ. Ovarian cancer cytoreductive surgery in the elderly. *Curr Treat Options Oncol.* 2009;10(3-4):171–179.
19. Nordin AJ, Chinn DJ, Moloney I, et al. Do elderly cancer patients care about cure? Attitudes to radical gynecologic oncology surgery in the elderly. *Gynecol Oncol.* 2001;81:447–455.
20. Cloven NG, Manetta A, Berman MI, et al. Management of ovarian cancer in patients older than 80 years of age. *Gynecol Oncol.* 1999;73:137–139.
21. Susini T, Scambia G, Margariti PA, et al. Gynecologic oncologic surgery in the elderly: retrospective analysis of 213 patients. *Gynecol Oncol.* 1999;75:437–443.
22. Norman GAV. Ethical challenges in the anesthetic care of the geriatric patient. *Syllabus on geriatric anesthesiology.* Washington, DC: ASA.
23. Salma, S. Anesthesia for the elderly patient. *J Pak Med Assoc.* 2007;57(4):196–201.
24. Francis J Jr. Surgery in the elderly. In Goldman DR, Brown FH, Guarneri DM (eds) *Peri-operative medicine*, 2nd edn (pp. 385–394). New York: McGraw Hill, Inc., 1994.
25. von Gruenigen VE, Gil K, Huang H, et al. Quality of life in ovarian cancer patients during chemotherapy: a gynecologic oncology group study. *Gynecol Oncol.* 2008;108:S28–S29.
26. von Gruenigen VE, Frasure HE, Grandon M, et al. Longitudinal assessment of quality of life and lifestyle in newly diagnosed ovarian cancer patients: the roles of surgery and chemotherapy. *Gynecol Oncol.* 2006;103:120–126.
27. Kim A, Fall P, Wang D. Palliative care: optimizing quality of life. *J Am Osteopath Assoc.* 2005;105(suppl 5):S9–S14.
28. Hawkins KA, Kalhan R. Pulmonary changes in the elderly. In Katlic MR (ed) *Cardiothoracic surgery in the elderly* (pp. 271–278). New York: Springer Science and Business Media LLC, 2011.
29. Barash PG, Cullen BF, Stoelting RK, Cahalan MK, Stock MC. *Clinical anesthesia*, 6th edn. Philadelphia, PA: Lippincott Williams & Wilkins, 2009.
30. Dzankic B, Pastor D, Gonzalec C, Leung JM. The prevalence and predictive value of abnormal preoperative laboratory testing in elderly surgical patients. *Anesth Analg.* 2001;93:301–308.
31. Raymond R. Anesthetic management of the elderly patient. *53rd ASA Annual Meeting Refresher Course Lectures #321.* 2002;1–7.
32. Schein OD, Katz J, Bass EB, et al. The value of routine preoperative medical testing before cataract surgery. *N Engl J Med.* 2000;342:168–175.
33. ACOG Committee on Ethics. ACOG committee opinion No 439. Informed consent. *Obstet Gynecol.* 2009;114:401–408.
34. Fleisher L. Should beta-adrenergic blocking agents be given routinely in noncardiac surgery? In Fleisher L (ed) *Evidence-based practice of anesthesiology* (pp. 163–167). Philadelphia, PA: Elsevier Inc., 2004.
35. Gulur P, Nishimori M, Ballantyne JC. Regional anaesthesia versus general anaesthesia, morbidity and mortality. *Best Pract Res Clin Anaesthesiol.* 2006;20(2):249–263.
36. Morgan GE, Mikhail MS, Murray MJ. *Clinical anesthesiology*, 4th edn. New York: Lange Medical Books/McGraw-Hill Medical Publishing, 2006.
37. Roy RC. *Anesthetic management of the elderly patient.* Education: Annual Meeting—American Society of Anesthesiologists, 2010. <http://www.wfubmc.edu/anesthesia>.

38. Aubrun F. Management of postoperative analgesia in the elderly. *Reg Anesth Pain Med.* 2005;30:363–379.

39. Morrison RS, Magaziner J, Gilbert M, *et al.* Relationship between pain and opioid analgesics on the development of delirium following hip fracture. *J Gerontol A Biol Sci Med Sci.* 2003;58:76–81.

40. Mann C, Pouzeratte Y, Bocarra G, *et al.* Comparison of intravenous or epidural patient-controlled analgesia in the elderly after major abdominal surgery. *Anesthesiology.* 2000;92(2):433–441.

CHAPTER 25

Anaesthesia for urological surgery in the elderly

Ian Whitehead and John Hughes

Introduction

Anaesthesia for urological surgery increasingly involves the management of large numbers of elderly patients. The elderly (>65 years) population is one of the fastest growing parts of the population in the developed world and advancing age increases the probability of a person requiring surgery.

The incidence of urological conditions increases with age.[1] In addition to the procedure itself; the older patient has a greater likelihood of having other pre-existing medical disease. Bladder cancer is associated with smoking and these patients are likely to have an element of coronary artery and obstructive airways disease.

Urological surgery performed in the elderly includes a wide range of procedures, ranging from outpatient or day case procedures to major interventions that may cause marked physiological disturbances.

Physiology

Even in the absence of other pre-existing medical disease, physiological changes occur as a normal consequence of ageing.[2] Those of particular reference to urological surgery include:

Renal function

Renal blood flow and kidney mass reduce with age. Glomerular filtration rate (GFR) decreases by 50 per cent by the age of 80. The plasma creatinine usually remains within the normal range as there is associated age related reduction in muscle mass. The elderly also have decreased concentrating and diluting ability along with impaired sodium handling.[3]

The underlying pathology for which the patient requires urological surgery can add to the deterioration in renal function, e.g. chronic renal tract obstruction.

Temperature control

See also Chapter 35.

Protection from hypothermia is an essential part of the care of the elderly patient. The elderly are particularly susceptible to hypothermia as they show a decreased ability to detect changes in environmental temperature.[1] Their capacity to respond to changes in body temperature is impaired by reduced muscle mass, impaired autonomic function and decreased basal metabolic rate (BMR). The elderly patient may therefore, not be able to restore themselves to a normal body temperature. Consideration of methods to maintain a patients temperature should occur at all stages of the perioperative pathway, from leaving the ward to the preoperative holding area, the operating theatre, recovery area, and back to the ward.[3]

All patients undergoing anaesthesia lose heat, with losses of 0.5–1.0°C being common within the first hour due to redistribution from core to periphery. In addition to heat loss via conduction, convection, evaporation, radiation, and respiratory losses, endoscopic urological procedures exacerbate the heat loss due to irrigation of the bladder with large volumes of often cold fluid.

Fluid balance

Total body water as a proportion of body weight decreases with age, the elderly patient having approximately 40 per cent body water in comparison to a young adult's 60 per cent. As stated earlier, the normal homeostatic mechanisms which control fluid and electrolyte balance are decreased, therefore reducing their concentrating ability. The ability to conserve sodium is reduced. Elderly patients are therefore at increased risk of dehydration.[4] The National Confidential Enquiry into Peri-Operative Deaths (NCEPOD) report *Extremes of Age* emphasized the need for careful management of fluid balance. Hypovolaemia was considered a major factor in morbidity resulting from hypotension during anaesthesia.

Hypervolemia is also poorly tolerated in the elderly and can occur as a result of overhydration with intravenous fluids or resulting from excess absorption of irrigation fluid. The kidney is unable to excrete excess water or salt with excess circulating volume precipitating cardiac failure and pulmonary oedema, this is often exacerbated as elderly patients often have impaired cardiac function.

Urological procedures

Non-tumour-related procedures performed commonly in the elderly are; transurethral resection of prostate (TURP), bladder neck incisions, urethral dilatation, meatoplasty, optical urethrotomy, insertion or change of ureteric stents, extraction of stones (bladder, kidney, or ureter), percutaneous nephrolithotomy (PCNL), transrectal ultrasound (TRUS), and prostatic biopsy and bladder washout.

Urological malignancies have a higher incidence in the elderly. Prostatic cancer has a significant relationship to age with 75 per cent of cases seen in men over the age of 75. Renal carcinoma increases with age, 75 per cent of cases occurring in men and women over the age of 60 and bladder cancer is the most frequent tumour occurring within the urological system with incidence increasing significantly in men over the age of 65.[5]

Procedures for these include transurethral resection of bladder tumour (TURBT), open cystectomy, prostatectomy, and nephrectomy. More recently laparoscopic surgery has been used for resection of bladder, kidney, or prostate.

Cystoscopy

This can be a 'flexible cystoscopy' which is usually performed under topical anaesthesia. Rigid cystoscopy requires either regional or general anaesthesia and is usually performed in the lithotomy position.

Surgery for renal tract stones

Renal stones are frequently idiopathic; however they can be caused by hypercalciuria from a variety of sources. Elderly patients may present with renal stones but the majority have had previous urological interventions for renal stones.

Stones in the lower ureters and bladder are treated with endoscopic procedures. These include flexible and rigid uretroscopy with basket stone extraction and laser lithotripsy. Stones in the upper ureters and kidneys are removed via extracorporeal shock-wave lithotripsy (ESWL) or percutaneous nephrolithotomy (PCNL). ESWL utilizes ultrasound to disintegrate the stones. The procedure may take up to 60 minutes and can be painful.

Many patients require or have had ureteric stents inserted as a temporizing procedure or to allow drainage of urine following the procedure.

Percutaneous nephrolithotomy

The removal of renal stones via PCNL is used in the treatment of large stones in the renal pelvis. The procedure requires general anaesthesia with the patient in the prone position.

A retrograde pyelogram is performed initially in order to locate the stone in the kidney and ureteral stent inserted to facilitate drainage following the procedure. The patient is then turned prone and a percutaneous sheath is inserted into the kidney using an endoscope, the stones are visualized and then broken up with ultrasound. The fragments are removed via irrigation through the endoscope.

Transurethral resection of prostate

Despite the development of alternative forms of treatment (Holmium-YAG laser resection or laser ablation; KTP-laser photoselective vaporization of the prostate) TURP remains a commonly performed procedure for benign prostatic hyperplasia. Indications include symptomatic bladder outlet obstruction in patients who have not responded to medical therapy, recurrent urinary infections, renal insufficiency, or gross persistent haematuria.[6] It is performed in the lithotomy position and involves the introduction into the bladder of a resectoscope and then resection of the prostatic tissue is performed via an electroresection technique that utilizes a monopolar, high-frequency current passed through a metal loop that acts as an electrode. This causes coagulation whilst cutting. The operation lasts up to an hour. During the procedure a continuous flow of irrigation fluid through the resectoscope is required to remove resected prostatic fragments and provide adequate visibility. The most commonly used irrigating fluid is glycine, the fluid chosen as it must not allow electrical conduction as this would cause dispersion of the diathermy current. Attempts to assess the quantity of glycine absorbed have used ethanol as a tracer. Breath-ethanol levels being compared to serum glycine levels. As the absorption of glycine is unpredictable, the use of this technique cannot accurately determine serum glycine levels.[7]

Up to 60 per cent of patients presenting for TURP have cardiovascular or respiratory comorbidities. Despite the increasing mean age of patients who present for TURP, morbidity is estimated as less than 1 per cent and mortality 0.25 per cent in large studies.[8] This has decreased significantly during the last few decades, as a result of improvements in the surgical technique and advances in anaesthesia.

The risk of complications increases with increased operative time especially with resections lasting greater than 60 minutes. TURP can be associated with several serious complications that that include:

TURP syndrome

The TURP syndrome is a clinical condition characterized by mental confusion, nausea, vomiting, hypertension, bradycardia, and visual disturbances.[7,9] It is caused by the absorption of the irrigation solution into the circulation from the prostatic venous sinuses. It is recognized that the amount of fluid absorbed correlates well with the duration of the resection and the height of the irrigation fluid above the bladder. Absorption is normally about 20 ml/min and 1.5 L is typically absorbed but can be as much as 5 L. Absorption of the fluid leads to hyponatraemia and fluid overload.[7] The type of anaesthesia also affects the quantities of irrigation fluid absorbed, those spontaneously breathing under spinal anaesthesia absorbing more than those who had a general anaesthetic with positive pressure ventilation.

The symptoms described are as a result of hyponatraemia and water intoxication. Hypervolaemia is likely to lead to pulmonary oedema especially in those patients with poor cardiovascular reserve. In combination with hyponatraemia it may lead to cerebral oedema and increased intracranial pressure. Patients under spinal anaesthesia may show agitation, cerebral disturbance or shivering as early signs. The incidence of TURP syndrome is approximately 1 per cent. As soon as the diagnosis of TURP syndrome is suspected then treatment should be instigated; this includes stopping the surgery as soon as is practical, replacement of the irrigating fluid with saline, administration of diuretics, and checking the serum electrolytes specifically sodium. Symptoms of hyponatraemia do not usually occur until the sodium concentration is <120 mmol/L. In most cases treatment with fluid restriction and diuretics will suffice. In severe hyponatraemia or in patients who develop neurological complications (e.g. fitting, coma) require treatment with hypertonic saline.

Infection—in the perioperative period

Infection of the urinary tract is common in patients with outflow obstruction. Recurrent infection is an indication for TURP. The prostate has a rich blood supply and can contain significant bacteria. Penetration of antibiotics into the prostatic tissue is poor. Instrumentation of the urinary tract in the presence of infection is likely to lead to bacteraemia and possibly septic shock. This may be confused in the elderly with TURP syndrome.

Preoperative urinalysis is performed and it is mandatory not to operate on patients who have an untreated urinary tract infection. All patients undergoing TURP surgery should receive prophylactic antibiotics at induction of anaesthesia.

Patients with indwelling catheters require careful consideration regarding antibiotic therapy prior to surgery. These patients frequently have chronic urinary colonization and it is impossible to render the urine 'sterile' whilst the catheter is *in situ*. These patients are treated with antibiotics tailored to the urine culture to reduce the risk of bacteraemia during surgery.

Bladder perforation

Accidental perforation of the bladder during TURP is rare. This occurs as a result of the resectoscope going through the bladder wall or due to over-distension of the bladder with irrigation fluid. In most cases the perforation is extra-retropertioneal and may initially be indicated by reduced return of irrigation fluid from the bladder. Later signs of bladder perforation include lower abdominal pain and distension, hypotension, and nausea.

Haemorrhage

Haemorrhage remains a major complication of both TURP and bladder tumour surgery. Significant blood loss can occur and is difficult to estimate as a result of the constant irrigation of the bladder. Clinical judgement and measurement of haematocrit gives a better estimate of blood loss and can be used as a guide for blood transfusion.[6] All patients undergoing TURP should have a 'Group and Save' so that blood can be rapidly cross matched if required. In the past a haemoglobin concentration of <10 g/dl would have been a trigger for transfusion, nowadays the clinical situation with regards to ongoing blood loss and the patients comorbidities must be considered with an individualized approach to blood transfusion.

The development of new surgical techniques (photoselective vaporization and laser resection) has almost eliminated significant blood loss during resection.

Transurethral resection of bladder tumour

This procedure can range from diathermy of a small lesion in the bladder to resection of large tumours. The larger resections have similar problems to TURP with regards blood loss, although the absorption of irrigation fluid is seldom a problem as the large venous sinuses of the prostate are not opened.

Laparoscopic surgery

Laparoscopic surgery is now increasingly utilized in urology. It is used for nephrectomy, pyeloplasty, prostatectomy with or without pelvic lymph node dissection, and retroperitoneal lymph node dissection. Anaesthesia is similar to that for other laparoscopic procedures.[10]

Radical cystectomy

This is a major operation often undertaken in patients with multiple comorbidities and may carry a significant mortality risk. It is not uncommon to see elderly patients listed. The procedure may have significant blood loss which may be rapid requiring transfusion and lasts between 4–6 hours. Invasive arterial monitoring is mandatory and most patients have central venous pressure monitoring if they have limited cardiorespiratory reserve. For an open cystectomy general anaesthesia is often supplemented with epidural anaesthesia that can be continued into the postoperative period.

Patients on anticoagulants and antiplatelet agents

See also Chapter 13.

Antiplatelet therapy has become a major treatment for both primary and secondary prevention of myocardial infarction or stroke and for the prevention of coronary stent thrombosis following percutaneous coronary intervention (PCI). As a result of this many patients and increasingly elderly patients are treated with these agents. More than 25 per cent of the elderly population are receiving aspirin.[9] It is therefore common for anaesthetists to be presented with an elderly patient on antiplatelet drugs for an endoscopic procedure.

The systemic inflammatory response syndrome and acute phase response associated with surgery are known to increase platelet adhesiveness and decrease fibrinolysis resulting in a hypercoagulable state. This combined with increased circulating endogenous catecholamines increases thrombosis risk.

Aspirin is recommended as a lifelong therapy and should not be interrupted for patients with cardiovascular disease. Clopidogrel therapy is mandatory for 6 weeks following the placement of bare metal cardiac stents, 3–6 months following MI, and at least 12 months following drug-eluting cardiac stent placement.[11]

After cessation of aspirin or clopidogrel, platelet aggregation returns to baseline in 5–7 days.[12] There is no difference in bleeding risk between the two drugs when given alone. A newer drug prasugrel increases risk of haemorrhage by 30 per cent. Cessation of these drugs is associated with increased cardiac complications, which for aspirin has a risk of death causing an acute coronary syndrome (ACS) leading to death or MI of two to four times greater than that of a patient continuing on the drug with the risk peaking at 10 days. Stopping clopidogrel is the most significant predictor of stent thrombosis (drug-eluting stents being greater risks than bare metal ones).[13] Stopping dual antiplatelet therapy within 6 weeks after angioplasty or stenting has a mortality of up to 71 per cent, compared with 5 per cent if it is continued throughout the perioperative period.

Overall urological surgery is associated with a 2 per cent risk of postoperative MI and cardiac-related mortality. Most perioperative MIs occurr within the first 3 days following surgery.

There is lack of consensus amongst urologists regarding the management of these patients in the perioperative period.[14] Patients are commonly advised to stop these drugs 7–10 days prior to surgery in order to decrease the haemorrhage risk that may occur if the drug is continued. The evidence suggests that this practice may be putting patients at significant risk of cardiovascular events during the perioperative period.

Patients on oral anticoagulants should always have these interrupted before urological surgery. If necessary they can be substituted with alternatives during the perioperative period depending on the indication for anticoagulation.

What are the bleeding risks?

Endoscopic urological procedures are not without risk of significant bleeding. If this continues into the postoperative period patients may require further surgery. The majority of published literature for urology in patients continuing on antiplatelet therapy surrounds aspirin and TURP. These followed two case reports of deaths after prostatectomy due to bleeding.[14] The results of these studies have been contradictory, some stating that there is increased risks of haemorrhage and others reporting no difference. A randomized controlled study looking at the effects of bleeding following TURP found no difference in operative blood loss or transfusion requirements but did find a higher postoperative blood loss in the aspirin group. This did not lead to higher morbidity or mortality.

A large meta-analysis looking at the effects of aspirin on surgical blood loss in non-cardiac surgery found that although the risk of interoperative blood loss increased by 1.5 times there was no increase in the severity of bleeding complications, surgical morbidity, or mortality with the exception of transurethral prostatectomy which was associated with higher morbidity and mortality.

The risk of cardiovascular complications following withdrawal of antiplatelet agents is higher than the risk of haemorrhage. Careful consideration should be given to continuing aspirin as a minimum in these situations and stopping clopidogrel for the minimum time possible (Fig. 25.1). In high-risk patients this requires close communication with the patient's cardiologist.[15]

Patient positioning

There are various patient positions used for urological surgery. The position chosen should allow optimal access by the surgeon to perform surgery without causing injury to the patient. Positioning may be more difficult in the elderly due to fixed posture or reduced mobility of joints. Extra care should be taken in those patients with joint replacements, especially hip and shoulder. Injuries caused as a result of positioning include: peripheral nerve injuries, ocular injuries, and pressure sores.[16]

Positions utilized in urological surgery include: supine, prone, lateral, flexed lateral, lithotomy. All these positions may also require a Trendelenburg tilt. It is important at the pre-assessment visit to consider the patient's ability to tolerate specific positions, e.g. a patient with respiratory disease may not tolerate steep Trendelenburg for a laparoscopic prostatectomy.

Lithotomy

The commonest position in urology as this allows surgical access to the perineum. The patient lies supine, the lower limbs are flexed at hip and knee and both legs are simultaneously elevated and separated. The legs are then supported either with straps or devices designed to hold the legs which can be adjusted. The leg supports are padded.

Injuries occurring as a result of the lithotomy position include: injury to the common peroneal nerve and saphenous nerve as a result of the leg straps, obturatror and femoral nerve damage as a result of excessive flexion of the thigh, and compartment syndrome of the lower limb.

The lithotomy position causes significant physiological disturbances in the elderly. The functional residual capacity (FRC), which is already reduced, falls further as a result of the increased intra-abdominal pressure resulting in hypoventilation, basal atelectasis, and hypoxia. Elevation of the legs increases venous return and may exacerbate heart failure. At the end of the procedure lowering of the legs leads to venous pooling, reduces venous return, and can result in hypotension. It is at this point that hypovolaemia as a result of intraoperative blood loss may be unmasked.

Trendelenburg

The patient lays supine and the operating table tilted head-down. This allows the viscera to gravitate cephalad and provides

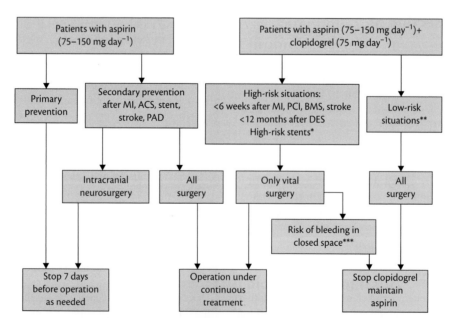

Fig. 25.1 Algorithm for preoperative management of patients under antiplatelet therapy. Reproduced from Chassot P, et al. 'Perioperative antiplatelet therapy: the case for continuing therapy in patients at risk of myocardial infarction', *British Journal of Anaesthesia*, 2007, 99, pp. 316–328, by permission of Oxford University Press and the Board of Management and Trustees of the British Journal of Anaesthesia.

better exposure to the pelvis. This may be used in combination with lithotomy.

Physiological effects of Trendelenburg include: decreased cardiac output, heart rate, and blood pressure as a result of baroreceptor activation; decreased lung capacities and ventilation–perfusion ratio as a result of the abdominal contents obstructing the movement of the diaphragm. There is also an increased risk of regurgitation especially in the elderly who have poor airway reflexes. Trendelenburg also causes intracranial venous congestion and raised ICP.

Prone

In the usual prone position, rolls or pillows are placed under the chest and pelvis, this elevates the trunk. The roles need to be firm enough to maintain elevation of the chest and pelvis and cover a sufficient surface area to avoid pressure areas. In PCNL a roll is also placed under the lower chest to push the kidney upwards and aid localization. This can interfere with the excursion of the diaphragm.

Care must also be taken with the head and neck and to avoid pressure on the eye which can cause retinal artery thrombosis and blindness. Care should also be taken with pressure on the ears and nose as well as positioning of the neck (particularly in an elderly population).

Brachial plexus injury is possible and care should be taken when positioning the arms. Padding should be used to protect the ulnar nerve at the elbow. The head of the humerus can also stretch and compress the axillary neurovascular bundle. The shoulders should not be beyond 90° in any direction to minimize the risk of brachial plexus injury.

Physiological effects of the prone position include a decrease in cardiac output and blood pressure as a result of abdominal compression and a reduction in lung compliance.

Lateral

The patient is placed with the operative side upmost. The patient is stabilized by flexion of the thigh and knee of the bottom leg. A pillow is placed between the legs and a back support prevents the patient rolling supine. The upper arm is usually supported in a gutter with care not to put pressure on the brachial plexus or nerves of the forearm. The patient is kept in position by tapes over the hips and chest.

In any of the positions mentioned the operating table may be 'broken' such that there is hyperextension of the lumber spine to facilitate access to the pelvis, lateral extension of the spine to open up the renal angle and improve access to the kidney, or in the prone position flexion of the spine to facilitate access for a PCNL. All these positions exacerbate the physiological changes mentioned previously. They also have the potential to put a strain on the axial skeleton and exacerbate any mechanical back pain the patient may have. This will settle postoperatively as the patient mobilizes and returns to normal activity. The elderly often have relatively fixed deformities or reduced range of movement of the axial skeleton and due care should be taken with positioning. Patients should also be warned of the potential for increased back pain postoperatively along with instructions on how to best manage it (mobilize).

Anaesthesia for urological surgery in the elderly

The choice of anaesthetic technique for urological surgery will depend on both the individual patient and the anaesthetist. Regional anaesthesia, more specifically spinal anaesthesia, has been advocated in patients who are to be positioned in the lithotomy position, due to the avoidance of central nervous system depressant drugs which reduces postoperative confusion and allows early detection of TURP syndrome.

Spinal anaesthesia potentially offers some advantages over general anaesthesia in that it prevents postoperative inhibition of fibrinolysis, reducing the incidence of deep venous thrombosis as well as the haemodynamic effects associated with reduced blood loss in pelvic operations. In all cases the potential risks and benefits of regional anaesthesia should be discussed with the patient and documented.

Epidural anaesthesia can provide adequate anaesthesia for the majority of endoscopic urological procedures. Satisfactory blockade takes longer to achieve with epidural compared to spinal anaesthesia and the technique is technically more difficult. The extent of blockade with epidural anaesthesia is, however, more controllable and the placement of a catheter allows analgesia to continue into the postoperative period.

Not all patients or operations are suited to regional anaesthesia and many patients continue to have general anaesthesia for urological surgery. This can be due to patient factors, anaesthetic factors, or surgical factors. Patients with poor cardiorespiratory reserve or cough tolerate lithotomy poorly. Patient movement increases the risk of bladder perforation. Haemodynamic stability is easier to maintain with general anaesthesia and allows these patients to tolerate the surgery and remain still, creating a clearer surgical field. Patients on anticoagulants or who continue on antiplatelet therapy may also require general anaesthesia.

The length and type of surgery may also influence choice of anaesthesia. Prolonged periods in lithotomy may result in backache or pain in the lower limbs which could be attributed to regional anaesthesia if this has been performed. Laparoscopic surgery necessitates a general anaesthetic.

The effect of age on the pharmacology of anaesthetic drugs is described in more detail in Chapter 3.

For general anaesthesia the choice lies between spontaneous breathing on a laryngeal mask airway or IPPV with muscle relaxation and intubation of the trachea. Fit elderly patients can breathe spontaneously on a LMA. Patients with pre-existing respiratory or cardiovascular disease should be formally ventilated. Anaesthesia can be maintained either via propofol target controlled infusion (TCI) or via volatile anaesthetic agents, e.g. sevoflurane or desflurane. Patients should be ventilated to normocapnia

In patients undergoing TURP there is no difference in perioperative mortality between those who had regional or general anaesthesia.

Postoperative analgesia is similar to that for any surgical procedure and with the same considerations to the normal age-related physiological changes. Care has to be taken when considering which agents to use and the potential risk of drug interactions as this group of patients are frequently on several medications.

As with any anaesthesia the aim has to be to maintain the patient's physiology as close to their normal as possible whilst providing optimal conditions for the surgery to progress. This is never more true than with an elderly population who have an normally reduced physiological reserve, have an altered response to medications (pharmacodynamic and pharmacokinetic), frequently have comorbidities, and may respond less predictably to our interventions. Positioning has to be balanced within the limitations set by the patient (fixed or reduced mobility). Postoperative and ward care requires as much attention to detail for the best outcome to be achieved.

Conclusion

Urological surgery ranges from minor 'office type' procedures to complex major operations with significant risks to fluid balance, temperature control, and from blood loss. As the population presenting for surgery continues to get older these considerations become all the more important. The need to place the patient into prone, lateral, or Trendelenburg positions and to have large areas of their trunk and abdomen exposed can be challenging for elderly patients with their reduced cardiovascular, respiratory, and renal reserves. Assessment, optimization, careful operative management, and attentive postoperative care are essential for satisfactory outcomes. As these procedures may be repeated frequently, detailed recording of their recovery and return to their previous quality of life becomes essential especially with regard to cognitive and functional ability. As with most interventions in the elderly, access to skilled and experienced practitioners, medical and nursing, is probably the most important determinant of reaching a successful outcome.

References

1. Ryall DM, Dodds C. Anaesthesia for urological surgery in the elderly. *Curr Anaesth Crit Care.* 1992;3.200–206.
2. Murray D, Dodds C. Perioperative care of the elderly. *Cont Educ Anaesth Crit Care Pain.* 2004;4(6).
3. Kanonidou Z. Karystianou G. Anaesthesia for the elderly. *Hippokratia.* 2007;11(4):175–177.
4. Cousins J, Howard J, Borra P. Principles of anaesthesia in urological surgery. *BJU Int.* 2005;96:223–229.
5. Office for National Statistics. *Cancer statistics: registrations series MB1.* <http://www.statistics.gov.uk>.
6. Cherian VT. Anaesthetic implications of urological surgery. *Ind J Urol.* 2006;22:194–200.
7. Collins JW, Macdermott S, Bradbrook RA, *et al.* Is using ethanol-glycine irrigating fluid monitoring and 'good surgical practice' enough to prevent harmful absorption during transurethral resection of the prostate? *BJU Int.* 2006;97(6):1247–1251.
8. Rassweiler J Teber D, *et al.* Complications of TURP—incidence, management, and prevention. *Eur Urol.* 2006;50:969–980.
9. Porter M. Anaesthesia for transurethral resection of the prostate (TURP). *Update Anaesth.* 2003;16:21–26. <http://www.nda.ox.ac.uk/wfsa/html/u16/u1608_01.htm>
10. Midgley S, Tolley D. Anaesthesia for laparoscopic surgery in urology. *EAU-EUB Update Series* 4, 2006;241–245.
11. Cook L, Cottrell AM. Anti-platelet agents in urology. *BJU Int.* 2010. <http://www.bjui.org/general/Urology_in_General.aspx>.
12. Weber A, Braun M, Hohlfeld T, *et al.* Recovery of platelet function after discontinuation of clopidogrel treatment in healthy volunteers. *Br J Clin Pharmacol.* 2001;52(3):333–336.
13. *Summary product characteristics clopidogrel.* Updated 25 September 2012. <http://www.medicines.org.uk/emc/medicine/23906>.
14. Pawan V, Goel A, Sengottayn VK, *et al.* Antiplatelet drugs in the perioperative period: what every urologist needs to know. *Ind J Urol.* 2009;25:3 296–301.
15. Douketis JD, Berger PB, Dunn AS, *et al.* The perioperative management of antithrombotic therapy. *Chest.* 2008;133;299S–339S.
16. Knight DJW, Mahajan RP. Patient positioning in anaesthesia. *Cont Educ Anaesth Crit Care Pain.* 2004;4(5):160–163.

CHAPTER 26

Pain management in the elderly

Andrew Severn and Joanne McGuire

Introduction

There are three dimensions in which the assessment of acute pain in the elderly has to be considered in a different light from that of younger patients subjected to similar operative or traumatic insult. It may be useful to remember at this point the definition of pain as formulated by the International Association for the Study of Pain (IASP), which states that pain is 'an unpleasant sensory and emotional experience associated with actual or potential tissue damage, or described in terms of such damage'. The critical issue here, for our consideration of the elderly is the way in which pain is 'described' or 'reported'.

- There are age-related alterations in the somatosensory system (see Chapters 5 and 11).
- There are differences in the affective and cognitive processing of the sensory information that are influenced by life experiences and these will be expected to increase with age.
- There may be changes in cognition, which mean that the normal ways of measuring pain and evaluating the response to intervention are either inaccurate or inappropriate. These may be a consequence of either normal age-related changes or disease.

Pain assessment in cognitive impairment

There are abundant data on pain and its treatment in elderly patients with cognitive disturbances. Understandably much of the literature on pain assessment and management in the elderly is derived from studies of populations residing in institutions such as nursing homes. The challenge of this chapter is to distil this data into a format which enables the practising hospital clinician to recognize and treat postsurgical or trauma pain when the normal assessment methods (self-reporting of symptoms) may be deemed to be unreliable.

The important issue is whether patients with cognitive disturbance can reliably report pain and if so, what tools may be of use. Which behavioural rating scales should be used in an acute hospital setting and whether it is more appropriate to listen to patients or observe their behaviour when assessing surgical or trauma pain.

The observation that simple analgesics can influence the restlessness of patients with dementia is reported[1] and has recently received renewed attention in a randomized controlled trial. Husebo et al.[2] investigated whether a simple stepwise protocol for pain management could reduce agitated behaviour in nursing home residents with dementia cared for in 60 different institutions. They assessed pain in 352 patients with a behavioural rating scale, the MOBID2, which had previously been validated for pain in dementia[3] and described this population as showing clinically relevant pain in over 55 per cent of patients.

Institutions were randomized to provide normal care or to provide a stepwise protocol using analgesia for the treatment of agitation whilst keeping doses of antipsychotic drugs unchanged. They found a reduction in agitated behaviour with analgesia that was as good as any of the reported controlled trials of the antipsychotic risperidone the only drug licensed for this agitation in dementia. Furthermore, the treatment effect reverted to the baseline within 4 weeks of stopping the analgesics. While the sceptical might argue that analgesics have a non-specific sedative effect that might confound analysis, examination of the analgesic regimen refutes this objection. Over two-thirds of the intervention group needed no more than 3 g of paracetamol a day. A further quarter needed only low doses of opioids (up to 20 mg of morphine or 10 mcg/hour of transdermal buprenorphine). A small proportion (7 per cent) received the maximum medication (up to 300 mg of pregabalin a day). Furthermore, where drowsiness or other side effect was a problem (up to 5 per cent of the original intervention group), the patients were taken out of the study and not included in the analysis. The elegance of the study design is further highlighted by the use of the pain rating scale through the period of study to demonstrate the correlation between reduction in agitation and the reduction in pain. The message for practice is clear: agitated behaviour may reflect undertreated pain in demented patients and responds to simple analgesic measures that can be implemented easily on surgical wards.

In considering the implications of this study, the reader who wishes to become acquainted with the extent of the literature on pain in dementia is directed to the clinical review by Scherder et al.[4] who, commenting of the state of the science of pain assessment in dementia, concluded that 'a final step in the process is the use of an analgesic trial to help validate if potential behavioural indicators of pain do respond top analgesic treatment'. It would appear that in the case of the MOBID2 scale, that this has now been done, and furthermore, that clinically relevant changes in this tool are mirrored with clinically relevant changes as measured with a tool to measure agitation.

We will now look further at the issue of the usefulness of pain behavioural rating scales versus self-reporting scales (verbal or other) in elderly patients with cognitive disturbance.

Verbal and self-reporting

In a review of 30 pain instruments [5] 60 per cent were verbal. This might imply that even in the cognitively impaired the patient's self-report of pain remains the most accurate. However, it was acknowledged that of these verbal rating tools none demonstrated excellent reliability or validity.

One early study examined the association between self-reported pain and cognitive impairment and concluded that verbal pain reports were no less valid in cognitive decline than those with no cognitive deficits.[6] However, the same study also identified that a substantial proportion of the participants were unable to understand and answer simple yes/no questions. This appears to suggest that reports of pain are valid but not all cognitively impaired people are able to report their pain. Ferrell et al.[7] suggested that pain reports in this population are reliable and valid: 83 per cent of those studied could complete one pain assessment tool and those who were unable to could identify pain presence by direct questioning. However, it was also acknowledged that those with moderate to severe impairment could not reliably or accurately communicate, which limits the applicability of their conclusions to the less severely affected.

The difficulty with interpreting the results of these studies is the poor correlation that seems to exist between the severity of dementia and the difficulty in reporting. A report of 154 participants described large numbers (a third of the group) who were unable to use any of four assessment tools but they could not identify a clear co-relation between difficulty and degree of dementia.[8]

Which self-rating technique works best for the elderly patients with a degree of cognitive impairment? Closs et al.[9] assessed the value of five instruments:

- Verbal Rating Scale (VRS)
- Horizontal Numeric Rating Scale (NRS)
- Faces Pictorial Scale (FPS)
- Colour Visual Analogue Scale (CVAS)
- Mechanical Visual Analogue Scale (MVAS).

They described that VRS was followed by the NRS as having better overall completion rates but noted that repeated explanations of the tools increased the completion rates for those with higher levels of cognitive impairment. This observation may be of considerable clinical value. The VRS was outperformed in a similar type of comparative study[10] by the McGill Word Scale, a tool which requires participants to choose a word to describe their pain. In addition to visual analogue and pain face scoring three 'pain location' instruments were also investigated: in this case by asking participants to describe pain with reference to a doll, a diagram or on themselves. Eighty-six per cent of the cognitively impaired participants were able to locate pain on their own body using one of these location instruments. Again, this could be a useful assessment strategy.

Observational (or behavioural) rating scales

For those people who are more severely affected by cognitive impairment, it is claimed that performing behavioural or observation based assessment is best practice.[11] This is based upon observation of patients' behaviour and function, providing an indirect, 'objective' measure of pain. Specific pain behaviours that have been identified in the literature include: rapid blinking and other facial expressions; agitation or aggression; crying or moaning; becoming withdrawn and quiet; guarding of a body part; noisy breathing; negative vocalizations and fidgeting.[12] These pain indicators have been used to produce assessment instruments that may be useful for patients with severe cognitive impairment. However, these behaviours may be culturally determined and judgments regarding them may be subjective.

A systematic review has compared the usefulness of 12 such tools and concluded that none of the tools were convincingly appropriate or preferable for assessing pain in people with dementia.[13]

Facial expression has been claimed to be a reliable and consistent indicator of pain.[14] One of the obvious difficulties in research is the ethical problem of causing pain sufficient to enable it to be assessed in this group of patients. This problem can be addressed by observing existing practice such as dressing a decubitus ulcer. Nurses and medical students can reliably identify pain from videotaped recordings of facial expression of demented patients undergoing a dressing change of ulcers. In a study of nine patients, the one patient whose expression did not suggest pain was using a fentanyl transdermal patch for analgesia.

The clinician who is faced with making an assessment of acute pain but is not completely familiar with the more subtle neuropsychiatric manifestations of the various causes of cognitive impairment may justifiably admit to a degree of confusion. Frontal lobe dementia might be characterized by more disinhibited pain responses.[15] The expression of pain may be a consequence of the disinhibition of behaviour due to the disease process rather than because of an increase in pain. Non-facial behavioural cues may also be exaggerated responses of affective distress because of an inability to comprehend what is happening when challenged with a moderately noxious stimulus.[16] Identified pain behaviours may overlap with symptoms of other states of discomfort and with syndromes such as delirium or depression whilst discomfort can be caused by other states such as thirst, hunger, frustration, loneliness, boredom, constipation, or infection.[17] These behaviours therefore might only be attributed to pain when a known procedure has been performed or painful condition exists. Conversely physical limitations such as contractures or immobility may limit the behavioural response. It must be also considered that in some types of advanced dementia facial expression is muted.

The challenge for the clinician attempting to assess pain in the surgical setting is to know the value and limitations of observational techniques and how they compare with self-rating. There is evidence that observers may underestimate pain[18] while family members may do the opposite.

Many behavioural pain assessment tools have been produced but there appears to be little research evidence to test validity and reliability and therefore support their introduction into clinical practice.[13] Only eight studies have attempted to validate behavioural tools by comparing them to the gold standard of

Table 26.1 Studies which have compared behavioural rating scores with self reports of pain in elderly patients with cognitive impairment

| Author | Tools | Results | | Significance |
		Verbal	Behavioural	
Krulewitch et al 2000	VAS, PIS & FPS vs Hospice Approach Discomfort Scale	PIS works	Poorest correlation with other caregiver reports	Poor correlation between behavioural and verbal reports of pain
Hadjistavropoulos et al, 2000	CVAS vs FACS & PBM	Sensitivity in variations of pain during different activities	Identified greater emotional distress associated with painful activity	Self-report not correlated with behavioural report
Alexander et al 2005	CVAS vs pain target behaviours list	Most participants unable to use CVAS	Led to increase in pain medication and reduction in pain behaviours over time	No correlation could be made between verbal and behavioural tools
Pautex et al, 2005	HVAS, VVAS, FPS,VRS vs DOLOPUS-2	VRS better for more severe dementia	Underestimated pain when compared to verbal report	Modest correlation between behavioural & verbal tools
Pautex et al 2006	VRS, HVAS, FPS vs DOLOPUS-2	Greater comprehension of VRS & FPS	Underestimated pain when compared to verbal report	Routine use of behavioural tools not justified
Leong et al 2006	VDS vs Nurse report VDS PAINAD	No correlation with nurse report or PAINAD tool	Strong correlation between nurse report and PAINAD	Questions the need for behavioural pain scales if nurse report is as accurate
Horgas et al, 2007	NRS & VDS vs PBM & NOPPAIN	Strong correlation in cognitively intact participants		Recommends assessment using both verbal and behavioural tools
Horgas, et al 2009	NRS vs PBM	Cognitively impaired reported less intense pain	Strong correlation between verbal and behavioural tools	Self-report less reliable in those with moderate to severe impairment

Verbal Tools: VRS – Verbal rating scale; NRS – Numerical rating Scale; VDS – Verbal descriptor scale; HVAS – Horizontal visual analogue scale; VVAS – Vertical visual analogue scale; FPS – Faces pain scale; CVAS – Coloured visual analogue scale; VAS – Visual analogue scale; PIS – Pain intensity scale. **Behavioural Tools:** FACS – Facial action coding system; PBM – Pain behaviour measure; NOPPAIN – Non-communicative patients pain assessment instrument; DOLOPUS 2 – A behavioural pain assessment scale; PAINAD – pain assessment in advanced dementia.

self-reporting (Table 26.1). The majority of the studies identified a poor to modest correlation between self-reporting and behavioural observation, which led to conclusions that they underestimate pain and that routine use of these tools could not be justified.[19] One study aimed to assess the construct validity of three measures of pain.[20] This compared self-reported pain to nurse report of pain and a behavioural tool. The first two assessments were completed by the patient and a nurse using the same verbal tool. The third assessment was performed by the same nurse using the PAINAD behavioural tool. Interestingly, whilst there was poor correlation between self-report and the other assessments, the strong correlation between the nurse assessment and the behavioural tool questioned the value of using these tools at all.

However, one study suggested that the behavioural tool was able to highlight evidence of greater emotional distress and pain experience which was not evident on the self-report measure.[21] By facilitating a programme of structured activity the researchers were able to compare the frequency of non-verbal behaviours such as grimacing, to the patients actual self-report of pain at that time. Correlation between the two assessments was poor leading to the suggestion that they measure very different parts of the pain experience and therefore should be used in conjunction as part of a comprehensive pain assessment. Alexander et al.[22] observed pain behaviours over a 6-month period in an elderly unit and found that this directly influenced an increase in pain medication and a reduction in pain

behaviours were noted over time. Acknowledging and acting upon the non-verbal displays of pain behaviour is important and the introduction of a behavioural tool increased awareness of staff.

Behavioural pain assessments are advocated by the British Pain Society and the British Geriatrics Society for use in people who are unable to self-report pain. They may also be beneficial, used alongside self-report, for all frail elderly with or without cognitive impairments. The Abbey Pain tool was created in Australia for people with end-stage dementia.[23] The tool was built upon the results of two previous studies published in 1992 and 1995[24,25] using indicators that had previously shown some validity and modified by pain and geriatric experts using a Delphi study. It is considered to be a short and easy to apply scale, which takes 1 minute to complete. This had made it a popular choice for consideration of introduction into clinical practice. However, it has been identified that there are still some problems with reliability and validity and that it lacks conceptual clarity in that there is no distinguishing between acute and chronic pain characteristics.[26]

Specific analgesic drugs

Paracetamol

The effect of a single dose of 1gm of intravenous paracetamol has been compared between the 80–90 age group and other age groups.[27] The relationship between paracetamol concentration and time, expressed as 'area under the curve' (AUC) indicated a higher exposure to paracetamol in the older patients and the same was true for conjugates with glucuronide and sulphate that were also raised, the very elderly being exposed up to 1.5 as much metabolite as younger patients. After regular dosing steady state pharmacokinetics are observed even in very elderly patients on multiple medications with mild renal impairment (creatinine clearance of 42 ml/min ± 12 ml/ min) at 5 days of dosing with 1 g three times a day.[28] The effect of regular paracetamol dosing on plasma levels and hepatoxicity has been investigated in an observational study comparing fit and frail elderly in-patients with a younger cohort.[29] Patients received paracetamol 3–4 g/day. On the fifth day the plasma level of alanine transferase (ALT) and paracetamol was measured. Frail patients had higher concentrations of paracetamol, but this did not correlate with a rise in ALT. Indeed the abnormalities in liver function as assessed by ALT concentrations were restricted to the younger patients and the fit elderly. There was an inverse relationship between frailty score and ALT concentration.

In animal studies age-related muscle atrophy is characterized by increased oxidative stress, and the consequent loss of activity of two enzyme pathways involved in the mRNA translation of muscle protein. Paracetamol is able to reverse this effect of oxidative stress.[30] It is noted that during exercise training in older adults, the concomitant use of paracetamol increases muscle volume. This phenomenon may reflect the role of cyclo-oxygenase pathways in regulating muscle protein turnover.[45]

Non-steroidal anti-inflammatory drugs

This class of drugs is commonly used in the management of musculoskeletal pain and has historically relieved much of the pain and suffering associated with it. It is not surprising that elderly patients presenting for surgery may have been taking them for years. The drugs have a number of systemic side effects which mean that vigilance must be exercised in detecting gastrointestinal, renal, and cardiovascular side effects. The same is true for the so-called COXIB drugs, anti-inflammatory drugs with a specific action on the type 2 cyclo-oxygenase (COX) enzyme (non-steroidal anti-inflammatory drugs (NSAIDs) act on both isozymes type 1 and 2 to different extents). Specific COX type 2 inhibitors have limited, but useful, gastrointestinal sparing properties but still have adverse cardiovascular and renal side effects. Creatinine clearance was reduced after intravenous administration of parecoxib but was unchanged in a similar group of elderly patients receiving paracetamol.[31]

Older patients have a higher incidence of gastrointestinal, renal, and cardiovascular pathology that may compound the presentation of symptoms of dyspepsia or haemorrhage, and renal or heart failure. Comorbidities such as atrial fibrillation may require the use of anticoagulants. The capacity of the gastric mucosa to protect itself is reduced with age: this being in part an explanation for the observation that age itself is an independent risk factor for complications of NSAID therapy.[32] In an attempt to address the long-term effects on the health of elderly patients a Canadian Consensus on NSAID prescribing[33] has produced guidelines on administration:

◆ Non-pharmacological or local therapies should be offered before considering NSAIDs.

◆ NSAIDs should be used with caution because of gastrointestinal risks.

◆ Creatinine clearance and blood pressure should be checked before starting NSAIDs or COXIBs.

◆ Proton pump inhibitor gastric protection is required if aspirin and NSAIDs are used together

The association between NSAIDs and cognitive impairment is of interest considering their widespread use in the elderly. It is tempting to argue that the link between dementia and non-use of NSAID is spurious, related to the fact that, in dementia, pain may be poorly treated and patients therefore receive less medication. However it is known that NSAID *in vitro* reduce production of beta amyloid, a protein that is associated with the pathological lesions of Alzheimer's disease. The suggestion that NSAIDs do indeed reduce the incidence of dementia has been confirmed in a study of 3229 individuals over the age of 65.[34] However the protection against dementia afforded by NSAID extends only to Alzheimer's disease, not vascular dementia, and only to those individuals with a certain genotype (APOE epsilon 4) associated with the condition. Furthermore, the relationship between Alzheimer risk reduction and NSAID is not related to the specific beta amyloid inhibitory actions of particular NSAID (different NSAID varying in their ability to inhibit its production).

It may be very difficult, on compassionate and ethical grounds, to restrict access to NSAID during the perioperative period if patients are already taking them for co-morbid conditions such as arthritis, unless specific steps have been taken in the preoperative period to rationalize usage or to provide alternative analgesia. Muzarelli et al.[35] investigated 197 elderly patients (mean age 80) with a history of heart failure and found that 22 per cent used NSAIDs. Of these, almost half were detected only after specific questioning designed to elicit the use of NSAIDs: the information was not offered during the initial consultation. It was possible to persuade two out of three patients to abandon NSAIDs after offering alternative treatments such as paracetamol and opioids.

Such a strategy may be useful for preoperative assessment clinics, and it is in these clinics that a detailed drug history is important, together with screening for the presence of gastrointestinal symptoms, or evidence of renal insufficiency, hypertension or heart failure that might indicate risk factors for the use of NSAIDs.

In surgical and anaesthetic practice the side effects of NSAIDs on gastrointestinal integrity are clearly important. Chronic blood loss leads to a patient presenting for surgery with iron deficient anaemia. The impact of a prolonged surgical stress, coupled with the routine use of anticoagulants for prophylaxis against deep venous thrombosis may precipitate a dangerous gastrointestinal haemorrhage in the patient who has already been exposed to NSAID.

The acute renal and cardiovascular side effects of NSAID are clearly of direct and immediate importance in the perioperative period, more so than the side effects on the gastrointestinal system. Inhibition of prostaglandin synthesis affects renal autoregulation and will result in a reduction of filtration when the renal afferent arteriolar pressure falls. The consequent stimulation of renin release leads to salt and water retention, with a reduction of urine output. The effects of NSAIDs are therefore compounded by falls in blood pressure due to hypovolaemia, major regional anaesthesia, or when cardiac output falls during general anaesthesia. The decision to deploy these drugs as part of a strategy of 'balanced analgesia' during the perioperative period may therefore be a difficult one, and the clinician needs to justify their use on an individual basis, depending on the circumstances and likelihood of complications.

Opioid drugs

The issues around the use of opioid drugs in the elderly surgical patient are multiple, complex and potentially serious. (For details on the pharmacology see Chapter 3.) Veering[36] has summarized electroencephalographic data pertaining to the use of fentanyl, alfentanil, and remifentanil and concluded that the elderly brain is itself intrinsically more sensitive to these agents, irrespective of any pharmacokinetic considerations. Aside from the presentation of acute respiratory depression, side effects with opioids in the elderly include the propensity to provoke delirium. To this problem must be added the difficulty of making a specific diagnosis of the cause of delirium, the observation that untreated acute pain may itself be responsible for delirium and the fact that many patients present with painful conditions for which they are already taking opioids. There are a few valuable literature resources that can help us understand the problem.

Pethidine

The case for (or rather against) pethidine, can be simply put. In 1987, it was said to be the most widely used opioid in the United States for postoperative pain. The danger of delirium in young patients taking large doses was blamed on its anticholinergic properties and interaction with anticholinergic drugs. It was claimed to be reversible by substituting with morphine.[37] A systematic review has confirmed the difficulties that pethidine poses as an analgesic.[38] Hip fracture patients (mean age over 80) treated with pethidine had a higher incidence of delirium (43.2 per cent) compared with those who received morphine (27.1 per cent) (odds ratio 2.5) and it was suggested that patients should be switched from pethidine to 'low-dose morphine'.[39] In a larger study of 541 fractures (65 per cent of the sample being over 80) pethidine was also associated with greater incidence of delirium.[49] Pethidine was implicated in postoperative delirium when case notes of delirious patients were compared with case notes of matched patients who did not suffer this complication, even when it was given by the epidural route.[40] The review concedes that the assessment of analgesia was inadequate in some of the studies, so it is hard to compare whether doses of different drugs were comparable. In summary, pethidine is an unsuitable analgesic drug for the elderly.

Postoperative surgical pain: techniques and factors in delivery

While the last two decades have seen a recognition of the importance of acute postoperative pain management, it is difficult to tease out specific lessons relevant to the elderly from the existing data as the age ranges under investigation are wide. Furthermore some study designs are frankly unhelpful, in that they have included an upper age limit, in some cases as low as 75.[41] The extrapolation of the techniques under investigation to an age group outside that in the study may not be appropriate. Indeed it has been argued that ethical permission should be withheld from research proposals that seek to impose an unjustifiable age limit.[42]

Many hospitals in the United Kingdom have adopted a model of an 'acute pain service' based on the leadership of a consultant anaesthetist supported by specialist nursing staff providing expert assistance to staff on general wards and specific clinical interventions in particularly challenging patients. It is of more than historical interest that the original description of a prototype UK acute pain service describes particular difficulties with older patients, such that they were not well served by the service as it existed [43]. More recent evidence supports this conclusion. For instance, a different model of care in which elderly patients presenting for major joint replacement were assessed and 'optimized' beforehand by a team led by a geriatrician demonstrated a number of postoperative benefits, one of which was a reduction in the number of visits from the acute pain service.[44] One of the ways in which this was achieved was by reviewing analgesic medication prior to elective surgery so that patients were able more easily to exercise and maintain muscle strength around a damaged joint prior to surgery (J Dhesi personal communication). Recent work linking paracetamol analgesia to muscle turnover provides a possible mechanism to support the use of regular analgesia prior to surgery.[45]

Such information is important when considering the recent media response to a report on the care of elderly surgical patients. The frame of reference of the 2010 NCEOPD report was to use the records from patients over the age of 80 who died within 30 days of a surgical procedure to ask questions about the quality of care and to make recommendations about future service provision based on questionnaires sent to institutions reporting a death. Of these institutions, a fraction, predominantly private sector providers and specialist surgical units reported that they did not have a formal 'acute pain service' as defined earlier. Such information, released in the public domain, provoked adverse media interest with newspaper headlines[46] proclaiming that patients were 'dying in agony' for want of a service.

Clearly the role of the acute pain service has to be appropriately tailored to the specific needs of the elderly patient if it is to deliver the right sort of service. Like any other service, however, its effectiveness is hampered by the current evidence base. Evidence, or lack of it, aside the problems are:

◆ Acute pain services provide and supervise safe delivery of high-technology controlled administration of drugs, including patient-controlled intravenous analgesia, epidural analgesia, and continuous plexus analgesia.

◆ Acute pain services have an educational and governance role that limits their personal responsibility to individual patients.

◆ There is currently no formal requirement for a member of an acute pain team, whether medically trained or not, to demonstrate understanding of the particular problems of elderly patients.

One way of addressing the problem of lack of data for the elderly is to consider specific procedures, such as surgery for hip fracture. There are several large studies which have specifically investigated postoperative pain after surgery for hip fracture. Their conclusions may usefully be applied to other older age groups undergoing different types of surgery.

Analysis of 117 elderly patients with hip fracture suggests that the type of operation performed is a factor for pain during mobilization, even when resting pain is controlled with an epidural infusion. Patients undergoing more extensive surgery such as dynamic hip screws or intramedullary nails have more postoperative pain than those undergoing lesser procedures such as hemiarthroplasty or parallel screw fixation.[47] It is difficult to extrapolate these findings to the more frail hip fracture patients, as the study patients were the most able bodied and cognitively intact patients of a total cohort of 981. The study, however, does demonstrate some of the difficulty in assessing the value of different analgesic regimens in isolation. As in many other types of surgery the type of operation performed has such an influence on postoperative pain.

The consequences of untreated pain after hip fracture are stated to be longer hospital stay, curtailment of physiotherapy sessions, delay in mobilization, functional disability (as measured by ability to negotiate past a bedside chair) and reduced mobility at 6 months.[48] In this study of 412 patients pain at rest was not significantly associated with post-operative complications, the need for nursing home admission, or residual pain at 6 months. Nor was survival to 6 months affected. A further study by the same authors on 541 patients with and without delirium claimed that cognitively intact patients were very vulnerable to developing delirium if pain control was inadequate. Further evidence for this was the observation that patients who received less than 10 mg of morphine were more likely to develop delirium than those who received larger doses over the perioperative period.[49]

The relationship between analgesia and acute cardiovascular events has been studied by randomizing hip fracture patients to either 'standard' or continuous epidural analgesia on arrival in the emergency department. In a study of 68 patients the 'standard' analgesia group sustained four fatal cardiac perioperative events and three other cardiac events. The epidural group were spared such complications.[50] While this is evidence of the value of good pain relief, it must be considered that the 'standard' analgesic was pethidine, a drug with an established reputation for side effects in the elderly[40] related to its anticholinergic action. Thus it is difficult to draw any firm conclusions about the specific value of epidural analgesia, as opposed to any other suitable analgesia, in these high-risk elderly patients.

Possibly of more value in answering this question is a systematic review[51] looking at the effectiveness of analgesia after hip fracture surgery. In limiting the search to literature published after 1990 the authors provide an up-to-date account which emphasizes the safety of modern general anaesthesia. Whilst systematic reviews have important influences on clinical practice, it is important to reflect on the difficulty that exists in interpreting the review, however rigorous the methodology may be. Only three trials, out of a total of 83 reviewed, compared different systemic drugs, and one of these trials had used pethidine. Almost half of the studies had explicitly excluded patients with cognitive impairment.

Fourteen studies that investigated the effectiveness of regional blockade in the treatment of postoperative pain are reported in the review. The nerve block techniques which contributed to the review are shown in Table 26.2 and Table 26.3.

The review concludes that nerve blocks reduce postoperative pain, and states that seven of the studies report reduced use of analgesic medication. Pain relief aside, improvement in delirium was noted, but no other complications could be reliably prevented by the use of nerve blocks. Mortality at 30 days and the incidence of cardiorespiratory complications were not influenced by the use of nerve block techniques.

Detailed examination, however, of this one promising area demonstrates the problems of extrapolating data from small studies into clinical practice. Take the studies reporting femoral nerve block for instance. A comparison between intravenous regional

Table 26.2 Distribution of patients in trials of nerve block for pain relief after hip fracture

Block type	n (intervention group)	n (controls)
3:1 block	65	87
Epidural	73	72
Fascia iliaca block	224	197
Femoral nerve block	47	62
Psoas compartment	20	20
'Combined techniques'	80	55

Adapted from AbouSetta et al[45].

analgesia and continuous femoral nerve block[52] excluded the over 80s: according to the statistics reported only six patients in each group would have been aged over 68 in the nerve block group or over 72.3 in the control group.

A 1995 study, on an older, more 'typical' sample, used a single dose of local anaesthetic administered onto the femoral nerve using anatomical landmarks.[53] While the technique worked, reduced requests for analgesia and the number of respiratory complications its conclusions have to be considered in the light of the appropriateness of the methods used in the control group: pethidine and diclofenac are probably not useful drugs to use in comparison. Considering the implications of these two studies for today's practice the technique of nerve location may be important in determining efficacy. Thus a 2006 study in which a nerve stimulator was used may provide more realistic conclusions: administered in this way at the right time, in this case in the emergency room, femoral nerve block reduces pain at rest and increases the range of painless movement.[54]

Conclusion

Postoperative pain control is an important indicator of the quality of care. A seminal textbook on the subject of anaesthesia and the elderly patient published in 1988 provided the reader of the day with general advice on the management of postoperative pain limiting specific comparisons with younger patients to a discussion of the effect of age on opioid pharmacokinetics.[55] A 1997 book devoted to the subject of pain in the elderly describes how and why the elderly may have atypical presentations of pain in acute conditions such as myocardial infarction and peritonitis. The conclusion is that the normal methods used in the assessment of acute pain are less useful in older patients as pain may be underreported.[56] This conclusion is still valid today. Its implications affect all of us charged with alleviating pain in a group of patients which will increase in number in future years.

Table 26.3 Patients in Tuncer's study did not faithfully represent the age group of patients who undergo surgery for hip fracture.[52]

Group	Mean age	SD	Age +1 SD
continuous femoral nerve block	57.2	10.8	68
patient controlled iv analgesia	61.1	11.2	72.3

Tuncer[46] used an age group that did not represent the population at risk.

References

1. Chibnall JT, Tait RC, Harman B, Luebbert RA. Effect of acetaminophen on behaviour, wellbeing, and psychotropic medication use in nursing home residents with moderate-to-severe dementia. *J Am Geriatr Soc.* 2005;53:1921–1929.

2. Husebo BS, Ballard C, Sandvik R, Nilsen OB, Aarsland D. Efficacy of treating pain to reduce behavioural disturbances in residents of nursing homes with dementia: cluster randomised trial. *Br Med J.* 2011;343:d4065.

3. Husebo BS, Strand LI, Moe-Nilssen R, Husebo SB, Ljunggren AE. Pain I Older persons with severe dementia. Psychometric properties of the Mobilization-Observation-Behaviour-Intensity-Dementia (MOBID2) Pain Scale in a clinical setting. *Scandinavian Journal of Caring Science* 2010;24:380–391.

4. Scherder E, Herr K, Pickering G, Gibson S, Benedetti, F, Lautenbacher S. Pain in Dementia. *Pain* (2009).

5. Stolee P, Hillier LM, Esbaugh J, Bol N, McKellor, L, Gauthier N. Instruments for the assessment of pain in older persons with cognitive impairment. *J Am Geriatr Soc.* 2005;53:319–326.

6. Parmalee P, Smith B, Katz I. Pain complaints and cognitive status among elderly institution residents. *J Am Geriatr Soc.* 1993;50: 517–522.

7. Ferrell BA, Ferrell BR, Rivera L. Pain in cognitively impaired nursing home patients. *J Pain Symptom Manage.* 1995;10:591–598.

8. Brummel-Smith K, London M, Drew N, Krulewitch H, Singer C, Hanson L. Outcomes of pain in frail older adults with dementia. *J Am Geriatr Soc.* 2002;50:1847–1851.

9. Closs SJ, Barr B, Briggs M, Cash K, Seers K. A comparison of five pain assessment scales for nursing home residents with varying degrees of cognitive impairment. *J Pain Symptom Manage.* 2004;27(3):196–205.

10. Wynne C, Ling S, Remsburg, R. Comparison of pain assessment instruments in cognitively impaired nursing home residents. *Geriatr Nurs.* 2000;21(1):20–23.

11. Buffum MD, Hutt E, Chang V, Craine MH, Snow AL. Cognitive impairment and pain management—review of issues and challenges. *J Rehabil Res Dev.* 2007;44(2):315–330.

12. Kaasalainen, S. Pain assessment in older adults with dementia: using behavioural methods in clinical practice. *J Gerontol Nurs.* 2007;June:6–10.

13. Zwakhalen S, Hamers J, Abu-Saad H, Berger M. Pain in elderly people with severe dementia: a systematic review of behavioural pain assessment tools. *BMC Geriatr.* 2006;6(3). <http://www.biomedcentral.com/1471-2318/6/3>.

14. Manfredi P, Breuer B, Meier D, Liblow L. Pain assessment in elderly patients with dementia. *J Pain Symptom Manage.* 2003;25 (1):48–52.

15. Fuchs-Lacelle S, Hadjistavropoulos, T. Development and preliminary validation of the pain assessment checklist for seniors with limited ability to communicate (PACSLAC). *Pain Manag Nurs.* 2004;5(1):37–49.

16. Villanueva M, Smith T, Erickson J, Lee A, Singer C. Pain assessment for the dementing elderly (PADE): reliability and validity of a new measure. *J Am Dir Assoc.* 2003;4:1–8.

17. Buffum MD, Haberfelde M. Moving to new settings: pilot study of families perceptions of professional caregivers' pain management in persons with dementia. *J Rehabil Res Dev.* 2007;44(2):295–304.

18. Snow AL, Weber J, O'Malley K, et al. NOPPAIN: a nursing assistant administered pain assessment instrument for use in dementia. *Dementia Cognit Disord.* 2004;17:240–246.

19. Pautex S, Michon A, Guedira M, et al. Pain in severe dementia: self assessment or observational scales? *J Am Geriatr Soc.* 2006;54:1040–1045.

20. Leong I, Chang, M, Gibson S. The use of a self-reported pain measure, a nurse-reported pain measure and the PAINAD in nursing home residents with moderate and severe dementia: a validation study. *Age Ageing.* 2006;35:252–256.

21. Hadjistavropoulos T, La Chapelle D, Macleod F, Snider B, Craig K. Measuring movement exacerbated pain in cognitively impaired frail elders. *Clin J Pain.* 2000;16:54–63.

22. Alexander B, Plank P, Carlson M, Hanson P, Picken K, Schwebke, K. Methods of pain assessment in residents of long term care facilities: a pilot study. *J Med Dir Assoc.* 2005;6:137–143.

23. Abbey J, Piller N, De Bellis A, et al. The Abbey pain scale: a one minute indicator for people with end-stage dementia. *Int J Palliat Nurs.* 2004;10(1):6–13.

24. Hurley A, Volicer B, Hanrahan P, Houde S, Volicer I. Assessment of discomfort in advanced Alzheimer patients. *Res Nurs Health.* 1992;15:369–377.

25. Simons W, Malabar R. Assessing pain in elderly patients who cannot respond verbally. *J Adv Nurs.* 1995;22:663–669.

26. Herr K, Bjoro, K, Decker, S. Tools for assessment of pain in non-verbal older adults with dementia: a state-of-the-science review. *J Pain Symptom Manage.* 2006;31:170–192.

27. Liukas A, Kuusniemi K, Aantaa R, et al. Pharmacokinetics of intravenous paracetamol in elderly patients. *Clin Pharmacokinet.* 2011;50(2):121–129.

28. Bannwarth B, Pehourcq F, Lagrange F, et al. Single and multiple dose pharmacokinetics of acetaminophen (paracetamol) in polymedicated very old patients with rheumatic pain. *J Rheumatol.* 2001;28(1):182–184.

29. Mitchell SJ, Hilmer SN, Murnion BP, Matthews S. Hepatotoxicity of therapeutic short-course paracetamol in hospital inpatients: impact of ageing and frailty. *J Clin Pharm Ther.* 2011;36(3):327–335.

30. Wu M, Liu H, Fannin J, et al. Acetaminophen improves protein translational signaling in aged skeletal muscle. *Rejuvenation Res.* 2010;13(5):571–579.

31. Koppert W, Frötsch K, Huzurudin N, et al. The effects of paracetamol and parecoxib on kidney function in elderly patients undergoing orthopedic surgery. *Anesth Analg.* 2006;103(5):1170–1176.

32. Zullo A, Hassan C, Campo SMA, Morini S. Bleeding peptic ulcer in the elderly risk factors and prevention strategies. *Drugs Aging.* 2007;24(10):815–828.

33. Duran-Barrigan S, Russell AS. Use of nonsteroidal antinflammatory drugs and coxibs in the elderly: are we following the guidelines? *Clinical Rheumatol.* 2008;27:1081–1082.

34. Szekely CA, Breitner JC, Fitzpatrick AL, et al. NSAID use and dementia risk in the Cardiovascular Health Study: role of APOE and NSAID type. *Neurology.* 2008;70(1):5–6.

35. Muzzarelli S, Tobler D, Leibundgut G, et al. Detection of intake of nonsteroidal anti-inflammatory drugs in elderly patients with heart failure. How to ask the patient? *Swiss Med Wkly.* 2009;139(33–34):481–485.

36. Veering BT. Management of anaesthesia is elderly patients. *Curr Opin Anaesthesiol.* 1999;12:333–336.

37. Eisendrath SJ, Goldman B, Douglas J, Dimatteo L, Van Dyke C. Meperidine-induced delirium. *Am J Psychiatry.* 1987;144:1062–1065.

38. Fong HK, Sands LP, Leung JM. The role of postoperative analgesia in delirium and cognitive decline in elderly patients: a systematic review. *Anesth Analg.* 2006;102:1255–1266.

39. Adunsky A, Levy R, Heim M, Mizrahi E, Arad M. Meperidine analgesia and delirium in aged hip fracture patients. *Arch Gerontol Geriatr.* 2002;35(3):253–259.

40. Marcantonio ER, Juarez G, Goldman L. The relationship of postoperative delirium with psychoactive medications. *JAMA.* 1994;272(19):1518–1522.

41. Bugeja G, Kumar A, Bannerjee AJ. Exclusion of elderly people from clinical research: a descriptive study of published reports. *British Medical Journal.* 1997;315:1059.

42. Bayer A, Tadd, W. Unjustified exclusion of elderly people from studies submitted to research ethics committee for approval: a descriptive study. *British Medical Journal.* 2000;321:992–993.

43. Wheatley, RG, Madej, TH, Jackson IJB, Hunter D. The First year's experience of an acute pain service. *British Journal of Anaesthesia.* 1991;67:353–359.

44. Harari D, Hopper A, Dhesi J, Babic-Illman G, Lockwood L, Martin F. Proactive care of older people undergoing surgery ('POPS'): designing, embedding, evaluating and funding a comprehensive geriatric

assessment service for older elective surgical patients. *Age Ageing.* 2007;36:190–196.

45. Trappe TA, Carroll CC, Dickinson JM, *et al.* Influence of acetaminophen and ibuprofen on skeletal muscle adaptations to resistance exercise in older adults. *Am J Physiol Regul Integr Comp Physiol.* 2011;300(3):R655–R662.

46. Commentary on NCEPOD Report—An Age Old Problem 2010. *Daily Mail.* 10 November 2010.

47. Foss NB, Kristensen MT, Palm H, Kehlet H. Postoperative pain after hip fracture is procedure specific. *Br J Anaesth.* 2009;102:111–116.

48. Morrison RS, Magaziner J, McLaughlin MA, *et al.* The impact of post-operative pain on outcomes following hip fracture. *Pain.* 2003;103(3):303–311.

49. Morrison RS, Magaziner J, Gilbert M, *et al.* Relationship between pain and opioid analgesics on the development of delirium following hip fracture. *J Gerontol A Biol Sci Med Sci.* 2003;58(1):76–81.

50. Matot I, Oppenheim-Eden A, Ratrot R, *et al.* Preoperative cardiac events in elderly patients with hip fracture randomized to epidural or conventional analgesia. *Anesthesiology.* 2003;98(1):156–163.

51. Abou-Setta AM, Beaupre LA, Rashiq S, *et al.* Comparative effectiveness of pain management interventions for hip fracture: a systematic review. *Ann Intern Med.* 2011;155:234–245.

52. Tuncer S, Sert OA, Yosunkaya A, Mutlu M, Çelik J, Ökesli S. Patient-controlled femoral nerve analgesia versus patient-controlled intravenous analgesia for postoperative analgesia after trochanteric fracture repair. *Acute Pain.* 2003;4:105–108.

53. Haddad FS, Williams RL. Femoral nerve block in extracapsular femoral neck fractures. *J Bone Joint Surg (Br).* 1995;77B:922–923.

54. Murgue D, Ehret B, Massacrier-Imbert S, *et al.* Equimolar nitrous oxide/oxygen combined with femoral nerve block for emergency analgesia of femoral neck fractures. *Journal Européen des Urgences.* 2006;19:9–14.

55. Dodson ME. Modifications of general anaesthesia for the aged. In Davenport HT (ed) *Anaesthesia and the aged patient* (pp. 204–230). Oxford: Blackwell Scientific, 1988.

56. Gaglieze L, Melzack R. The assessment of pain in the elderly. In Mostofsky DI, Lomranz J (eds) *Handbook of pain and aging* (pp. 83–85). Plenum Series in Adult Development and Aging. New York: Plenum Press, 1997.

CHAPTER 27

Palliative care and the elderly

Shahla Siddiqui

Introduction

More people are living longer and the proportion of those living beyond 60 years has increased, and will continue to increase further until 2050. The very oldest people (e.g. those aged 85+) often experience multiple chronic diseases, and in developed countries, are often cared for in long-term care facilities such as nursing or residential homes. Palliative care patients are admitted increasingly to care homes if their prognosis is too prolonged for inpatient hospice care or acute palliative care beds. Although it is still a minority, a significant proportion of people die in these settings: ranging from 13 per cent in Austria, 20 per cent in England, to 39 per cent in Canada. When people move to a care home they frequently experience multiple losses: physical, mental, social, and spiritual. Although death may not necessarily be imminent, residents of care homes are highly likely to die there, making these settings where high-quality palliative care is needed.

Older people are often overlooked in the design of care provision, and yet they usually have the greatest and most complex needs. In this chapter we seek to understand and determine the needs of older people with progressive illnesses, and to assess interventional strategies to improve palliative care for this globally rapidly growing population. Palliative (from Latin *palliare*, to cloak) care, is a specialized area of healthcare that focuses on relieving and preventing the suffering of patients. Palliative medicine utilizes a multidisciplinary approach to patient care, relying on input from physicians, pharmacists, nurses, chaplains, social workers, psychologists, and other allied health professionals in formulating a plan of care to relieve suffering in all areas of a patient's life. This multidisciplinary approach allows the palliative care team to address physical, emotional, spiritual, and social concerns that arise with advanced illness.

Medications and treatments are said to have a palliative effect if they relieve symptoms without having a curative effect on the underlying disease or cause. This can include treating nausea related to chemotherapy or something as simple as morphine to treat a broken leg. Although the concept of palliative care is not new, most physicians have traditionally concentrated on trying to cure patients. Treatments for the alleviation of symptoms were viewed as hazardous and seen as inviting addiction and other unwanted side effects. The focus on a patient's quality of life has increased greatly during the past 20 years. In the United States today, 55 per cent of hospitals with more than 100 beds offer a palliative care programme, and nearly one-fifth of community hospitals have palliative care programmes. A relatively recent development is the concept of a dedicated healthcare team that is entirely geared toward palliative treatment: a palliative care team.

In a nutshell, palliative care is appropriate and possible regardless of which disease process a person has, what the prognosis is, or what cure-directed treatment choices a person makes. Palliative care should be interwoven concurrently with cure-directed treatment. It can either be used with treatment intended to cure or as the sole form of treatment. Palliative care (regardless of other treatment plans being used) optimizes quality of life and when your energies are not spent coping with pain, nausea, breathlessness, fatigue, and the immobility (among other things) resulting from this, there is more energy to cope with the manifestations of the disease. When a person is comfortable, they eat more, sleep better, are not as fatigued, not as depressed and at least have the possibility of enjoying their day. Jerant and colleagues,[1] in 'The TLC Model of Palliative Care in the Elderly: Preliminary Application in the Assisted Living Setting' published in the *Annals of Family Medicine*, describe five barriers to palliative care with the elderly who live in assisted living facilities. Basically, the five barriers to palliative care for them are: the perception that palliative care is only terminal care; palliative care is defined as mutually exclusive of cure-directed treatment; the decision, if palliative care should be the sole form of care, is not '...negotiated among patients, family members, and providers...'; making treatment choices is given more importance than discussing the reality of life with a chronic debilitating illness; and palliative care is treated as an either/or decision instead of an integrated part of the treatment plan.

Presently, palliative care in the elderly relies on three principles:

1. Fostering dignity for older people at the end of life

A study exploring the views on maintaining dignity of older people in care homes has broadly supported a model of dignity at the end of life developed for people with advanced cancer and canvassed their views and highlighted a number of challenges to conducting research in care homes for older people;[2] 'People respond to the way you treat them...dignity is a two-way thing'.

2. The effectiveness of interventions to improve palliative care for older people

There is a need to develop and evaluate more ways to improve palliative care for older people. There are several such initiatives currently underway around the world. *Better Palliative Care for Older People*[3] is an example of such a publication which expresses a European viewpoint but may reflect relevant issues in other parts of the world. It targets policy- and decision-makers within government health and social care, the non-governmental, academic, and private sectors, and health professionals working with older people. All these groups will need to work to integrate palliative care more widely across health services, and policy-makers need to be aware of the proven benefits of palliative care in the elderly. The booklet aims to provide information that will help this task.

3. Symptom burden and quality of life for older people in care homes and intensive care units (ICUs)

Although it is assumed that the symptom burden on older people in care homes and ICUs in high, there is relatively little good quality research on their symptoms, in particular psychological and spiritual problems, and their quality of life. The suitability of many standardized measures for older people in such places is not known.

Definitions
Palliative care

The World Health Organization's (WHO) definition is 'an approach that improves the quality of life of patients and their families facing the problem associated with life-threatening illness, through the prevention and relief of suffering by means of early identification and impeccable assessment and treatment of pain and other physical, psychosocial, and spiritual problems'.[4]

Palliative care provides relief from pain and other distressing symptoms, affirms life and regards dying as a normal process, intends neither to hasten nor postpone death, integrates the psychological and spiritual aspects of patient care, offers a support system to help patients live as actively as possible until death, offers a support system to help the family cope during the patient's illness and in their own bereavement, uses a team approach to address the needs of patients and their families, including bereavement counselling, if indicated, will enhance quality of life, and may also positively influence the course of illness.

It is applicable early in the course of illness, in conjunction with other therapies that are intended to prolong life, such as chemotherapy or radiation therapy, and includes those investigations needed to better understand and manage distressing clinical complications.

Geriatric palliative care

'The approach to care for the chronically ill and frail elderly.' The focus is on quality of life, support for functional independence, and centrality of the patient's values and experiences in determining the goals of medical care.[5] Geriatric palliative care is integrative using interdisciplinary delivery of care. The goal is to relieve pain and suffering and to improve the quality of life for elderly patients and their families. The core principles are a comprehensive, patient/family unit-centred approach that enhances functional independence and quality of life transitioning between levels of care.[5]

Symptom management

'Recognition and treatment of physical and nonphysical symptoms to prevent suffering and improve quality of life.'[6]

Goal of palliative care

The goal of palliative care is 'to prevent and relieve suffering and to support the best possible quality of life for patients and their families regardless of the stage of disease'.[7]

Background of geriatric palliative care

Although people over the age of 80 years have fewer interventions for symptom management they are more likely to suffer and die from chronic illnesses preceded by a lengthy period of decline and functional impairment.[8] Older persons are at higher risk for developing multiple chronic, life-threatening diseases (cancer, stroke, heart disease, respiratory diseases). Alzheimer's disease is the 14th leading cause of death in older adults;[9] yet 80 per cent of Medicare patients enrolled in hospice have cancer. Only 3 per cent have chronic obstructive pulmonary disease (COPD) and less than 3 per cent of nation's hospice census is made up of Alzheimer's patients.[10] Patients over 80 referred for palliative care consultation have fewer interventions for pain, nausea, anxiety, and other symptoms.[8] Persons 65 years and over often have undertreated or untreated pain and other symptoms.

Markers for initiation of palliative care in geriatrics

1. *Core end-stage indicators* indicating terminal phase of chronic illness are physical decline, weight loss, multiple comorbidities, and a serum albumin of <2.5 g/dl. Dependence on assistance with most activities of daily living (ADLs) and a Karnofsky Performance score of less than 50 per cent.[9,11] The Karnofsky Performance Scale Index allows patients to be classified as to their functional impairment from 0–100. This can be used to compare effectiveness of different therapies and to assess the prognosis in individual patients. The lower the Karnofsky score, the worse the survival for most serious illnesses.

2. *Non-disease specific indicators* such as:

   Frailty—extreme vulnerability to morbidity and mortality due to progressive decline in function and physiological reserve. Frequent falls, disability, susceptibility to acute illness, and reduced ability to recover are examples of frailty.

   Functional dependence—dependence on others to perform activities of daily life.

   Cognitive impairment—changes in memory, attention, thinking, language, praxis, and executive function.

   Family support needs—emotional support, information and educational support unique to each patient/family and/or caregivers.

3. *Disease-specific markers*: include symptomatic congestive heart failure (CHF), dementia, stroke, cancer, recurrent infections, and degenerative joint disease causing functional impairment and chronic pain.

Needs of the geriatric palliative care patient

For patients with active, progressive, far-advanced disease, the goals of palliative care are to provide relief from pain and other physical symptoms, to maximize the quality of life, to provide psychosocial and spiritual care, and to provide support to help the family during the patient's illness and bereavement.

Their specific needs are: continuity and coordination of care that responds to episodic and long-term chronic illnesses and transitioning between levels of care, management of multiple chronic illnesses, and assistance in navigating a complex medical system. Other needs include maintaining functional independence, decision-making regarding care and treatment decisions, pain and symptom control, determining risk versus benefit of treatment, home support for family caregivers, and the need for community resource information and access assistance.

Principles of palliative care

Palliative care incorporates the whole spectrum of care—medical, nursing, psychological, social, cultural, and spiritual. A holistic approach, incorporating these wider aspects of care, is good medical practice and in palliative care it is essential. The principles of palliative care might simply be regarded as those of good medical practice such as the following:

A caring attitude that involves sensitivity, empathy and compassion, and demonstrates concern for the individual, and ensures that there is concern for all aspects of a patient's suffering, not just the medical problems. There is a non-judgemental approach in which personality, intellect, ethnic origin, religious belief, or any other individual factors do not prejudice the delivery of optimal care.

The consideration of individuality; the practice of categorizing patients by their underlying disease, based on the similarity of the medical problems encountered, fails to recognize the psychosocial features and problems that make every patient a unique individual. These unique characteristics can greatly influence suffering and need to be taken into account when planning the palliative care for individual patients.

Cultural considerations including ethnic, racial, religious, and other cultural factors may have a profound effect on a patient's suffering. Cultural differences are to be respected and treatment planned in a culturally sensitive manner. The consent of a patient, or those to whom the responsibility is delegated, is necessary before any treatment is given or withdrawn. It is mostly the case that the majority of patients want shared decision-making although physicians tend to underestimate this, therefore having assessed what treatment is appropriate or inappropriate, this needs to be discussed with the patient. In most instances, adequately informed patients will accept the recommendations made.

The choice of site of care is also important. The patient and family need to be included in any discussion about the site of care. Patients with a terminal illness should be managed at home whenever possible.

Good communication between all the healthcare professionals involved in a patient's care is essential and is fundamental to many aspects of palliative care. Good communication with patients and families is also essential.

The clinical context and appropriate treatment is also very important. All palliative treatment should be appropriate to the stage of the patient's disease and the prognosis. Over-enthusiastic therapy that is inappropriate and patient neglect are equally deplorable. Palliative care has been accused of the 'medicalization' of death, and care must be taken to balance technical interventions

with a humanistic orientation to dying patients. The prescription of appropriate treatment is particularly important in palliative care because of the unnecessary additional suffering that may be caused by inappropriately active therapy or by lack of treatment. When palliative care includes active therapy for the underlying disease, limits should be observed, appropriate to the patient's condition and prognosis. The treatment known to be futile, given because 'you have to do something', is unethical and where only symptomatic and supportive palliative measures are employed, all efforts are directed at the relief of suffering and the quality of life, and not necessarily at the prolongation of life. The provision of total or comprehensive inter-professional care for all aspects of a patient's suffering requires an interdisciplinary team. Palliative care should deliver the best possible medical, nursing, and allied healthcare that is available and appropriate.

Consistent medical management requires that an overall plan of care be established, and regularly reviewed, for each patient as this will reduce the likelihood of sudden or unexpected alterations, which can be distressing for the patient and family. Coordinated care involves the effective organization of the work of the members of the interprofessional team, to provide maximal support and care to the patient and family. Planning meetings, to which all members of the team can contribute, and at which the views of the patient and the family are presented, are used to develop a plan of care for each individual patient. The provision of continuous symptomatic and supportive care from the time the patient is first referred until death is basic to the aims of palliative care. Problems most frequently arise when patients are moved from one place of care to another and ensuring continuity of all aspects of care is most important. Good palliative care involves careful planning to prevent the physical and emotional crises that occur with progressive disease. Many of the clinical problems can be anticipated and some can be prevented by appropriate management and the patients and their families should be forewarned of likely problems, and contingency plans made to minimize physical and emotional distress. The relatives of patients with advanced disease are subject to considerable emotional and physical distress, especially if the patient is being managed at home and particular attention must be paid to their needs as the success or failure of palliative care may depend on the caregivers' ability to cope. Continued reassessment is a necessity for all patients with advanced disease for whom increasing and new clinical problems are to be expected and this applies as much to psychosocial issues as it does to pain and other physical symptoms.

Advance care planning

The principle of advance care planning is not new; it is common for patients aware of approaching death to discuss with their carers how they wish to be treated, however, these wishes have not always been respected, especially if the patient is urgently taken to hospital and if there is disagreement amongst family members about what is appropriate treatment.[11]

Criteria for hospice eligibility for persons with dementia

It is important for medical providers to be familiar with the criteria for hospice eligibility. Hospice is often under-utilized in end-stage dementia and often times not utilized until the last days or weeks of life. In fact, less than 3 per cent of the nation's hospice census comprises patients with Alzheimer's dementia (the most prevalent form of dementia), according to the Virginia-based National Hospice and Palliative Care Organization (NHPCO).[13]

General assessment and interventions in symptom management

Symptom management in palliative care

Research indicates that people near the end of life, those who are frail, and those who have multiple chronic symptoms suffer symptoms of distress.[6–8] Research also indicates that ageing persons are often undertreated if treated at all for distressing symptoms. Clearly, assessment and management of distressing symptoms is paramount for quality of life in ageing persons.

There is useful information available on the Internet to help with the assessment of these patients, usually with intervention strategies provided, these include the Edmonton Symptom Assessment Scale,[14] the Palliative Performance Scale,[15,] and the Karnofsky Performance Scale.[11]

The following are common symptoms in geriatric palliative care: dyspnoea, depression, fatigue, gastrointestinal symptoms: constipation, anorexia, dysphagia, and pain.

Dyspnoea

Dyspnoea is a subjective experience described as an uncomfortable awareness of breathing, breathlessness, or severe shortness of breath.[17] It is one of the most common symptoms experienced by patients with all types of advanced lung disease, including cancer, interstitial lung disease, and particularly COPD. Dyspnoea is more common, and often more severe in the last few weeks before death.[4] Dyspnoea, like pain, is a multidimensional experience with multiple layers of meaning: physiological, emotional, cognitive, behavioural dimensions. It is more prevalent in ageing persons and does not only occur only in the end stages of life. Research indicates dyspnoea is inadequately assessed at the end of life.[16] Dyspnoea is a *highly prevalent* symptom in older adults and increases with age regardless of the type of illness or community in which they live.[18]

The potential causes of dyspnoea are many[5] and include the following:

♦ Debilitating conditions associated with ageing such as anaemia, atelectasis, pulmonary embolism, pneumonia, emphysema, cachexia-anorexia syndrome, or weakness (asthenia).

♦ Those concurrent diseases often associated with increased age: COPD, asthma, CHF, acidosis, angina, respiratory infection, cancer complications, pleural effusions, bronchial obstruction, metastasis, superior vena cava syndrome, tumour replacing normal lung tissue, lymphangitis carcinomatosis, mediastinal obstruction, pericardial effusion, massive ascites, or abdominal distention.

♦ They may be complications of treatment for a primary disease such as CHF secondary to chemotherapy or constrictive pericarditis related to radiation therapy, radiation induced fibrosis, or anaemia secondary to chemotherapy,

♦ Finally they may be due to psychological disorders: anxiety, depression, panic disorders.[19]

Assessment of dyspnoea

Assessment should start with using the patient's descriptor of how they are feeling, e.g. breathlessness, need to gasp or pant, unable to get enough air, feeling like suffocating,[5,6] and asking the following questions: when was the onset (in days, weeks, hours)? Is it acute or more chronic, what makes it better or worse, what does it feel like? Do other symptoms occurr with it: pain, chest tightness, palpitations, cough, fever, lightheadedness? How severe is it (using a scale such as a visual or verbal analogue scale)? How much does it interfere with daily life and function? When is it at its worst? Is it always present or does it come and go? Are there any temporal factors (night or daytime)?

If the patient is unable to answer ask a caregiver their observations for these questions. Review their the past history for potential underlying causes of dyspnoea, e.g. COPD, CHF, renal failure, or lung cancer[6] and review their list of medications. On physical examination note the general appearance including their mental status (is it different than normal?). Can the patient speak a complete sentence without stopping? Count the respiratory rate accurately, note use of accessory muscles or not, examine the skin, cardiac system (is there an S_3 or murmur?), respiratory status (are breath sound decreased, crackles or rhonchi/is wheezing present?) and look for signs of infection or dehydration. Look at the oxygen saturation whilst resting and after walking (if able).

Management of the symptoms of dyspnoea

It is often helpful to reduce the need for exertion by arranging for readily available help (e.g. access to call light, caregiver at bedside), reposition, usually more upright position or with the compromised lung down. Improve air circulation: provide draft-fans, open windows. Adjust the humidity with humidifier or air conditioner. Identify and address situational components that trigger dyspnoea. Address anxiety (consider anti-anxiety agent) and provide reassurance. Discuss the meaning of symptoms and other patient and family concerns. Discuss family concerns about use of opioids to relieve dyspnoea and most importantly provide oxygen if there is a likelihood of mild hypoxia as many patients will feel better with a saturation of over 90 per cent.

It is important to offer a Foley catheter if there is dyspnoea with voiding or patient is on diuretics for dyspnoea. Pursed lip breathing is an ominous sign pathognomonic of CHF. Complementary therapies include: imagery, massage, breathing exercises, therapeutic touch, music, aromatherapy, relaxation exercises.

Specific causes and treatment

BREATH AIR is a useful mnemonic:[19]

B: Bronchospasm—where appropriate treat with corticosteroids, bronchodilators, nebulized or inhaler delivered salbutamol, and/or oral steroids for COPD, asthma. If CHF is present a review of their medications, i.e. digoxin, antiarrhythmics, nitrates, dobutamine, antitussives, to help with cough would be warranted.

R: Rales—if volume overload is present, reduce artificial feeding or stop intravenous fluid, diuretics such as frusemide, are occasionally needed. If pneumonia is present, decide whether antibiotics will be effective or simply prolong the dying process. Patient and family participation in this process is essential.

E: Effusions—thoracentesis is effective and if the effusion reoccurs and patient is ambulatory, chest tube pleurodesis or placing an indwelling drainage catheter may be beneficial, paracentesis for severe ascites is also effective. If the patient is close to death then palliation with opioids and benzodiazepines may be more appropriate.

A: Airway obstruction—make sure that tracheostomy appliances are cleaned regularly. If aspirating food use pureed and thickened liquids. Instruct family on positioning patient during feeding and suctioning if necessary.

T: Thick secretions—if the cough reflex is still strong the use of nebulized saline and expectorants as needed may work. If the cough is weak and ineffective, drying the secretions with hyoscyamine, or transdermal scopolamine or glycopyrrolate is useful

H: Haemoglobin—a blood transfusion may improve energy and reduce dyspnoea for a few weeks. Erythropoietin should be considered for patients who are likely to improve to a higher level of function. Haemorrhage or marrow failure may be part of the dying process and is best palliated with opioids, benzodiazepines, and other symptomatic treatments.

A: Anxiety—treat initially with a short-acting opioid, such as morphine, if that is less effective a trial of a short-acting benzodiazepine may be needed, for instance, lorazepam. If there is a tremor, reducing the dose of theophylline or adrenergic agents may help. If the patient is already being treated with an opioid, increase the dose by 25–50 per cent. If the dose is limited by drowsiness, reduce the benzodiazepine intake and increase the opioid. Antidepressants for anxiety related to depression may be beneficial

I: Interpersonal issues—there may be social and financial problems which contribute to dyspnoea. Counselling with social workers and other members of the interdisciplinary team may bring relief. When family relationships exacerbate the problem, a few days in an inpatient unit as respite from family may help to relieve the patient symptoms.

R: Religious concerns—some beliefs, such as 'God is punishing me' or 'God will heal me if I have enough faith' can precipitate or exacerbate symptoms. Taking time to listen may help and can offer other ways for the patient to explore to reconnect with God, higher being, self, others. Ensure that there is coordination between the various people offering spiritual advice, be they chaplains, counsellors, or other healthcare professionals and family members.

Patient and family education and follow-up

Leave clear instructions for the family and patient on non-pharmacological interventions and on possible signs and symptoms of exacerbations. Discuss how to prioritize activities whilst minimizing unnecessary activities. Maximize the usefulness of medications as far as possible and do not leave patients in distress alone. They should be able to monitor their self-care activities and know when and how to seek additional assistance.

Depression in palliative care

The overlap of physical illness symptoms with signs and symptoms of depression often affects the reliability of diagnosis. The incidence of depression increases with higher levels of disability, advanced illness and pain.[5] Persistent feelings of helplessness, hopelessness, inadequacy, depression, and suicidal ideation are not normal at the end of life or in ageing and should be aggressively evaluated and treated.[5]

Amongst hospitalized geriatric patients, 10–20 per cent suffer from major depression, and 30 per cent from minor degrees of depression. In elderly communities depression coexists about 10–20 per cent in Alzheimer's patients, 33 per cent with other forms of dementia, and 36 per cent in rehabilitation facilities.

In nursing homes 60 per cent of residents suffer from depression, especially those with cancer. Among patients with cancer and the terminally ill, 20–25 per cent of patients suffer from depression. Palliative care patients have a higher risk of developing depression because of their chronically deteriorating health, made worse with a recent diagnosis of a life threatening illness. The presence of chronic or life threatening illness may certainly cause increased dependence, helplessness, uncertainty, and a negative self-critical view.[17]

Assess for depression risk factors

Factors such as uncontrolled pain, multiple comorbid issues and associated deficits—inability to walk, loss of bowel and bladder control, amputation, inability to eat or swallow, sensory loss, exhaustion—can all cause depression.[19] Patients with a serious medical comorbidity such as cancer are at the highest risk, especially those that are diagnosed with oral, pharyngeal, or lung cancer. Other factors indicative of likely depression include recent family conflicts or a loss of significant relationship; prior episodes of depression or a suicide attempt; lack of social support and feelings of being a burden to family.

Assessment and screening tools for depression are available. Examples include the EPERC Fast Fact,[20] or the Geriatric Depression Scale.[21]

Fatigue

Fatigue is an overwhelming, sustained sense of exhaustion and decreased capacity for physical or emotional work.[22] It is often described by the patients as feeling worn out, exhausted, sleepiness, tired, of low energy and by care providers as being lethargic or suffering from malaise.[5] There has been no consensus on the definition of fatigue in palliative care; however the following criteria were delineated by Dean and Anderson:[23] it is a subjective perception with alteration in neuromuscular and metabolic processes and a decrease in physical performance with deterioration in mental and physical activities.

Fatigue is often erroneously seen as inevitable and as a normal consequence of ageing by patients and care providers alike. It is often reported to medical providers because of this belief. It occurs in diseases that commonly afflict the older adult, such as cardiac failure or coronary disease. It is often difficult to ascertain whether the fatigue is due to the treatment or the chronic disease processes such as CHF or depression themselves. Many causes of fatigue can be treated and improve quality of life by teaching coping mechanisms and lifestyle changes.

Gastrointestinal symptoms

Constipation is common in those requiring palliative care and increases in prevalence with advancing years. Sixty-three per cent of the elderly in hospitals suffer from it as compared to 22 per cent of the elderly in the home as well as 95 per cent of people taking opioids.

Causes

Cancer-related causes may be directly related to the tumour site: bowel cancers, secondary bowel cancers, pelvic cancers. There may be hypercalcaemia, and surgical interruption of bowel integrity, inactivity, weakness and/or inability to reach toilet, poor nutrition, and dehydration related to nausea and vomiting, polyuria, or fever are all likely causes. Hypocalcaemia causes decreased absorption leading to constipation. Concurrent diseases such as diabetes, hypothyroidism, hypokalaemia, diverticular disease, haemorrhoids, colitis, or chronic neurological diseases are all causes of constipation. Medication with opioids, anticholinergic effects, tricyclic antidepressants, antiparkinson medications, antihypertensives, antihistamines, antacids, diuretics, the vinca alkaloids, NSAIDs, or anticholinergics are also likely to precipitate constipation.

Non-pharmacological interventions for constipation include increasing dietary fibre, improving mobility as much as tolerated, encouraging fluids and eliminating constipating drugs as feasible.[24] Many studies do not recommend one specific treatment over another. Combinations of stimulant and softening laxatives have shown fewer adverse effects.

Anorexia/cachexia

A loss of appetite is common in the end stages of illness. However, it needs to be differentiated from potential reversible causes such as medication-induced constipation. Reversible causes should be evaluated in ageing people before adding more medication. Anorexia accompanies physical deterioration and frequently causes significant concern in patients and families.[5] It also contributes to the cachexia syndrome (which is not due to inadequate food intake—see following sections). Weight loss often ensues before anorexia and the only treatment is to reverse the underlying cause where possible. Potential reversible causes include poor oral hygiene, mucositis or other oral problems, nausea, medications, dysphagia where treatment is beneficial and desired, depression and/or anxiety. It may simply be that the dietary choices available are not what the patient desires or likes.

Dysphagia

Dysphagia affected 12 per cent in one study of 800 palliative care patients[24] and 30 per cent of these were not confirmed by assessment to have a direct physical cause and it was attributed to possible anxiety and poor appetite. A dry mouth or inadequate chewing in edentulous patients can also cause dysphagia when no obstruction or neuro deficit exists.[5]

Oral health

Mouth problems left untreated can lead to further problems, including difficulties with nutritional intake, infections, pain, and in communicating. These problems may also include a dry mouth, infections, or mucositis (due to chemotherapy).

Pain

Pain is the most distressing and feared symptom near the end of life.[5] Older people tend to underreport pain and are often undertreated for pain.[8] In addition, ageing patients often have complications from treatment; however, pain can be relieved in the elderly if managed appropriately. Medical personnel have a moral obligation to provide effective pain relief and prevent unnecessary suffering, particularly in those at the end of life.[25]

Models of care

There is no one right or wrong model for the provision of palliative care. The best model is determined by local needs and resources, in consultation with the local healthcare providers and authorities. It is important to differentiate between palliative care principles, which apply to all care, whatever the disease suffered by a patient, palliative techniques or therapies which include medical and surgical therapies (e.g. stenting, paracentesis, internal fixation of fractures and radiotherapy) that are employed to palliate symptoms and ease suffering but are only a small part of the spectrum of care known as palliative care, and specialist palliative care which in some countries is delivered in units operated exclusively for palliative care by doctors and nurses who are accredited specialists in palliative care. Whether such specialization is important or essential is something that can only be debated in the context of national needs and resources.

Palliative care services operate in one or more of the following ways, reflecting local practice and needs, but there is no 'right' or 'wrong' type of service.

Inpatient beds

An inpatient palliative care unit may be part of an acute hospital or be an independent free-standing unit. A hospital unit may be either a special ward within the hospital or a separate unit built in the hospital grounds or may be physically separate from the hospital, but still be able to access its staff and services. Patients may be admitted for symptom management (physical or psychosocial), terminal care, short duration rehabilitation/convalescence as well as to provide a period of respite for family carers. In the UK, most units have few beds (6–30), an average length of stay of 2 weeks or less, and a discharge rate of 40–60 per cent. These figures vary greatly around the world and depend on local needs and resources, the relationship to other services.

Community services

There are various models for community-based palliative care services providing specialist advice and support for the family doctors and community nurses managing the patients. There are also services providing 'hands-on' nursing and allied health services to patients at home, in cooperation with the patient's own doctor and comprehensive services providing medical, nursing and allied healthcare to patients and their families at home. In view of their dependence on care home staff for most aspects of their lives, it is not surprising that the perceptions of attitudes of care home staff impacts on residents' sense of dignity. Care tenor is linked to other dignity themes, for example, attitudes that foster dignity are reflected when care home staff encourage independence, respect privacy, provide social support and care in such a way that residents maintain a sense of pride and do not feel that they are a burden.

Day units

These are known as day care, day hospice, day palliative care units and usually form part of a hospital or inpatient palliative care unit. They provide care, rehabilitation, support, and respite during the day for people under care at home, who are still well enough to be transported to and from the day care unit, often by volunteer transport.

Hospital palliative care teams

These operate in general and specialist hospitals and are staffed by doctors and palliative care nurses. Some also have a social worker or a pastoral care specialist to provide consultative advice on patients referred to them in any department of the hospital. They advise on every aspect of palliation, provide support for family members, and provide support and education for the staff. They also facilitate the provision of high-quality palliative care in all wards where the patient is familiar with the staff and surroundings without the need to be transferred to another unit; they also help educate the ward staff about matters pertaining to palliative care.

Communication with patients

Important and potentially difficult discussions are frequently necessary with palliative care patients who have active, progressive, far-advanced disease, regarding breaking of bad news, further treatment of the underlying disease, communicating prognoses, planning admission to a palliative care programme, artificial nutrition, artificial hydration, medications such as antibiotics and 'do not attempt resuscitate' (DNAR) orders. Decisions must be individualized for each patient and should be made in discussion with the patient and family.

Important questions to discuss are:

◆ Would you be surprised if this patient died of their disease within 6 months?

This may provide a better guide for decision-making, as attempting to prognosticate may be difficult and inaccurate. Alternatively, assess how much the patient's condition has deteriorated in the last month or 6 weeks, using observations by the team and objective measures such as X-rays and biochemistry.

◆ What specific therapies are available to treat the underlying disease?

Where known information on the percentage chances of significant clinical improvement and does that take into account the patient's age and any other diseases/comorbidities? Is it known how long would the improvement last, is it likely to be days, weeks or months. What are the percentage chances of serious adverse effects and on balance, do the potential benefits outweigh the potential burdens?

About the patient and family

What is their understanding of the state of the disease and the prognosis? Do they understand the goal of any treatments to be discussed, i.e. palliative, not curative and do they understand the potential benefits and burdens of the treatment options? What are their expectations and what do you think their preferences are?

An appropriate setting should be chosen for these discussions and they should be held in person and not by telephone, except when face-to-face meetings are not possible for geographic reasons. Privacy and uninterrupted time must be ensured, preferably sitting down face to face with the relatives or the patient/resident. Enough time should be given for the discussion and appropriate (non-technical) language should be used, with an interpreter if necessary. It is important to get a feeling of what they understand and expect. Direct but open questioning is best, for example: 'Tell me what you understand about your illness at the moment', 'Tell me what you see happening with this illness in the future', and 'Tell me what things are important for you'. Provide medical information, if necessary in a caring and sympathetic way, not abruptly or bluntly. Make it clear what treatments can be offered and the possible benefits and adverse effects of any treatments offered.

Discuss realistic possibilities in the context of their view of the present and future

Most research indicates that people prefer informed choices and decision-making rather than being incorrectly reassured. Discussing further active treatment for the underlying disease is important with a truthful discussion of what therapy is or is not available and the benefits and burdens of any therapies. Do *not* say 'there is nothing more that can be done' as patients interpret this to mean no treatment for anything. It is rarely true and patients and families will feel abandoned. Patients may be told there is no further therapy for the underlying disease, but the provision of continuing care and symptom control should be stressed. If further active therapy for the underlying disease is not appropriate, the positive aspects of symptomatic and supportive palliative care should be emphasized.

Discussing prognoses

The uncertainty in estimating an individual patient's prognosis needs to be explained and precise prognostication avoided. It is recommended to give a realistic time range, provide realistic hope—helping them to achieve what is important for them, recommend that family relationships and worldly affairs be attended to, be prepared to answer questions about the process of dying, provide on-going support and counselling and provide reassurance about continuity of care.

Discussing appropriate medical care

Issues related to the appropriateness of artificial hydration and nutrition, antibiotics, and other medications are important and need clarification. It is advisable to explain the possible benefits and burdens (or futility) of any intervention.

Discussing 'do not attempt resuscitate' orders

Experts recommend introducing the discussion in the context of the patient's view of their future. If necessary, futility of cardiopulmonary resuscitation (CPR) (chances of surviving to discharge), indignity of CPR, and being on a respirator in ICU and unable to communicate must be discussed. Of course it is essential to respond sympathetically to emotional reactions and reassure the patient that all other medical care will continue. If a patient clearly understands that they are dying and that the only care that they will receive is directed to their comfort, it may not be necessary to discuss DNAR orders. If this is the case, it must be recorded in case-notes.

Agree on a plan, with provision that it can be modified if circumstances change. *Remember, death is the natural end to life and is not a failure of medicine.*

Advance care planning

Advance care planning is a means for patients to record their end-of-life values and preferences, including their wishes regarding future treatments (or avoidance of them). Advance care planning involves a number of processes; including informing the patient, eliciting preferences, and identifying a surrogate decision maker—to act if the patient is no longer able to make decisions about their own care.

The principle of advance care planning is not new. It is common for patients aware of approaching death to discuss with their carers how they wish to be treated; however, these wishes have not always been respected, especially if the patient is urgently taken to hospital or if there is disagreement amongst family members about what is appropriate treatment.

The 'Respecting Choices' programme developed in Wisconsin is an example of advance care planning and employs trained personnel to facilitate the discussions and record the outcomes, which are in writing and signed, and kept in the front of the patient's file. The surrogate decision-maker is involved in the discussions so that they have explicit knowledge of the patient's wishes; otherwise they may feel burdened by the responsibility and there is less conflict between patients and their families if advance care planning has been discussed.[12]

Conclusion

A multicomponent palliative care service aims to improve the quality of life for people reaching the end of their life by providing relief from their pain and other distressing symptoms. They also help patients' families cope with the illness and bereavement. Substantial shortfalls in the quality of palliative care of the elderly can be attributed to five fundamental flaws in the way end-of-life care is currently delivered. Firstly, palliative care is viewed as a terminal event rather than a longitudinal process, resulting in a reactive approach and unnecessary pre-terminal distress in elderly patients suffering from chronic, slowly progressive illnesses. Secondly, palliative care is defined in terms of a false dichotomy between symptomatic and disease-focused treatment, which distracts attention from the proper focus on healing illness. Thirdly, the decision about whether the focus of care should be palliative is not negotiated among patients, family members, and providers. Fourthly, patient autonomy in making treatment choices is accorded undue prominence relative to more salient patient choices, such as coming to terms with their place in the trajectory of chronic illness. Finally, palliative care remains a parallel system rather than an integrated primary and secondary care process.

Palliative care is appropriate and possible regardless of which disease process a person has, what the prognosis is or what cure directed treatment choices a person makes. Palliative care should be interwoven concurrently with cure directed treatment. It can either be used with treatment intended to cure or as the sole form of treatment.

Palliative care (regardless of other treatment plans being used) optimizes the quality of life and when patients are not having to cope with pain, nausea, breathlessness, fatigue and the immobility (among other things) resulting from this, they are more able to cope with the manifestations of the disease. When a person is comfortable, they eat more, sleep better, are not as fatigued, not as depressed and at least have the possibility of enjoying their day. Delivering palliative care to elderly, dying patients is a present and future challenge. In Germany, this has been underlined by legislation in 2009 implementing palliative care as compulsory in the medical curriculum. While the number of elderly patients is increasing in many Western countries, multiple morbidities, dementia, and frailty complicate care. Teaching palliative care of the elderly to an interprofessional group of medical and nursing students can help to provide better care as acknowledged by the ministry of health

and its expert panels. Patient and family input, 24/7 access to key members of the team, and physician, social worker, and nurse collaboration in care plan development and review are hallmarks of interdisciplinary involvement in palliative care. Several such models exist globally; however, it is important not to let the patient or their family feel abandoned by the primary care team once palliative care is initiated.

A palliative care plan includes the periodic assessment, review and revision with regard to functionality (including ADL self-care and medication/treatment administration), falls risk, emotional and mental status, follow-up after hospitalization and new diagnoses, goals of care and realistic outcomes, arrangements for necessary interventions, staff education to implement the plan of care, and management of episodic instability or exacerbation.

There are multiple barriers to palliative care. Many patients with advanced disease do not receive palliative care because some are referred too late in the course of their disease to benefit from treatment. The reasons for this may relate to the physician, the patient, or to social factors. Physician factors include late referral due to prognostication or lack of communication skills for end of life issues, a reluctance to refer; or lack of understanding or belief in palliative care due to loss of control or financial loss; or lack of institutional standards for end of life. Patient factors include disbelieving their poor prognosis, unrealistic expectations of disease response, patient—family disagreement about treatment options and lack of advanced care planning. Social factors include ethnic minorities with language barriers, rural communities and groups that are poor or underprivileged which precludes them from access to costly treatment and medication. At present there may be no government subsidies for healthcare such as in developing countries, or major limitations in funding in even the most affluent countries.

Palliative care should be available to all as the most humane delivery of medical care.

References

1. Jerant AF, Azari RS, Nesbitt TS, Meyers FJ. The TLC model of palliative care in the elderly: preliminary application in the assisted living setting. *Ann Fam Med.* 2004;2(1):54–60.
2. Henwood M. *Community Care and Elderly People.* London: Family Policy Studies Centre, 1990.
3. Davies E, Higginson I. *Better palliative care for older people.* Geneva: World Health Organization, 2004.
4. World Health Organization (WHO). *Definition of palliative care.* 2005. <http://www.who.int/cancer/palliative/definition/en/>.
5. Morrison RS, Meier DE (eds). *Geriatric palliative care.* New York: Oxford University Press, 2003.
6. Kazanowski MK. Symptoms management in palliative care. In Mazo ML, Sherman DW (eds) *Palliative care nursing: quality care to the end of life* (pp. 327–361). New York: Springer Publishing Company, 2003.
7. National Consensus Project for Quality Palliative Care. American Academy of Hospice and Palliative Medicine & Hospice and Palliative Nursing Association Task Force. *Clinical practice guideline for quality palliative care.* 2004. <http://www.nationalconsensusproject.org/> (accessed 29 October 2005).
8. Evers MM, Meier DE, Morrison RS. Assessing differences in care needs and service utilization in geriatric palliative care patients. *J Pain Symptom Manage.* 2002;23(5):424–432.
9. Hoyert DL, Rosenberg HM. Alzheimer's disease as a cause of death in the United States. *Public Health Rep.* 1997;112(6):497–505.
10. Matzo ML. Palliative care: prognostication and the chronically ill. *Am J Nurs.* 2004;104(9):40–49.

11. Karnofsky Performance Status Scale definitions rating (%) criteria. <http://www.hospicepatients.org/karnofsky.html>

12. Doyle D, Woodruff R. *The IAHPC manual of palliative care*, 2nd edn. Houston, TX: IAHPC Press, 2008.

13. Miller KE. *Predicting life expectancy in patients with dementia*. 2003. View eligibility criteria at: <http://www.aafp.org/afp/2003/1015/p1639.html>.

14. Victoria Hospice Society. *The Edmonton Symptom Assessment Scale*. <http://www.palliative.org/PC/ClinicalInfo/AssessmentTools/esas.pdf>.

15. Victoria Hospice Society. *Palliative Performance Scale Relevant to palliative care function*. 2001. <http://www.palliative.org/PC/ClinicalInfo/AssessmentTools/PPS.pdf>.

16. Sykes NP. A volunteer model for the comparison of laxatives in opioid-induces constipation. *J Pain Symptom Manage*. 1997;11:363–369.

17. Hospice and Palliative Nurses Association (HPNA). *Clinical practice protocol: Dyspnea*. Pittsburgh, PA: HPNA, 1996.

18. Bednash G, Ferrell B. *End-of-Life Nursing Education Consortium (ELNEC)*. Washington, DC: Association of Colleges of Nursing, 2001.

19. Dickerson D, Benedetti C, Davis M, *et al. Palliative care pocket consultant*. Dubuque, IA: Kendall-Hunt Publishing Company, 2001.

20. Periyakoil VJ. *Fast Facts and Concepts #43: Is it grief or depression?* (2nd ed.). End-of-Life Physician Education Resource Center, 2005. <http://www.eperc.mcw.edu/fastFact/ff_43.htm>.

21. The Geriatric Depression Scale (GDS). <http://psychology-tools.com/geriatric-depression-scale/>.

22. Tiesinag LJ, Dassen TW, Halfens RJ. Fatigue: a summary of the definitions, dimensions and indicators. *Nurs Diagnos*. 1996;7:51–56.

23. Dean GE, Anderson PR. Fatigue. In Ferrel BR, Coyle N (eds) *The textbook of palliative nursing* (pp. 91–100). New York: Oxford University Press, 2001.

24. Sykes NP, Baines M, Carter RL. Clinical and pathological study of dysphagia conservatively managed in patients with advanced malignant disease. *Lancet*. 1998;ii:726–728.

25. AGS Ethics Committee. The care of dying patients: a position statement. *J Am Geriatr Soc*. 2003;43:577–578.

CHAPTER 28

Day case anaesthesia and the elderly

Uma Shridhar Iyer

Introduction

The geriatric population needs access to healthcare more frequently than younger age groups. According to the United Nations population division, the ratio of the elderly to children will rise to 1:2 by 2050 and the overall elderly population will rise to 32 per cent of the world population.[1] This huge challenge to healthcare systems needs to be dealt with by advance planning to provide safe and effective healthcare to the ageing population. The most common operations performed on the elderly include ophthalmic surgery followed by urology, orthopaedics, and other surgical procedures.

All of these are being increasingly undertaken in the ambulatory setting.[2] This group of patients presents challenges to anaesthetists due to the limited time constraints of ambulatory surgery and the elderly's vulnerability and fragile disposition.

Day surgery is not without its disadvantages. We are now seeing increasing claims in the elderly population, even under monitored anaesthetic care.[3] Complications, especially of the severe nature are noted to be more frequent in the elderly patient.[4,5] The needs of the geriatric patient are very different from the regular adult patient, and we need to tailor our practice patterns to adapt to the physiological, pathological, and psychological requirements of this subgroup of patients, with particular relevance to the ambulatory setting. We shall review the pathophysiology of ageing and the challenges of surgery and anaesthesia especially as day surgery, in this otherwise vulnerable population.

Day surgery

Surgical procedures

The scope of day surgery is constantly expanding. Patients with complex medical problems and elderly patients are being increasingly considered for day surgery. Economic factors are also titling the scales in favour of day surgery with increasing pressure on the anaesthetist to balance the risk effectively and safely.

Benefits of day surgery are established and include lower risk of morbidity, mortality, and infection, greater efficiency, lesser waiting time, and lower overall procedure costs. Thus day surgery has clear benefits. For the geriatric patient, it offers an attractive prospect of less disruption from daily schedules. Same day discharge to the home environment reduces the impact of the procedure on daily activities and separation from the familiar home environment. The reduction in the incidence of infection is especially important to the geriatric patient as they may have a compromised immune system associated with ageing and day surgery may help avoid the devastating effects of a postoperative infection. Day surgery also encourages early resumption of regular activities and mobility which may be easily sacrificed in an inpatient setting.

The types of surgeries that can be undertaken in the ambulatory setting are expanding but follow the same underlying principle that the postoperative physiological changes must be minimal and recovery should be uncomplicated.[6] Surgeries previously requiring large incisions are now being undertaken safely in the outpatient setting with the use of minimally invasive techniques and therefore less pain and physiological derangements. Surgery not associated with large fluid shifts, prolonged immobilization or severe postoperative pain is suitable for day surgery. Surgical duration of less than 90 minutes was one of the early requirements for suitability for day surgery, but now longer surgical times of 3–4 hours are also being undertaken. Common procedures undertaken in an ambulatory setting include cataract and other ophthalmic procedures, inguinal hernia repair, gynaecological, urological, orthopaedic, and general surgical procedures.[7]

Patient selection

As the geriatric population is represented by a very heterogeneous population, specific guidelines are lacking and there is limited evidence for making generalized recommendations. A comprehensive preoperative assessment focusing on identification of coexisting diseases, its severity and extent, and determination of the existing functional reserve of the systems is crucial to safe and favourable outcomes. American Society of Anesthesiologists (ASA) Class 1, 2, and stable 3 patients are considered suitable for day surgery and it is being recognized that ASA status cannot be looked at in isolation to determine suitability for day surgery.[8] Morbidity in ASA 3 patients has been shown to be no different from that in ASA 1 and ASA 2 patients and it is attributed to good patient selection, preoperative assessment, and perioperative planning. In addition, many patients understand their diabetes and chronic conditions better than a new doctor or nurse and hence are best left to manage their conditions independently. Even some ASA 4 patients are being operated upon in the ambulatory setting, under local anaesthesia safely, mostly cataract surgery or inguinal hernia repair surgery.[9] It is important to bear in mind that not all procedures and patients are suitable to surgery in day surgery setting and some are best undertaken in the inhospital setting. They include those patients with unstable diseases, like unstable angina, brittle diabetes, morbid obesity complicated by cardiorespiratory problems, and those patients with no suitable caregivers at home or no quick access to medical care facility.

Age is rightfully not a restriction to undertaking surgery in an ambulatory setting. The evidence on influence of age on perioperative outcome has been conflicting. Some studies show an increased incidence of adverse cardiovascular events in the elderly patients in an ambulatory setting when compared to their younger counterparts.[10] The study showed increase in changes in haemodynamic variables with increasing age, but these patients were far less likely to suffer adverse events postoperatively. Another prospective study on 15 000 patients did not show any association with postoperative adverse events and age.[11] Another study by Fleisher et al., a series of 564 000 patients for day surgery showed that risk is low for elderly patients, even though it may become important at extremes of age, above 85 years.[12,13] Though age greater than 85 seems to be strongly associated with readmission or increase in postoperative complications, it does not mean that outpatient surgery is contraindicated in this group. Instead, age greater than 85 should be a flag to institute additional care and attention to ensure their safe outcome.[14] The selection of patients for suitability for day surgery thus should be regardless of age. The biological rather than the chronological age defines the fitness and ability of the individual to withstand additional physiological challenges to the various organ systems. Another problem noted frequently in the elderly is lack of medication compliance, which may be linked to their cognitive skills and this can compromise the degree of disease optimization.[15]

Day surgery and its associated reduction in disruption from daily schedules and separation from the familiar home environment may reduce the incidence of postoperative cognitive disorders. One of the requirements of being able to carry out surgery in an ambulatory setting mandates the presence of a suitable caregiver. Often elderly patients are cared for by elderly people themselves. Such a scenario places the added burden of enhanced caring for an elderly person on another elderly person. Hence it is necessary to assess the suitability of the patient for day surgery from the caregiver's point of view as well. Some elderly patients live alone and therefore are not suitable for consideration for same day discharges after surgery despite satisfying all other criteria.

Preparation for day surgery

Preoperative assessment and preparation is the key to successful and safe outcomes. In keeping with the pathophysiological changes associated with ageing as described earlier, comorbidities are noted more frequently in the elderly patient.[16] A detailed assessment focusing on assessing the severity of the coexisting diseases, the physiological reserve and functional abilities is necessary. While the value of preoperative assessment few days prior to surgery has its distinct benefits of being able to critically assess, counsel and prepare the patient, there is a role for healthy patients undergoing surgical procedures of low risk or complexity to be seen on the day of surgery with the relevant information available for review in advance, should all concerned parties be comfortable with this kind of arrangement.[17] But high-risk patients scheduled for complex surgery will benefit from pre-anaesthetic evaluation ahead of time. Common diseases in the elderly like cardiovascular diseases, diabetes, respiratory disorders, etc. need to be worked up and evaluated depending on their severity and the complexity of surgery, as with inpatient surgery. Metabolic equivalent testing to determine the cardiorespiratory fitness may be difficult to evaluate due to other motor disorders or joint afflictions and therefore pose diagnostic and therapeutic dilemmas. Diabetes, hypertension, hyperlipidaemia, and vascular diseases are associated with an increased risk of coronary artery disease. There is a need to be aware and screen at risk patients for evidence of ischaemia, even if it is rare for the patient to require further evaluation before day surgery. We have moved from an era of routine preoperative testing to indicated testing. In a randomized, single-blinded, prospective controlled pilot study, it was shown that the abnormal preoperative electrolyte values and full blood counts were not predictive of adverse outcomes postoperatively and hence should not be carried out on the basis of age alone, rather on the patient's medical status.[18] In another study, Chung et al. all studied the incidence of adverse events in day surgery in 1061 patients with and without preoperative blood testing and found no increase in adverse events in the group that was not subjected to any testing.[19] But this was a pilot study with limited power and the exclusion criteria eliminated sicker and older patients and hence the results cannot be extrapolated to all patients undergoing day surgery for now.

Tests for assessing cognitive skills and any pre-existing cognitive decline with the use of questionnaires may be considered. Use of testing with questionnaires like Mini Mental State Examination, Sweet 16 or Confusion Assessment method are reproducible tests to assess the degree of pre-existing delirium or cognitive compromise.[20,21] Recognition of existing cognitive deficit is the first step towards preventing the occurrence and management of postoperative delirium and postoperative cognitive dysfunction (POCD) or at the least, reduces its severity and impact. In summary, preoperative assessment provides the opportunity to assess the patient, the need for investigations and carry out any necessary optimization.

After assessing suitability, the patients must be prepared for the surgery by explaining to them the information in a clear and simple format that is paced to their cognitive levels. Explanations may have to be provided to them in their own native language for improved comprehension. All the information should be provided to the patient and family members before surgery in a written format as patient comprehension may be compromised after surgery, especially those who received a general anaesthetic or a sedative.[22] Any written information that is provided may require use of larger fonts and further explanation. Audiovisual aids are greatly helpful in conveying information, but information in the forms of CDs or discs or URLs may be of little use to the less educated elderly who is not very familiar to newer technology. Information related to the risks and benefits of surgery and anaesthesia, the preoperative instructions, and likely complications must be thus conveyed to the patient. The consent for the procedure must include the surgical procedure, anaesthesia risk and the postoperative phase. The importance of assessing the cognitive level of the patients becomes imperative in order to be able to convey the information effectively. In the event of proven incapacity, the family and care givers must be detailed all of the details just mentioned. The possibility of POCD and delirium must be highlighted to the patient and their family as it impacts the care and support the patient will then require after surgery.

Intraoperative care

The options of local, regional, and general anaesthesia, or monitored anaesthetic care, are available depending on the suitability of the anaesthetic plan to the proposed surgical procedure and patient preferences.

Local anaesthesia

This may be more suitable than general anaesthesia to enhance recovery profiles.[23] Local anaesthesia is often combined with sedation (monitored anaesthetic care). But the possibility of complications and larger than anticipated depths of sedation achieved is a distinct reality and therefore sedation in the elderly cannot be taken lightly. Miniscule doses of sedatives may cause unexpected deep and prolonged sedation levels and occasional disinhibition. Careful calculation of drug doses with titration to effect is mandatory and strongly recommended as complications and litigation is often associated with sedation, especially in the elderly population.[3] Administration of sedation requires expertise and most centres have guidelines in place for administering sedation, especially by non-anaesthetists. The need for training and licensing for administering sedation is increasingly being recognized.[24] Commonly used drugs for sedation are propofol, midazolam, dexmedetomidine, remifentanil, or fentanyl singly or in combination.[25]

General anaesthesia

Drug dose titration is imperative when general anaesthesia is planned. Laboratory studies indicate that general anaesthetic agents are toxic to nervous tissue and function.[26,27] The evidence in favour of regional anaesthesia over general anaesthesia, at least in terms of cognitive impairment seems lacking. In a study by Williams- Ruso, a prospective study comparing the effects of epidural versus general anaesthesia in elective unilateral knee replacement, revealed an overall 5 per cent decline in cognitive function 6 months after surgery, but no statistical significant differences between the two anaesthesia groups.[28] The lack of benefit may be attributed to the use of sedation in regional anaesthesia techniques thereby skewing results away from an expected benefit. Adequate preoxygenation is critical since the patients are vulnerable to hypoxia and hypoxia related cardiac events. As explained earlier, there is a need to calculate doses, reduction in median effective dose requirements for drugs, especially those acting on the central nervous system, regardless of the route of administration. In keeping with the reduction in minimum alveolar concentration (MAC) of inhaled anaesthetics with advancing age, by the age of 80 years, they require MAC one-third than that of a young adult. Concurrent use of different classes of sedatives or hypnotics requires further downward titration of doses. Use of short-acting agents like propofol, desflurane, and sevoflurane, in conjunction with Bispectral Index monitoring may result in early awakening and reduce recovery time.[29,30] In addition to the need for reduced dosing, reduced cardiac reserve and output may lead to delayed onset of action of induction agents, prolonged induction times and lesser ability to compensate for any associated hypotension. The time required to recover from neuromuscular blockade is also increased, especially for drugs that rely on organs for clearance. Hence it may be advisable to use equipment to monitor neuromuscular blockade and recovery in the elderly patient when non-depolarizing neuromuscular blocking agents are used.

Regional anaesthesia

While this is an attractive option, it is important to bear in mind that elderly patients who receive a central or peripheral nerve block technique are at an increased risk of postoperative numbness or nerve injury. Nerve fibres are especially vulnerable to local anaesthetic agents in the elderly leading to prolonged motor and sensory blockade.[31] Central neuraxial blocks are associated with higher levels of blocks for the same volume of drugs as well as a higher degree and incidence of hypotension and bradycardia.[32] This may be of a grave concern in the elderly who have a compromised cardiovascular reserve to begin with. It is also this need for reduction in drug dosages and anticipated prolongation in its effects that makes rapid recovery profile of day surgery difficult. The technical skills required to administer a pain-free spinal to the elderly patient with an ossified spinal canal and interspinous spaces add to the challenges. Low-dose spinal anaesthesia with bupivacaine or lignocaine may be well tolerated for certain surgical procedures like transurethral prostatectomy, but bupivacaine is associated with significantly longer block duration and postoperative room stay.[33] Recently 2-chloroprocaine has generated considerable interest as a suitable local anaesthetic of choice especially in the ambulatory setting.[34,35] Concerns of prolonged operating room time with regional anaesthesia have been quelled with efficient block room setups even in an ambulatory setting.[36] The safety profile and economic benefits have shown to be favouring spinal anaesthesia with short-acting agent in comparison to general anaesthesia.[37] Nerve blocks have the added advantage of providing prolonged postoperative analgesia.

Intraoperatively, meticulous attention must be adhered to positioning, avoidance of hypothermia, and hydration needs of the elderly patients. The fragile condition of their skin means that special care should be instituted when applying tapes and dressings and during positioning. Joints may be stiff due to arthritic joints and due considerations must be given to them mandating innovation in optimally positioning the patient.

Surgical time also needs to be minimized to the best extent possible, since duration of surgery can affect the outcomes adversely. Minimally invasive techniques can decrease the metabolic response to surgery and facilitate faster recovery.[38]

Postoperative care

It is important to appreciate that desaturation occurs faster in the elderly patients. Prophylactic oxygen supplementation is recommended after sedation or anaesthesia. Fast-track protocols may be used to improve efficiency and maximize resources without compromising patient safety, but elderly patients and sicker patients may not always be suited for fast tracking.[39] In a recent study it was shown that general anaesthesia, in comparison to spinal anaesthesia, was associated with reduction in anaesthesia preparation time, length of surgery, start time of surgery, time to sit or walk, but time to fast track eligibility, phase 1 recovery time and discharge time were similar in both groups.[40] Spontaneous voiding before discharge after neuraxial blockade may take longer to achieve and must be borne in mind when used in the outpatient setting. The inability to void and subsequent possible need for urinary catheterization after a spinal anaesthetic is higher in patients over the age of 60 years.[41] While this criterion is relaxed in the day surgery setting occasionally, in the elderly it is recommended to ensure ability to void before discharge and maintain a high index of suspicion for the need for urinary catheterization.[42,43] Male patients may be especially prone to urine retention due to concomitant prostatic hypertrophy.[44]

Postoperative pain is often undertreated in the elderly though untreated pain has the potential to lead to tachycardia, hypertension, myocardial ischaemia, and adverse cardiac outcomes. Fear of side effects, drug interactions, or cognitive issues often leads to underdosing. Pain may be persistent for as long as 3 days after surgery, compromising the quality of life even longer.[45] Multimodal approaches to pain management are recommended to reduce the dose of individual class of drugs. Local infiltration, nerve blocks in conjunction with paracetamol, non-steroidal anti-inflammatory drug (NSAIDs), opioids are commonly used pain management options. But caution must be exercised with the use of NSAIDs and opioids in the elderly. Among opioids, tramadol and oxycodone are widely used, but still mandate the same degree of caution in their use.[46] The postoperative pain can be better managed by providing clear instructions about the analgesic regimen, options, and postoperative course over the first few days after surgery.[47]

Effective communication to manage expectations also goes a long way to manage pain and improve patient satisfaction.[48] POCD is possible after day surgery and requires appropriate management. It may take several days for full recovery. It may reflect worsening of pre-existing subclinical compromise in cognitive status.

Postoperative follow-up after surgery must be detailed and carefully individualized. In addition to written postoperative instruction and telephonic follow-ups, home visits by trained personnel are ideal and must be considered in select patients.

Audits on preoperative assessments, intraoperative and postoperative course and events are necessary to assess efficacy of current systems. This will lead to eventual improvement of care provided. A multidisciplinary approach incorporating surgeons, nurses, and clerical staff should also be encouraged to improve all round involvement and commitment in the care of the elderly.

Conclusion

Age is not a contraindication for day surgery. It is important to weigh the scales of risk and benefit. Day surgery appears to be more of an opportunity for the elderly patient than a danger. But assessment of physiological, psychological, functional, and social factors is crucial to ensure success and safety in this vulnerable population. The future holds a distinct possibility of increase in surgical care for the elderly in the ambulatory setting. With few newer anaesthetic options potentially available for better choice, the focus should be a better understanding of the pathophysiology of the ageing process, designing and implementation of protocols and multidisciplinary care for the elderly patient, and focused training in this important subspecialty.

References

1. United Nations. 'Major' rise in world's elderly population: DESA report, 28 January 2010. <http://www.un.org/en/development/desa/news/population/major-rise-in.html>(accessed 15 December 2010).
2. Etzioni DA, Liu JH, O'Connell JB, Maggard MA, Ko CY. Elderly patients in surgical workloads: a population- based analysis. Am Surg. 2003;69(11):961–964.
3. Bhananker SM, Posner KL, Cheney FW, Caplan RA, Lee RA, Domino KB. Injury and liability associated with Monitored Anaesthesia Care: ASA Closed Claims Analysis. Anesthesiology. 2006;104(2):228–234.
4. Forrest JB, Rehder K, Cahalan MK, Goldsmith CH. Multicentre study of general anaesthesia. III. Predictors of severe perioperative adverse outcomes. Anesthesiology. 1992;76(1):3–15.
5. Forster MC, Calthorpe D. Mortality following surgery for proximal femoral fractures in centenarians. Injury. 2000;31(7):537–539.
6. Liu MC, Chen CC. Postoperative care after geriatric ambulatory surgery: several specific considerations. Int J Gerontology. 2008;2(3):98–102.
7. Bettelli G. Anaesthesia for the elderly outpatient: preoperative assessment and evaluation, anaesthetic technique and postoperative pain management. Curr Opinion in Anesth. 2010;23:726–731.
8. Ansell GL, Montgomery JE. Outcome of ASA III patients undergoing day case surgery. Br J Anaesth. 2004;92(1):71–74.
9. P Sanjay, P Jones, Woodward A. Inguinal hernia repairs: are ASA grades 3 and 4 patients suitable for day case hernia repair? Hernia. 2006;10(4):299–302.
10. Chung F, Mezei G, Tong D. Adverse events in ambulatory surgery: a comparison between elderly and younger patients, Can J Anaesth. 1999;46(4):309–321.
11. Fortier J, Chung F, Su J. Unanticipated admission after ambulatory surgery – a prospective study. Can J Anaesth 1998;45(7):612–619.
12. Fleisher LE, Pasternak LR, Herbert R, Anderson GF. Inpatient hospital admission and death after outpatient surgery in elderly patients. Arch Surg. 2004;139(1):67–72.
13. Lermitte J, Chung F. Patient selection in ambulatory surgery. Curr Opin Anaesth. 2005;18(6):598–602.
14. Stierer T, Fleisher LA. Challenging patients in an ambulatory setting. Anesthesiol Clin North Am. 2003;21(2):243–261.
15. Insel K, Morrow D, Brewer B, Figueredo A. Executive function, working memory and medication adherence among older adults. J Gerontol B Psychol Sci Soc Sci. 2006;61(2):102–107.
16. Repetto L, Venturino A, Vercelli M, et al. Performance status and comorbidity in elderly cancer patients compared with young patients with neoplasia and elderly patients without neoplasia conditions. Cancer. 1998;82(4):760–765.
17. Pasternak R. Risk assessment in ambulatory surgery: challenges and new trends. Can J Anesth. 2004;51(6):R1–R5.
18. Dzankic S, Pastor D, Gonzalez C, Leung JM. The prevalence and predictive value of abnormal preoperative laboratory tests in elderly surgical patients. Anesth Analg. 2001;93(2):301–308.
19. Chung F, Hongbo Y, Ling Yin, Vairavanathan S. Elimination of preoperative testing in ambulatory surgery. Anesth Analg. 2009;108(2):467–475.
20. Flinn DR, Diehl KM, Sevfried LS, Malani PN. Prevention, diagnosis and management of postoperative delirium in older adults. J Am Coll Surg. 2009;209(2):261–268.
21. Fong TG, Jones RN, Rudolph JL, et al. Development and validation of a brief cognitive assessment tool: the sweet 16. Arch Intern Med. 2011;171(5):432–437.
22. Blandford CM, Gupta BC, Montgomery J, Stocker ME. Ability of patients to retain and recall new information in the post anaesthetic recovery period: a prospective clinical study in day surgery. Anaesthesia. 2011;66(12):1088–1092.
23. Kurzer M, Kark A, Hussain ST. Day-case inguinal hernia repair in the elderly: a surgical priority. Hernia. 2009;13(2):131–136.
24. American Society of Anesthesiologists Task Force on Sedation and Analgesia by non-anesthesiologists. Practice guidelines for sedation and analgesia by non-anesthesiologists. Anesthesiology. 2002;96:1004–1017.
25. Hohener D, Blumenthal S, Borgeat A. Sedation and regional anaesthesia in the adult patient. Br J Anaesth. 2008;100(1):8–16.
26. Culley DJ, Baxter MG, Crosby CA, Yukhanov R, Crosby G. Impaired acquisition of spatial memory 2 weeks after isoflurane and isoflurane-nitrous oxide anaesthesia in aged rats. Anesth Analg. 2004;99(5):1393–1397.

27. Eckenohoff RG, Johansson JS, Wei H, *et al.* Inhaled anesthetic enhancement of amyloid-beta oligomerization and cytotoxicity. *Anesthesiology.* 2004;101(3):703–709.

28. Williams-Ruso P, Sharrock NE, Mattis S, Szatrowski TP, Charlson ME. Cognitive effects after epidural vs general anaesthesia in older adults: a randomized trial. *JAMA.* 1995;274(1):44–50.

29. Heavner JE, Kaye AD, Lin BK, King T. Recovery of elderly patients from two or more hours of desflurane or sevoflurane anaesthesia. *Br J Anaesth.* 2003;91(4):502–506.

30. Fredman B, Sheffer O, Zohar E, *et al.* Fast track eligibility of geriatric patients undergoing short urologic procedures. *Anesth Analg.* 2002;94(3):560–564.

31. Pagueron X, Boccaran G, Bendahou M, *et al.* Brachial plexus nerve block exhibits prolonged duration in the elderly. *Anesthesiology.* 2002;94:1245–1249.

32. Simon MJG, Veering BT, Stienstra R, Van Kleef JW, Burm AG. The effects of age on neural blockade and hemodynamic changes after epidural anaesthesia with ropivacaine. *Anesth Analg.* 2002;94(5):1325–1330.

33. Sirivanasandha B, Lennox PH, Vaghadia H. Transurethral resection of the prostrate (TURP) with low dose spinal anaesthesia in outpatients: a 5 year review. *Can J Urol.* 2011;18(3):5705–5709.

34. Hejtmanek MR, Pollock JE. Chloroprocaine for spinal anaesthesia: a retrospective analysis. *Acta Anaesthesiol Scand.* 2011;55(3):267–272.

35. Lacasse MA, Roy JD, Forget J, *et al.* Comparison of bupivacaine and 2-chloroprocaine for spinal anesthesia for outpatient surgery: a double-blind randomized trial. *Can J Anaesth.* 2011;58(4):384–391.

36. Mariano E, Chu L, Peinado C, *et al.* Anaesthesia controlled time and turnover time for ambulatory upper extremity surgery performed with regional versus general anaesthesia. *J Clin Anesth.* 2009;21(4):253–257.

37. Nishikawa K, Yoshida S, Shimodate Y, Igarashi M, Namiki A. A comparison of spinal anaesthesia with small dose lidocaine and general anaesthesia with fentanyl and propofol for ambulatory prostrate biopsy procedures in elderly patients. *J Clin Anesth.* 2007;19(1):25–29.

38. Kehlet H. Multimodal approach to control postoperative pathophysiology and rehabilitation. *Br J Anaesth.* 71997;8:606–617.

39. Twersky R, Sapozhnikova, Toure B. Risk factors associated with fast track ineligibility after monitored anesthesia care in ambulatory surgery patients. *Anesth Analg.* 2008;106:1421–1426.

40. Dilsen O, Seyhan M, Serpil D, *et al.* The influence of various anesthesia techniques on postoperative recovery and discharge criteria among geriatric patients. *Clinics.* 2010;65(10):941–946.

41. Kreutziger J, Frankenberger B, Luger TJ, Richard S, Zbinden S. Urinary retention after spinal anaesthesia with hyperbaric prilocaine 2% in an ambulatory setting. *Br J Anaesth.* 2010;104(5):582–586.

42. Ruhl M. Postoperative voiding criteria for ambulatory surgery patients. *AORN J.* 2009;8 (5):871–874.

43. Mulroy MF, Salinas FV, Larkin KL, Polissar NL. Ambulatory surgery may be discharged before voiding after short acting spinal and epidural anesthesia. *Anesthesiology.* 2002;97(2):315–319.

44. Sarasin SM, Walton MJ, Singh HP, Clark DI. Can a urinary tract symptom score predict the development of postoperative urinary retention in patients undergoing lower limb arthroplasty under spinal anaesthesia? A prospective study. *Ann R Coll Surg Engl.* 2006;88(4):394–398.

45. Beauregard L, Pomp A, Chinrie M. Severity and impact of pain after day surgery. *Can J Anaesth.* 1998;45:304–311.

46. Okkola KT, Hagelberg NM. Oxycodone: a new 'old' drug. *Curr Opin Anesthesiol.* 2009;22:459–462.

47. McHugh GA, Thoms GM. The management of pain following day case surgery. *Anaesthesia.* 2002;57(3):270–275.

48. Lemos P, Pinto A, Morais G, *et al.* Patient satisfaction following day surgery. *J Clin Anesth.* 2009;21(3):200–205.

CHAPTER 29

Ophthalmic anaesthesia in the elderly

Chandra M. Kumar

Introduction

Patients requiring anaesthesia for ophthalmology in the elderly are challenging. These elderly patients have increased morbidity and they receive multiple drugs that make anaesthesia risky even for minor surgery. Eye surgical procedures range from simple cataract surgery to major procedures lasting several hours. It is essential to understand the intricate relationship between ophthalmic physiological and pathological changes associated with the ageing. The elderly may also receive drugs which can interact with drugs employed during anaesthesia. There has been a shift in the delivery of anaesthesia towards local anaesthesia with general anaesthesia being used for more complex cases. A careful preoperative assessment and preparation of these patients are important towards safe outcome regardless of technique. The choice and preferences for anaesthesia and techniques vary worldwide and several factors play an important part in choosing the type of anaesthesia. Routine postoperative care in a proper postoperative recovery unit is desirable.

There are many age-related physiological changes. Although the basic functions of most organs are largely unchanged, the functional reserve and ability to compensate for physiological stress is reduced. Decreased basal metabolic rate leads to an overall increase in percentage of body fat. Muscle mass decreases with time due to inactivity. Total body water decreases by 20–30 per cent with age resulting in decreased total blood volume. These age-related changes have a bearing on the anaesthetic management especially during general anaesthesia. These changes are covered elsewhere in this book see Chapters 1 and 5–11.

It is important to understand how the intraocular pressure (IOP), which can increase up to 40 mmHg during coughing and bucking, can affect anaesthetic management and vision. Injection of local anaesthetic agents behind the globe during needle based blocks is known to increase the IOP and the return of the IOP to baseline can take 5–10 min. An increase in arterial carbon dioxide tension (pulmonary arterial carbon dioxide tension) also increases the IOP. Spontaneous respiration with inhalational agent increases ends tidal carbon dioxide resulting in a clinically significant increase in the IOP. It is important therefore to assist or control ventilation in patients with raised IOP undergoing intraocular surgery to prevent a further rise. During clinical anaesthesia rises in IOP also occur with hypoxia, hypertension, and venous congestion. It is important to know that barbiturates, benzodiazepines and propofol decrease IOP. All inhalational agents including sevoflurane and desflurane are also known to decrease IOP during normocapnia. Non-depolarizing muscle relaxants do not have any effect on IOP.

Assessment and preparation

Preoperative assessment is carried out for all patients irrespective of the type of anaesthesia they are likely to receive. However, if the patient is to undergo general anaesthesia, a full preoperative assessment and investigations are performed as for any other major surgery. Investigations should be considered based on the relevant examination findings and national guidelines.[1] Age, comorbidity (such as cardiorespiratory disease), and chronic drug treatments make routine investigations such as electrocardiogram, full blood count, and urea and electrolytes potentially useful tests. Multiprofessional teamwork is the norm and the Joint Royal Colleges guidelines (2012) offer appropriate guidance for patients undergoing local anaesthesia.[2] If local anaesthesia is planned, investigations are usually reserved for very specific indications such as hypertension, ischaemic heart disease, diabetes mellitus, and chronic obstructive pulmonary disease. Patients are not fasted and this especially helpful in managing patients with diabetes mellitus. They can therefore receive all of their normal medications and achieve better glycaemic control in the perioperative period. The blood sugar level must be checked. It is important that the preoperative preparation includes checking that these patients are able to lie flat for up to an hour without becoming uncomfortable, claustrophobic, and worse still hypoxic or suffering ischaemic cardiac problems. Patients receiving anticoagulants pose problems that are more relevant to the surgeon but the choice of local anaesthesia is limited to topical or blunt cannula based technique sub-Tenon's block. Patients receiving anticoagulants and antiplatelet agents are advised to continue their usual medications unless told otherwise.[3,4] Warfarin therapy is not considered an absolute contraindication to local anaesthesia provided that preoperative INR (international normalized ratio) values are in the therapeutic target range.

Choosing type of anaesthesia

Risks and benefits of the technique used include considerations of important factors such as the urgency of the procedure, the length of surgical procedures, age, American Society of Anesthesiology (ASA) status of the patient, surgical conditions, preferences of the surgeon, and patient's choice all influence the technique used. Local or regional anaesthesia is preferred in the elderly patients with comorbidities to reduce the stress response to surgery and avoid postoperative complications such as nausea, vomiting, confusion, and urinary retention. The duration of the procedure and the patient's ability to lie still for a longer period is an important consideration. General anaesthesia is indicated for patient choice, and, for example, many 'training' procedures, poorly cooperative patients, or those with unpredictable movement disorders.

General anaesthesia

Indication for general anaesthesia

General anaesthesia is indicated in a patient who is unwilling or unable to tolerate local anaesthesia. The length and complexity of the operation is an important determinant influencing the surgeon's and the patient's requests. There are other more pressing reasons for general anaesthesia such as severe Parkinson's disease, mentally challenged patients, and very claustrophobic patient. The list of indications for general anaesthesia is becoming smaller.

Contraindications to general anaesthesia

There is no absolute contraindications and it is not uncommon for patients with serious comorbidities, which are not improvable, to safely undergo general anaesthesia. However, it should be remembered that cardiovascular, respiratory, and neurological diseases increase in frequency with age and there is an increased incidence of adverse cardiac outcome, respiratory failure, and postoperative cognitive dysfunction. Although impairment or decline in cognitive dysfunction is feared in the elderly after general anaesthesia, there is little or no evidence of a difference between regional or general anaesthesia following cataract surgery.

Induction agent

A smooth induction is the goal and this is even more important during ophthalmic surgery. Coughing, straining, accidental increases in intrathoracic pressure, and venous congestion are to be avoided at all costs. Propofol has a number of advantages especially related to the ease of insertion of a laryngeal mask airway (LMA). Propofol has a greater depressant effect on IOP and blood pressure than thiopentone in equipotent doses. Ketamine probably has little effect on the IOP. Short-acting opioids such as fentanyl or alfentanil act synergistically with the induction agent and obtund responses to airway manipulation.

Choice of airway

The airway is likely to remain inaccessible during surgery and any need to adjust or reposition the airway during surgery could cause disruption to surgery with potentially sight-threatening consequences. Thus, the safest option is to secure the airway with an endotracheal tube and the use of a muscle relaxant if desired. A south facing Ring–Adair–Elwyn (RAE) or other preformed endotracheal tube is the best option, and together with mechanical ventilation provides ideal conditions for nearly all ophthalmic surgery. Intubation is associated with an increase in IOP related to coughing and bucking during induction, the pressor response to laryngoscopy and intubation, laryngospasm during extubation or coughing, as well as postoperative nausea and vomiting related to the use of reversal. These complications have much greater importance in open eye surgery.

LMA with propofol as the induction agent is popular, especially for short ophthalmic procedures. It reduces some of the risks but there is an increased risk of losing the airway if LMA is not secured or positioned properly in patients who are edentulous and covered under the surgical drape. Neuromuscular blocking agent aids LMA and makes mechanical ventilation easier but at the expense of increased risk of aspiration.

Anaesthesia maintenance and postoperative care

Volatile anaesthetic agents are commonly used due to their familiarity of use, controllability, and cost, and it has a dose-dependent effect on reducing the IOP. There is little academic difference between any individual inhalational agents.

Nitrous oxide use may depend on local availability of medical air and personal preference. The benefits of nitrous oxide are well known but it brings two particular risks. There is an increased incidence of postoperative nausea and vomiting as well as the potentially catastrophic rise in IOP when intraocular gas mixtures are used for vitrectomy. Total intravenous techniques are increasingly used but its use is limited to short surgical procedure such as phacoemulsification surgery.

The physiological challenge of most eye surgery can be considered to be low. Care should be taken in administering intravenous fluid in an elderly patient fasting too long for surgery and care should be taken not to be too liberal with intravenous fluids in case of overloading the myocardium or inducing urinary retention in the elderly population. The elderly are prone to hypothermia especially if the surgical procedure takes more than an hour. Venous thromboembolism prevention measures should be in place with mechanical compression device. In diabetic patients local euglycaemia protocols must be followed. Analgesia requirements are not usually a great problem postoperatively and intraoperative short-acting opioids usually suffice. Paracetamol and non-steroidal anti-inflammatory drugs may be useful if there are no contraindications. Local anaesthesia injection in conjunction with general anaesthesia is particularly useful. Ophthalmic patients are particularly prone to suffer from nausea and vomiting despite the absence of long-acting opioid and prophylaxis with dexamethasone and/or ondansetron are useful.

Local anaesthesia for eye surgery

Local anaesthesia can be achieved in three ways: as topical drops, local infiltration, and nerve blocks.

Topical anaesthesia

If local anaesthetic drops are applied to the conjunctival sac they will anaesthetize the conjunctiva and corneal surface. This may be sufficient for minor surgical and diagnostic procedures, for instance, removing corneal foreign bodies or checking IOPs or routine simple and non-complicated cataract extraction surgery. Various topical local agents are available which include amethocaine 1 per cent, oxybuprocaine 0.4 per cent, proxymetacaine 0.5 per cent, lidocaine 4 per cent, lidocaine gel 2 per cent. The anaesthesia will be short-lived but the effect of topical drops can be increased if a small swab is soaked in the local anaesthetic agent and left for a minute on the conjunctiva.

Local infiltration

Local infiltration involves injection of local anaesthetic into the tissues to produce anaesthesia in the region where it is injected. This is the usual method of anaesthesia for surgery to the eyelids or conjunctiva. Lidocaine 1–2 per cent is the most popular agent. Simple cataract surgery can also be performed under this technique.

Orbital nerve blocks

Nerve blocks are performed by injecting the anaesthetic agent close to the main trunk of a nerve or its branches so that its sensory or motor function is blocked. This is the usual way of giving local anaesthesia for intraocular surgery. With a nerve block a relatively small injection can achieve a large effect. A detailed knowledge of the anatomy of the eye is of paramount importance before performing a block. A brief description of orbital anatomy is described here and readers are encouraged to read the full detail in authoritative textbooks of anatomy.[5,6]

The orbit is a four-sided irregular pyramid with its apex pointing posteromedially and its base anteriorly. The eye movements are controlled by six extraocular muscles: inferior, lateral, medial, superior recti, and the superior oblique and inferior oblique muscles. These muscles form an incomplete muscle cone. The optic nerve (II), oculomotor nerves (III containing both superior and inferior branches), abducens nerve (VI nerve), nasociliary nerve (a branch of V nerve), ciliary ganglion, and vessels lie within the cone. The ophthalmic division of the oculomotor nerve (III) divides into superior and inferior branches before emerging from the superior orbital fissure. The superior branch supplies the superior rectus and the levator palpebrae superioris. The inferior branch divides into three to supply the medial rectus, the inferior rectus, and the inferior oblique muscles. The abducens nerve (VI) supplies the lateral rectus muscle. The trochlear nerve (IV nerve) courses mostly supplies the superior oblique muscle. Squeezing and closing of the eyelids outside the cone are controlled by the zygomatic branch of the facial nerve (VII), which supplies the motor innervation to the orbicularis oculi muscle.

Tenon's capsule or bulbar fascia is a membrane that envelops the eyeball from the optic nerve to the sclerocorneal junction separating it from the orbital fat and forming a socket in which it moves. The capsule originates at the limbus and extends posteriorly to the optic nerve and as sleeves along the extraocular muscles. Tenon's capsule is arbitrarily divided by the equator of the globe into anterior and posterior portions. Anterior Tenon's capsule is adherent to episcleral tissue from the limbus posteriorly for about 5–10 mm and is fused with the intermuscluar septum of the extraocular muscles and overlying bulbar conjunctiva. Posteriorly, the sheath fuses with the openings around the optic nerve.

Sensation to the globe is supplied through the ophthalmic division of the trigeminal nerve (V). Just before entering the orbit, it divides into three branches: lacrimal, frontal, and nasociliary. The nasociliary nerve is sensory to the entire globe. Two long ciliary nerves give branches to the ciliary ganglion and, with the short ciliary nerves, transmit sensation from the cornea, iris and ciliary muscle. Some sensation from the lateral conjunctiva is transmitted through the lacrimal nerve and from the upper palpebral conjunctiva via the frontal nerve. Both nerves are outside the cone.

The superomedial and superotemporal quadrants have abundant blood vessels but the inferotemporal and medial quadrants are relatively avascular and are the safer places to insert needles or cannulae.

Selection of patients for orbital nerve block

Numerous published studies confirm the preference of ophthalmologists, anaesthetists, and patients for local techniques but the decision is largely made by the person performing the block. The decision is based on factors which influence the choice of a particular technique. The preferred technique varies from topical anaesthesia, cannula-based block to needle-based blocks. The technique chosen should depend on a balance between the patient's wishes, the operative needs of the surgeon, the skills of the anaesthetist, and the type of surgery.

Insertion of an intravenous cannula is good clinical practice and must be established if a sharp needle technique is planned.[2] Full cardiopulmonary resuscitation equipment and trained staff should be immediately available. Appropriate cardiorespiratory monitoring should be used.

Orbital nerve blocks

The terminology used for ophthalmic blocks varies and terminology based on the anatomical placement of the needle is widely accepted.[7] The injection of local anaesthetic agent into the muscle cone behind the globe formed by four recti muscles and the superior and inferior oblique muscles is termed as intraconal (retrobulbar) block whereas in the extraconal (peribulbar) block the needle tip remains outside the muscle cone. Multiple communications exist between the two compartments and the injected local anaesthetic agent diffuses easily across compartments and depending on its spread, anaesthesia and akinesia may occur.[8] A combination of intraconal and extraconal block is described as the combined retro-peribulbar block.[9] In sub-Tenon's block, local anaesthetic agent is injected under the Tenon's capsule[10] and this block is also known as parabulbar block,[11] pinpoint anaesthesia,[12] or medial episcleral block.[13] A detailed description of local anaesthetic technique is beyond the scope of this book and readers are advised to consult an authoritative textbook on ophthalmic anaesthesia.[14]

Complications of local anaesthesia

Topical anaesthesia is devoid of serious complication but this technique is not suitable for all patients. Complications of needle blocks range from mild to serious.[15] It can manifest locally into the eye (globe or areas around the globe) or systemically. Complications arising to the globe and surrounding structures include failure of the block, corneal abrasion, chemosis, subconjunctival haemorrhage, orbital haemorrhage, globe damage, optic nerve damage, and extraocular muscle malfunction. These complications are very well documented. Systemic manifestations include local anaesthetic agent toxicity, brainstem anaesthesia, and cardio-respiratory arrest may occur due to intravenous or spread or misplacement of drug in the orbit during or immediately after injection.

Although the cannula block (sub-Tenon's) is considered a safe alternative to needle block, a number of complications, both minor and major, have been reported.[16] Minor complications are frequent, such as pain during injection, reflux of local anaesthetic, chemosis, and subconjunctival haemorrhage. Subconjunctival haemorrhage is considered unacceptable by many surgeons and arises more in patients receiving clopidogrel, warfarin, and aspirin.[17] Occurrence can be reduced with careful dissection, application of topical adrenaline or controversially the use of handheld cautery.[18,19] All major complications which have been reported following needle blocks can occur during sub-Tenon's block but they are very infrequent indeed.

Sedation during local anaesthesia

Sedation is commonly used during topical anaesthesia.[20] Explanation and reassurance are usually adequate but some patients may benefit from sedation. Short-acting benzodiazepines, opioids, or small doses of an intravenous anaesthetic induction agent such as propofol are favoured.[21] The routine use of sedation is unnecessary because there is an increased incidence of adverse intraoperative events.[22]

Anaesthesia for specific procedures

Cataract surgery

Surgical techniques for cataract have undergone recent changes and the surgery has become less invasive. Phacoemulsification surgery is increasingly performed with much smaller phaco probes. The procedure is increasingly performed under topical anaesthesia but many surgeons prefer a block technique. The use of sub-Tenon's block is common and needle-based blocks which may have devastating complications are avoided. General anaesthesia is now administered for specific indications as described earlier.

Glaucoma surgery

Local anaesthesia is commonly used. If general anaesthesia is required many of the considerations are the same as for cataract surgery. Balanced anaesthesia technique requiring neuromuscular blockade and good anaesthetic control over IOP produces the best operating conditions.

Vitreoretinal surgery

Vitreoretinal (VR) surgery covers a range of intra- and extraocular procedures requiring a longer period of surgery, usually in a dark environment. The procedures are usually more frequently performed in younger patients with comorbidities but if the procedure is performed in elderly patients, they are likely to have serious comorbidities of relatively longer duration. Procedures are categorized as detachment surgery, anterior vitrectomy, and pars plana vitrectomy (repairing break in retina, peeling of membranes, use of gases for temponading, firing of laser beams, cryotherapy and others). Detachment surgery can also be performed from outside the sclera. Buckling, bands, cryotherapy, and laser therapies are used to repair breaks. The eye requires a lot of surgical manipulation during these procedures and the oculocardiac reflex can be triggered. Vitrectomy removes the vitreous from the eye for the purpose of clearing cloudy or bloody vitreous, as well as to perform intraocular procedures on the retina. The cavity may then be filled with an air/gas mixture (commonly perfluoropropane or sulphur hexafluoride) or silicone. The use of a local anaesthesia block is common and both needle and cannula-based blocks are in use. General anaesthesia may be required in selected patients. The surgeon may make a decision on which of these agents to use for tamponade towards the end of surgery and as such it is sensible to avoid nitrous

oxide use for vitrectomy surgery due to the fact that nitrous oxide in equilibrium in the eye cavity may diffuse out quickly leaving a lower pressure in the eye than surgically intended causing detachment or re-detachment of the retina. If nitrous oxide has been used it should be switched off well before the insertion of surgical gas into the vitreal cavity. Gases may persist for up to 3 months postoperatively, therefore a wrist band may be placed on the patient after surgery to alert any subsequent anaesthetist to avoid nitrous oxide for subsequent anaesthesia. Nitrous oxide may diffuse into the cavity faster than any nitrogen would diffuse out and the IOP could rise with serious consequences.[23]

Squint surgery

General anaesthesia is the norm but in selected patients, the surgery can be performed under local anaesthesia. Airway considerations of head and neck procedures apply but a laryngeal mask is the most commonly chosen. Many surgeons request the avoidance of muscle relaxants if adjustable sutures are used. Long-acting opioids are not required and are only likely to increase an already high risk of postoperative nausea and vomiting.

Dacrocystorhinostomy

Dacrocystorhinostomy (DCR) is a procedure performed for watering eyes usually due to lacrimal duct stenosis. The surgical procedure involves exposure of the tear duct and a new opening is created into the nasal cavity. Surgery can be performed with an open technique or by nasal endoscopy. Usually general anaesthesia is requested although local anaesthesia (with or without sedation) has gained popularity.[24] All normal ophthalmic anaesthetic considerations apply. There is a risk of blood in the airway during and immediately after the procedure hence endotracheal intubation and the safe use of a throat pack offer airway protection. Endoscopic laser DCR is another surgical operation and the anaesthetist should have additional training in the practicalities of laser airway surgery.

Eye trauma

A penetrating open eye injury can happen in any patient and the elderly are no exception. The extent of injury may be difficult to ascertain due to swelling and pain. An eye injury may be associated with other major injuries. As with any case of trauma there may be a short fasting time prior to the injury and subsequent delay in gastric emptying. If a penetrating eye injury is associated with other trauma, general anaesthesia is routine. Orbital regional anaesthesia has been used successfully in selected centres.[25] The use of suxamethonium is considered essential to prevent aspiration pneumonitis especially in patients with full stomach but there is a risk of increased IOP associated with suxamethonium causing loss of eye contents. The overwhelming importance is to choose the anaesthetic technique that prevents aspiration most effectively throughout the perioperative period and that thought must also be given to reducing the IOP until the eye is made safe. Large retrospective studies of penetrating eye injury have not shown vitreous loss to be clinically significant.[25]

Other procedures

These procedures include surgery relates to the lid, socket or adnexae. Many procedures are short and lid surgery is generally performed under local anaesthesia. Longer procedures such as enucleation and tumour surgery are generally performed under general anaesthesia and appropriate measures are taken to control postoperative pain relief.

Conclusion

The practice of anaesthesia has seen preferences for local or general anaesthesia for ophthalmology swing in both directions. Currently the preference is firmly in favour of local anaesthesia considering age-related pathophysiological changes and their implications on ageing body.

References

1. National Institute for Clinical Excellence. *Preoperative tests. The use of routine preoperative tests for elective surgery.* CG 3. Developed by the National Collaborating Centre for Acute Care. London: NICE, 2003. <http://www.nice.org.uk/nicemedia/pdf/CG3NICEguideline.pdf> (accessed 1 October 2012).

2. Kumar CM, Eke T, Dodds C, *et al.* Local anaesthesia for ophthalmic surgery—new guidelines from the Royal College of Anaesthetists and the Royal College of Ophthalmologists. *Eye.* 2012;26:897–898.

3. Koopmans SA, van Rij G. Cataract surgery and anticoagulants. *Doc Ophthalmol.* 1996–1997;92:11–16.

4. Konstantatos A. Anticoagulation and cataract surgery: a review of the current literature. *Anaesth Intensive Care.* 2001;29:11–18.

5. Dutton JJ. *Atlas of clinical and surgical orbital anatomy.* Philadelphia, PA: Saunders, 1994.

6. Snell RS, Lemp MA. *Clinical anatomy of the eye.* Boston, MA: Blackwell Scientific Publications, 1989.

7. Fanning GL. Orbital regional anesthesia: let's be precise. *J Cataract Refract Surg.* 2003;29:1846–1847.

8. Ripart J, Lefrant JY, de La Coussaye JE, Prat-Pradal D, Vivien B, Eledjam JJ. Peribulbar versus retrobulbar anesthesia for ophthalmic surgery: an anatomical comparison of extraconal and intraconal injections. *Anesthesiology.* 2001;94:56–62.

9. Hamilton RC. Retrobulbar block revisited and revised. *J Cataract Refract Surg.* 1996;22:1147–1150.

10. Stevens J. A new local anaesthesia technique for cataract extraction by one quadrant sub-Tenon's infiltration. *Br J Ophthalmol.* 1992;76:620–624.

11. Greenbaum S. Parabulbar anesthesia. *Am J Ophthalmol.* 1992;114:776.

12. Fukasaku H, Marron JA. Sub-Tenon's pinpoint anesthesia. *J Cataract Refract Surg.* 1994;20:468–471.

13. Ripart J, Prat-Pradal D, Charavel P, Eledjam JJ. Medial canthus single injection episcleral (sub-Tenon) anesthesia anatomic imaging. *Clin Anat.* 1998;11:390–395.

14. Kumar CM, Dodds C, Gayer S. *Ophthalmic anaesthesia.* Oxford: Oxford University Press, 2012.

15. Kumar CM, Dowd TC. Complications of ophthalmic regional blocks: their treatment and prevention. *Ophthalmologica.* 2006;220:73–82.

16. Kumar CM, Eid H, Dodds C. Sub-Tenon's anaesthesia: complications and their prevention. *Eye.* 2011;25:694–703.

17. Kumar N, Jivan S, Thomas P, McLure H. Sub-Tenon's anesthesia with aspirin, warfarin, and clopidogrel. *Cataract Refract Surg.* 2006;32:1022–1025.

18. Kumar CM, Williamson S. Diathermy does not reduce subconjunctival haemorrhage during sub-Tenon's block. *Br J Anaesth.* 2005;95:562.

19. Gauba V, Saleh GM, Watson K, Chung A. Sub-Tenon anaesthesia: reduction in subconjunctival haemorrhage with controlled bipolar conjunctival cautery. *Eye.* 2007;21:1387–1390.

20. Leaming DV. Practice styles and preferences of ASCRS members – 2003 survey. *J Cataract Refract Surg.* 2004;30:892–900.

21. Greenhalgh DL, Kumar CM. Sedation during ophthalmic surgery. *Eur J Anaesthesiol.* 2008;25:701–707.

22. Katz J, Feldman MA, Bass EB, *et al.* Adverse intraoperative medical events and their association with anesthesia management strategies in cataract surgery. *Ophthalmology.* 2001;108:1721–1726.

23. Yang YF, Herbert L, Rüschen H, Cooling RJ. Nitrous oxide anaesthesia in the presence of intraocular gas can cause irreversible blindness. *BMJ.* 2002;325:532–533.

24. McNab AA, Simmie RJ. Effectiveness of local anaesthesia for external dacryocystorhinostomy. *Clin Exp Ophthalmol.* 2002;30:270–272.

25. Scott IU, Mccabe CM, Flynn HW, *et al.* Local anesthesia with intravenous sedation for surgical repair of selected open globe injuries. *Am J Ophthalmol.* 2002;134:707–711.

CHAPTER 30

Frailty in the peri-surgical context

Peter Crome and Frank Lally

Introduction

The proportion of the population aged over 65 years in the United Kingdom is projected to increase to 23 per cent by 2033.[1] Surgery in this age group is now considered routine and in no way exceptional. However, although surgical and anaesthetic advances have reduced the risk from surgery in old age, this group of patients continue to have the highest mortality as well as longer hospital stays and more adverse health outcomes than those in younger people.

Much research has suggested that age in itself is not indicative of higher risk in surgical procedures,[1–4] but if age does not increase surgical mortality in older people then what does? Several factors have been identified as important considerations in the context of surgery in the older population (Table 30.1).

All of these factors are clearly important in dealing with older patients in the perioperative setting but the last of these, frailty, is a concept that appears to be emerging as a new 'geriatric giant' and may in itself have an important and complex relationship to the care of the older person undergoing surgery.[11]

Definitions

The word 'frailty' has many meanings in a general context and until relatively recently this was also true within the clinical setting. However, the 'idea' of frailty has clearly been around for quite a long time—Sheldon in his seminal work on the state of older people in the 1940s wrote 'An even more incapacitating symptom of old age is weakness...Its nature and delineation from states such as heart disease are difficult and uncertain; but there is little doubt that it is true clinical entity'.[12]

In the last few years frailty has attracted a great deal of interest within the geriatric medicine community not least because defining the term is challenging but also because it appears to be relevant to other specialities of medicine and has important clinical and financial connotations. It may also help define for which section of the older population geriatricians should take responsibility. A universally accepted definition of frailty has, however, yet to be established. This uncertainty is also reflected in the surgical literature where frailty is identified as a factor that can adversely affect surgical outcome but is defined in many different ways by different authors or on occasions given no definition at all. Table 30.2 illustrates this diversity by providing some definitions of frailty derived from the surgical literature. Physiological reserve is a common theme as a possible underlying factor. Palmer[5] stated that 'frailty, in which there is impaired homeostasis, is also is common in older adults...may predispose older patients to severe and multiorgan system failure even from a relatively minor perturbation of surgery that would not affect the average younger patient'. While Christmas[9] thought it was due to a 'decreased physiologic reserve to handle stress' and that this 'ultimately may be shown to be an important independent risk factor for poor surgical outcomes in the elderly'. Equally Audisio et al.[13] also believed that frailty was 'representing the dependency of someone with poor physiological reserve who has a high occurrence of repeated chronic illness and hospital admissions and where there may be complex medical and psychosocial problems'. This has led to the use of scoring systems to try to quantitate the degree of frailty and the patient's ability to manage their activities of daily living, for instance, Herrick[14] used 'a modified PPT [PPT: physical performance test] score between 12 and 28...requirement for assistance in one or more ADLs [activities of daily living]...' as a definition of frailty and Makary et al.[10] also used a validated frailty scoring system that included weakness, shrinking, exhaustion, low physical activity, and a slowed walking speed.

This chapter will provide an overview of frailty including epidemiology and how the medical community is attempting to define it in terms of the currently proposed models of frailty. In addition we will discuss the importance of frailty as a predictor of poor surgical outcome and the application of models of frailty in the clinical setting.

Table 30.1 Perioperative risk factors for adverse outcomes in older surgical patients

• Decreased reserve due to reduction in functional capacity of organs[5]
• Coexisting disease
• Confusion[3] and can lead to cognitive deficit[6]
• Nutritional state[5,7]
• Heterogeneity of ageing
• Physiological and pharmacological stress[8]
• Frailty[9,10]

Table 30.2 Definitions of frailty from papers on surgery

- 'Frailty, in which there is impaired homeostasis, is also is common in older adults...Frailty may predispose older patients to severe and multiorgan system failure even from a relatively minor perturbation of surgery that would not affect the average younger patient.'[5]
- '....decreased physiologic reserve to handle stress.... ultimately may be shown to be an important independent risk factor for poor surgical outcomes in the elderly.'[9]
- 'It has been described as representing the dependency of someone with poor physiological reserve who has a high occurrence of repeated chronic illness and hospital admissions and where there may be complex medical and psychosocial problems.'[13]
- '...a modified PPT (PPT: Physical Performance Test) score between 12 and 28...requirement for assistance in one or more ADLs.'[14]
- 'We measured frailty using a validated frailty scoring system based on weakness, shrinking, exhaustion, low physical activity, and slowed walking speed.'[10]

What is frailty?

The term itself 'frailty' may be seen as having pejorative connotations and this has led some researchers, particularly in the social sciences, to prefer to describe the concept in terms of its opposite using words such as resilience, robustness, or vigour. However, frailty appears to have stuck, at least in the medical setting. We can begin to think of frailty in a medical context as a combination of factors that influence an individual's physiological state in a manner that reduces reserve and increases vulnerability to external stressors, potentially leading to disability, cognitive impairment, hospitalization, institutionalization, and increased mortality.

Only a subset of older people are frail or are at imminent risk of becoming frail but these groups are important because of their potential for dependency and reduced life expectancy. Frailty also needs to be differentiated from multiple pathologies and from disability although both of the latter types of conditions can cause perioperative issues of their own. Participants in the Paralympics are by definition disabled but could in no way be described as frail.

Despite attempts to reach a consensus there is as yet no single internationally agreed definition of frailty. The majority view from the medical literature is essentially that frailty is the consequence of a collection of biomedical factors which influences an individual's physiological state in such a way as to reduce their capacity to withstand environmental stresses and thereby become dependent. A person who is not frail, on the other hand, can withstand such a stressor without undue sequelae. A surgical procedure could constitute such a stressor. This bio-medical approach has been challenged by others who propose that psychological and sociological factors acting alone or in conjunction with biomedical factors may also lead to dependency. Fig. 30.1 illustrates the proposed pathways.

Models of frailty

Several models of frailty have been proposed but those most often cited in the medical literature are those by Fried and by Rockwood. In Fried's model the presence of three or more of unintended weight loss, tiredness, weak grip strength, slow walking speed, and physical inactivity predicted a range of adverse outcomes including falls, disability, hospitalizations, and death[15]. Fried refers to these elements as a 'phenotype of frailty' and operationalized it using data from the Cardiovascular Health Study (CHS) (Table 30.3).[16]

Fried used follow-up data from the same cohort to validate the predictive ability of the model and another large prospective study[17] supported the concept of the model as a predictor of poor outcomes. Fried reported that people who were categorized as frail using the criteria in (Table 30.1) were at risk of adverse outcomes such as falls disability and death. Further, Fried identified an intermediate group of pre-frail individuals who were at increased risk of becoming frail compared to non-frail counterparts. It is notable

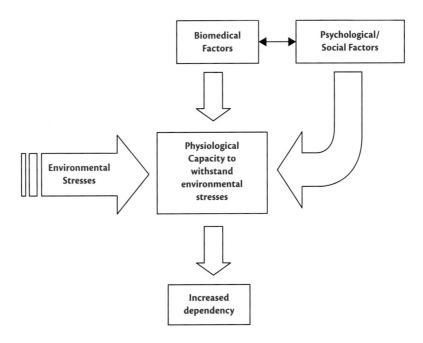

Fig. 30.1 Pathways leading to dependency and frailty.

Table 30.3 The Fried criteria

Characteristic	Measure
Shrinking: weight loss, sarcopenia	Unintentional weight loss: ≥10 lbs, ≥5% body weight in prior year
Weakness	Grip strength, adjusted for gender and BMI
Poor endurance and energy	Self-report exhaustion
Slowness	Slowness: time to walk 15 ft adjusted for gender and standing height
Low physical activity	Weighted score of kilocalories/week

Reproduced from Fried, LP, et al., 'Frailty in older adults: evidence for a phenotype', *Journal of Gerontology, Series A: Biological Sciences and Medical Sciences*, 2001, 56, 3, pp. M146–156, by permission of Oxford University Press and The Gerontological Society of America.

Table 30.4 Indicators/criteria proposed in two alternate frailty measures

Hubbard et al.	Romero-Ortuna et al.
Weight loss >5 kg preceding year (PFI)	Weight loss—self report (PFI)
Grip strength ≤16 kg (PFI)	Grip strength—dynamometer (PFI)
Mini Mental State Examination (MMSE) Score ≤24 (CDI)	Exhaustion—self report (PFI)
Timed get-up-and-go (CDI) ≥17 s	Slowness—self report (PFI)
Forced expiratory volume in 1 s (FEV$_1$) ≤30% (CDI)	Low activity—self report (PFI)

Derived from: Fried's phenotypic frailty index (PFI), Rockwood's cumulative deficit index (CDI).

Data from Hubbard RE, O'Mahony MS, Woodhouse KW. Characterising frailty in the clinical setting a comparison of different approaches. *Age Ageing* 2009; 38 (1):115-9 and Romero-Ortuno R, Walsh CD, Lawlor BA, Kenny RA. A frailty instrument for primary care: findings from the Survey of Health, Ageing and Retirement in Europe (SHARE). *BMC Geriatr* 2010; 10 :57.

that the Fried criteria do not specifically include direct measurements of mental health or psycho-social status which are felt to be an important part of the definition by some clinicians[18,19] and older people themselves[20] and which in a subsequent paper,[21] Fried and colleagues also suggested was related to frailty. In addition some clinicians believe that models/definitions of frailty also need to include association with ageing and inclusion of individual's biological, clinical, and environmental factors.[19,22,23] The 'diagnosis' of frailty by using defined cut-off values is attractive although the Fried criteria are difficult to apply to all groups, e.g. those who are acutely ill and those who are the most dependent. For example a small prospective study characterizing frailty in a clinical setting found that none of a group of continuing care patients (n=30) could perform timed get-up-and-go or 6-minute walk and 13 per cent could not be assessed for grip strength.[24]

An alternative model has been suggested by Rockwood and colleagues in which frailty has been defined as the accumulation of deficits and takes a mathematical approach.[25,26] Essentially Rockwood and colleagues propose that the risk of becoming frail increases with certain deficits. These may be based on multisystem physiological or cognitive changes that need not necessarily reach disease status and can be drawn from clinical data such as symptoms, disease, and laboratory reports. The deficits are on a continuous scale and can be indexed, the more deficits that are present the higher the index and the greater risk of the individual becoming frail. Unlike the Fried model, the Rockwood model allows for mental health or psycho-social issues such as sleep disturbances to be incorporated since the model covers multisystem impairment.[22] Rockwood has further developed the accumulated deficit approach in a recent paper[27] in which he showed that the number of these deficits predicted mortality across the lifespan although, as would be expected, the prevalence of frailty was much lower in younger patients. The deficits approach has not been fully accepted in the clinical setting, possibly due to its complex nature and the authors have tried to address this by introducing a simpler seven-point clinical scale to measure frailty.[28] This latter scale is judgement-based and includes decisions on fitness, wellness, comorbidity, and three levels of frailty based on dependency.

Evidence that the Fried and Rockwood approaches may have similarities can be seen from an analysis of the Women's Health and Aging Studies[29] in which it was found that the number of abnormal physiological systems, based on the measurements of biomarkers (e.g. haemoglobin, inflammatory markers) was associated with an increased risk of frailty in the same way as Rockwood's accumulated deficits.

Although the Fried and Rockwood models have both been validated as predictors of frailty in several studies neither has been entirely accepted. Indeed, Rockwood and colleagues themselves indicated that it may be too early to select one or the other but instead explore both as an aid to further understanding the concept.[30] A study based on the Cardiovascular Health Study (CHS) using a deficit index (DI) and a phenotypic frailty index (PFI)[31] concluded that although the DI better identified susceptibility to death an integration of both indices may increase precision in vulnerable older people. Two studies have compared Fried's PFI and Rockwood's cumulative deficit index (CDI).[30,31] The conclusions are that although each has good predictability for frailty Fried's is easier in the clinical setting and Rockwood's for indicating risk of death and the most vulnerable.

Other studies have proposed alternatives based on one or other of the Fried and Rockwood models but in keeping with clinical practice or geographical location. For example, a UK prospective study of frailty[24] proposed an alternative frailty score consisting of five indicators drawn from the Fried and Rockwood criteria (Table 30.4). The study compared the proposed model with those of Fried and Rockwood in the same cohort. The authors of the study reported that the proposed frailty score correlated highly with both existing measures. Similarly, a recent study aimed at producing an instrument for identifying frailty in European primary care institutions was claimed by the authors to be a valid alternative to the Fried criteria.[32] The authors of this study used the five Fried criteria but in a context that was suited to European primary care institutions and also gender orientated. This was also reported to be consistent with the results of the original Fried study. The outcomes of these two studies in terms of frailty prevalence are discussed briefly in the epidemiology section.

Epidemiology of frailty

Because there is a lack of consensus on what exactly defines frailty the epidemiology of frailty is also unknown accurately. In the original Fried study[15] the overall prevalence of frailty was 6.9 per cent (7.3 per cent females and 4.9 per cent males) with a 4-year incidence of between 7 and 11 per cent depending on cohort. In the latter study women and people of lower socioeconomic status were more likely to be frail. A recent 10-year study[33] of almost 2000 Mexican Americans reported 7.8 per cent frail and 47.3 per cent pre-frail using the Fried criteria. Those categorized as frail or pre-frail at baseline were at greater risk of mortality (odds ratio (OR) 1.8/1.3 respectively) compared to those who were not frail. Another recent study[32] using criteria similar to Fried, reported frailty in 7.3 per cent of women and 3.1 per cent men which was in close agreement to the original Fried study although the overall prevalence in this study was 5.4 per cent compared to 6.9 per cent in the Fried study.

Assessment of frailty in the surgical context

The use of preoperative risk assessment scales such as the Society of Thoracic Surgeons Score (STS), assessment of fitness for anaesthesia and surgery (American Society of Anesthesiologists: ASA grade), and European System for Cardiac Operative Risk Evaluation (EuroSCORE) have been integrated into clinical practice. A criticism of these assessment systems is that they do not take physiological reserve into account leading to overestimated operative risks in healthy older people and underestimated operative risk in frail older patients.[34] Several authors have suggested improving such scales by including biological information from patients or using scales aimed at identifying frailty.

Frailty and surgical outcome

There have been numerous publications reviewing the influence of chronological age on the outcome of surgical procedures. On the other hand there have only been a few papers which have investigated the link between frailty and outcome. This is not surprising given the relative newness of the frailty concept and the unresolved issues that surround its definition. However, where frailty has been investigated it has been shown to influence outcome and may be a more powerful predictor than the more standard risk assessment scales mentioned earlier.

Dasgupta et al.[35] examined the validity of the Edmonton Rating Scale as a predictor of postoperative complication risk in patients undergoing non-cardiac elective surgery (mainly orthopaedic). Frailty was assessed preoperatively using the Edmonton rating Scale which is a composite measure recording cognition, health status, function, social support, medicine use, nutrition, mood, continence, and mobility. The scale itself was developed in medical rather than in surgical patients. The scale runs from 0 to 17 with higher scores indicating worsening frailty. A potentially limiting fact was that postoperative complications were recorded by chart review rather than by direct observation of the patient. In a multiple logistic regression analysis only age and total Edmonton Frailty Score were associated with the chance of developing postoperative complications with ORs of 1.14 (95 per cent CI 1.05–1.24) and 1.22 (95 per cent CI 1.02–1.46) respectively. Both of these variables were also associated with being discharged to an institution and prolonged hospital stay. The authors also found that cut-off scores of <4 and >7 had utility for predicting both lower and higher rates of postoperative complications. The age-adjusted OR (95 per cent confidence intervals) for any complication for the two cut-off scores respectively were 0.27 (0.09–0.80) and 5.02 (1.55–16.25).

A similar composite approach to the recording of frailty was employed by Kristjannson et al.[36] in their study of patients undergoing elective colorectal surgery for cancer. The domains included personal and instrumental activities of daily living, comorbidity, polypharmacy, nutritional status, cognition, and depression. Patients were then classified as fit, intermediate or frail based on whether they met cut-off scores in the individual domains. Details of complications were collected from case notes using a specific case report form and were supplemented by other sources of information as necessary. In bivariate analysis, comprehensive geriatric assessment but not ASA class or age were associated with increased frequency of both serious and any complications. In a multivariate analysis the adjusted odds ratio for severe complications in the frail group were 3.13 (95 per cent CI 1.65–5.92). The relative risk of type of complications including anastomotic leakage, delirium and readmission were also higher in the frail group. In a sub-group of this population, Rønning et al.[37] studied the impact of inflammatory bio-markers on the development of postoperative complications. They found that of the biomarkers studied interleukin (IL)-6 was an independent predictor of severe complications (OR 2.4, 95 per cent CI 1.14–5.06) when adjusted for tumour location and comprehensive geriatric assessment score. They concluded that biomarkers may add validity to comprehensive geriatric assessment in assessing risk for older surgical patients. This topic is expanded upon in the section on immunosenescence.

Sündermann[38] also used an augmented Fried approach to the quantification of frailty. These authors' comprehensive assessment of frailty (CAF) score included the Fried criteria supplemented by measures of physical performance, albumin, creatinine, brain natriuretic peptide, and forced expiratory volume in 1 s (FEV_1). The primary outcome measure was 30-day mortality which was 21.7 per cent, 7.8 per cent, and 3.6 per cent in the severely frail, moderately frail, and not frail groups respectively. The authors commented that the accuracy of the CAF test was as good as but not better than the EuroSCORE and STS tests which were also measured.

A more limited approach to the definition of frailty was employed by Lee et al.[39] who assessed the impact of any ADL impairment (measured by the Katz scale) or mobility restriction or the presence of documented dementia on the primary outcomes on both hospital and post-hospital mortality and institutionalization on adult patients undergoing elective or emergency cardiac surgery. The study centre was the only cardiac surgery centre in the Province and 85 per cent of patients were linked to a provincial database which allowed for post-hospital discharge mortality to be measured. Less than 5 per cent of the total study population were recorded as frail. Unadjusted in-hospital mortality, discharge to an institution and a range of secondary outcomes were all higher in the frail group. For example, unadjusted in-hospital mortality was 4.5 per cent in the non-frail group and 14.7 per cent in the frail group. The percentages of patients discharged home were 91 per cent in the non-frail group compared to only 51 per cent in the frail group.

In the largest of these studies, Makaray et al.[40] classified patients as frail, intermediately frail, or non-frail using the Fried criteria (weight loss, reduced grip strength, tiredness, low physical activity, and slow walking speed) as measured in a preoperative assessment clinic. Three other widely used risk indices (ASA, Lee, and Eagle) were also measured preoperatively. Outcomes were surgical complications, length of stay and discharge to a skilled or assisted-care facility in those previously living at home, although it was not stated whether the latter was on a short-term or a permanent basis. Frailty was an independent risk factor for postoperative complications with odds ratios for intermediately frail patients being 2.06 (95 per cent CI 1.18–3.60) whilst for those classified as frail the odds ratio was 2.64 (95 per cent CI 1.78–2.13). Frailty also predicted length of stay, the odds ratios being 1.69 (95 per cent CI 1.28–2.23) equating to a 65–89 per cent increase in hospitalization. The predictive power for determining transfer to a supported environment was even greater with an odds ratio of 20.48 (5.54–75.68). Even allowing for the wide confidence intervals the predictive power of frailty in predicting place of discharge is impressive. Those who were intermediately frail had lower but still statistically significant increased likelihoods for these eventualities. The inclusion of frailty improved the predictive ability of the other risk indices (ASA, Lee, and Eagle) significantly.

One of the components of the Fried frailty model (slow walking speed) was assessed by Afilalo et al.[41] as a potential predictive factor for poor outcomes in patients over 70 undergoing cardiac surgery. They found that a slow walking speed defined as taking 6 s or more to cover 5 m), was associated with poorer outcomes in terms of mortality, length of stay and discharge to a supported care environment. The odds ratio for a composite endpoint of postoperative mortality and major morbidity was 3.05 (95 per cent CI 1.23–7.54) after adjusting for the STS risk score. 43.2 per cent of patients with a high STS risk score and a slow gait speed experienced a major morbidity or death compared to only 18.9 per cent with a high STS risk score and normal gait speed.

It can be concluded from these studies that frailty appears to have validity as a concept for predicting outcome in surgical patients (Table 30.5).

Immunosenescence and frailty

As shown in Fig. 30.1, biomedical factors have been linked to frailty and may be important in both the initiation of the frailty process and its diagnosis. Proponents of the biomedical model have sought to identify diagnostic markers that may indicate predisposition to individuals becoming frail. Although other markers have been studied the main focus has been on the role of pro-inflammatory markers such as cytokines. However, the potential role of such compounds needs to be seen in the context of normal age-related changes to the immune system and any differences that there are between the frail and non-frail individuals.

There is now strong evidence from multiple sources to indicate that as people age there are associated changes to the immune system that may increase susceptibility to diseases and lower response to vaccines, see Weiskopf et al. for review.[42] The term immunosenescence has been coined to describe the decreased responsiveness in the immune system of older people and it is proposed that viral infections in younger years may predispose to immunosenescence in later life.[43] Interest has been generated by the observation that older people who are sera-positive for cytomegalovirus (CMV) appear to be more at risk of manifesting immune system disorders than CMV negative individuals of the same age group. Independent longitudinal studies of a population-based cohort of the very old in Sweden over a decade have led to the concept of an 'immune risk phenotype' (IRP)[44] that may predict non survival in a similar way to the Fried frailty phenotype. Individuals with this phenotype

had a poor proliferative response, reduced CD4 and increased CD8 lymphocytes (normally a ratio of 1). A similar CD4/CD8 inversion was reported in a UK healthy ageing study[45] where it was associated with an increased risk of death (HR = 1.56) when adjusted for age but not gender. Interestingly, a Swedish follow-on study[46] to the one just described, confirmed the findings of the original and also a prevalence (>90 per cent) of persistent CMV infection in those with the inversion.

IL6, an important pro-inflammatory cytokine, has been termed 'a cytokine for gerontologists'.[47] The reason for this is that from middle age on IL6, normally only detectable when there is infection, becomes detectable in serum in the absence of inflammatory stimuli and concentrations rise with increasing age.

Several studies have reported increases in the acute phase C-reactive protein (CRP) and pro-inflammatory tumour necrosis factor-alpha (TNFα) in older people with or without obvious underlying pathology. However, this is more controversial than the IL6 findings since some studies have not been able to confirm these findings.[48]

The underpinning mechanism for the increase in these pro-inflammatory mediators with age is unclear however, several authors have suggested such factors as a reduction in sex steroids, growth hormones, and vitamin D levels as possible candidates since these may normally regulate IL6.

Taken as a whole, the weight of evidence indicates that there are one or more identifiable changes to the immune systems of older people; we will examine how these changes are associated with frailty. The association of IL6 and many diseases such as Alzheimer's, cancer, and osteoporosis has been well documented.[49] IL6 has also been related to functional decline,[50] higher risk of mortality,[51] and poor physical performance and loss of muscle strength in older people.[52] Taken together these factors broadly fit either of the two main definitions (Fried and Rockwood) of frailty in that they may lead to multiple deficit accumulation and/or weight loss reduced muscle mass and lowered physical activity.

IL6 levels have been reported as being independently associated with frailty (Fried criteria) in two studies.[53,54] CMV seropositivity and increased IL6 levels have also been associated with frailty.[55] Increased CRP levels have been linked to frailty and as a predictor of postoperative complications in older people.[37] Increased levels of IL6, CRP, and TNFα have also been reported with increasing levels of frailty using the Fried criteria.[56] Increased levels of IL6, TNFα, and CRP have also been reported[57,58] with associated declines in muscle mass and strength which have in turn been associated with frailty.

For these reasons increased levels of IL6, CRP, and TNFα amongst others have been actively studied in the frail population in recent years. Hubbard et al.[59] reported that in three different populations of older people with increasing degrees of frailty, both CRP and IL6 significantly increased with greater frailty which in turn was associated with greater reliance on care.

There is an unanswered question surrounding presence of pro-inflammatory markers in older people. Ageing has been described in the literature as successful or unsuccessful. In successful ageing there are no obvious diseases or frailty and in unsuccessful ageing individuals are frail with multiple pathologies. But if there are pro-inflammatory cytokines such as IL6 in the sera of all older people why are some more successful at ageing than others? For now there is no clear answer to this question but there have

Table 30.5 Summary of studies that have investigated the relationship between frailty and outcome

Study	Country	Setting	Number and age of Patients	Definition of frailty	Effect of frailty	Comments
Afilalo et al. (2010)	Canada and USA	Elective cardiac surgery	131 Mean age 75.8 (SD 4.5)	5-metre walking speed	Slow walking speed was an independent risk factor for a composite end point of morbidity/mortality (OR 3.05 95% CI 1.23–7.54)	Only used walking speed as a marker of frailty
Dasgupta et al. (2009)	Canada	Elective non-cardiac surgery	125. Mean age 77 (range 70–92	Edmonton Frailty Score	Independently associated with discharge to an institution and prolonged hospital stay	Age also associated independently with discharge to an institution and prolonged hospital stay Used chart review to record complications
Kristjansson et al. (2010)	Norway	Elective surgery for colorectal cancer	178 Mean age 79.6 (range 70–94)	Fit, intermediate, or frail using criteria based on comprehensive geriatric assessment	Increased risk of serious complications 62% in frail group, and 33% and 36% in fit and intermediate groups respectively	Age and ASA classification not associated with complications
Lee et al. (2011)	Canada	Elective cardiac surgery	3826 Median age frail 66 Median age non-frail 71 Age range (frail and non-frail 15-94	Frailty defined as deficiency in Katz ADL, ambulation or previous diagnosis of dementia	Frailty was independent predictor of in-hospital mortality (odds ratio 1.8, 95% CI 1.1–3.0) and institutional discharge (odds ratio 6.3 95%CI 1.1–2.2).	Includes all ages. Post-discharge mortality also recorded
Makary et al. (2010)	USA	Elective surgery	594 Mean age 72.8 (range 65–94)	Fried criteria	Makary et al. (2010)	Frailty measured by Fried criteria improved predictive power of ASA, Lee, and Eagle score
Sündermann et al. (2011)	Not stated	Elective cardiac surgery	400 Mean age 80.1	Comprehensive assessment of frailty (Fried criteria with additional physical performance and laboratory measurements)	Mortality 21% in severely frail group compared to 7.8% and 3.6% in the moderately and not frail groups respectively	EuroSCORE and STS scores also measured

been some suggestions offered. One is that lifestyle factors such as smoking, obesity and decreased physical activity may in some way leave an individual at risk of increased pro-inflammatory assault that may not occur otherwise.[48] Another is that polymorphisms in pro-inflammatory alleles such as receptors involved in antigen recognition may be involved.[60] So depending on the individual's particular genetic profile successful ageing may occur or onset of disease such as Alzheimer's or atherosclerosis which in turn may contribute to deficits leading to frailty.

Treatment/management of frailty in the surgical setting

There are no evidence-based treatments for the frailty phenotype per se. Any medical interventions are based on the identification of individual components of the syndrome or co-morbidities. These can be identified by comprehensive geriatric assessment as part of the preoperative assessment and, depending on the urgency of the surgical intervention, there may be opportunity to improve a patient's frailty status.

More specific therapies have been suggested. Anti-inflammatory drugs may help to reduce the effects of frailty in cases that are thought to have inflammatory components although the use of these agents needs to be balanced against their increased risk in older people. There is no evidence that such an approach is effective and they cannot be recommended outside the specialist or research setting.

An anabolic approach such as that suggested for cancer patients[61] may be beneficial for frail patients exhibiting low body weight and decreased muscle mass. This integrated approach has increased the chances of successful outcome in cancer patients and involves a triad of nutritional, hormonal, and exercise factors designed for the individual patient. It has also been suggested that a combined approach of anti-inflammatory agents and nutritional support may be beneficial in the treatment of frail older people with cachexia and warrants further study.[62,63]

Finally, many studies on frailty have concluded that exercise can be beneficial for frail subjects. Exercise can help to increase lean muscle mass and improve balance. In addition exercise may also help to lower IL6 levels and so may have an anti-inflammatory component.[64] Since exercise is cheap, efficacious, and readily available it should be part of any therapeutic approach that may be considered and may also be beneficial in postoperative recovery.

Conclusion

The principal driver for the study of frailty in the surgical context has been the concern that neither chronological age nor the existing prognostic scales were sufficiently precise for routine use in assessing postoperative risk. Incorporating measures of frailty, which have been shown to have validity in medical patients, seemed a logical next step for investigation. A range of new and established frailty scores have been shown to predict both complications and mortality. Which, if any, of the scales is the most predictive of risk remains to be determined and it is possible that different frailty scales may be needed in different surgical populations. The incorporation of measures of frailty into preoperative assessment may help medical staff, patients and their families in decision making prior to surgery and to identify patients at greater risk of postoperative complications. In time it may be possible that more specific medical interventions, possibly related to immunological changes may also be developed. It is also important to review the continued validity of any particular frailty score in the light of developments in anaesthetic, surgical, and postoperative care. What may be a reliable prediction score now may not be in 10 years' time. A key aim for the treatment of older people is always the reduction of risk in those identified as being at high risk rather than the identification of high-risk patients being used as continuing justification for non-intervention.

References

1. Office for National Statistics. *National population projections.* Office for National Statistics. <http://www.statistics.gov.uk/cci/nugget.asp?id=1352>
2. Kazumata K, Kamiyama H, Ishikawa T. Reference table predicting the outcome of subarachnoid hemorrhage in the elderly, stratified by age. *J Stroke Cerebrovasc Dis.* 2006;15(1):14–17.
3. Merchant RA, Lui KL, Ismail NH, Wong HP, Sitoh YY. The relationship between postoperative complications and outcomes after hip fracture surgery. *Ann Acad Med Singapore.* 2005;34(2):163–168.
4. Shimada H, Shiratori T, Okazumi S, et al. Surgical outcome of elderly patients 75 years of age and older with thoracic esophageal carcinoma. *World J Surg.* 2007; 31(4):773–779.
5. Palmer RM. Perioperative care of the elderly patient. *Cleve Clin J Med.* 2006;73(Suppl 1):S106–S110.
6. Dodds C, Allison J. Postoperative cognitive deficit in the elderly surgical patient. *Br J Anaesth.* 1998;81(3):449–462.
7. Dalliere O, Blanchon MA, Blanc P, Presles E, Gonthier R. Impact des facteurs de fragilite sur le devenir des sujets ages de 75 ans et plus operes d'une prothese de hanche. *Ann Readapt Med Phys.* 2004;47(9):627–633.
8. Jin F, Chung F. Minimizing perioperative adverse events in the elderly. *Br J Anaesth.* 2001;87(4):608–624.
9. Christmas C, Makary MA, Burton JR. Medical considerations in older surgical patients. *J Am Coll Surg.* 2006;203(5):746–751.
10. Makary MA, Takenaga RK, Pronovost PJ, et al. Frailty in elderly surgical patients: Implications for operative risk assessment. *J Surg Res.* 2006;130(2):212.
11. Crome P, Lally F. Frailty: joining the giants. *CMAJ.* 2011;183(8):889–890.
12. Sheldon JH. *The social medicine of old age: report of an enquiry in Wolverhampton.* London: Oxford University Press for the trustees of the Nuffield Foundation, 1948.
13. Audisio RA, Ramesh H, Longo WE, Zbar AP, Pope D. Preoperative assessment of surgical risk in oncogeriatric patients. *Oncologist.* 2005;10(4):262–268.
14. Herrick C, Steger-May K, Sinacore DR, et al. Persistent pain in frail older adults after hip fracture repair. *J Am Geriatr Soc.* 2004;52(12):2062–2068.
15. Fried LP, Tangen CM, Walston J, et al. Frailty in older adults: evidence for a phenotype. *J Gerontol A Biol Sci Med Sci.* 2001; 56 (3):M146–M157.
16. Fried LP, Borhani NO, Enright P, et al. The Cardiovascular Health Study: design and rationale. *Ann Epidemiol.* 1991;1(3):263–276.
17. Woods NF, LaCroix AZ, Gray SL, et al. Frailty: emergence and consequences in women aged 65 and older in the women's health initiative observational study. *J Am Geriatr Soc.* 2005;53(8):1321–1330.
18. Fillit H, Butler RN. The frailty identity crisis. *J Am Geriatr Soc.* 2009;57(2):348–352.
19. Hogan DB, MacKnight C, Bergman H. Models, definitions, and criteria of frailty. *Aging Clin Exp Res.* 2003;15(3 Suppl):1–29.
20. Puts MTE, Shekary N, Widdershoven G, Heldens J, Deeg DJH. The meaning of frailty according to Dutch older frail and non-frail persons. *J Aging Stud.* 2009;23(4):258–266.
21. Szanton SL, Seplaki CL, Thorpe RJ, Allen JK, Fried LP. Socioeconomic status is associated with frailty: the Women's Health and Aging Studies. *J Epidemiol Community Health.* 2010;64(01):63–67.
22. Rockwood K, Hogan D, MacKnight C. Conceptualisation and measurement of frailty in elderly people. *Drugs Aging.* 2000;17(4):295–302.
23. Walston J, Hadley EC, Ferrucci L, et al. Research agenda for frailty in older adults: toward a better understanding of physiology and etiology: summary from the American Geriatrics Society/National Institute on Aging Research Conference on Frailty in Older Adults. *J Am Geriatr Soc.* 2006;54(6):991–1001.
24. Hubbard RE, O'Mahony MS, Woodhouse KW. Characterising frailty in the clinical setting a comparison of different approaches. *Age Ageing.* 2009;38(1):115–119.
25. Mitnitski AB, Mogilner AJ, Rockwood K. Accumulation of deficits as a proxy measure of aging. *Scientific World Journal.* 2001;1:323–336.
26. Rockwood K, Mitnitski A. Frailty in relation to the accumulation of deficits. *J Gerontol A Biol Sci Med Sci.* 2007;62(7):722–727.
27. Rockwood K, Song X, Mitnitski A. Changes in relative fitness and frailty across the adult lifespan: evidence from the Canadian National Population Health Survey. *CMAJ.* 2011;183(8):E487–E494.
28. Rockwood K, Song X, MacKnight C, et al. A global clinical measure of fitness and frailty in elderly people. *CMAJ.* 2005;173(5):489–495.
29. Fried LP, Xue QL, Cappola AR, et al. Nonlinear multisystem physiological dysregulation associated with frailty in older women: implications for etiology and treatment. *J Gerontol A Biol Sci Med Sci.* 2009;64A(10):1049–1057.
30. Rockwood K, Andrew M, Mitnitski A. A comparison of two approaches to measuring frailty in elderly people. *J Gerontol A Biol Sci Med Sci.* 2007;62(7):738–743.
31. Kulminski AM, Ukraintseva SV, Kulminskaya IV, et al. Cumulative deficits better characterize susceptibility to death in elderly people than phenotypic frailty: lessons from the cardiovascular health study. *J Am Geriatr Soc.* 2008;56(5):898–903.
32. Romero-Ortuno R, Walsh CD, Lawlor BA, Kenny RA. A frailty instrument for primary care: findings from the Survey of Health, Ageing and Retirement in Europe (SHARE). *BMC Geriatr.* 2010;10:57.
33. Graham JE, Snih SA, Berges IM, et al. Frailty and 10-year mortality in community-living Mexican American older adults. *Gerontology.* 2009;55(6):644–651.
34. Chikwe J, Adams DH. Frailty: The missing element in predicting operative mortality. *Semin Thorac Cardiovasc Surg.* 2010;22(2):109–110.

35. Dasgupta M, Rolfson DB, Stolee P, Borrie MJ, Speechley M. Frailty is associated with postoperative complications in older adults with medical problems. *Arch Gerontol Geriatr.* 2001;48(1):78–83.

36. Kristjansson SR, Nesbakken A, Jordhøy MS, *et al.* Comprehensive geriatric assessment can predict complications in elderly patients after elective surgery for colorectal cancer: A prospective observational cohort study. *Crit Rev Oncol Hematol.* 2010;76(3):208–217.

37. Rønning B, Wyller TB, Seljeflot I, *et al.* Frailty measures, inflammatory biomarkers and post-operative complications in older surgical patients. *Age Ageing.* 2010;39(6):758–761.

38. Sündermann S, Dademasch A, Praetorius J, *et al.* Comprehensive assessment of frailty for elderly high-risk patients undergoing cardiac surgery. *Eur J Cardiothorac Surg.* 2011;39(1):33–37.

39. Lee DH, Buth KJ, Martin BJ, Yip AM, Hirsch GM. Frail patients are at increased risk for mortality and prolonged institutional care after cardiac surgery. *Circulation.* 2010;121(8):973–978.

40. Makary MA, Segev DL, Pronovost PJ, *et al.* Frailty as a predictor of surgical outcomes in older patients. *J Am Coll Surg.* 2010;210(6):901–908.

41. Afilalo J, Eisenberg MJ, Morin JF, *et al.* Gait speed as an incremental predictor of mortality and major morbidity in elderly patients undergoing cardiac surgery. *J Am Coll Cardiol.* 2010;56(20):1668–1676.

42. Weiskopf D, Weinberger B, Grubeck-Loebenstein B. The aging of the immune system. *Transpl Int.* 2009;22(11):1041–1050.

43. Pawelec G. Immunosenescence and vaccination. *Immun Ageing.* 2005;2(1):16.

44. Ferguson FG, Wikby A, Maxson P, Olsson J, Johansson B. Immune parameters in a longitudinal study of a very old population of Swedish people: a comparison between survivors and nonsurvivors. *J Gerontol A Biol Sci Med Sci.* 1995;50(6):B378–B382.

45. Huppert FA, Pinto EM, Morgan K. Survival in a population sample is predicted by proportions of lymphocyte subsets. *Mech Ageing Dev.* 2003;124(4):449–451.

46. Wikby A, Ferguson F, Forsey R, *et al.* An immune risk phenotype, cognitive impairment, and survival in very late life: impact of allostatic load in Swedish octogenarian and nonagenarian humans. *J Gerontol A Biol Sci Med Sci.* 2005;60(5):556–565.

47. Ershler WB. Interleukin-6: a cytokine for gerontologists. *J Am Geriatr Soc.* 1993;41(2):176–181.

48. Krabbe KS, Pedersen M, Bruunsgaard H. Inflammatory mediators in the elderly. *Exp Gerontol.* 2004;39(5):687–699.

49. Ershler WB, Keller ET. Age-associated increased interleukin-6 gene expression, late-life diseases, and frailty. *Ann Rev Med.* 2000;51:245–270.

50. Cohen HJ, Pieper CF, Harris T, Rao KM, Currie MS. The association of plasma IL-6 levels with functional disability in community-dwelling elderly. *J Gerontol A Biol Sci Med Sci.* 1997;52(4):M201–M208.

51. Harris TB, Ferrucci L, Tracy RP, *et al.* Associations of elevated interleukin-6 and c-reactive protein levels with mortality in the elderly. *Am J Med.* 1999;106(5):506–512.

52. Cesari M, Penninx BWJH, Pahor M, *et al.* Inflammatory markers and physical performance in older persons: the InCHIANTI Study. *J Gerontol A Biol Sci Med Sci.* 2004;59(3):M242–M248.

53. Leng SX, Xue QL, Tian J, Walston JD, Fried LP. Inflammation and frailty in older women. *J Am Geriatr Soc.* 2007;55(6):864–871.

54. Leng SX, Tian X, Matteini A, *et al.* IL-6-independent association of elevated serum neopterin levels with prevalent frailty in community-dwelling older adults. *Age Ageing.* 2011;40(4):475–481.

55. Schmaltz HN, Fried LP, Xue QL *et al.* Chronic cytomegalovirus infection and inflammation are associated with prevalent frailty in community-dwelling older women. *J Am Geriatr Soc.* 2005;53(5):747–754.

56. Hubbard R, O'Mahony M, Calver B, Woodhouse K. Plasma esterases and inflammation in ageing and frailty. *Eur J Clin Pharmacol.* 2008;64(9):895–900.

57. Schaap LA, Pluijm SMF, Deeg DJH, Visser M. Inflammatory markers and loss of muscle mass (sarcopenia) and strength. *Am J Med.* 2006;119(6):526.

58. Schaap LA, Pluijm SMF, Deeg DJH, *et al.* higher inflammatory marker levels in older persons: associations with 5-year change in muscle mass and muscle strength. *J Gerontol A Biol Sci Med Sci.* 2009;64A(11):1183–1189.

59. Hubbard RE, O'Mahony MS, Calver BL, Woodhouse KW. Nutrition, inflammation, and leptin levels in aging and frailty. *J Am Geriatr Soc.* 2008;56(2):279–284.

60. Balistreri C, Colonna-Romano G, Lio D, Candore G, Caruso C. TLR4 polymorphisms and ageing: implications for the pathophysiology of age-related diseases. *J Clin Immunol.* 2009;29(4):406–415.

61. Langer CJ, Hoffman JP, Ottery FD. Clinical significance of weight loss in cancer patients: rationale for the use of anabolic agents in the treatment of cancer-related cachexia. *Nutrition.* 2001;17(1, Suppl 1):S1–S21.

62. Hubbard RE, O'Mahony MS, Calver BL, Woodhouse KW. Nutrition, inflammation, and leptin levels in aging and frailty. *J Am Geriatr Soc.* 2008;56 (2):279–284.

63. Baracos VE. Cancer-associated cachexia and underlying biological mechanisms. *Annu Rev Nutr.* 2006;26:435–461.

64. Taaffe DR, Harris TB, Ferrucci L, Rowe J, Seeman TE. Cross-sectional and prospective relationships of interleukin-6 and C-reactive protein with physical performance in elderly persons: MacArthur studies of successful aging. *J Gerontol A Biol Sci Med Sci.* 2000;55(12):M709–M715.

CHAPTER 31

Anaesthesia in the elderly obese

Samuel R. Grodofsky and Ashish C. Sinha

Introduction

The global prevalence of obesity and overweight has reached pandemic levels.[1] The standard Western diet is characterized by affordable, enticing, accessible and calorically dense food and this is combined with predominantly sedentary lifestyles. This cultural paradigm has been made possible by modern industrial advances, but it has resulted in unheralded imbalances between caloric intake and energy expenditure. Unfortunately, the human body does not have effective means of metabolizing and storing these excess calories. Increased adiposity is linked to the development of various chronic diseases such as diabetes, hypertension, coronary artery disease, and many more. It may be appropriate to consider obesity as a disease itself.[2] A tremendous amount of healthcare services are dedicated to these problems. It has been estimated that the United States spends about $150 billion annually to care for obesity-related health issues.[3] As populations continue to grow older, the prevalence of obesity in the elderly has also grown. In 1960–1962, the prevalence of obesity in people aged 65–74 in the United States was estimated at 10.4 per cent and this trend increased to 33.4 per cent between 1999 and 2002 according to the National Health and Nutrition Examination Surveys (NHANES).[4]

In the past, patients with the excesses of age and weight were not considered as elective operative candidates. There is some evidence to support this claim, as Medicare patients over the age of 65 years of age has been identified to increase the risk of adverse events in patients undergoing bariatric surgery in multiple centres,[5] however, it is met with conflicting data[6] and is currently not an accepted contraindication to the procedure. The combined stress of ageing and increased body mass present a distinct set of technical and multi-organ system problems to anaesthetists. This chapter will review the pathophysiology and important considerations related to obesity in the elderly and its pertinent anaesthetic care.

Assessing fat deposition in the elderly

The body mass index (BMI) or Quetelet index is an inexpensive and broadly accepted approximation of an individual's body fat based on height and weight. It was devised in the nineteenth century as a tool to conduct population-based studies, but has since crept into clinical practice. It is defined as weight (kg) divided by the square of height (m²). The World Health Organization (WHO) has stratified individuals to underweight (BMI $\leq$18.5 kg/m²), normal weight (BMI 18.5–24.9 kg/m²), overweight (BMI 25–29.9 kg/m²), obese class I (BMI 30–34.9 kg/m²), obese class II or morbidly obese (BMI 35–39.9 kg/m²) and obese class III or ultra/extreme obese (BMI $\geq$40 kg/m²) (see Table 31.1). It is a useful metric in the clinical setting because a male patient who is 5′3″ (160 cm) and weighs 230 lbs (104 kg) (BMI 40.7 kg/m²) presents greater challenges to the anaesthetist than another patient of the same weight but is 6′2″ (188 cm) (BMI 29.5 kg/m²).

Epidemiological surveys have shown a positive linear relationship with the prevalence of obesity and age from 20 to 60 years of age and then a subsequent decline after this period. In fact, the prevalence of obesity in 80 year olds is half the rate of those aged 50–59 years.[7] These observational, cross-sectional studies are clearly influenced by a survival advantage for patients with a BMI less than 35 m/kg².[8] Nevertheless, longitudinal cohort studies have shown modest declines in BMI as the elderly are followed over time despite concomitant declines in height due to vertebral body compression.[9,10]

There are substantial changes in body composition and metabolism as a person ages. The basal metabolic rate declines in the elderly.[11] This is partly due to decreased physical activity but also to other biological changes that occur with age such as decreased serum testosterone and growth hormone levels, decreased responsiveness to thyroid hormone and resistance to leptin.[7] The elderly demonstrate a lower ratio of lean body mass to adipose tissue. After the age of 20–30 years old, lean body mass primarily from skeletal muscle progressively declines, with a 40 per cent decrease from 20 to 70 years of age. At the same time, fat mass increases with age and reaches its highest levels between 60 and 70 years of age.[7,12] (See Fig. 31.1.) There are also marked changes in fat distribution with an

Table 31.1 WHO body mass index classification

Classification	BMI (kg/m²)
Underweight	<18.5
Normal weight	18.5–24.9
Overweight	25–29.9
Obese Class I	30–34.9
Obese Class II (morbidly obese)	35–39.9
Obese Class III (Ultra obese)	>40

Reproduced with permission from World Health Organization.

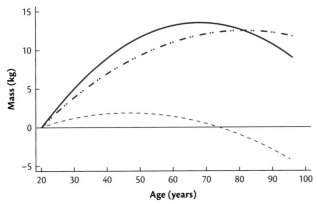

Fig. 31.1 Model of the longitudinal changes in body mass (—), fat mass (– – – – –) and lean body mass (– –). Reproduced from Villareal, D.T., Apovian, C.M., Kushner, R.F., Klein, S., American Society for Nutrition & NAASO, T.O.S. 2005, 'Obesity in older adults: technical review and position statement of the American Society for Nutrition and NAASO, The Obesity Society', *Obesity*, 13, 11, pp. 1849–1863, Copyright 2005 North American Association for the Study of Obesity (NAASO), with permission.

increased deposition of visceral fat (omental and mesenteric), subcutaneous abdominal fat, intramuscular fat and intrahepatic fat, which all increase the risk for insulin resistance and metabolic diseases.[13,14] There are also gender differences with respect to age-related adipose accumulation as post-menopausal women tend to demonstrate a greater tendency to increase fat compared to men.[4,15]

Returning to the use of BMI as a proxy for a person's 'fatness', this index has been argued to be an unsatisfactory clinical tool, especially for the elderly.[15] Age-dependent changes may reflect a lower mass, but increased adiposity leading to various metabolic problems that cannot be measured by BMI. In addition, studies have shown no increase in operative mortality in overweight and moderately obese elderly based on BMI.[16,17] There are more quantitative techniques such as CT scan or bio-impedence measurements that can provide a more precise measure of both adipose tissue and lean body mass. In addition, approximation of the level of central obesity by measurement of the waist circumference, or waist:hip circumference ratio, is a better indicator of morbidity and mortality when compared to BMI.[18,19]

Metabolic syndrome

The metabolic syndrome is a constellation of chronic health illnesses related to the abnormal accumulation of adipose tissue. There are several diagnostic criteria recommended by various organizations (see Table 31.2) but all incorporate the presence of insulin resistance, central obesity, dyslipidaemia and hypertension. The aetiology of metabolic syndrome is poorly understood. It has been described as a complex interaction involving high levels of circulating free fatty acids, the accumulation of lipid in non-adipose cells, increase in local and systemic inflammatory markers (CRP, TNF-α, IL-6, homocystein) decreased insulin sensitivity with reduced function of adiponectin and leptin that are involved in insulin sensitivity and tissue fuel oxidation.[20] In the latter, adiponectin levels become reduced, while leptin levels are increased due to resistance.

The development of the metabolic syndrome increases with ageing. In fact, in people aged 65 years or older, the prevalence of obesity defined by BMI ≥30 is estimated at 33 per cent while metabolic syndrome has been reported as >40 per cent.[20] Metabolic syndrome, when compared to isolated obesity, has been associated with a greater risk of coronary artery disease, hypercoagulability, pulmonary dysfunction, and obstructive sleep apnoea.[21] (The significance of this phenomenon means that the insidious metabolic effects of adipose tissue may be present in patients with a BMI <30 kg/m^2 and go unrecognized, especially in the elderly.)

Airway

Maintaining airway patency during all aspects of perioperative care is one of the major anaesthetic difficulties of patients with a large body habitus. Age greater than 55 years old and BMI ≥ 30 kg/m^2 are independent predictors of difficult mask ventilation.[22–24] There is no consensus of agreement that BMI is an independent predictor for difficult intubation with some studies claiming an increased risk[25,26] and others refuting one.[27–29] This controversy may be related to positioning as the conventional 'sniff' position cannot be achieved in morbidly obese patients with excessive accumulation of fat tissue in the suboccipital and nuchal area.[30] Instead, patients with a large body habitus should

Table 31.2 Diagnostic Criteria for metabolic syndrome according to the International Diabetes Federation (IDF, 2006), National Cholesterol Education Program Adult Treatment Panel (NCEP ATP, 2001) and the World Health Organization (WHO, 1999)

Criteria	Diagnostic criteria	Central obesity	Insulin resistance*	Lipid profile*	Hypertension	Others
IDF (2006)	Ethnicity specific waist circumference values and ≥ t2 of the following:	Waist circumference: M≥94 cm, F ≥80 cm	Fasting glucose > 100 or diagnosis of diabetes mellitus type II	HDL M <40, F <50 or treatment of HDL dyslipidaemia	SAP >130, or DAP >85, or previous treatment of hypertension	
NCEP ATP (2001)	≥3 of the following:	Waist circumference: M> 102 cm, F >88 cm	Fasting glucose >110	TG >150, HDK: M <40, F <50	SAP >130, or DAP >85	
WHO (1999)	Diabetes mellitus or insulin resistance and ≥2 of the following:	Waist-to-hip ratio M >0.9, F >0.85, BMI >30		TG >150 and/or HDL: M <35, F <39	> 140/90	Urine Alb >20 mcg/min or Alb: Cr ≥30 mg/g

Data from K. G. M. M. Alberti, P. Zimmet, J. Shaw Metabolic syndrome—a new world-wide definition. A Consensus Statement from the International Diabetes Federation 20 APR 2006, National Cholesterol Education Program National Heart, Lung, and Blood Institute, National Institutes of Health NIH Publication No. 01-3670 May 2001, and Alberti, KGMM; Zimmet). Definition, Diagnosis, and Classification of Diabetes Mellitus and its Complications World Health Organization 1999 pp. 32–33.

be positioned in the 'ramped' position with the head, shoulders and upper body elevated above the chest. In one series, patients presenting for bariatric bypass surgery undergoing direct laryngoscopy with a ramp have shown no relationship with BMI and difficult intubation.[29] While an awake fibreoptic intubation may not be necessary, there is some suggestion that videoscopic intubation in obese patients provides a better visualization of the larynx and facilitates intubation.[31]

There is conflicting evidence as to whether morbidly obese patients are at a greater risk for gastric aspiration upon induction and intubation as various studies have refuted or demonstrated a higher rate of gastro-oesophageal reflux, increased gastric volume and decreased pH in the stomach.[32–34] The decision to employ rapid sequence induction to reduce the risk of aspiration should be based on the preoperative evaluation of known factors such as gastro-oesophageal reflux or recent oral intake, rather than obesity alone.

Obstructive sleep apnoea (OSA) is a common sleep disorder that is caused by occlusion of the airway by soft tissue when the negative pressure generated by inspiratory muscles exceeds the positive pressure from pharyngeal dilator musculature.[35] OSA is diagnosed by physiological monitoring during sleep which may extend to full polysomnography, where, various measures factor into an apnoea/hypopnea index (AHI) that describe the total number of apnoeic (complete cessation of airflow lasting ≥ 10 seconds) or hypoponeic (>50 per cent reduction of airflow lasting ≥ 10 seconds) episodes divided by the total sleep time. OSA can be classified as mild with an AHI of 5–15 events per hour, moderate 15–30 events per hour, or severe >30 events per hour. Increased AHI has been associated with age, BMI and waist:hip ratio among other factors. Men, especially with a BMI ≥ 35 typically demonstrate an increased risk during adulthood with respect to women, yet at age 60 years or older, obese men and women show a similar risk of OSA.[36] With obesity, fat deposits may reduce the diameter of the airway and favour collapsibility and the elderly are predisposed to a reduced upper airway muscle tone. In addition, the inflammatory effects of adipose tissue have been speculated to contribute to the development of OSA. The influence of hypnotics, narcotics, and sedatives provide further depression of these airway reflexes.[35]

A related sleep disorder to OSA is obesity hypoventilation syndrome (OHS), which is characterized by the combination of obesity (BMI >30 kg/m^2) and awake hypercapnia (PaCO$_2$ >45 mmHg). The exact aetiology of OHS is not fully elucidated, but there is a blunting of the brainstem central chemoreceptors and diminished responsiveness to both hypercapnia and hypoxia. As a result, these patients may demonstrate a compensatory polycythaemia and renal retention of bicarbonate.[37]

Most patients with OSA are undiagnosed and many have limited access to overnight physiological monitoring and therefore a clinical diagnosis and effective treatment. The 'STOP-BANG' questionnaire is a useful tool that asks patients about the presence of snoring, tiredness during daytime, observed apnoea, high blood pressure. This is then combined with the following factors: BMI >35 kg/m^2, age >50 years old, neck circumference >40 cm, and male gender. The presence of three or more of these features is a sensitive indicator for a high probability for OSA (see Table 31.3).[38,39] Preoperative care is centred on the use of continuous positive airway pressure (CPAP) therapy that for at least a month before surgery is scheduled and that should be demonstrated to be both effective and that

Table 31.3 STOP BANG Questionnaire

Snore	Have you been told that you snore?
Tired	Are you often tired during the day?
Obstruction	Has anyone witnessed an episode where you stopped breathing while you were asleep?
Pressure	Do you have high blood pressure?
BMI	BMI >35 kg/m^2
Age	Age >50 years
Neck	Neck circumference >40 cm
Gender	male gender

Reproduced from Ogunnaike, B.O., et al., 'Anesthetic considerations for bariatric surgery', *Anesthesia and Analgesia*, 95, 6, pp. 1793–1805, with permission from International Anesthesia Research Society and Wolters Kluwer.

the patient is compliant. Immediate preanaesthetic management includes pre-oxygenation with either the home CPAP settings or pressure support with 10 cmH$_2$O and positive end expiratory pressure (PEEP) of 5 cmH$_2$O and then intubation in the ramped position. There is no strong evidence to justify the routine use of awake fibreoptic intubation unless other signs of difficult intubation are present.[29,40] More problematic complications present in the postoperative care as patients with OSA are at higher risk to hypoxaemia, ICU transfers and longer hospital stays.[41] In particular, patients with OSA are very sensitive to the respiratory depressing effects of anaesthetic medications which are compounded in the elderly. It is important to reduce high doses of opiate use during the operative period, by utilizing a multi-modal analgesia.

Pulmonary

There are multiple age-related declines in pulmonary function that are further diminished as a result of obesity creating a tendency to oxygen desaturation and hypercapnia. This requires constant vigilance during all the stages of perioperative care.

Obesity is a well demonstrated cause of restrictive respiratory physiology. There is a linear relationship between BMI and reductions in total lung capacity (TLC) and vital capacity (VC) and an exponential relationship with BMI and reductions in functional residual capacity (FRC) and expiratory reserve volume (ERV).[42] In obese patients, TLC is reduced due to the limitations of inspiratory lung inflation caused by the static load of extra adipose tissue on the rib cage, abdomen, and thorocoabdomnial viscera and when supine increased abdominal pressure preventing diaphragamatic excursion. FRC is determined by the equilibrium between the inward elastic recoil of lung parenchyma and the outward elastic expansion of the chest wall. In obese elderly patients, the compliance of both components is affected. With increasing age, diminished elastic recoil related to a decrease in elastic fibres and changes in crosslinking and fibre orientation leads to reductions of pulmonary compliance.[43] In obesity, decreases in pulmonary compliance have been well demonstrated and it has been felt that this was related to an increase in total blood volume in the lung and closure of dependent alveoli.[44–48] These studies have shown no or a small relationship with BMI and chest wall compliance but there are other studies that have shown that decreases in total respiratory compliance are a result of chest wall rigidity.[48] Age, however, has been demonstrated to increase chest wall stiffness due to age-related changes in shape, calcification and articulations of the rib cage.[49,50]

In obese elderly patients, as FRC approaches residual volume, the external pleural pressure may be greater than internal airway pressure which leads to a tendency towards alveolar collapse. This process has also been described as an increase in closing capacity, where both elderly and obese patients are greatly predisposed to atelectasis and air trapping. In fact, the closing capacity may be increased (or described in another way, FRC reduced) to the point that atelectasis occurs with tidal volume breathing.[51,52] Under anaesthesia, the loss of diaphragmatic tone and increased intra-abdominal pressure along with structural forces from the thoracic spine and rib cage places a greater load on the dependent lung regions.[45] This decreased ventilation of persistently perfused lung segments leads to venous blood mixing and ultimately oxygen desaturation. In addition, as dependent segments close, there is a shift in regional ventilation as gas is preferentially distributed to the poorly perfused upper lung zones, leading to further ventilation–perfusion mismatch.[53–55]

Hypoxaemia occurs more frequently in obese patients despite preoxygenation.[26] There are several approaches that may be taken to reduce desaturation upon induction. During pre-induction denitrogenation, the use of CPAP or pressure support ventilation with PEEP, as described for airway management of OSA, may decrease atelectatic lung tissue and has been shown to increase the non-hypoxic apnoeic time.[56,57] Ventilator strategies employed to reduce atelectasis and pulmonary shunts have also been demonstrated. The use of room air to create a fractional inspired oxygen ratio of 0.3–0.4 may prevent the early formation of atelectasis.[58,59] The ventilator should be set to achieve a tidal volume of 6–10 mL/kg of ideal body weight with a PEEP of 5–10 cm H_2O.[60–63] Atelectasis can be decreased in obese patients through alveolar recruitment manoeuvres, which is performed under manual ventilation mode by holding pressure on the bag with the pressure release valve partially closed to achieve static vital capacity tidal volumes for a certain period of time.[58,61,64,65] The exact protocol for vital capacity manoeuvres varies between studies, but it has been suggested, and it is the practice at our institution, to hold 30 cm H_2O for 30 seconds in normovolaemic patients.[66]

Postoperative care is complicated by the impaired work of breathing and respiratory drive associated with ageing and obesity. Obese patients have decreased power from their respiratory musculature that may be related to increased adipose tissue deposition and from overloading diaphragm muscle fibres leading to length-tension inefficiency.[67,68] Age related declines in respiratory muscle function and decreased physical condition further diminish spontaneous negative pressure respiratory mechanics.[69] As a result, the breathing patterns are typically characterized by an increased respiratory rate and decreased tidal volume. Obese and elderly patients are also particularly sensitive to the respiratory depressing effects of opiates, benzodiazepines, volatile agents, and paralytics and require careful dosing particularly at the end of a case. Patients should have monitored, full reversal of neuromuscular blocking agents and be weaned off of pressure support ventilation before being placed on spontaneous ventilation mode. Upon extubation and during recovery, the patient should be placed in the beach chair or reverse Trendelenburg position to allow for gravitational forces to assist in generating adequate tidal volumes. All patients with OSA should have their CPAP support from the time of extubation, with supplemental oxygen as required. There must be great vigilance in monitoring for signs of respiratory distress such as the use of accessory

Table 31.4 Airway and respiratory management recommendations

Pre-induction

- High suspicion of OSA, use STOP-BANG questionnaire
- CPAP therapy in holding area or in operating room denitrogenation

Induction

- Ramp positioning
- Reduce apnoeic time
- Prepare for difficult mask ventilation
- Unclear recommendations for routine fibreoptic or video laryngoscopes

Maintenance

- Use of 6–10 ml/kg of ideal body weight plus 5–10 mmHg of PEEP
- Use room air combination of gas with an FIO_2 goal of 0.4 as tolerated
- Perform alveolar recruitment manoeuvres periodically during case

Extubation

- Extubate in back up or reverse Trendelenburg position
- Wean off pressure support ventilation only after full reversal of paralytic
- Low threshold to use Bousignac CPAP mask in PACU or immediately after extubation
- Aggressive monitoring for decreased respiratory drive due to residual anaesthetics

neck muscles or paradoxical chest movement. Aggressive chest physical therapy and a low threshold to employ CPAP or other non-invasive respiratory support are valuable strategies to employ during PACU care.[62] Recommendations of perioperative airway and respiratory management are listed in Table 31.4.

Cardiac

Obesity and ageing are linked to an increased risk of developing dyslipidaemia, coronary artery disease, cardiac arrhythmias, hypertension, cerebrovascular disease, peripheral vascular disease, and congestive heart failure.[7] While the pathophysiology of these disease processes and their impact on anaesthetic care is well described, there are unique cardiac abnormalities specific to obesity. This includes obesity cardiomyopathy, the increase risk of sudden cardiac death and the increased survivorship phenomenon described as the obesity paradox.

Adipose tissue is metabolically active and demands significant vascularization. Obese patients have a rise in total body blood volume and necessarily, increased stroke volume and cardiac output from Frank–Starling forces due to an increased stretch of myocardial fibres. With a greater preload, there also comes an increased afterload as the link between obesity and hypertension is well known and exerts its effects from multiple pathways. The excessive mass of adipose tissue exerts a physical compression on the kidneys which leads to increased renal sodium reabsorption and may explain the associated risk of chronic kidney disease. In addition, by incompletely understood mechanisms, adipose tissue exerts a hormonal influence by activation of the sympathetic nervous system and renin–angiotensin–aldosterone system that further impairs pressure natriuresis.[70–72]

These physiological changes raise transmural stress placed on the left and possibly right ventricle leading to a dilation of tissue. Over time this may lead to a compensatory eccentric hypertrophy of the myocardium, which typically keeps ejection fraction within normal limits if the level of hypertrophy keeps pace with the amount of dilatation. Adipocytes also influence serum hormone levels, such as various cytokines, angiotensin-II, leptin, resisten, and others which may further lead to myocyte hypertrophy and the development of interstitial fibrosis.[73] This may result in a diastolic dysfunction, or if the hypertrophy is unable to match the increased wall stress, then systolic dysfunction with an elevation in pulmonary arterial pressures and/or central venous pressures.[74] In addition, the effects of chronic hypoxia related to OSA and OHS elevate pulmonary vascular resistance which may lead to, or contribute to, right ventricular dysfunction. The development of these hypertropic changes has been described as obesity cardiomyopathy.[75]

In addition to ventricular strain as evidenced by heart failure, there is an associated atrial dilation and this accounts for the higher prevalence of atrial fibrillation and other dysthymias found in obesity. In fact, it has been demonstrated that obesity increased the risk of atrial fibrillation by 49 per cent and that this risk shows a direct relationship with BMI.[76] The ventricular pathological changes in addition to abnormalities in sympathovagal balance, leads to increased cardiac electrical excitability. Obesity is related to a higher heart rate and more frequent and complex dysthymias.[77] In fact, the Framingham Heart Study has shown a 40 times higher rate of sudden cardiac death in in obese patients.[78]

It is quite clear that the accumulative effects of excessive adiposity and weight lead to a significant predisposition to cardiovascular morbidities. Yet, evidence from multiple observational studies has demonstrated surprisingly greater survival in overweight and moderately obese patients with hypertension,[17] heart failure,[79–81] and coronary artery disease.[82,83] This phenomenon has also been replicated in surgical patients undergoing coronary artery bypass surgery.[84,85] It appears that this relationship between longevity and body habitus shows a U-shaped distribution with the underweight and morbidly obese having the poorest prognoses. This phenomenon has been described as the obesity paradox and it is clearly present in the elderly as well.[16,86,87] Although it is quite possible this may be a statistical anomaly caused by the increased mortality in patients with unintentional weight loss from other morbid conditions, but it has generated speculation into a protective cardiovascular effect of obesity.[74,88]

Currently, there are no specific recommendations for anaesthetic care to address cardiovascular abnormalities due to obesity in the elderly as an independent phenomenon. Nevertheless, during preoperative evaluation, it seems prudent that anaesthetists should have a high index of suspicion for the presence of cardiovascular comorbidities.

Renal

While obesity related chronic diseases such as hypertension and type 2 diabetes are known risk factors for the development of chronic kidney disease, obesity in itself has been etiologically linked to renal damage. In fact, after adjusting for co-factors, obesity demonstrated a threefold increase in the risk of developing chronic kidney disease.[89] The mechanisms of renal damage may be due to an increased excretory load due to the increased body mass leading to glomerular capillary hypertension, hyperinsulinaemia leading to preglomerular vasodilation that worsens glomerular hypertension and lipotoxicity from excess adipose tissue. These adverse physiological adaptations are related to the development of proteinuria,

glomerulomegaly, tubular interstitial nephritis and obesity-related focal segmental glomerulosclerosis.[20] These effects are cumulative and elderly patients with a long history of obesity are more likely to manifest renal insufficiency. Kidney dysfunction also affects dosing frequencies of renally cleared drugs.[90] Medications with renally cleared harmful metabolites such as meperidine should be avoided. In addition, the amount of crystalloid fluid administered should be carefully monitored to avoid fluid overload.

Hepatological

Obesity is associated with extremely high rates of non-alcoholic fatty liver disease (NAFLD), which has been measured in up to 80–90 per cent of patients. NAFLD describes a spectrum of liver pathology from fat accumulation (hepatic steatosis) to the more advanced steatohepatitis which is characterized by inflammatory changes that can progress to fibrosis and cirrhosis. The gold standard for diagnosis is a liver biopsy, although imaging by CT scan or ultrasonography can be performed if abnormal synthetic liver function or elevated liver aminotransferaces are present. Extensive liver pathology can affect the metabolism of certain medications and should be recognized by anaesthetists.[91]

Endocrine

It has been thought that age is an independent risk factor for the development of type 2 diabetes mellitus and glucose intolerance; however data has demonstrated that this association is more specifically linked to abdominal obesity rather than healthy ageing.[92] Obesity-associated type 2 diabetes is related to insulin insensitivity in the liver and skeletal muscles with a resultant increase in insulin synthesis that eventually fails to bring euglycaemia. Excessive adipocyte deposition in the liver and skeletal muscle is associated with chronic inflammatory cytokine production including tumour necrosis factor-α, interleukin-6 (IL6), and interleukin-1β (IL1β) that have been implicated in the decreased sensitivity to insulin.[93] The subsequent hyperglycaemia leads to vascular and neural damage which increases the risk for myocardial ischemia, cerebrovascular infarction, renal ischemia and postoperative pain due to neuropathies.

Musculoskeletal and neurological

Age and obesity are well-known constitutional factors for the development of fractures, osteoarthritis and soft-tissue injury.[94,95] The excessive loading from increased weight stresses bones and joints leading to the development of these orthopaedic disorders, however other poorly understood factors related to biomechanics and bone metabolism contribute to the predisposition of obese patients to the development of joint disorders.[95,96] There is strong data demonstrating a positive relationship with body mass and bone mineral density and a decreased incidence of osteoporosis and hip fractures.[97–99] This has been suggested to be related to both increased bone turnover and the hormonal influences through oestrogen conversion in adipose tissue.[100] Recent studies have shown no statistically significant increase in mortality or complication rate from total hip replacements with morbidly obese patients based on BMI.[101,102] However, other studies have identified age and increased BMI as risk factors for adverse events, but not in mortality.[103]

With the increased incidence of musculoskeletal disorders in the obese and elderly, there exists a predisposition to pain, both chronic and acute. In a cohort of elderly subjects, chronic pain was found twice as likely with moderate obesity (BMI 30–34.9) and four times with severe obesity (BMI >35).[104] While the source of pain is related to musculoskeletal degeneration, obesity also carries an increased risk for neuropathic pain[105] and migraine headaches.[106]

Haematological

Obesity and age are independent risk factors for the development of deep vein thromboembolism (DVT).[107-110] Patients who have limited physical activity, nursing home residents and those with symptomatic congestive heart failure have an added risk factor due to venous stasis. Surgery, particularly orthopaedic hip, knee, spine and oncological procedures are associated with a higher incidence of DVT. When clinically allowable, patients should receive mechanical compression stockings and prophylactic heparin therapy, either low-molecular-weight heparin (LMWH) or unfractionated heparin.[111] Dosing poses a particular concern in obese patients. LMWH uses weight-based dosing and in the severely obese weighing more than 190 kg, there is a theoretical concern that due to a non-linear relationship between intravascular volume and total body weight, these patients may pose an increased risk of bleeding. It has been considered reasonable to test anti-factor Xa activity 4 hours after administration.[112] It has also been suggested that for certain procedures, particularly orthopaedic, regional anaesthesia as an alternative to general anaesthesia may provide an additional protection against venous thromboembolism.[111] It has been recommended that with the diagnosis of a DVT, elective surgery should be delayed for up to 1 month and the patient placed on anticoagulant therapy in the interim.[113]

Pharmacology

Obesity affects the pharmacokinetics and pharmacodynamics primarily by alterations of the volume of distribution through increases in lean and fat body weight and increases in cardiac output and by alterations in drug clearance. Morbidly obese patients are typically excluded from clinical trials making little data available for optimal dosing. Dosing based on total body weight in obese patients may lead to excessive administration of anaesthetics that especially with elderly patients may lead to undesirable effects such as hypotension or respiratory depression.

Drug distribution is different in the morbidly obese as the fat tissue increases proportionally with total body weight (TBW), while lean body weight decreases proportionally despite an overall weight increase. Age-related changes further compound this affect. While the use of an adjusted body weight (ABW) scale has been commonly used for dosing to correct for these metabolic changes, the estimation of lean body weight (LBW) has been demonstrated to be the optimal weight scale in morbidly obese patients.[114-116] The equations developed by Janmahasatian et al.[117] have been the most verified in the extremes of obesity are shown as follows:[117]

For males: LBW (kg) = $9270 \times$ weight (kg) / $6680 + 216 \times$ BMI (kg/m^2)

For females: LBW (kg) = $9270 \times$ weight (kg) / $8780 + 244 \times$ BMI (kg/m^2)

The use of routine anaesthetics should be approached with care in obese elderly patients. Midazolam has a twofold increased half-life and decreased total clearance in the elderly versus young individuals and obese subjects demonstrated a greater volume of distribution due to adipose deposition which further prolongs the half-life.[118] Propofol is highly lipophilic, but is has been shown that it does not accumulate in morbidly obese patients because clearance and volume of distribution were similar to lean subjects. It has been suggested that induction doses based on LBW be used while maintenance infusions should be based on TBW.[119] Studies have suggested that fentanyl, sufentanil, and remifentanil should be dosed based on lean body weight, but extra care should be taken to titrate the dose to patient need as obesity and advanced age predispose patients to postoperative hypoxia. For neuromuscular blocking agents, it has been suggested that succinylcholine be dosed based on TBW due to increased pseudocholinesterase synthesis, while non-depolarizing agents such as vecuronium, rocuronium, and pancuronium should be dosed on ideal body weight to avoid a prolonged duration of action. Cisatracurium could be dosed based on TBW. Obese patients have classically shown

Table 31.5 Weight-based dosing of common anaesthetic drugs[123]

Drug	Dosing	Comments
Propofol	Induction: LBW Maintenance: TBW	When reaching steady state, clearance (hepatic metabolism) and V$_D$ correlate with TBW
Midazolam	TBW	If used for induction, expect prolonged sedation
Fentanyl	LBW	While the V$_D$ is increased, elimination half-time also increases which places risk for respiratory depression
Sufentanil	Bolus: LBW Maintenance: LBW	There is increased distribution in excess body mass, however elimination half-time is increased
Remifentanil	Bolus: LBW Maintenance: LBW	
Succinylcholine	TBW	Plasma cholinesterase activity is increased with body mass
Vecuronium, Rocuronium, Pancuronium	LBW	Alterations of clearance may predispose to prolonged recovery
Cisatracurium, atracurium	TBW	Metabolism by organ-independent processes allows for unaltered dose per body weight dosing

TBW= total body weight, LBW= lean body weight.

increased emergence times due to increased fat tissue distribution of volatile agents. Desflurane has been suggested as the preferred inhaled anaesthetic due to its lower fat solubility and it has been shown that lean patients have similar recovery times as obese patients.[120,121] Currently, there is insufficient evidence for dosing recommendations for ketamine, etomidate, dexmetomidine, and lignocaine.[114,122] See Table 31.5.

Conclusion

Greater numbers of obese elderly patients are presenting for surgery, whether it is for elective bariatric, cardiac, orthopaedic procedures, or after trauma. While the anaesthetist usually considers the technical and physiological effects of obesity based on BMI, in elderly patients there must be a broader threshold for consideration of the multi-organ effects of adiposity. The metabolic alterations that lead to a lower lean body mass to fat tissue ratio and the accumulative impact of excess adiposity that come with ageing will affect the elderly more profoundly and the anaesthetic plan should reflect the wide-ranging effects even when the BMI is not excessively high.

References

1. World Health Organization. *Obesity: preventing and managing the global epidemic.* Report of a WHO consultation. World Health Organization technical report series. 894. Geneva: WHO, 2000.
2. Conway B, Rene, A. Obesity as a disease: no lightweight matter. *Obesity Rev.* 2004;5(3):145–151.
3. Finkelstein EA, Trogdon JG, Cohen JW, Dietz W. Annual medical spending attributable to obesity: payer-and service-specific estimates. *Health Affairs.* 2009;28(5):w822–831.
4. Wang Y, Beydoun MA. The obesity epidemic in the United States—gender, age, socioeconomic, racial/ethnic, and geographic characteristics: a systematic review and meta-regression analysis. *Epidemiol Rev.* 2007;29:6–28.
5. Livingston EH, Langert J. The impact of age and Medicare status on bariatric surgical outcomes. *Arch Surg.* 2006;141(11):1115–1120.
6. Buchwald H, Estok R, Fahrbach K, Banel D, Sledge I. Trends in mortality in bariatric surgery: a systematic review and meta-analysis. *Surgery.* 2007;142(4):621–632.
7. Villareal DT, Apovian CM, Kushner RF, *et al.* Obesity in older adults: technical review and position statement of the American Society for Nutrition and NAASO, The Obesity Society. *Obesity Res.* 2005;13(11):1849–1863.
8. Solomon CG, Manson JE. Obesity and mortality: a review of the epidemiologic data. *Am J Clin Nutr.* 1997;66(4 Suppl):1044S–1050S.
9. Dey DK, Rothenberg E, Sundh V, Bosaeus I, Steen B. Height and body weight in the elderly. I. A 25-year longitudinal study of a population aged 70 to 95 years. *Eur J Clin Nutr.* 1999;53(12):905–914.
10. Fogelholm M, Kujala U, Kaprio J, Sarna S. Predictors of weight change in middle-aged and old men. *Obesity Res.* 2000;8(5):367–373.
11. Vaughan L, Zurlo F, Ravussin E. Aging and energy expenditure. *Am J Clin Nutr.* 1991;53(4):821–825.
12. Dzien A, Winner H, Theurl E, Dzien-Bischinger C, Lechleitner M. Body mass index in a large cohort of patients assigned to age decades between <20 and ≥80 years: relationship with cardiovascular morbidity and medication. *J Nutr Health Aging.* 2011;15(7):536–541.
13. Beaufrere B, Morio B. Fat and protein redistribution with aging: metabolic considerations. *Eur J Nutr.* 2000;54(Suppl 3):S48–S53.
14. Zamboni M, Mazzali G, Zoico E, *et al.* Health consequences of obesity in the elderly: a review of four unresolved questions. *Int J Obesity.* 2005;29(9):1011–1029.
15. Perissinotto E, Pisent C, Sergi G, Grigoletto F, ILSA Working Group (Italian Longitudinal Study on Ageing). Anthropometric measurements in the elderly: age and gender differences. *Br J Nutr.* 2002;87(2):177–186.
16. Chapman IM. Obesity paradox during aging. *Interdiscip Top Gerontol.* 2010;37:20–36.
17. Uretsky S, Messerli FH, Bangalore S, *et al.* Obesity paradox in patients with hypertension and coronary artery disease. *Am J Med.* 2007;120(10):863–870.
18. Goel K, Thomas RJ, Squires RW, *et al.* Combined effect of cardiorespiratory fitness and adiposity on mortality in patients with coronary artery disease. *Am Heart J.* 2011;161(3):590–597.
19. Yusuf, S, Hawken, S, Ounpuu, S, *et al.* Obesity and the risk of myocardial infarction in 27,000 participants from 52 countries: a case-control study. *Lancet.* 2005;366(9497):1640–1649.
20. Bagby SP. Obesity-initiated metabolic syndrome and the kidney: a recipe for chronic kidney disease? *J Am Soc Nephrol.* 2004;15(11):2775–2791.
21. Tung A. Anaesthetic considerations with the metabolic syndrome. *Br J Anaesth.* 2010;105(Suppl 1):i24–i33.
22. El-Orbany M, Woehlck HJ. Difficult mask ventilation. *Anesth Analg.* 2009;109(6):1870–1880.
23. Kheterpal S, Han R, Tremper KK, *et al.* Incidence and predictors of difficult and impossible mask ventilation. *Anesthesiology.* 2006;105(5):885–891.
24. Langeron O, Masso E, Huraux C, *et al.* Prediction of difficult mask ventilation. *Anesthesiology.* 2000;92(5):1229–1236.
25. Lundstrom LH, Moller AM, Rosenstock C, Astrup G, Wetterslev J. High body mass index is a weak predictor for difficult and failed tracheal intubation: a cohort study of 91,332 consecutive patients scheduled for direct laryngoscopy registered in the Danish Anesthesia Database. *Anesthesiology.* 2009;110(2):266–274.
26. Juvin P, Lavaut E, Dupont H, *et al.* Difficult tracheal intubation is more common in obese than in lean patients. *Anesth Analg.* 2003;97(2):595–600.
27. Brodsky JB, Lemmens HJ, Brock-Utne JG, Vierra M, Saidman LJ. Morbid obesity and tracheal intubation. *Anesth Analg.* 2002;94(3):732–736.
28. Ezri T, Medalion B, Weisenberg M, Szmuk P, Warters RD, Charuzi I. Increased body mass index per se is not a predictor of difficult laryngoscopy. *Can J Anaesth.* 2003;50(2):179–183.
29. Neligan PJ, Porter S, Max B, *et al.* Obstructive sleep apnea is not a risk factor for difficult intubation in morbidly obese patients. *Anesth Analg.* 2009;109(4):1182–1186.
30. Neligan PJ. Metabolic syndrome: anesthesia for morbid obesity. *Curr Opin Anaesthesiol.* 2010;23(3):375–383.
31. Sinha AC. Some anesthetic aspects of morbid obesity. *Curr Opin Anaesthesiol.* 2009;22(3):442–446.
32. Freid EB. The rapid sequence induction revisited: obesity and sleep apnea syndrome. *Anesthesiol Clin North Am.* 2009;23(3):551–564, viii.
33. Harter RL, Kelly WB, Kramer MG, Perez CE, Dzwonczyk RR. A comparison of the volume and pH of gastric contents of obese and lean surgical patients. *Anesth Analg.* 1998;86(1):147–152.
34. Juvin P, Fevre G, Merouche M, Vallot T, Desmonts JM. Gastric residue is not more copious in obese patients. *Anesth Analg.* 2001;93(6):1621–1622.
35. Chung SA, Yuan H, Chung F. A systemic review of obstructive sleep apnea and its implications for anesthesiologists. *Anesth Analg.* 2008;107(5):1543–1563.
36. Tishler PV, Larkin EK, Schluchter MD, Redline S. Incidence of sleep-disordered breathing in an urban adult population: the relative importance of risk factors in the development of sleep-disordered breathing. *JAMA.* 2003;289(17):2230–2237.
37. Olson AL, Zwillich C. The obesity hypoventilation syndrome. *Am J Med.* 2005;118(9):948–956.
38. Chung F, Yegneswaran B, Liao P, *et al.* STOP questionnaire: a tool to screen patients for obstructive sleep apnea. *Anesthesiology.* 2008;108(5):812–821.
39. Chung F, Elsaid H. Screening for obstructive sleep apnea before surgery: why is it important? *Curr Opin Anaesthesiol.* 2009;22(3):405–411.

40. Valenza F, Vagginelli F, Tiby A, *et al*. Effects of the beach chair position, positive end-expiratory pressure, and pneumoperitoneum on respiratory function in morbidly obese patients during anesthesia and paralysis. *Anesthesiology*. 2007;107(5):725–732.

41. Kaw R, Pasupuleti V, Walker E, Ramaswamy A, Foldvary-Schafer N. Postoperative complications in patients with obstructive sleep apnea. *Chest*. 2012;141(2):436–441.

42. Jones RL, Nzekwu MM. The effects of body mass index on lung volumes. *Chest*. 2006;130(3):827–833.

43. D'Errico A, Scarani P, Colosimo E, Spina M, Grigioni WF, Mancini AM. Changes in the alveolar connective tissue of the ageing lung. An immunohistochemical study. *Virchows Archiv*. 1989;415(2):137–144.

44. Behazin N, Jones SB, Cohen RI, Loring SH. Respiratory restriction and elevated pleural and esophageal pressures in morbid obesity. *J Appl Physiol*. 2010;108(1):212–218.

45. Pelosi P, Croci M, Ravagnan I, *et al*. The effects of body mass on lung volumes, respiratory mechanics, and gas exchange during general anesthesia. *Anesth Analg*. 1998;87(3):654–660.

46. Hedenstierna G, Santesson J. Breathing mechanics, dead space and gas exchange in the extremely obese, breathing spontaneously and during anaesthesia with intermittent positive pressure ventilation. *Acta Anaesthesiol Scandinav*. 1976;20(3):248–254.

47. Van Lith P, Johnson FN, Sharp JT. Respiratory elastances in relaxed and paralyzed states in normal and abnormal men. *J Appl Physiol*. 1967;23(4):475–486.

48. Naimark A, Cherniack RM. Compliance of the respiratory system and its components in health and obesity. *J Appl Physiol*. 1960;15:377–382.

49. Berend N. Normal ageing of the lung: implications for diagnosis and monitoring of asthma in older people. *Med J Aust*. 2005;183(1 Suppl):S28–29.

50. Oskvig RM. Special problems in the elderly. *Chest*. 1999;115(5 Suppl):158S–164S.

51. Milic-Emili J, Torchio R, D'Angelo E. Closing volume: a reappraisal (1967-2007). *Eur J Appl Physiol*. 2007;99(6):567–583.

52. Hakala K, Mustajoki P, Aittomaki J, Sovijarvi AR. Effect of weight loss and body position on pulmonary function and gas exchange abnormalities in morbid obesity. *Int J Obes Relat Metab Disord*. 1995;19(5):343–346.

53. Salome CM, King GG, Berend N. Physiology of obesity and effects on lung function. *J Appl Physiol*. 2010;108(1):206–211.

54. Holland J, Milic-Emili J, Macklem PT, Bates DV. Regional distribution of pulmonary ventilation and perfusion in elderly subjects. *J Clin Invest*. 1968;47(1):81–92.

55. Holley HS, Milic-Emili J, Becklake MR, Bates DV. Regional distribution of pulmonary ventilation and perfusion in obesity. *J Clin Invest*. 1967;46(4):475–481.

56. Herriger A, Frascarolo P, Spahn DR, Magnusson L. The effect of positive airway pressure during pre-oxygenation and induction of anaesthesia upon duration of non-hypoxic apnoea. *Anaesthesia*. 2004;59(3):243–247.

57. Gander S, Frascarolo P, Suter M, Spahn DR, Magnusson L. Positive end-expiratory pressure during induction of general anesthesia increases duration of nonhypoxic apnea in morbidly obese patients. *Anesth Analg*. 2005;100(2):580–584.

58. Hedenstierna G, Rothen HU. Atelectasis formation during anesthesia: causes and measures to prevent it. *J Clin Monitor Comput*. 2000;16(5-6):329–335.

59. Rothen HU, Sporre B, Engberg G, Wegenius G, Reber A, Hedenstierna G. Atelectasis and pulmonary shunting during induction of general anaesthesia—can they be avoided?. *Acta Anaesthesiol Scandinav*. 1996;40(5):524–529.

60. Neumann P, Rothen HU, Berglund JE, Valtysson J, Magnusson A, Hedenstierna G. Positive end-expiratory pressure prevents atelectasis during general anaesthesia even in the presence of a high inspired oxygen concentration. *Acta Anaesthesiol Scandinav*. 1999;43(3):295–301.

61. Talab HF, Zabani IA, Abdelrahman HS, *et al*. Intraoperative ventilatory strategies for prevention of pulmonary atelectasis in obese patients undergoing laparoscopic bariatric surgery. *Anesth Analg*. 2009;109(5):1511–1516.

62. Pelosi P, Gregoretti C. Perioperative management of obese patients. *Best Pract Res Clin Anaesthesiol*. 2010;24(2):211–225.

63. Coussa M, Proietti S, Schnyder P, *et al*. Prevention of atelectasis formation during the induction of general anesthesia in morbidly obese patients. *Anesth Analg*. 2004;98(5):1491–1495.

64. Reinius H, Jonsson L, Gustafsson S, *et al*. Prevention of atelectasis in morbidly obese patients during general anesthesia and paralysis: a computerized tomography study. *Anesthesiology*. 2009;111(5):979–987.

65. Chalhoub V, Yazigi A, Sleilaty G, *et al*. Effect of vital capacity manoeuvres on arterial oxygenation in morbidly obese patients undergoing open bariatric surgery. *Eur J Anaesthesiol*. 2007;24(3):283–288.

66. Neumann P. Airway pressure settings during general anaesthesia. *Anasthesiol Intensivmed Notfallmed Schmerzther*. 2007;42(7):538–546.

67. Sharp JT, Druz WS, Kondragunta VR. Diaphragmatic responses to body position changes in obese patients with obstructive sleep apnea. *Am Rev Respir Dis*. 1986;133(1):32–37.

68. Parameswaran K, Todd DC, Soth M. Altered respiratory physiology in obesity. *Can Respir J*. 2006;13(4):203–210.

69. Watsford ML, Murphy AJ, Pine MJ. The effects of ageing on respiratory muscle function and performance in older adults. *J Sci Med Sport*. 2007;10(1):36–44.

70. Wofford MR, Hall JE. Pathophysiology and treatment of obesity hypertension. *Curr Pharmaceut Design*. 2004;10(29):3621–3637.

71. da Silva AA, do Carmo J, Dubinion J, Hall JE. The role of the sympathetic nervous system in obesity-related hypertension. *Curr Hypertens Rep*. 2009;11(3):206–211.

72. Hall JE, da Silva AA, do Carmo JM, *et al*. Obesity-induced hypertension: role of sympathetic nervous system, leptin, and melanocortins. *J Biol Chem*. 2010;285(23):17271–17276.

73. Galinier M, Pathak A, Roncalli J, Massabuau P. Obesity and cardiac failure. *Archives des Maladies du Coeur et des Vaisseaux*. 2005;98(1):39–45.

74. Lavie CJ, Milani RV, Ventura HO. Obesity and cardiovascular disease: risk factor, paradox, and impact of weight loss. *J Am Coll Cardiol*. 2009;53(21):1925–1932.

75. Alpert MA. Obesity cardiomyopathy: pathophysiology and evolution of the clinical syndrome. *Am J Med Sci*. 2001;321(4):225–236.

76. Wanahita N, Messerli FH, Bangalore S, Gami AS, Somers VK, Steinberg JS. Atrial fibrillation and obesity—results of a meta-analysis. *Am Heart J*. 2008;155(2):310–315.

77. Klein S, Burke LE, Bray GA, *et al*. Clinical implications of obesity with specific focus on cardiovascular disease: a statement for professionals from the American Heart Association Council on Nutrition, Physical Activity, and Metabolism: endorsed by the American College of Cardiology Foundation. *Circulation*. 2004;110(18):2952–2967.

78. Messerli FH, Nunez BD, Ventura HO, Snyder DW. Overweight and sudden death. Increased ventricular ectopy in cardiopathy of obesity. *Arch Intern Med*. 1987;147(10):1725–1728.

79. Oreopoulos A, Padwal R, Kalantar-Zadeh K, Fonarow GC, Norris CM, McAlister FA. Body mass index and mortality in heart failure: a meta-analysis. *Am Heart J*. 2008;156(1):13–22.

80. Horwich TB, Fonarow GC, Hamilton MA, MacLellan WR, Woo MA, Tillisch JH. The relationship between obesity and mortality in patients with heart failure. *J Am Coll Cardiol*. 2001;38(3):789–795.

81. Fonarow GC, Srikanthan P, Costanzo MR, Cintron GB, Lopatin M, ADHERE Scientific Advisory Committee and Investigator. An obesity paradox in acute heart failure: analysis of body mass index and inhospital mortality for 108,927 patients in the Acute Decompensated Heart Failure National Registry. *Am Heart J*. 2007;153(1):74–81.

82. Romero-Corral A, Montori VM, Somers VK, *et al*. Association of bodyweight with total mortality and with cardiovascular events in coronary artery disease: a systematic review of cohort studies. *Lancet*. 2006;368(9536):666–678.

83. Aursulesei V, Cozma A, Datcu MD. Obesity paradox. *Revista medico-chirurgicala a Societatii de Medici si Naturalisti din Iasi.* 2009;113(4):1006–1015.

84. Sung SH, Wu TC, Huang CH, Lin SJ, Chen JW. Prognostic impact of body mass index in patients undergoing coronary artery bypass surgery. *Heart.* 2011;97(8):648–654.

85. Le-Bert G, Santana O, Pineda AM, Zamora C, Lamas GA, Lamelas J. The obesity paradox in elderly obese patients undergoing coronary artery bypass surgery. *Interactive Cardiovasc Thorac Surg.* 2011;13(2):124–127.

86. Wassertheil-Smoller S, Fann C, Allman RM, *et al.* Relation of low body mass to death and stroke in the systolic hypertension in the elderly program. The SHEP Cooperative Research Group. *Arch Intern Med.* 2000;160(4):494–500.

87. Dorner TE, Rieder A. Obesity paradox in elderly patients with cardiovascular diseases. *Int J Cardiol.* 2012;155(1):56–65.

88. Habbu A, Lakkis NM, Dokainish H. The obesity paradox: fact or fiction? *Am J Cardiol.* 2006;98(7):944–948.

89. Ejerblad E, Fored CM, Lindblad P, Fryzek J, McLaughlin JK, Nyren O. Obesity and risk for chronic renal failure. *J Am Soc Nephrol.* 2006;17(6):1695–1702.

90. Sinha AC, Eckmann, DM. Anesthesia for Bariatric Surgery. In Miller RD (ed) *Miller's anesthesia,* 7th edn (pp. 2089–2104). Philadelphia, PA: Churchill Livingstone Elsevier, 2010.

91. Collazo-Clavell ML, Clark MM, McAlpine DE, Jensen MD. Assessment and preparation of patients for bariatric surgery. *Mayo Clinic Proc.* 2006;81(10 Suppl):S11–S17.

92. Cefalu WT, Wang ZQ, Werbel S, *et al.* Contribution of visceral fat mass to the insulin resistance of aging. *Metabolism.* 1995;44(7):954–959.

93. Martyn JA, Kaneki M, Yasuhara S. Obesity-induced insulin resistance and hyperglycemia: etiologic factors and molecular mechanisms. *Anesthesiology.* 2008;109(1):137–148.

94. Hart DJ, Spector TD. The relationship of obesity, fat distribution and osteoarthritis in women in the general population: the Chingford Study. *J Rheumatol.* 1993;20(2):331–335.

95. Wearing SC, Hennig EM, Byrne NM, Steele JR, Hills AP. Musculoskeletal disorders associated with obesity: a biomechanical perspective. *Obesity Rev.* 2006;7(3):239–250.

96. Malnick SD, Knobler H. The medical complications of obesity. *QJM.* 2006;99(9):565–579.

97. Morin S, Leslie WD, Manitoba Bone Density Program. High bone mineral density is associated with high body mass index. *Osteoporos Int.* 2009;20(7):1267–1271.

98. Morin S, Tsang JF, Leslie WD. Weight and body mass index predict bone mineral density and fractures in women aged 40 to 59 years. *Osteoporos Int.* 2009;20(3):363–370.

99. Pocock N, Eisman J, Gwinn T, *et al.* Muscle strength, physical fitness, and weight but not age predict femoral neck bone mass. *J Bone Mineral Res.* 1989;4(3):441–448.

100. Felson DT, Zhang Y, Hannan MT, Anderson JJ. Effects of weight and body mass index on bone mineral density in men and women: the Framingham study. *J Bone Mineral Res.* 1993;8(5):567–573.

101. Andrew JG, Palan J, Kurup HV, *et al.* Obesity in total hip replacement. *J Bone Joint Surg (Br).* 2008;90(4):424–429.

102. McCalden RW, Charron KD, MacDonald SJ, Bourne RB, Naudie DD. Does morbid obesity affect the outcome of total hip replacement?: an analysis of 3290 THRs. *J Bone Joint Surg (Br).* 2011;93(3):321–325.

103. Huddleston JI, Wang Y, Uquillas C, Herndon JH, Maloney WJ. Age and obesity are risk factors for adverse events after total hip arthroplasty. *Clin Orthop Relat Res.* 2012;470(2):490–496.

104. McCarthy LH, Bigal ME, Katz M, Derby C, Lipton RB. Chronic pain and obesity in elderly people: results from the Einstein aging study. *J Am Geriatr Soc.* 2009;57(1):115–119.

105. Miscio G, Guastamacchia G, Brunani A, Priano L, Baudo S, Mauro A. Obesity and peripheral neuropathy risk: a dangerous liaison. *JPNS.* 2005;10(4):354–358.

106. Winter AC, Berger K, Buring JE, Kurth T. 2009. Body mass index, migraine, migraine frequency and migraine features in women. *Cephalalgia.* 2009;29(2):269–278.

107. Pomp ER, le Cessie S, Rosendaal FR, Doggen CJ. Risk of venous thrombosis: obesity and its joint effect with oral contraceptive use and prothrombotic mutations. *Br J Haematol.* 2007;139(2):289–296.

108. Abdollahi M, Cushman M, Rosendaal FR. Obesity: risk of venous thrombosis and the interaction with coagulation factor levels and oral contraceptive use. *Thromb Haemost.* 2003;89(3):493–498.

109. Tsai AW, Cushman M, Rosamond WD, Heckbert SR, Polak JF, Folsom AR. Cardiovascular risk factors and venous thromboembolism incidence: the longitudinal investigation of thromboembolism etiology. *Arch Intern Med.* 2002;162(10):1182–1189.

110. Edmonds MJ, Crichton TJ, Runciman WB, Pradhan M. Evidence-based risk factors for postoperative deep vein thrombosis. *ANZ Journal of Surgery.* 2004;74(12):1082–1097.

111. Roderick P, Ferris G, Wilson K, *et al.* Towards evidence-based guidelines for the prevention of venous thromboembolism: systematic reviews of mechanical methods, oral anticoagulation, dextran and regional anaesthesia as thromboprophylaxis. *Health Technol Assess.* 2005;9(49):iii–iv, ix–x, 1–78.

112. Hirsh J, Raschke R. Heparin and low-molecular-weight heparin: the Seventh ACCP Conference on Antithrombotic and Thrombolytic Therapy. *Chest.* 2004;126(3 Suppl):188S–203S.

113. Kearon C, Hirsh J. Management of anticoagulation before and after elective surgery. *N Engl J Med.* 1997;336(21):1506–1511.

114. Lemmens HJ. Perioperative pharmacology in morbid obesity. *Curr Opin Anaesthesiol.* 2010;23(4):485–491.

115. Han PY, Duffull SB, Kirkpatrick CM, Green B. Dosing in obesity: a simple solution to a big problem. *Clin Pharmacol Therapeut.* 2007;82(5):505–508.

116. Green B, Duffull SB. What is the best size descriptor to use for pharmacokinetic studies in the obese? *Br J Clin Pharmacol.* 2004;58(2):119–133.

117. Janmahasatian S, Duffull SB, Ash S, *et al.* Quantification of lean bodyweight. *Clin Pharmacokinet.* 2005;44(10):1051–1065.

118. Greenblatt DJ, Abernethy DR, Locniskar A, *et al.* Effect of age, gender, and obesity on midazolam kinetics. *Anesthesiology.* 1984;61(1):27–35.

119. Ingrande J, Brodsky JB, Lemmens HJ. Lean body weight scalar for the anesthetic induction dose of propofol in morbidly obese subjects. *Anesth Analg.* 2011;113(1):57–62.

120. La Colla G, La Colla L, Turi S, *et al.* Effect of morbid obesity on kinetic of desflurane: wash-in wash-out curves and recovery times. *Minerva Anestesiol.* 2007;73(5):275–279.

121. La Colla L, Albertin A, La Colla G, Mangano A. Faster wash-out and recovery for desflurane vs sevoflurane in morbidly obese patients when no premedication is used. *Br J Anaesth.* 2007;99(3):353–358.

122. Ingrande J, Lemmens HJ. Dose adjustment of anaesthetics in the morbidly obese. *Br J Anaesth.* 2010;105(Suppl 1):i16–i23.

123. Ogunnaike BO, Jones SB, Jones DB, Provost D, Whitten CW. Anesthetic considerations for bariatric surgery. *Anesth Analg.* 2002;95(6):1793–1805.

PART 5

Other Important Aspects

CHAPTER 32

Training in geriatrics for anaesthesiologists

Sheila Ryan Barnett

Introduction

In the United States alone the number of individuals over 65 years is expected to double from 35 million in 2010 to 78 million by 2050. Furthermore by 2030 the number of persons over 65 years will outnumber those aged 15 years or less by 2:1.

Within hospitals the number of older patients undergoing invasive procedures is also steadily rising. One-third of admissions following trauma involve older patients, and 40% of surgical procedures are performed on geriatric patients. Older patients are more likely to have complications, and have increased morbidity and mortality following emergency procedures (Table 32.1).

Despite these impressive numbers, it remains challenging to create a sustainable training programme covering the unique issues encountered in the elderly patient. The importance of competence for anaesthetists and other specialists in matters related to the elderly is readily acknowledged, but poorly executed. Integrating geriatrics into the curriculum at multiple stages of medical education has been recognized as critical to the success of an integrated ageing programme.[1–4] Several individual programmes in geriatric anaesthesia have been successful at a local level, however the establishment of a widely disseminated, sustainable geriatric curriculum in anaesthesia remains elusive.

There are multiple reasons contributing to the difficulty in creating a lasting geriatric curriculum. The sheer number of geriatric patients actually fosters complacency in the surgical workforce. When presented with opportunities to receive additional education on geriatrics, specialists are often reluctant, commenting, 'I look after older patients already'. In addition, changes in medical education and healthcare have led to new challenges for medical educators in all fields. When considering these barriers, it is not surprising that geriatric education for the surgical specialist is under-represented compared with the demographics in healthcare in general.[5]

Undergraduate education

As stated in the introduction, the ageing population is an important part of our society and education in geriatrics starts in medical school. In the United States, the Association of American Medical Colleges (AAMC) recently added multiple geriatric required competencies to the medical school curriculum.[6,7] Graduating medical students must be 'competent' in these areas. The range of competencies is substantial including topics on medication management to discussion about end of life and the role of palliative care (Table 32.2). The addition of these competencies and other similar requirements in other countries provides a baseline of minimum knowledge all residents should have when entering specialty-training programmes. However, it is not clear that these competencies or types of changes in curricula lead to changes in outcomes for older patients or future engagement by the training physician in geriatric education in general.

Opportunities and resources for education in geriatric anaesthesia

Significant strides have been made in education on important age-related areas for anaesthesia and perioperative physicians in general. Delirium and postoperative cognitive function are excellent examples of important clinic geriatric syndromes that are clinically relevant to anaesthetists. In addition, these areas represent a major focus of both basic and clinical anaesthesia research.

Many advances in the area of geriatric anaesthesia have occurred through the development and cooperation of various funding agencies and societies. For example, the Society for the Advancement of Geriatric Anesthesia was established in 2000.[8] This US-based society provides education on geriatric anaesthesia and represents a valuable networking opportunity for faculty. In the United Kingdom, a similar society, the Age Anaesthesia Association formed in 1987,[9] hosts regular annual scientific meeting featuring key topics in geriatric anaesthesia.

The most significant US champions of geriatric education in the surgical specialties are the American Geriatrics Society, the John A Hartford Foundation, and the Reynolds Foundation (Table 32.3). These agencies, through collaboration with academic institutions and specialty societies, have established several excellent educational multidisciplinary programmes across many of the surgical specialties, including anaesthesia. However sustaining educational initiatives beyond the funding period has been a major challenge.[2,3,10]

Table 32.1 Commonly encountered challenges in geriatric care

- Heterogeneous population
- High disease burden
- Atypical disease presentation
- Unpredictable organ reserve
- Emergent procedures poorly tolerated
- Minor complications can rapidly escalate

Table 32.2 AAMC geriatric competencies: relevance to anaesthesia

- Medication management: dose reduction, polypharmacy
- Cognitive and behavioural disorders: delirium, POCD
- Self-care capacity: outpatient assessment in the frail elderly
- Falls, balance and gait disorders: preoperative functional assessment
- Health planning and promotion: consent, 'do not attempt resuscitation' orders, healthcare proxy
- Atypical presentation of disease: cardiac and pulmonary complications, recognition of impaired cognition

Data from Leipzig RM, Granville L, Simpson D, Anderson MB, Sauvigné K, Soriano RP. Keeping granny safe on July 1: a consensus on minimum geriatrics competencies for graduating medical students. Acad Med. 2009 May;84(5):604–10.

An example of a valuable resource for the clinician educator is the Portal of Geriatric Online Education (POGOe).[11] This is a public website that has a substantial collection of geriatric educational materials. The educational products are frequently updated and provide easy to access teaching tools in many different formats. Examples of the types of products that can be downloaded for use include PBLDs, virtual patients, and didactic lectures. Submissions are also encouraged and can contribute to a trainee or faculty member's educational portfolio. These products are not specific to anaesthesia and there is a wide range in the content of materials available.

In addition to the products available online through POGOe; the American Society of Anesthesiologists (ASA) also has several products on geriatric anaesthesia. Examples of products include a curriculum composed of extensive literature recommendations and also a 'Frequently asked question' booklet addressing common problems for encountered in elderly patients by practising anaesthesiologists.[12]

Fortunately through the advocacy, dedication, and work of many 'geriatric' anaesthetists the number of textbooks and references devoted to geriatric anaesthesia and surgical specialties has steadily increased in the last decade.[13–15] In addition most anaesthesia textbooks now include at least one chapter on the elderly patient. Sustainability of programmes in geriatric anaesthesia is one of the biggest challenges to overcome within anaesthesia, and hopefully the steady increase in educational materials and their broad distribution through the Internet will help establish geriatrics as an important area for education.

Table 32.3 Goals of the Geriatrics for Specialists Project: also known as the Section for enhancing geriatric understanding and expertise amongst surgical and medical specialists[a] (SEGUE).

- Improve the amount and quality of *geriatric education* medical and surgical residents receive
- Develop *faculty leaders* to promote geriatric training and research within their specialities
- Encourage and enable *professional societies and their boards* to recognize geriatrics as an important aspect of patient care

[a] The ten surgical and medical specialties: Anaesthesiology, Emergency Medicine, General Surgery, Gynaecology, Ophthalmology, Orthopaedic Surgery, Otolaryngology, Physical Medicine and Rehabilitation, Thoracic Surgery, and Urology.

Data from Heflin MT, Bragg EJ, Fernandez H, Christmas C, Osterweil D, Sauvigné K, Warshaw G, Cohen HJ, Leipzig R, Reuben DB, Durso SC The Donald W. Reynolds Consortium for Faculty Development to Advance Geriatrics Education (FD~AGE): a model for dissemination of subspecialty educational expertise. *Acad Med.* 2012 May;87(5):618-26, and Williams BC, Weber V, Babbott SF, Kirk LM, Heflin MT, O'toole E, Schapira MM, Eckstrom E, Tulsky A, Wolf AM, Landefeld S. Faculty development for the 21stcentury: lessons from the Society of General Internal Medicine – Hartford Collaborative Centers for the Care of the Older Adults *J Am Geriatr Soc.* 2007 Jun;55(6):941–7.

Postgraduate framework

In recent years there has been an increased regulation and oversight of postgraduate medical training. This has led to the establishment of national frameworks upon which post graduate and in some instances professional training are accomplished and maintained.

In the USA, the Accreditation Council for Graduate Medical Education (ACGME)[16] working together with the American Board of Anesthesiology (ABA) has established required competencies and a broad programme anaesthesiology curriculum. All residents must demonstrate proficiency within the competencies, and training programmes are regularly reviewed to ensure appropriate educational standards are being upheld. Competency-based residency-training uses an outcomes based approach. Assessment and evaluation of trainees is a core component of a well-functioning competency-based curriculum. The relatively new shift towards outcomes has created new challenges for education programmes.[17,18] These programmes tend to be resource heavy, especially for individual teachers. In addition outcomes-based programmes can be difficult to implement in an era of diminishing resources and financial constraints. One advantage for geriatric anaesthesia is the sheer volume of elderly patients, which can lend itself to these types of clinically intense education programmes.

Basic knowledge in ageing physiology, pharmacology, and evidence of management of elderly patients is required by both the ACGME (Table 32.4) and the ABA. However the actual requirements for education in geriatric anaesthesia are limited. Essentially the ACGME requires that residents receive appropriate didactic instruction and clinical experience managing geriatric patients. The ABA publishes content outlines for training programmes and this does include geriatrics pharmacology and ageing physiology. Canada has a similar competency-based requirements for curricula development, referred to as CanMEDS (Table 32.5).[19] These competencies are slightly different than those proposed by the ACGME, but again provide a framework for postgraduate medical education. It is striking that both in the United States and Canada the ability of the current workforce to appropriately care for the growing elderly population has been questioned.

Irrespective of the actual framework in place, there is an opportunity to review current guidelines and make recommendations to include geriatrics as a required field of study for anaesthesia. The importance of establishing geriatrics as an important entity is the key issue.[2,3,5,20]

Developing a curriculum in geriatric anaesthesia

As more programmes embark on developing geriatric curricula it is important to consider which topics are important to cover.

Table 32.4 ACGME competencies

1. Patient care
2. Medical knowledge
3. Practice-based learning and improvement
4. Interpersonal and communication skills
5. Professionalism
6. Systems-based practice

Data from ACGME Program Requirements for Graduate Medical Education in Geriatric Medicine ACGME Approved: September 28, 2004; Effective July 1, 2005 Editorial Revision: July 1, 2009 Revised Common Program Requirements Effective: July 1, 2011 ACGME Approved Categorization: September 30, 2012; Effective: July 1, 2013.

Table 32.5 Canadian Medical Education Directives for Specialists (CanMEDS)

1. Medical Expert
2. Communicator
3. Collaborator
4. Manager
5. Health Advocate
6. Scholar
7. Professional

Data from http://www.collaborativecurriculum.ca/en/modules/CanMEDS

The most successful endeavours will focus on areas in which there is specific geriatric research and a depth of knowledge is required.[21] For example, simply adding an older age to a case stem and discussing the management of myocardial ischemia in a 90-year-old patient does not in itself promote geriatric anaesthesia. However, a case discussion on myocardial ischaemia in an extremely old patient that thoroughly explores the age-related changes in cardiovascular physiology that may mandate changes in care would be a valuable experience. The challenges and obstacles facing the integration of geriatrics into a curriculum are not unique to anaesthesia, surgery and others have faced similar problems.[22–24]

The following section contains recommended areas to cover when establishing a curriculum in anaesthesia.[25,26] These should not be considered a final list and all curricula should be constantly evolving and changing as new evidence emerges.

Physiology

A geriatric anaesthesia curriculum must include material on expected age-related physiological changes and the potential impact of these changes on the administration of anaesthesia. Age-related changes contribute to the vulnerability of the older patient by reducing their basic reserve function even before the impact of comorbidities is considered. Although all systems undergo some degree of physiology decline, the key areas to include in a basic syllabus are the cardiopulmonary, central nervous, and metabolic/renal systems. The challenge is to make this an interesting topic, avoiding the temptation to present a 'laundry list' of age-related physiological changes. Cases-based discussion (CBDs) highlighting the impact of the underlying lack of physiological reserves can help to emphasize important physiology changes.[3]

Preanaesthetic assessment

The growing trend in preoperative assessment is 'less is better'. The elderly population provides a rich environment to teach appropriate and targeted preoperative assessments. The involvement of a geriatrician in the preoperative setting can also provide a multidisciplinary approach, adding additional expertise in complex elderly patients.

Pharmacology

The selection and administration of medications is central to the practice of anaesthesia. Inadvertent overdosing of an older patient due to a lack of appreciation of the pathophysiology can lead to devastating consequences in the frail older patient. Creative

ways to emphasize the importance of appropriate using might be through the use of simulation, or case reviews. Information on appropriate dosing is readily available in several of the basic anaesthesia textbooks (see also Chapter 3).

Pain control

Pain control in the perioperative period presents a major challenge at all ages and the elderly are particularly vulnerable from developing complications related to either under- or overtreatment of pain. Involving pain and regional anaesthesia specialists in teaching pain control of the elderly patient may enhance the visibility of geriatrics within the anaesthesia curriculum.

Perioperative cognitive dysfunction

Central nervous system complications in the elderly are a significant source of morbidity and mortality. A curriculum for geriatrics must include a robust section on postoperative cognitive dysfunction and delirium. In addition to clinical material, this area is also an exciting area for both basic and clinical research by anaesthetists.

Choosing the anaesthetic

This is an incredibly important section for any curriculum. It will demand an appreciation of the common comorbidities and basic age-related changes. It should be used as an opportunity to review a wide range of geriatric issues and the impact on the anaesthesia delivery. For example, a discussion on the pros and cons of regional anaesthesia in the context of cognitive dysfunction can be used to highlight many key geriatric concepts. This area clearly lends itself to CBDs.

Geriatric syndromes

The geriatricians have identified several important 'geriatric' syndromes (Table 32.6). Syndromes refer to the presence of a collection of comorbidities that are common in older patients. These are not specific diseases and yet in many instances they are directly related to mortality. Although not all of these are relevant for anaesthesia, some of the concepts and new literature emerging are important for perioperative care. For example, 'frailty' is becoming increasingly recognized as an important predictor of poor perioperative outcomes in the older patient. Thus a greater understanding of geriatric syndromes such as frailty and impaired homeostasis, can lead to improved patient care and collaboration.[27]

Table 32.6 Geriatric syndromes

1. Multiple comorbidities
2. Cognitive impairment
3. Frailty
4. Disability
5. Malnutrition
6. Impaired homeostasis
7. Chronic inflammation
8. Sarcopenia

Data from Kane RL, Shamliyan T, Talley K, PacalaJ The association between geriatric Syndromes and Survival J AM Geriatric Soc 2012; 60: 896–904.

What tools to use during curriculum development

When developing a curriculum in geriatric anaesthesia it is especially important to acknowledge and respond to the needs of the audience. In stark contrast to geriatric medicine itself, anaesthesia is a fast paced and highly procedural area of medicine. Technical expertise is highly valued and training technical prowess is a major focus of training; especially early in a programme. Without an appropriate understanding of the viewpoint of the anaesthetist or a proceduralist, a geriatrician may not engage the curiosity of trainees in anaesthesia. However, a geriatrician can offer significant value to an anaesthesia programme. For example, discussion on code status and advanced health directives can be complementary to critical care training. Similarly a discussion on polypharmacy can expand a trainee's knowledge of preoperative medications and reinforce the important age-related changes surrounding geriatric pharmacology and physiology.

When designing a curriculum it is important to include popular and effective teaching venues. The integration of simulation into the anaesthesia curriculum has been both popular and effective. Simulation can be utilized to teach an array of skills from procedures to communication. Including geriatric issues in simulation sessions can be extremely valuable. For example, a simulation involving a delirious elderly patient in the post-anesthesia care unit can integrate both physiology and treatment. Using other creative teaching tools is also important, for example, CBDs, team training, interdepartmental sessions with surgeons and geriatricians to promote collaboration and shared expertise. Internet-based educational products are becoming more popular and allow interactive distant learning. Using different types of forum such as gaming can make the curriculum more engaging for residents and faculty.[28-30]

Barriers to establishing a sustainable geriatric anaesthesia curriculum

Geriatric medicine in crisis

When attempting to integrate geriatrics successfully into an anaesthesia or other surgical specialty curriculum, the first obstacle encountered lies within the practice of geriatrics itself. Geriatric medicine itself is a field that has struggled to maintain its identity and value in medicine. For example, in the United States geriatrics is the one of the few fields where a practitioner will earn less upon completing a fellowship than they might have done without the specialized training. It is perhaps not surprising then that only 44 per cent of available geriatric fellowship positions are filled and there is a marked shortage of geriatricians in the workforce. The lack of available geriatricians leads to difficulty with visibility to surgical specialists and accessibility for patients, resulting in lost opportunities for collaboration and education about ageing. A lack of understanding of the expertise offered by geriatricians adds to the barriers encountered in establishing geriatric anaesthesia as a significant part of anaesthesia education.[1,31]

Despite the lack of a powerful workforce, there is ample literature illustrating the utility of geriatric specific care. In the field of geriatrics there have been many advances in patient care including the identification of frailty as an important syndrome, the treatment of delirium, the risks and dangers of polypharmacy, and other commonly recognized geriatric issues. Multiple studies have demonstrated improved outcomes when a comprehensive geriatric assessment model is used in hospitalized elders. These multidisciplinary team approaches have reduced delirium and length of stay and mortality in vulnerable elderly patents. There are other multiple examples of programmes that bring value to elders. The Hospital Elder programme was able to demonstrate a decrease in the incidence of delirium, institutionalization, and hospitalization. Other programmes have focused on reducing falls in older patients, and treating depression appropriately. Unfortunately the value provided through collaboration with geriatricians is frequently overlooked.

The older patient

Geriatric medicine presents many challenges for all physicians. The patients are complex, have multiple comorbidities, and limited reserve function. Visits with patients can take longer due to difficulties with mobility and communication. Hospitalizations are often prolonged and complications can result in significant increases in length of stay, institutionalization, and mortality.

In anaesthesia, the older patient carries a higher risk, especially for major operations, even a small perioperative complication can lead to a dramatic increase in morbidity and mortality. Complex medical histories can make preoperative assessments more difficult, and procedures more complex. Some of the more 'classic' geriatric cases, such as cataract eye surgery and urological procedures may not be viewed by trainees as 'exciting' compared with 'bigger' cases such as lobectomies and craniotomies. This can lead to a perception that geriatric cases are not as valuable for education.

Financing

Limited reimbursement for taking care of older complex patients can create disincentives for physicians, especially those practising in fee for service areas that reward high-volume procedural-based practices. Geriatric patients can require more follow-up visits and experience more complications following a surgery or procedure. These and overall lower reimbursement rates can discourage physicians for making geriatrics a significant focus of a practice. As health care reform is embraced some of these finical disincentives may be removed as more countries move towards the creation of collaborative work forces.[32]

Leadership

A major obstacle facing geriatrics within the subspecialties and anaesthesia in particular is a lack of a geriatric champion within individual departments. Although on a national level in the United States, the AGS has created several leadership opportunities and grant funding for research for geriatrics, there are still not enough geriatric champions within the specialty of anaesthesia to guarantee high penetration across training programmes. The lack of leadership impacts the development of geriatrics for both trainees and for faculty. Faculty development in geriatric anaesthesia is needed.

Hours/competition in the medical curriculum

Medical education has changed substantially in recent years. In the past medical education was based largely on a didactic/apprenticeship model. Residents and house officers would spend a limited amount of time in didactic sessions and most of the learning was

Table 32.7 Future directions for geriatric anaesthesia

- Development of age-specific risk reduction strategies
- Inclusion of a cognitive examination in the preoperative assessment
- Assessment of functional outcomes
- Encourage perioperative and team ageing interventions
- Develop guidelines for age-specific treatment
- Greater education for entire healthcare workforce

expected to occur at the patient's bedside. For procedures especially this led to the familiar 'see one, do one, teach one' approach to training. As medical training moves towards a competency-based system, an increase in unallowable hours has also contributed to a premium on teachable hours.[3,18,28]

In anaesthesia there has been tremendous growth in the field, the addition of significant critical care training, expansion of pain and regional anaesthesia, the addition of transoesophageal echo-cardiography. These changes and the expanding curricula have led to significant competition amongst all specialists for time with the residents. The limited teaching time really emphasizes the need for a geriatric champion.

Conclusion

The specialty of geriatric anaesthesia should be considered an emerging field (Table 32.7). The importance of a sound knowledge and an understanding of the unique issues that pertain to the older person undergoing anaesthesia cannot be underestimated. As the demographics of our patient population age, there will be many opportunities to use the knowledge gained on the elderly in our operating rooms and intensive care units and pain clinics. There are many different approaches to educating our workforce; each situation may need to be handled differently. Every health care entity is unique and an important aspect developing a successful curriculum geriatric anaesthesia will be playing the strengths of a particular department or institution.

References

1. Bardach SH, Rowles GD. Geriatric Education in the health professions: are we making progress? *Gerontologist*. 2012;52(5):607–618.
2. Heflin MT, Bragg EJ, Fernandez H, *et al.* The Donald W. Reynolds Consortium for Faculty Development to Advance Geriatrics Education (FD~AGE): a model for dissemination of subspecialty educational expertise. *Acad Med.* 2012;87(5):618–626.
3. Potter JF, Burton JR, Drach GW, Eisner J, Lundebjerg NE, Solomon DH. Geriatrics for residents in the surgical and medical specialties: implementation of curricula and training experiences. *J Am Geriatr Soc.* 2005;53(3):511–515.
4. Pinheiro SO, Heflin MT. The geriatrics excellence in teaching series: an integrated educational skills curriculum for faculty and fellows development. *J Am Geriatr Soc.* 2008;56(4):750–756.
5. Retooling for an Aging America: Building the Healthcare Workforce. White paper. Section for enhancing geriatric understanding and expertise amongst surgical and medical specialists (SEGUE). *J Am Geriatr Soc.* 2011;59:1537–1539.
6. Leipzig RM, Granville L, Simpson D, Anderson MB, Sauvigné K, Soriano RP. Keeping granny safe on July 1: a consensus on minimum geriatrics competencies for graduating medical students. *Acad Med.* 2009;84(5):604–610.
7. Leipzig RM, Hall WJ, Fried LP. Treating our societal scotoma: the case for investing in geriatrics, our nation's future, and our patients. *Ann Intern Med.* 2012;156(9):657–659.
8. Society for the Advancement of Geriatric Anesthesia. <http://www.sagahq.org>.
9. Age Anaesthesia Association. <http://www.ageanaesthesia.com>.
10. Williams BC, Weber V, Babbott SF, *et al.* Faculty development for the 21st century: lessons from the Society of General Internal Medicine—Hartford Collaborative Centers for the Care of the Older Adults. *J Am Geriatr Soc.* 2007;55(6):941–947.
11. Portal of Geriatrics Online Education. <http://www.pogoe.org>.
12. <http://www.asahq.org>.
13. Silverstein JH, Rooke GA, Reves JG, Mclesky CH. *Geriatric anesthesiology, 2nd edn.* New York: Springer, 2008.
14. Sieber FE. *Geriatric anesthesia.* New York: McGraw-Hill, 2007.
15. Rosenthal R. *Surgery for the elderly.* 2nd edn. New York: Springer, 2010.
16. Accreditation Council for Graduate Medical Education. <http://www.acgme.org>.
17. Bould MD, Naik VN, Hamstra SJ. Review article: New directions in medical education related to anesthesiology and perioperative medicine 2012. *Canadian J Anesth.* 2012; 59(2):136–150.
18. Glavin R, Flin R. Review article: the influence of psychology and human factors on education in anesthesiology. *Can J Anaesth.* 2012;59(2):151–158.
19. Canadian Medical Education Directives for Specialists (CanMEDS). <http://www.collaborativecurriculum.ca/en/modules/CanMEDS>.
20. Shield RR, Besdine RW. Education in gerontology and geriatrics comes of age. *Gerontol Geriatr Educ.* 2011;32(4):291–294.
21. Supiano MA, Alessi C, Chernoff R, *et al.* Department of veterans affairs geriatric research, education and clinical centers: translating aging research into clinical geriatrics. *J Am Geriatr Soc.* 2012;60(7):1347–1356.
22. Faulk CE, Lee TJ, Musick D. Implementing a multidimensional geriatric curriculum in a physical medicine and rehabilitation residency program. *Am J Med Rehabil.* 2012;91(10):883–889.
23. Webb TP, Duthie E Jr. Geriatrics for surgeons: infusing life into an aging subject. *J Surg Educ.* 2008;65(2):91–94.
24. Williams BC, Warshaw G, Fabiny AR, *et al.* Medicine in the 21st century: recommended essential geriatrics competencies for internal medicine and family medicine residents. *J Grad Med Educ.* 2010;2(3):373–383.
25. Smith AF, Glavin R, Greaves JD. Defining excellence in anaesthesia: the role of personal qualities and practice environment. *Br J Anaesth.* 2011;106(1):38–43.
26. Callahan EH, Leipzig RM. Geriatric practices: review and update. *Mt Sinai J Med.* 2011;78(4):483–484.
27. Kane RL, Shamliyan T, Talley K, Pacala J. The association between geriatric syndromes and survival. *J Am Geriatr Soc.* 2012;60:896–904.
28. Leblanc VR. Review article: simulation in anesthesia: state of the science and looking forward. *Can J Anesth.* 2012;59(2):193–202.
29. Webb TP, Simpson D, Denson S, Duthie E Jr. Gaming used as an informal instructional technique: effects on learner knowledge and satisfaction. *J Surg Educ.* 2012;69(3):330–334.
30. Chao SH, Brett B, Wiecha JM, Norton LE, Levine SA. Use of an online curriculum to teach delirium to fourth-year medical students: a comparison with lecture format. *J Am Geriatr Soc.* 2012;60(7):1328–1332.
31. Golden AG, Silverman MA, Mintzer MJ. Is geriatric medicine terminally ill? *Ann Intern Med.* 2012;156(9):654–656.
32. *Institute of Medicine. Retooling for an aging America: building the healthcare workforce.* Washington, DC: The National Academies Press, 2008.

CHAPTER 33

Non-theatre environments (imaging, cardiac catheterization laboratory, and emergency department)

Naville Chia and Edwin Seet

Introduction

In recent times, and with increasing frequency, anaesthetists are expected to provide an integrated anaesthetic care service outside the traditional environment of the operating theatre. This may be due to advances in procedural techniques, demand for procedural sedation and anaesthesia for a widened spectrum of diagnostic and interventional procedures, cost-effectiveness, and patient preference for comfort and analgesia. These outside the operating theatre locations or non-theatre environments pose considerable challenges, as they do not often provide the anaesthetists and other healthcare providers with the support they are familiar with. Patients are at an increased risk of adverse outcomes, including oversedation, desaturation, and inadequate ventilation and even death.[1]

The increasing diversity and difficulty of cases have also made it more challenging. For example, interventional radiological procedures such as endovascular repair of aortic aneurysm can now replace major surgical procedures, and transcatheter aortic valve implantation can substitute for open aortic valve replacement. The patient population has also expanded to include those who may not have been routinely considered previously. The acceleration of population ageing associated with sicker, more elderly patients further compounds this difficult journey of providing adequate and safe care in non-theatre environments. Because of this rapidly developing trend, this practice has attracted a great deal of attention from anaesthetists, proceduralists, and hospital safety task groups alike.

Anaesthesia for such procedures outside the operating theatre encompasses a wide variation in location, procedure complexity, and anaesthetic technique. To mitigate risk and maintain patient safety, there is a clarion call to standardize care and monitoring for anaesthesia or procedural sedation in non-theatre environments.[2]

The various procedures undertaken in non-theatre environments can be carried out under any of the following techniques:

- No sedation or analgesia (monitoring only).

- Light sedation and/or analgesia. It is defined as the level of anaesthesia at which patients are able to tolerate unpleasant procedures through relief of anxiety, discomfort, or pain and at which uncooperative patients are able to tolerate procedures that require that they not move.

- Moderate sedation and/or analgesia. It is defined as the level of anaesthesia at which the patient retains purposeful responses to stimulation, requires no airway intervention, and can maintain adequate ventilation and cardiovascular function.

- Deep sedation.

- General anaesthesia.

- Regional anaesthesia.

Most procedures conducted in non-theatre locations can be performed under minimal to moderate sedation/analgesia. Non-anaesthesia personnel may care for patients undergoing procedures that require minimal to moderate sedation/analgesia, provided that they are trained to rescue patients from deep sedation. Deeper levels of sedation, general anaesthesia, or patients with complex underlying conditions require the presence of appropriately trained anaesthesia personnel.

Safe sedation of elderly patients includes maintaining appropriate practice standards in all areas where sedative/analgesic agents are administered. Institutions should develop sedation policies and procedures and anaesthetists should be directly involved in the establishment of these hospital policies since they possess domain knowledge on sedation, anaesthesia and patient safety.

Non-theatre environment (remote location)

In the context of anaesthesia, a non-theatre or remote site refers to a location, which is distant from the main operating theatre complex. Remote sites can be classified as follows:

- A location *not designed* for the administration of anaesthesia (e.g. emergency department, psychiatric ward for electroconvulsive therapy, and wards where cardioversion is performed).

◆ A location with *fixed equipment* (e.g. computed tomography (CT) scan, magnetic resonance imaging (MRI) and radiation therapy equipment).

◆ *Specially designed operating theatres* outside the main operating theatre (e.g. dental surgery, obstetric, and burns operating theatres).

◆ *Specialized suites* (e.g. interventional cardiology, radiology and endoscopy suites).

Many intrinsic features of the remote sites or non-theatre environment may render delivery of quality sedation and anaesthesia care difficult. These locations are frequently designed for their primary role, with provision for the requirements of anaesthesia being an afterthought.

Concerns for the anaesthetists covering a remote location

The concerns of anaesthetists covering a remote location can be related to monitoring, equipment, environmental, staff, patient, procedural, drug pharmacology, and radiological factors. Each of these will be dealt with in the following sections in the context of providing sedation and anaesthesia for the elderly patient.

Monitoring

Mandatory monitoring should be as for any location where anaesthesia is conducted. Monitoring at remote locations for the elderly should follow exactly the same standards as those observed in the main operating theatre complex. The prerequisites of safe care should include the monitoring of haemodynamics and respiration.[2]

Haemodynamic monitoring

Basic hemodynamic monitoring includes an electrocardiogram (ECG) and non-invasive blood pressure (NIBP) measurement. A three-lead ECG is standard monitoring for any patient without a history of cardiac events or cardiac risk. Elderly patients who have a history of congestive heart failure, ischaemic heart disease, or severe hypertension are recommended to have five-lead ECG monitoring with the ST segment analysis enabled. Every patient who is being monitored during a procedure should have an NIBP measured at least at 5-minute intervals. Difficulty or errors of measurement are encountered in patients with obese arms, use of inappropriately sized cuffs, uncooperative, moving or shivering patients, and patients with either a very high or low blood pressure. As more invasive procedures are being carried out in remote locations (e.g. endovascular stents, pacemaker/defibrillator insertions, or transjugular portocaval shunt), and the type of patients presenting for such procedures expected to have multiple comorbidities, the attendant procedural risk and/or the potential haemodynamic instability of such patients make it necessary to have an invasive monitoring of arterial blood pressure. Some of these patients may already have invasive blood pressure monitoring commenced in the intensive care units.

Monitoring of respiration

Respiratory depression is a significant concern in the elderly undergoing procedural sedation and anaesthesia as they are more sensitive to drugs than the younger patients due to altered physiology and pharmacokinetics. Recognizing hypoxia and hypercarbia early

is imperative in these susceptible older patients. Monitoring by clinical means such as observing chest excursions and auscultation of breath sounds is imprecise and of limited value. A more accurate monitoring of oxygenation and ventilation is recommended. The measurement of inspiratory oxygen concentration should be coupled with a low oxygen concentration limit alarm. The pulse oximeter is used to measure the haemoglobin oxygen saturation (SpO_2). There are limitations to the use and accuracy of pulse oximetry, which include situations of vasoconstriction (e.g. shock, hypothermia), excessive movement, where synthetic fingernails and nail polish are used (not common among the elderly), severe anaemia and abnormal haemoglobins (e.g. methaemoglobinaemia or carboxyhaemoglobinaemia). Desaturation is more likely to occur in patients with reduced functional residual capacity such as the elderly. Supplemental oxygen during procedural sedation and anaesthesia should be administered; the anaesthesiologist must be cognizant that it could mask the early detection of apnoea.

End-tidal carbon dioxide ($EtCO_2$) or capnography monitoring aids the detection of apnoea in cases where oxygen administration fails to reveal it. Continuous capnography monitoring detects clinically occult hypoventilation. It constitutes an indispensable part of monitoring for patients undergoing deep sedation or general anaesthesia. For patients with significant pre-existing pulmonary disease, cardiac diseases, or obstructive sleep apnoea, $EtCO_2$ should be monitored even for light sedation. During mechanical ventilation, disconnection from the ventilator has to be monitored continuously.

Although capnography is not currently a worldwide standard requirement for sedation and/or anaesthesia in non-theatre locations, its importance is supported by several published studies. Soto et al. found that episodes of apnoea for at least 20 seconds are frequent during monitored anaesthesia care and these go undetected by even anaesthesia care providers.[3] Qadeer et al. found that endoscopists who were blinded to capnography during moderate sedation with an opioid and benzodiazepine failed to recognize apnoea lasting more than 30 s in about two-thirds of the patients.[4] Capnography identified all cases of hypoxia before onset; and the median time from capnographic evidence of respiratory depression to hypoxia was 1 minute. The Anesthesia Patient Safety Foundation advises that capnography should be monitored for the detection of hypoventilation when supplemental oxygen is delivered.[5]

Temperature monitoring

Remote procedural locations are typically air-conditioned for comfort and to avoid overheating of technical equipment. Elderly patients are less able to regulate their body temperature as a result of alteration in responses to changes in body temperature. Therefore, both sedation and anaesthesia compromise the physiological thermal homeostatic mechanisms and put the elderly patients at a greater risk of hypothermia. Moderate hypothermia may be harmful, causing coagulopathy, shivering, and patient discomfort. More significantly, hypothermia has been associated with severe perioperative adverse outcomes including increased incidence of blood loss, wound infection and even in-hospital mortality[6]. Hypothermia, in addition to being more pronounced, lasts longer in the geriatric patients than it does in younger patients because of their low metabolic rate. For these reasons, any patient, especially the elderly, who is undergoing prolonged anaesthesia or sedation should have temperature monitoring. This could take the form of a temperature probe in the nasopharynx or oropharynx or even integrated into a Foley catheter. The use of active warming devices for prolonged cases should be considered irrespective of the location.

Brain function monitors

Brain function monitors (e.g. bispectral index monitor) are currently being evaluated as a level of consciousness monitoring. The processed electroencephalography signal is quantitated and used as an indicator of sedation level or anaesthesia depth. By allowing the titration of sedatives, it may help to minimise the usage of agents, thus speeding up recovery time.

Summarizing the need for monitoring in the elderly patient—pulse oximetry, NIBP monitors, ECG, and capnography are minimum requirements for any location where anaesthesia or deep sedation is conducted. Where muscle relaxants are used, a peripheral nerve stimulator should be available. During prolonged procedures, a temperature probe is recommended. Brain function monitoring may be useful in avoiding delayed awakening in the elderly patient.

Equipment

The safe care of the elderly for sedation and anaesthesia at a remote location should include all appropriate and readily available equipment and anaesthesia support staff necessary for monitored anaesthesia care, deep sedation, general anaesthesia, and cardiorespiratory emergencies.

Equipment (e.g. the anaesthesia machine) should be regularly serviced with the valid service date indicated on them. The anaesthesia gas should be delivered with recognized safety devices such as oxygen analysers, indexed gas connection systems, reserve supply for oxygen, oxygen supply failure alarm, multiple gas analysers, a volatile anaesthetic agent monitor, a breathing system disconnection alarm, and a scavenging system. It is not uncommon for out of date but still functioning equipment to be used at remote sites. Where the anaesthetic machine or monitoring in not the same as used in the general operating theatre complex, users should be signed off as competent to use the available equipment before use. The monitors used should follow the same standard as in the operating theatre complex. Visible parameters coupled to sufficiently audible alarms with appropriate settings should be activated when limits are breached. The anaesthesia work cart should be stocked as per operating theatre standards—including anaesthesia drugs, self-inflating resuscitator bags, and a range of intravenous equipment. Face masks, endotracheal tubes, laryngeal masks, and adjuncts to difficult intubation should be available. A good and functioning suction apparatus should be present. Importantly, there should be a ready access to a defibrillator and a fully stocked emergency cart with emergency drugs.

Environment

The space should be adequate in size and uncluttered with good access to the patient. In some medical facilities, space may be a premium and it is not uncommon to find anaesthetic equipment tucked away in corners. Access to the patient could be restricted in the MRI and CT scan suites. This compromised proximity to

the patient makes clinical observation, monitoring application, and airway management difficult in times of crisis.

In some MRI suites, long, extended breathing hoses or cables can be found on the floor as connections between the patient and the oxygen source or equipment need to take into account the distance travelled by the table during imaging so as to give adequate slack to prevent a disconnection. This could pose a danger of falls to healthcare worker. Since radiology tables are not specifically designed for anaesthesia, there should be an operating table, trolley or chair which can be readily tilted into Trendelenburg position when the need arises. All tables and trolleys should be able to allow effective cardiopulmonary resuscitation (CPR) without undue time loss due to repositioning.

There should be sufficient electrical outlets including clearly marked electrical outlets connected to an emergency back-up source. All electrical equipment must be routinely checked to mitigate the risk of electrocution and burns. In the radiology suites, exposure to radiation is always a concern. Therefore, there is a need to protect oneself and the patient from the effects of ionizing radiation. Lead protection including aprons and thyroid shields should be available and worn by personnel within the radiation field. In addition, there should also be movable lead shield panels for those who might want to stand behind them for protection during imaging. Lastly, for recovery of the patient, a suitable clinical area with oxygen, suction, resuscitation drugs and equipment is required.

Staff

Healthcare workers should be trained in the pre-sedation and pre-anaesthesia clinical assessment of patients. They should also be trained and experienced in airway management and cardiopulmonary resuscitation and in the use of anaesthetic and resuscitation drugs and equipment, and must ensure that equipment is present and functional prior to induction. As in the operating theatre, they should be dedicated to the continuous monitoring of the patient's physiological parameters and be vigilant at all times.

The non-anaesthesia staff should be appropriately trained to help deal with a cardiopulmonary emergency and be an assistant for the anaesthesiologist. Therefore, this person must be familiar with the anaesthetic procedures and equipment and also be able to help with the positioning of the patient. Provision should be made for the absence of anaesthesia personnel from the immediate vicinity of the patient if required for safety (i.e. in the presence of radiation hazards), provided that adequate patient monitoring is continued despite the physical separation of the anaesthesiologist from the patient. The staff should also be trained in post procedure observation and resuscitation.

One of the findings by the American Society of Anesthesiologists Closed Claims revealed that a higher proportion of patients in non-operating theatre anaesthesia claims underwent monitored anaesthesia care (58 per cent vs 6 per cent) and were at the extremes of age (50 per cent vs 19 per cent) than in operating theatre claims.[7] Half of the non-operating theatre anaesthesia claims occurred in the gastrointestinal suite. Inadequate oxygenation/ventilation was the most common specific damaging event in non-operating theatre anaesthesia claims (33 per cent vs 2 per cent in operating theatre claims).[7] The death proportion was increased in non-operating theatre anaesthesia claims (54 per cent vs 24 per cent). Non-operating theatre anaesthesia claims were more often judged as having sub-standard care preventable by better monitoring.[7]

Sedation progressing to general anaesthesia is a continuum; therefore sedation has the potential to become a general anaesthetic at any point. Complications from oversedation, compromised oxygenation, and ventilation may be more frequent in the hands of inexperienced care providers. Therefore, anaesthetist-led anaesthesia care teams may be the safest method for providing such a service.[8] Advance planning and effective communication with all involved personnel (including the procedurist and the anaesthetist) are important and necessary in providing safe sedation and anaesthetic care to patients in non-theatre locations. Finally, an emergency back-up call system should be prearranged to summon assistance from the main operating theatre complex in crisis situations.

Patient

The patients undergoing procedures outside the operating theatre are often older and medically higher-risk patients. It is estimated that in the latter half of the current decade 20–40 per cent of anaesthetic cases may be performed outside the operating theatre, with surveys showing the elderly preferring more ambulatory settings. This expansion of outpatient procedures for the elderly must be viewed with caution because perioperative complications may increase with age, most likely as a function of associated concurrent diseases. Ambulatory surgery for the elderly patient has to also be weighed against patient-cum-family comprehension and caregiver availability.[9,10]

One must be cognizant that geriatric patients have limited physiological reserves.[11] There is less heart rate responsiveness in response to hypotension. Ventilatory responses to hypoxia and hypercarbia are attenuated, with greater apnoea risk. Thermoregulation is impaired and water balance limited leading to an increased vulnerability for hypovolaemia and hypothermia. Changes in volume of distribution, bioavailablity, and receptor sensitivity lead to alterations in drug pharmacodynamics. Limitations in renal clearance and hepatic and hepatic function require reduction of dosage. Since many elderly have prolonged circulation time, longer periods are required for interval dosing. Titration to effect is an important principle.

Postoperative cognitive dysfunction and postoperative delirium occur in a high percentage of elderly surgical patients. Despite its prevalence, these conditions are often undiagnosed and may be associated with higher morbidity and even mortality rates.[12] Procedures in remote locations often have anaesthetic requirements that rival many operating theatre procedures. The risk of delirium may be increased with agents such as midazolam, pethidine, and anticholinergics. Immobilization and prolonged fasting status are prominent contributing factors for peri-procedure delirium. As with most elderly patients, pethidine has little to recommend it in this setting. See Chapter 26.

When sedating the geriatric patient, the agent of choice should have a short half-life, with minimal active metabolites and limited side effects. By avoiding pre-calculated dosing based on a weight basis and by slower administration of an agent to allow more time for peak effects, the desired end points could often be achieved with smaller quantities of drugs. Several novel approaches to sedation have evolved, and a few may prove useful in enhancing the care of geriatric patients undergoing procedures in remote locations. Similar to patient-controlled analgesia, the concept of patient-controlled sedation is being explored. Studies have demonstrated its safe and efficacious use for conscious sedation in colonoscopy patients.[13]

Among various other logistic considerations, geriatric patients take longer to accomplish tasks. More time must be allocated for pre-procedure preparation. The older patient's skin may be fragile, so adhesive tape should be used with caution to avoid torn skin. Extra padding should be used on procedure tables to prevent compression sores. The elderly are less agile and may require equipment aids (e.g. chair raiser or footstools). Many elderly are hearing impaired, so verbal and written post procedure instructions may foster comprehension.

Older studies have documented that perioperative complications increase with age. A large prospective study by Tiret et al. surveyed the outcomes of approximately 200 000 anaesthetics in France from 1978 to 1982 and demonstrated an almost tenfold increase in the rate of complications specifically attributed to anaesthesia as patient age increased from 30 to 80 years old.[14] This finding may not be surprising since the prevalence of significant comorbidities increase with increasing age. It is however still unclear whether the increased frequency of complications can be attributed to these comorbidities or whether age itself is an independent risk factor. Although the overall frequency of perioperative complications is increased in the elderly, it is still relatively low. In Tiret et al.'s study, the frequency of complications related to anaesthesia was 0.5 per cent in patients greater than 80 years old.[14] These findings suggest that appropriate surgery should not be denied simply on the basis of age alone. It is also believed that the functional status of the elderly may play an important role in predicting risk. Functional status is defined as behaviours necessary to maintain daily life (e.g. activities of daily living) and includes social and cognitive functioning. These functional measures may be even more important or relevant in predicting mortality in hospitalized patients than the standard indices such as acute physiological scores.

The preoperative assessment of the elderly must therefore be aimed at identifying the presence of coexisting illness, and also at determining their 'physiological age'. Specific scoring systems have been developed to assess risk in particular groups of patients, although their value in determining risk for an individual is disputed. Relevant questions about their normal activity levels may be of more use in this context. For example, it is well known that patients with chronic illness may increasingly limit their activity in order to prevent symptoms. Enquiring about the normal daily activities is thus a good way to determine their exercise tolerance. It is also important to bear in mind that disease in the elderly may present with a different spectrum of symptoms to those found in younger patients. A good history with regard to the patient's daily activities can be extremely useful, as this can be expressed in terms of metabolic equivalent tasks. However, it needs to be borne in mind that activity in the elderly can be reduced by factors which limit mobility, such as arthritis or claudication, as opposed to poor physiological reserve.

Once the pre-procedural assessment is complete, the sedationist should judge the suitability of the patient for the proposed procedure with sedation and taking into account the possible risks. Any suggestion of excess risk may warrant the presence of an anaesthesiologist during the procedure. It may be advisable to either postpone or defer the procedure; and even perform it in the main operating theatre where support is better.

Sedative and analgesic medications

Geriatric patients are sensitive to drugs, especially those used in the perioperative period.[15] This increased sensitivity is due to altered pharmacodynamics and pharmacokinetics. The elderly patient has more adipose tissue, decreased muscle mass, and less body water than a younger patient. These factors increase the plasma concentration of water soluble drugs, whereas increased adipose tissue provides for binding of lipid soluble drugs, which might decrease the plasma concentration of a lipid soluble drug.

When administering anaesthetics, it is worth remembering that the geriatric patients are more sensitive to these drugs than the younger patients. The minimum alveolar concentration (MAC) has been shown to decrease with increasing age. For each year above 40 years, MAC decreases by about 0.6 pe rcent. The anaesthetic concentrations needed to produce unconsciousness decrease during ageing. Elderly patients require approximately a third less inhalational agents to produce similar bispectral index levels when compared to younger patients.[16] Geriatric patients are also more sensitive to intravenous anaesthetics, such as propofol, etomidate and thiopental. Intravenous drug dosages should be reduced by up to 20–50 per cent in the elderly.

Combinations of sedative and analgesic medications such as midazolam and fentanyl are commonly used for conscious sedation. It is recommended that the drugs be administered individually and the doses carefully titrated to achieve the desired effect in a given patient while recognizing that combination of sedative and analgesic agents may cause more than additive respiratory depression. In the elderly, due to increased sensitivity and decreased clearance of these agents, smaller doses and more delayed increments must be used. The risk of delirium may also be increased with the use of midazolam in the elderly.

Remifentanil is an ultra-short-acting agent. It offers potent and rapid analgesia, but its rapid offset may prove a disadvantage in situations where postoperative analgesia is required. In the elderly, its use appears to be associated with an increased incidence of hypoventilation. While clearance is quite rapid and independent of age, the dosage required for clinical effect in the elderly is at most 50 per cent of the amount recommended for younger patients.

Propofol is a short acting induction agent with few side effects. Smaller induction doses in the elderly (approximately 1.5 mg/kg) produce a rapid onset of anaesthesia (<2 minutes) lasting 5–10 minutes. There is an age related decrease in propofol clearance, resulting in a decreased maintenance anaesthetic requirement in the elderly patient. Propofol produces dose-dependent cardiovascular and respiratory depression, leading to greater decreases in systemic blood pressure than thiopental when used for induction in elderly patients. This effect can be minimized by injecting propofol slowly to allow sufficient time for the achievement of the full effect, thereby decreasing the total dose. Nevertheless, propofol is a good choice for many elderly patients because it offers quick recovery with few side effects. The use of propofol can result in rapid onset of general anaesthesia; therefore propofol are best reserved for the use by persons trained in the administration of general anaesthesia.[17]

Imaging procedures

The frequency with which complex procedures are carried out in the radiology suite is increasing. Radiological procedures that may require sedation/analgesia include a number of imaging modalities such as X-rays, ultrasonography, CT and MRI, as well as various interventions guided by the imaging modalities. Such interventions include percutaneous placement of tubes, catheters and drains in the chest or abdomen, placement of intravascular access catheters, thrombolysis, embolization of tumours or arteriovenous malformations and others.

During a radiological procedure, whether diagnostic or therapeutic, patients may be expected to remain still for a prolonged period. While the cooperative patients may be able to undergo the procedure with no or minimal sedation, the confused or uncooperative patients will require some form of sedation and/or analgesia. In some instances, because of anxiety, claustrophobia or pain, even the normally cooperative patients may require sedation and /or analgesia to better tolerate the procedure. The situation gets more complicated when dealing with elderly patients where communication could be lost due to hearing impairment, inability to understand or any form of disorientation.

Among the elderly, it is not uncommon to find patients, brought to the radiology suite, who may have severe underlying medical conditions such as cardiovascular, pulmonary or neurological disease, which in the first place have precluded them from surgical interventions. Not surprising, anaesthesiologists on many occasions have been called to assist at a relatively late stage after failure of sedation/analgesia by the radiologist or non-anaesthesia personnel. The unfamiliar work environment in the radiology suite compounds the problem further. Clearly, this situation is unacceptable from a patient safety perspective, and open communication between the departments of radiology and anaesthesia is important. Familiarity of the anaesthesia personnel with the environment in the anaesthetizing location of the radiology suite is essential to providing safe patient care.

Radiation hazard safety

A real concern in the radiology suite is the hazard of radiation exposure. Anaesthesia personnel must be aware of radiation safety and take precautions when possible to avoid unnecessary radiation exposure. Ideally, dosimeters should be worn to monitor exposure. The maximum permissible radiation dose for occupationally exposed persons is 50 millisieverts (mSv) per year. Radiation exposure can be limited by wearing appropriate lead aprons with thyroid shields, using movable leaded glass screens, and allowing remote conduct of anaesthesia—with video monitoring and remote mirroring of monitor data.

Iodinated contrast media

Iodinated contrast agents are often used in diagnostic and therapeutic radiological procedures such as CT to assist imaging. X-rays are absorbed by the soluble contrast agents using iodine (atomic number 53). As older ionized contrast media were hyperosmolar and relatively toxic, non-ionized contrast media with low osmolality and improved side effect profiles are being used increasingly.

Adverse reactions to contrast media range from mild to life threatening. The causes include direct toxicity, idiosyncratic reactions, and allergic reactions—either anaphylactic or anaphylactoid. Predisposing factors include a history of bronchospasm, history of allergy, underlying cardiac disease, renal dysfunction, extremes of age and medications such as β-blockers, aspirin, and non-steroidal anti-inflammatory drugs. Notably, elderly patient commonly have several of these predisposing conditions. Treatment is symptomatic such as the administration of oxygen and bronchodilators, and in severe cases, adrenaline administration. Corticosteroids and antihistamines may also be given to symptomatic patients assuming an immunological basis for the reaction.

Contrast-induced nephropathy is a significant complication of radiological procedures and a leading cause of hospital-acquired acute renal failure. High osmolality contrast agents are associated with greater nephrotoxicity than low osmolality agents. Most of these cases are self-limiting, resolving usually within 2 weeks although in some patients, dialysis may be required. Prevention of renal dysfunction includes hydration before, during and after the procedure, the use of low-osmolality contrast media and the administration of acetylcysteine or ascorbic acid. In view of the possibility of life-threatening lactic acidosis, extra care is needed when patients taking metformin receive contrast media.

Other issues confronting the anaesthesiologists in the CT scan room include inaccessibility of the patient during the procedure and control of movement artefact. Care needs to be taken to ensure that the sides of the scanning tunnel do not occlude or dislodge the breathing circuit or monitoring leads during the procedure. Dealing with difficult airways, whether anticipated or not, can be problematic outside the operating theatre. It is recommended that such anticipated difficult intubations be performed in the operating theatre to take advantage of the skilled assistance and specialized equipment. Once the airway is secured, the patient can be transferred to the site of the planned procedure. Even then, equipment for induction, maintenance and emergence from routine general anaesthesia should be available at all times in the radiology suites and of similar quality to that available in the main operating theatre complex. Tables in the radiology suite do not tilt into a head-down position. Therefore, the patient may require induction or emergence from anaesthesia on a tipping trolley.

Magnetic resonance imaging

Complex imaging technology such as the MRI has dramatically improved diagnostic capabilities but it has given rise to new challenges in ensuring safe patient care. Advantages of MRI includes the ability of obtaining transverse, sagittal, coronal, or oblique sections, provision of excellent soft tissue contrast, minimal preparation requirements, and that MRI does not produce deleterious ionizing radiation.

Concerns during MRI: limitations and hazards

MRI imaging takes time, anywhere from 20 minutes to more than 1 hour. Patient movement can affect imaging by producing artefacts. Patient's access and visibility is also limited because of the depth of the magnet of nearly 2 metres. This makes it near impossible to visualize the patient's face and chest for adequacy of ventilation during scanning. Though acceptance of MRI examination is generally high among patients, keeping still for long periods inside the narrow confines of the magnet (50 to 65 cm in diameter) can trigger a sense of claustrophobia in the already nervous or unprepared patient, and in the obese. The loud noises (>90 dB) produced, equivalent to light road work, during scanning could further unsettle such patients. Therefore, hearing protection in the form of ear plugs is necessary for both the patient and healthcare personnel who must be in the room. Sedation/analgesia may also be required in the uncooperative elderly patient. Anaesthesia personnel should preferably be on hand to decide when it becomes necessary to protect the patient's airway and control the ventilation if sedation fails. This conduct is fraught with difficulties given the unfamiliarity of the environment, the suitability of equipment used and the limited access to the patient.

The most significant hazard in the MRI suite is the magnetic field generated by the imaging equipment itself and its effect on ferrous objects. Although newer MRI machines are shielded so that the effects of the field decrease significantly, it is strongly advised that no equipment be brought into vicinity of the MRI without approval from the biomedical engineering department. At the 30–50 gauss line, some ferromagnetic equipment may be used safely.

Dislodgement and malfunction of implanted biological devices or objects containing ferromagnetic material also pose real concerns. The list of items includes vascular clips and shunts, pacemakers, automatic implantable cardioverter defibrillators, mechanical heart valves, implanted biological pumps and others. Death from torque of a vascular clip within the MRI field has been reported. More commonly, small frequently used items become projectiles including scissors, forceps, pens and so forth. Not only are injuries to patients and personnel reported but the magnet might need to be turned off to remove the items from the magnetic bore. Restarting the magnet might take several days and at a great cost. For this reason, the MRI suite is divided into four zones. Barriers to access have been identified for zones III and IV (the scanner room) where the magnetic field is apparent. The introduction of ferromagnetic objects within these zones may be hazardous.

Although heating of the whole patient is not quite a concern, the potential exists for heat generation within monitoring wires from electromagnetic induction, circuit resonance, or an 'antenna effect'. Injury from such manner of heating has been reported in the area of ECG electrodes and pulse oximeter probes. For this reason, coils in wires should be avoided and conductors should not touch the patient at more than one location.

MRI seems to be intrinsically safe for patients from the standpoint that no adverse biological effects of the MRI field have been known to occur; however, other hazards and risks from MRI scanning exist. Suffice to say that adherence to standard monitoring recommendations for only MRI compatible equipment from ventilators, ECG electrodes, pulse oximeters to infusion pumps, and being familiar with the environment and the patient, and being vigilant in attending to the patient, whether from the annexed room or the scanner room during the procedure, are essential for ensuring safety for elderly patients requiring sedation or anaesthesia in the MRI suite.

Cardiac catheterization laboratory

See also Chapter 21.

The expanding role of interventions in the cardiac catheterization laboratory has resulted in anaesthesia teams having to conduct anaesthesia in remote or non-theatre environments, which demand great flexibility in coping with different complications, types of patients and challenges.[18] Transcatheter aortic valve implantation (TAVI) is becoming routine practice in elderly patients affected by significant aortic valve stenosis who also have serious comorbidity prohibiting an open heart operation.

There are serious anaesthetic challenges confronting the anaesthesia team in catering and adapting to this expanding high-risk patient population undergoing such procedures. These challenges are further exaggerated by the catheterization laboratory itself, often a setting not intentionally designed for the requirements of the anaesthesia teams. Unfamiliarity and limitations with the setting can lead to potentially serious patient safety issues. Many other routine interventions in the cardiac laboratory such as percutaneous coronary intervention and electrophysiological procedures are carried out by the cardiology team in conscious patients.

Transcatheter aortic valve implantation

TAVI is an increasingly routine option for treatment of significant and limiting aortic valve stenosis in a patient population who, owing to advanced age in combination with either extreme co-morbidities (logistic EuroSCORE >20 or Society of Thoracic Surgeons Predicted Risk of Mortality Score-STS - PROM ≥10) or other factors (e.g. porcelain aorta, previous sternotomy, significant cirrhosis, severe kyphoscoliosis, or extensive mediastinal therapy), are at too high a risk to undergo an open heart operation and traditional aortic valve replacement.[18] Contraindications include life expectancy of less than 12 months, existing mechanical aortic valve or endocarditis, severe organic mitral regurgitation, coronary artery disease requiring surgical intervention, and no suitable access route.

TAVI is a less invasive therapeutic alternative when surgical aortic valve replacement is contraindicated because of technical limitations or when comorbid states amount to prohibitive surgical risk. The current technique of TAVI is now well established using two devices—the balloon-expanded Edwards SAPIEN® valve stent (Edwards Life Sciences, Irvine, CA, USA) and the self—expanding Medtronic CoreValve ReValving® system (Medtronic Inc., Minneapolis, MN, USA). The former consists of a metal stent (made of steel or cobalt-chromium) which secures the device in its intended position inside the valve and valve leaflets (made of biological material derived from cows) to direct the flow of blood out of the heart. It is commonly undertaken using a retrograde approach via the femoral or other major artery, or by an antegrade transapical approach through the apex of the left ventricle via an anterolateral thoracotomy. Implantation involves crossing the stenosed native aortic valve with a wire followed by balloon valvuloplasty and then deployment of the bioprosthesis within the annulus.

In the majority of TAVI cases, general anaesthesia is administered. A possible alternative is the use of local anaesthesia with sedation for the transfemoral approach. With either technique, a detailed cardiovascular preoperative assessment of the patient is crucial to evaluate whether TAVI is possible and which of the two techniques for TAVI (transfemoral or transapical route) is more suitable.

Preoperative investigations may include an ECG, angiogram, blood tests, chest X-ray, and CT scan. Determination of renal function is important as nephrotoxicity from intravenous fluoroscopic contrast is a potential complication, especially in elderly patients with pre-existing compromised renal function. Further

investigations relevant to the intervention itself include measurement of the aortic valve annulus, distance between the aortic valve and the coronary ostiae and screening the extent of possible atherosclerotic arterial disease both peripherally in the femoral and iliac vessels and centrally in the ascending aorta and aortic arch. It is also important to exclude a recent stroke.

Convening a discussion with all medical specialties involved; explaining the approach, the possible complications, and the course of action to take in the event of an acute life threatening complication during the procedure can facilitate teamwork during the actual procedure and avoid delay and confusion during a crisis. TAVI is ideally undertaken in a hybrid operating cum angiography suite with the patient in a supine position with arms by the side and the left chest slightly elevated if a transapical TAVI approach is used. Theatre personnel usually include a cardiac anaesthetic team, surgical team, perfusionist, and an echocardiographer.

Standard monitoring equipment may include five-lead ECG, invasive arterial line, central venous line, transoesophageal echocardiography (TOE), temperature probe, urine catheter and ACT monitor. Procedure specific equipment may include cardiac angiography table with mobile gantry, large-bore intravenous access, rapid infusion warming device, pacemaker, cell saver, heated blanket device, and external defibrillation pads.

Anaesthesia for TAVI

TAVI is still in its infancy in many parts of the world. Experienced anaesthetic involvement is critical to reduce patient morbidity and mortality.[19]

Although the transfemoral TAVI could be attempted under local anaesthesia with sedation to minimize haemodynamic instability and shorten procedure times, it makes patient immobility during valvuloplasty and valve deployment less reliable, managing major complications more difficult, and the use of echocardiography during the procedure more challenging. Emergency conversion to anaesthesia must be planned for. For transapical TAVI, patients frequently receive perioperative anticoagulation with aspirin, clopidogrel, and heparin, and the procedure is performed under general anaesthesia with a single-lumen tracheal tube.

Before induction, large-bore intravenous access is obtained, a rapid infusion warming device connected, and an arterial line in place. As the cardiac catheterization suite does not usually install waste gas scavenging systems, a total intravenous anaesthesia technique is performed with propofol and remifentanil.

After induction, central venous access is obtained, a TOE probe introduced and external defibrillation pads are placed. The temperature of the patient is maintained with heated blankets and air warming devices. A cell saving equipment should be readied for use and a perfusionist is on standby with extracorporeal circulation equipment.

In both approaches, a pacing wire is first introduced and connected to a pacemaker under the control of the anaesthetist. The native aortic valve is dilated by balloon valvuloplasty and the transcatheter aortic valve subsequently placed under the conditions of rapid ventricular pacing and a cessation of ventilation. During TAVI, temporarily minimizing cardiac motion and reducing left ventricular output with rapid ventricular transvenous pacing aids device positioning and minimizes displacement during balloon valvuloplasty and device deployment. Haemodynamic complications of rapid ventricular pacing are minimized by ensuring adequate pre-pacing arterial pressure and pre-emptive vasopressor in particularly fragile patients. During transapical TAVI, echocardiography is used to identify the left ventricular apex, a small incision made and the left ventricular cavity accessed with a Seldinger technique.

In emergency cases or in patients with an ejection fraction less than 20 per cent, consideration of initiating elective femoral–femoral bypass should be discussed because significant haemodynamic instability should be expected. A plan for initiation of rescue cardiopulmonary bypass or open heart surgery should be rehearsed by the perioperative team.

Perioperative concerns and management

Hypovolaemia, hypotension, cardiac ischaemia, and arrhythmia are all poorly tolerated and must be vigilantly observed. Resuscitation should include early identification of the cause and consideration of emergency cardiopulmonary bypass. Arterial injury can include tearing or avulsion near the access point, aortic dissection, or annulus rupture. Manipulation of wires can interfere with the mitral valve apparatus or cause poorly tolerated arrhythmias or tamponade. Neurological events including delirium, seizure and stroke, caused by atheroma, calcific or air embolization, dissection or hypotension are more easily assessed with awake patients.

The majority of patients undergoing TAVI will be extubated at the end of procedure and may be able to return to a cardiac ward or a high dependency unit. Patient-controlled analgesia, intercostal blocks, and paracetamol all provide satisfactory analgesia.

Recently, hybrid operating theatres have been developed to facilitate direct open heart operations with use of cardiopulmonary bypass in the same location as cardiac catheterization. If the two locations remain distinct, transport and relevant logistical problems will have to be negotiated to transfer the patient to the operating theatre. Meticulous planning is essential to ensure a smooth workflow.

Periprocedural mortality from TAVI may be about 6 per cent. Following TAVI, 30-day mortality rate was about 8–12 per cent, and serious morbidity was reported as occurring in about 24–32 per cent of patients.[19]

Coronary angiography and percutaneous coronary intervention

The great majority of percutaneous coronary diagnostic and intervention procedures take place without the presence of an anaesthesia team.[18] However, performing the procedure in patients in cardiogenic shock following an ischaemic event often requires endotracheal intubation to secure the airway and optimize oxygenation and ventilation and to some extent, aid a failing LV by reducing LV afterload. It may even be appropriate to consider the implantation of an intra-aortic counterpulsation device to optimize coronary perfusion and decrease the afterload of the failing LV or the percutaneous implantation of ventricular assist devices for refractory shock to inotropic therapy.

The role of the anaesthesia teams in the care of patients in cardiogenic shock is challenging owing to the acute and emergent nature of the situation. The conditions are less than optimal for safe patient care, effective resuscitation and coordinated teamwork. Centres offering an acute coronary interventional service should

ensure that anaesthetic equipment is readily installed and drugs are promptly stocked and easily available.

Limitations of the cardiac catheterization suite to anaesthesia

There are certain differences between a cardiac catheterization suite and a standard operating theatre which makes the environment in the former far less conducive to anaesthesia practice. The presence of the large C-arm of the fluoroscopy equipment may limit access to the patient and adds the risk of ventilation tubing and airway dislodgements. Central venous access may be difficult to obtain as the cardiac table can often not be placed in the Trendelenburg position. Access may be facilitated though by the use of ultrasound. Connections to pressure lines and intravenous pumps may also have to be extended to allow for the lack of space in the vicinity. The potential lack of space around the patient also limits the work environment of the anaesthesia team. Such issues can be greatly improved by the development of hybrid operating theatres which gives room for the increased number of staff and equipment necessary during such procedures.

The complex nature of the cardiac patient and intervention procedure demands meticulous planning by all involved to ensure a reasonable plan for the anaesthesia, monitoring, venous access, additional equipment, and complications anticipation. The formulation of a prearranged plan detailing potential emergency actions in the event of complications may greatly improve teamwork during the procedure itself.

Emergencies

Anaesthesia and airway management in emergency situations may save a life in critically ill or injured patients.[20] However, it may also increase morbidity and mortality if not performed properly. This is more so in the context of elderly patients. In some countries, emergency airway management and ventilatory support start from the prehospital phase when transfer time to the next hospital is undesirably long. An important consideration is the airway management skills of the attending healthcare personnel. In the event that the first medical rescuer is not adequately trained in tracheal intubation, the patient may benefit from a supraglottic airway device such as the laryngeal mask airway or non-invasive ventilatory support with a positive airway pressure mask.

Prehospital phase

See also Chapter 16.

Emergency physicians experienced in airway management in France had problems in only approximately 3 per cent of prehospital admissions.[21] However, in Miami, it was reported that paramedics encountered intubation difficulties in 31 per cent of patients.[22] In a German study observing prehospital intubations performed by primary emergency physicians, an approximately 15 per cent rate of bronchially and oesophageally positioned tubes were reported.[23] The incidence of unrecognized oesophageal intubation was associated with a high mortality rate. As illustrated here, the incidence of difficult prehospital intubation may vary from country to country and according to the varying experience of the healthcare personnel involved in the intubation attempt. As a result, the Association of Anaesthetists of Great Britain and Ireland recommended prehospital anaesthesia only for appropriately trained and competent practitioners.[24]

A three-level airway management skills model has been suggested by Braun et al.[20] in a recent review article, which could serve as a decision guide for a given rescuer. For instance, a highly skilled 'gold' level rescuer could decide freely how to oxygenate and ventilate a patient. A moderately skilled 'silver' level rescuer could attempt endotracheal intubation twice and then switch to an alternative supraglottic airway device or bag-valve-mask ventilation. A less skilled 'bronze' level rescuer should completely refrain from endotracheal intubation and try to optimize oxygenation, hasten hospital transfer and employ a supraglottic airway device or bag-valve-mask ventilation only in patients in life-threatening situations.[20]

According to Braun and colleagues, the decision as to whether a patient should be anaesthetized in the field or later in the hospital's emergency department depends on several parameters. Indications for prehospital anaesthesia include gold level rescue with experienced team members, in patients who have severe head trauma or have fast deteriorating respiratory failure, when long transport time to the hospital is anticipated, and where good equipment is available in a safe and appropriate environment (e.g. terrain, temperature, and light).

Emergency department anaesthesia and airway management

Patients requiring anaesthesia in the emergency department are frequently critically ill, severely injured, or in extremis. Their pathophysiological changes, sensitivity to anaesthetic drugs, together with the potential for increased difficult intubation, require the presence of a trained airway specialist. In most places, this role would be delegated to the anaesthetist, who has the competence to manage these challenges in a timely and effective manner. The College of Emergency Medicine has also recognized that emergency physicians should have the requisite skills to manage an airway in the first 30 minutes of admission.[25] Many emergency patients are initially managed with rapid sequence induction and intubation. This procedure should only be undertaken by doctors with adequate training and experience in anaesthetic agents and airway management. For instance, if bag mask ventilation should prove difficult in the elderly such as in the edentulous or those with sunken cheeks where mask fit may not be optimal, desaturation can easily set in.

The National Confidential Enquiry into Patient Outcome and Death reported in 2007 that inexperienced doctors may compromise care for the critically ill or injured patients. This may be compounded by lack of trained assistance, inadequate supervision, and problems with drug and equipment availability.[26] Failed intubation is more common in the emergency department. There should be a particular focus on adequate preoxygenation, the availability of difficult intubation equipment (e.g. intubating laryngeal mask airways and video laryngoscopes), capnography, and training for the management of the emergency surgical airway. Therefore the safe management of these vulnerable emergency patients depends on close collaboration between emergency physicians and anaesthesiologists to ensure that clear institutional policies and procedures are in place, and that audit and discussion of complications are undertaken regularly. A designated consultant anaesthesiologist should be responsible for ensuring that services meet the recommendations laid out in the hospital policies.

Drugs for sedation and anaesthesia in the emergency department

The emergency department has its own sedation practice governed by the Academy of Emergency Medicine. Although their experience with drugs such as propofol, ketamine, and various analgesics (fentanyl and morphine) is extensive, adverse events can still occur in the most versatile of settings. A good understanding of the pharmacokinetics and pharmacodynamics of such agents by emergency physicians in the elderly is important. An overzealous administration of drugs without due consideration for the differences between the elderly and the adult could lead to a disastrous fall in blood pressure and prolonged apnoea. Reversal agents including flumazenil and naloxone have to be within easy reach.

Hospitals need to ensure that their anaesthesia and/or intensive care services are staffed to a level which allows them to respond in a timely manner to care for emergency patients in the emergency department. The Royal Colleague of Anaesthetists Audit guidelines make recommendations about response times for anaesthetists to the emergency department.[27] Institutional response times should be audited and standards set.

Conclusion

Anaesthesia and sedation by anaesthesiologists in non-theatre environments are poised to rise exponentially on the backdrop of procedural advancement in technology and call for greater patient safety. Advanced diagnostic imaging, interventional radiology, and cardiac catheterization laboratory procedures will contribute to the increasing numbers. Adverse outcomes may occur without proper institutional procedures, healthcare personnel education, and training. Minimum monitoring standards, availability of equipment, trained healthcare workers, institution-specific guidelines, and appropriate patient selection are the components necessary to mitigate these risks and promote patient safety for sedation and anaesthesia in non-theatre environments.

References

1. Metzner J, Posner KL, Domino KB. The risk and safety of anesthesia at remote locations: the US closed claims analysis. *Curr Opinion Anaesthesiol.* 2009;22(4):502–508.
2. Eichhorn V, Henzler D, Murphy MF. Standardizing care and monitoring for anesthesia or procedural sedation delivered outside the operating theatre. *Curr Opin Anaesthesiol.* 2010;23:494–499.
3. Soto RG, Fu ES, Vila H, Miguel RV. Capnography accurately detects apnoea during monitored anesthesia care. *Anesth Analg.* 2004;99:379–382.
4. Qadeer MA, Vargo JJ, Dumot JA, et al. Capnographic monitoring of respiratory activity improves safety of sedation for endoscopic cholangiopancreatography and ultrasonography. *Gastroenterology.* 2009;136:1568–1576.
5. Weinger MB, Lee LA. 'No patient shall be harmed by opioid-induced respiratory depression'. In Proceedings of 'Essential monitoring strategies to detect clinically significant drug-induced respiratory depression in the postoperative period' conference. *APSF Newsletter.* 2011;26(2):21,26–28.
6. Karalapillai D, Story DA, Calzavacca P, et al. Inadvertent hypothermia and mortality in postoperative intensive care patients: retrospective audit of 5050 patients. *Anaesthesia.* 2009;64:968–972.

7. Robbertze R, Posner K, Domino KB. Closed claims review of anesthesia for procedures outside the operating theatre. *Curr Opin Anaesthesiol.* 2006;19(4):436–442.

8. Silber JH, Kennedy SK, Even-Shoshan O, *et al.* Anesthesiologist direction and patient outcomes. *Anesthesiology.* 2000;93:152–163.

9. Bettelli G. Anaesthesia for the elderly outpatient: preoperative assessment and evaluation, anaesthetic technique and postoperative pain management. *Curr Opin Anaesthesiol.* 2010;23:726–731.

10. Bryson GL, Chung F, Finegan BA, *et al.* Patient selection in ambulatory anesthesia—an evidence-based review: part I. *Can J Anesth.* 2004;51:768–781.

11. Silverstein J. Problems with geriatric anesthesia patients. *Anesthesiology Clin* 2009;27:xv–xvi.

12. Steinmetz J, Christensen KB, Lund T, *et al*; ISPOCD Group. Long-term consequences of postoperative cognitive dysfunction. *Anesthesiology.* 2009;110:548–555.

13. Ng JM, Kong CF, Nyam D. Patient-controlled sedation with propofol for colonoscopy. *Gastrointest Endosc.* 2001;54(1):8–13.

14. Tiret L, Desmonts JM, Hatton F, *et al.* Complications associated with anaesthesia: a prospective survey in France. *Can Anesth Soc J.* 1986;33:336–344.

15. Singh A, Antognini JF. Perioperative pharmacology in elderly patients. *Curr Opin Anaesthesiol.* 2010;23:449–454.

16. Matsuura T, Oda Y, Tanaka K, *et al.* Advance of age decrease the minimum alveolar concentration of isoflurane and sevoflurane for maintaining bispectral index below 50. *Br J Anaesth.* 2009;102:331–335.

17. Statement on safe use of propofol (amended by ASA House of Delegates Oct 21, 2009). <http://www.asahq.org/publicationsAndServices/standards/37.pdf>.

18. Braithwaite S, Kluin J, Buhre WF, *et al.* Anaesthesia in the cardiac catheterisation laboratory. *Curr Opin Anaesthesia.* 2010;23:507–512.

19. Klein AA, Webb ST, Tsui S, *et al.* Transcatheter aortic valve insertion: anaesthetic implications of emerging new technology. *Br J Anaesth.* 2009;103(6):792–799.

20. Braun P, Wenzel V, Paal P. Anesthesia in Prehospital emergencies and in the emergency department. *Curr Opin Anaesthesiol.* 2010;23:500–506.

21. Tentillier E, Heydenreich C, Cros AM, *et al.* Use of the intubating laryngeal mask airway in emergency prehospital difficult intubation. *Resuscitation.* 2008;77:30–34.

22. Cobas MA, De la Pena MA, Manning R, *et al.* Prehospital intubation and mortality: a level 1 trauma center perspective. *Anesth Analg.* 2009;109:489–493.

23. Timmermann A, Russo SG, Eich C, *et al.* The out-of-hospital esophageal and endobronchial intubation performed by emergency physicians. *Anesth Analg.* 2007;104:619–623.

24. The Association of Anaesthetists of Great Britain and Ireland (AAGBI). *Safety guideline for prehospital anaesthesia.* <http://www.aagbi.org/publications/guidelines/docs/prehospital_glossary09.pdf:2009>.

25. Nolan J, Clancy M. Airway management in the emergency department. *Br J Anaesth.* 2002; 88:9–11.

26. NCEPOD. *Trauma: Who cares? A report of the National Confidential Enquiry into Patient Outcomes and Death.* London: NCEPOD, 2007. <http://www.ncepod.org.uk/2007report2/Dwonload/SIP_summary.pdf>.

27. Oakley P. Anaesthesia in the accident and emergency department. In Jackson I (ed) *Raising the standard. A compendium of audit recipes,* 3rd edn. London: RCoA, 2012. <http://http://www.rcoa.ac.uk/system/files/CSQ-ARB-section6.pdf>.

CHAPTER 34

Heat balance and anaesthetic implications in the elderly

Amjad Maniar and Kwong Fah Koh

Introduction

The number of elderly patients presenting for complex and prolonged surgical procedures has been rapidly increasing. Elderly patients with their often compromised physiology and comorbidities have to endure longer hospital stays, costs, and complications as compared to younger patients. Thus, the focus of optimal anaesthesia care in this population is to ensure that preventable intraoperative events do not contribute significantly to the patient's recovery in the postoperative period.

Hyperthermia, as well as hypothermia, more commonly affect the elderly patient, the latter being the most common heat disturbance that we are likely to encounter during the perioperative period which may lead to increased morbidity. Alterations in physiology, environmental factors of the operating room, and the conduct of anaesthesia and surgery have a profound impact on heat regulation in an elderly patient. While maintenance of normothermia is desirable, this may not always be easily achieved and hence elderly patients may be subject to differential body temperatures while undergoing surgery.

Physiology of heat regulation

Normal body temperature regulation

The human body maintains a stable core temperature independent of external influence. This is essential for the metabolic and enzymatic processes within the body. Normal core body temperature can vary between healthy individuals, with differences between measurement sites.[1] The observed normal range for oral temperature is 33.2–38.2°C (92–101°F), for rectal 34.4–37.8°C (94–100°F), for the tympanic cavity it is 35.4–37.8°C (96–100°F), and for the axilla it is 35.5–37.0°C (96–99°F).[2] It is unclear if the baseline core temperature is decreased in the elderly, with some reports supporting this observation[2,3] while others indicate that a temperature decrease does not occur.[4] However it is well known that the elderly are susceptible to the deleterious effects of swings in temperature.

External and internal heat sources influence body temperature. Heavy exercise, illness, and hot and cold environments alter body temperature. Ambient temperature, humidity, air movement, and radiant heat from the sun, as well as warm and cold surfaces, contribute to climatic heat stress.

Heat exchange between the body and the surrounding environment occurs in unidirectional and bidirectional routes. Unidirectional routes imply that only either heat gain or heat loss can occur, but not both during that process. Examples of these are heat production within the core compartment by metabolism and heat loss from the skin by evaporation. Bidirectional heat exchange allows for heat to be gained and lost through that particular route. Examples of this are convection, conduction, and radiation.

Heat is produced within the body as a product of the various metabolic reactions within. Heat production from metabolic energy occurs almost immediately. Several factors determine the rate of heat production.

- Basal rate of metabolism of all the cells of the body.
- Metabolism caused by muscle activity, including muscle contractions caused by shivering.
- Metabolism caused by the effect of substances like thyroxine, and catecholamines, and the effect of meals.

About 70 per cent of energy production at rest occurs in the 'body core', which is the trunk and the brain. Most of the heat requirements of the human body are produced at these sites and this is effective in maintaining normal temperature when the ambient temperature is comfortable. The ratio of metabolic rate to surface area is highest in infancy and declines with age.

Heat exchange

Four mechanisms are responsible for heat exchange at the skin surface.[5]

Conduction

Conduction has a minimal effect on body heat transfer, as it depends upon direct contact between the skin and a cooler object. This process accounts for about 5 per cent of the heat loss in the perioperative period and is proportional to the area of the body exposed, the relative difference in temperature between the mediums or surfaces, and the thermal conductivity of these. Heat loss by this method is quite negligible in the operating room as most patients are usually insulated or in contact with materials that are poor thermal conductors (gowns, sheets, etc.).

Convection

Convection is responsible for transferring heat from working muscles and the skin surface. In operating rooms with laminar flow, the air around the body is in constant motion and it sweeps away the warmed air molecules close to the skin surface. This results in about 25 per cent of the heat loss in the operating room environment. It is dependent upon the temperature differential between skin and the environment and the heat transfer coefficient, which varies with available body surface area and wind velocity. Heat loss by convection could be accentuated in ultraclean operating rooms where the air changes can be high as 300/hour (as compared to 20–25 in plenum type rooms).

Radiation

Radiation is the primary method for discharging the body's excess heat at rest. Every surface emits energy as electromagnetic radiation. Losses via this mechanism are related to surface property (emissivity) and the difference to the fourth power of exposed skin and wall temperature (in degrees Kelvin). Since each body emits radiation with an intensity that depends on its temperature, the net heat flow is from the warmer to the cooler body. The heat is given off in the form of infrared rays. Radiation heat loss or gain depends upon the temperature gradient between the skin and the environment. Radiation accounts for 60 per cent of heat loss in humans. Loss of radiant heat is generally dependent on cutaneous blood flow and the body's exposed surfaces to the environment.

Evaporation

Evaporation normally occurs when the ambient temperature is hotter than the skin, and this phenomenon results when the environment is warmer than 36°C. However, in the operating room environment, heat loss by evaporation may not contribute significantly to hypothermia. Heat loss by evaporation can occur during normal or controlled respiration (respiratory heat loss). Skin disinfection with antiseptic solutions prior to surgery can also contribute (minimally) to evaporative heat losses. It can also occur in operations where the skin incision is large and prolonged exposure contributes to heat and moisture loss. Lamke[6] showed that the surface temperature of the bowel fell by 3.5°C in major exposure operations. More recently, it was shown in simulated study that the heat lost through the surgical wound in orthopaedic procedures was 6 per cent.[7] Heat loss may increase up to 280 per cent if contact with wet surgical drapes moistens the skin.

Maintenance of body temperature can thereby be represented by the net heat storage formula:

$$S = M \pm Cv \pm Cd \pm R - E$$

where S = net heat storage, M = metabolic heat, Cv = convection, Cd = conduction, R = radiation, and E = evaporation.

When the net heat storage (S) is positive, body temperature will rise and will reduce when negative.

Neural regulation of temperature

Homeothermy is maintained in the human body by a complex system of afferent inputs, central processing, and efferent responses.

Afferent system

The afferent system conducts warm and cold impulses to the central thermoregulatory system. Warm signals are transported through non-myelinated C fibres while cold signals are conducted through the thinly myelinated A-delta fibres.[8] Signals from these fibres ascend through the spinothalamic tract in the anterior spinal cord. Early processing of the signals may begin to occur at the level of the spinal cord.[9]

Central thermoregulation

It has been known for more than a century that the hypothalamus is the central structure within the brain that is involved in thermoregulation. The preoptic area that contains the anterior hypothalamus, the medial and lateral parts of the preoptic nucleus, and the septal regions are synaptically linked to the brainstem. Preoptic cooling can produce shivering, an increase in heat production, as well as non-shivering thermogenesis. Preoptic warming may elicit responses that are helpful in heat loss, such as sweating, panting, and cutaneous vasodilation.

In a completely intact nervous system, the modulation of the thermoregulatory response is precise as compared to a system where there is a lesion interrupting the pathways. The spinal cord and neuraxis may also provide outputs to the efferent response system if there is disruption of the normal pathways.

Efferent response

Thermal disturbances elicit varied responses that are dependent on the type of temperature change.

Hyperthermia

The eccrine (sweat) glands, which are distributed over nearly the entire body surface, are primarily responsible for thermoregulatory sweating in humans. Postganglionic non-myelinated C fibres pass through the grey ramus communicans, combine with peripheral nerves, and innervate sweat glands. Sweating allows for evaporation which cools the skin surface. Additionally, heat transfer from deeper tissues to the surface occurs by capillary vasodilatation.

Hypothermia

The normal responses to hypothermia include initial vasoconstriction and subsequent initiation of shivering. Shivering is only initiated when the body temperature drops 1°C below the temperature required to initiate vasoconstriction.[10] Vasoconstriction is a highly effective method of heat conservation which restricts blood flow into the peripheries, thereby minimizing heat loss. Vasoconstriction of the superficial limb veins diverts venous blood to the deep limb veins, which lie close to the major arteries of the limbs and do not constrict in the cold. As blood traverses in close proximity to the warm major arteries, it picks up heat which is transported back to the core. The marginally cooled arterial blood thereby loses less heat as it circulates closer to the surface. This mechanism is known as 'counter current heat exchange'.[11] The reverse of this phenomenon occurs when the body attempts to cool itself. Together, these are important methods of non-shivering thermogenesis.

As vasoconstriction peaks and the core temperature drops, shivering is initiated. Shivering is an involuntary, oscillatory muscular activity that augments metabolic heat production.[10] Shivering in adults can double metabolism at rest and subsequently increase it to more than 600 per cent[12] and may provide up to one-third of the heat production during cold exposure.

When the hypothalamus is cooled, thermally induced changes in neuronal activity in the mesencephalic reticular formation and the dorsolateral pontine and medullary reticular formation increase muscle tone. Spinal α motor neurons and their axons are the final common path for both coordinated movement and shivering.

Variations in the elderly affecting heat regulation

There is evidence in the literature that the effects of hypothermia may contribute to adverse outcomes in this age group both within and outside the hospital settings.[13] It is important to understand changes in the elderly which may affect temperature regulation and then consider other factors.

Thermal tolerance

In the elderly, the response to heat challenges may be impaired. Deterioration in thermal toleration does not seem to occur linearly with age, but may be most pronounced in individuals over the age of 80.

Changes in skin structure

With age, the number of eccrine (sweat) glands in the skin is markedly decreased along with the response in sweat output per gland. These results in an overall decrease in sweat production thereby impairing the principal cooling mechanism activated during hyperthermia.

Loss of perception

Cognitive decline may influence behavioural responses towards cold. Behavioural responses are absent under general anaesthesia or reduced under sedation. It may be of value to the clinician using regional anaesthesia as an indicator of thermal comfort (e.g. patient attempting to cover himself with the blanket during surgery).

Loss of skeletal muscle mass

The loss of skeletal muscle mass with ageing (sarcopenia) may affect body temperature and thermoregulation in both hot and cold environmental conditions. Sarcopenia alters the thermal properties of the body due to differences in water content, and thus specific heat, of muscle and adipose tissue. Loss of muscle mass may also contribute to reductions in insulator properties. There is an increased reliance on peripheral vasoconstriction to minimize heat loss which may already be affected in the elderly individual. These changes may lead to relatively lower body temperatures and an increased risk of hypothermia during cold stress.

Effect of medications

Some pharmacological agents, including the barbiturates, tricyclic antidepressants and benzodiazepines, can cause central thermoregulatory failure. Phenothiazines can impair central thermoregulation and inhibit peripheral vasoconstriction to cold by their alpha-blocking activity. Prazosin, an alpha blocker, can cause hypothermia, especially in the elderly. Alcohol consumption can lead to peripheral dilatation, impaired shivering, hypoglycaemia and environmental exposure to cold, as well as having a direct effect on the hypothalamus, by which it lowers the thermoregulatory set point, resulting in a fall in core temperature.

Coexisting illnesses

Certain medical diseases, commonly found in the elderly can impair central thermoregulatory control. Of particular note are neurological conditions such as stroke, central nervous system (CNS) trauma, infection, tumours, haemorrhage, Parkinson's disease, multiple sclerosis, and Wernicke's syndrome. Sepsis may predispose to hypothermia by causing failure of vasoconstriction or by causing an abnormal hypothalamic response. Long-term diabetes can cause autonomic dysfunction impairing the peripheral vasculature thereby disrupting normal thermoregulation. Endocrine disorders such as hypothyroidism, hypoadrenalism, and hypopituitarism, and hypoglycaemia alone can predispose to hypothermia. Age- or disease-related hepatic and renal impairment can reduce the clearance time of anaesthetic drugs in the elderly, prolonging the risk of hypothermia.

Anaesthetic influences on thermoregulation

Heat loss under anaesthesia

Phase 1

On induction of general anaesthesia, there is an initial rapid decline in core temperature during the first 30 minutes. The accompanying vasodilation and hypothalamic influences produced by the anaesthetic drugs causes redistribution of the body heat from the warmer core to the cooler peripheries. Redistribution under anaesthesia occurs when there is inhibition of tonic thermoregulatory vasoconstriction. This allows heat to flow from the relatively warm core thermal compartment to cooler peripheral tissues. Redistribution is the most important form of heat loss under anaesthesia.

Phase 2

After about 1 hour, with the gradual suppression of metabolism (which is a constant source of heat production), the core temperature begins to decline at a slower rate causing heat loss by eventual radiation from the skin. Heat loss occurs faster than heat production. Core temperature may drop by 1–2°C at this time and this phase may extend for 2–3 hours.

Phase 3

After about 3–4 hours, the body temperature drops to a level where it equals that of heat production, causing the core temperature to plateau. The plateau phase may be achieved in patients who are relatively warm (thereby maintaining a steady thermal state) as well as those with continually declining temperatures. As core temperatures reach 33–35°C, peripheral thermoregulatory vasoconstriction occurs. This mechanism attempts to decrease cutaneous heat loss as well as heat exchange between the core compartments. Body heat produced in the core compartments does not get redistributed outwards, thereby maintaining the plateau. However, cooling at the peripheries continues to occur.[14]

General anaesthesia

General anaesthesia causes an increase in warm response thresholds and a decrease in cold response thresholds. Modern volatile anaesthetics decrease the vasoconstriction and shivering thresholds. The thresholds for warm responses like sweating and vasodilation are increased by inhalational anaesthetics.[15] These responses are further exaggerated in the elderly by as much as 1°C.[16] Nitrous oxide's effects on vasoconstriction and shivering thresholds are marginal when compared to that of other inhalational agents.[17]

Propofol can cause vasodilation that is significant enough to produce core hypothermia, and to a greater degree when compared to sevoflurane.[18] Opioids promote heat loss by vasodilation as well as a direct influence on the hypothalamus. Opioids may influence the thermoregulatory set point.[19] Incidentally, it is this mechanism of action that is taken advantage of when meperidine and tramadol are used to treat postoperative shivering. Clonidine, ketanserin, nefopam, and doxapram also have similar effects.

Midazolam alters thermoregulatory control, but to a lesser degree when compared to the other agents.[20] Muscle relaxants do not influence the thermoregulatory centre but suppress shivering due to their obvious effects. Premedication with anticholinergics including glycopyrrolate and hyoscine can increase the incidence of shivering.

General anaesthesia is the most powerful inhibitor of the thermoregulatory centre. So much so that these drugs may be used to induce hypothermia in some clinical situations.[21]

Regional anaesthesia

Regional anaesthesia does not appear to directly inhibit the central thermoregulatory centres. Regional anaesthesia interferes with the afferent and efferent pathways thereby contributing to hypothermia. Regional anaesthesia may contribute to hypothermia to the same extent as general anaesthesia in the elderly.[22]

Both epidural and spinal anaesthesia can decrease the triggering thresholds for vasoconstriction and shivering by about 0.6°C at levels above the block. The administration of additional drugs may contribute to hypothermia by influencing thermoregulatory control. The disproportionate blockade of afferent signals from the cold peripheries influences the hypothalamus to receive predominantly warm signals. Skin temperature contributes 5–20 per cent to the thermoregulatory control. Increased apparent temperature produces a complementary decrease in the core temperature triggering thermoregulatory shivering.[23] This may be the reason why some patients manifest with shivering despite having a sensation of warmth after initiation of epidural anaesthesia. Furthermore, the efferent responses to cold are lost and vasoconstriction and shivering do not occur below the level of the block. The level of the block can also influence the degree of hypothermia that may result. More core hypothermia is to be expected during higher levels of blockade.[24]

In the postoperative period, the core temperature recovers in a much slower manner than after general anaesthesia due to the residual sympathectomy and the associated heat loss.

Despite comparable heat loss experienced during regional anaesthesia, temperature monitoring is frequently not performed by clinicians as an awake patient is assumed to remain normothermic or exhibit behavioural thermoregulation. Hypothermia in these situations may go unnoticed.

Combined regional and general anaesthesia

Combined regional and general anaesthesia techniques can cause the greatest drop in temperature as compared to either technique alone.[25] Peripheral thermoregulatory vasoconstriction during combined regional/general anaesthesia is triggered at a core temperature approximately 1°C lower than during general anaesthesia alone. Once triggered, vasoconstriction produces a core temperature plateau during general anaesthesia alone but not during combined regional and general anaesthesia. The result is that core temperature during combined regional and general anaesthesia continues to decrease throughout surgery. This highlights the importance of thermal management while using such anaesthetic techniques.

Implications of hypothermia
Neurological protection

Hypothermia may provide neurological protection in times of transient reductions of blood flow to the brain and spinal cord (Fig. 34.1).[26] For every 1° reduction in temperature, the metabolic rate drops by 6–7 percent.[27] Apart from reducing the metabolic rate, mild hypothermia may suppress free radical production and the release of excitatory amino acids or calcium shifts which are associated with reperfusion and may lead to cell death.[28] Whether this mechanism is applicable to clinical practice remains controversial as a recent trial on 1001 patients found no benefit of hypothermia in patients undergoing cerebral aneurysm clippling.[29] Mild induced hypothermia (32–34°C) appears to have some benefit in the neurological protection of patients resuscitated from cardiac arrest[30] and is currently being investigated at various levels.

Shivering

Shivering is the most common and easily identifiable indicator of a hypothermic disturbance. Shivering is also an unexpected and unpleasant sensation for the patient. Most patients appear overtly anxious when they are subject to a shivering episode. Earlier studies reported an increase in oxygen consumption of 100–730 per cent during a shivering episode. More recent data suggests that the actual figures may be between 40–100 per cent in younger patients. This value may be further reduced in the elderly because, due to lower vasoconstriction thresholds, they do not shiver as much. This impaired thermoregulatory response results in an increase in oxygen consumption by about 38 per cent in the elderly.[31]

Shivering is more likely if the initial core temperature is high and affects males more than females. It was previously believed that such large changes in oxygen consumption could result in myocardial ischaemia if oxygen demands were not met. Intraoperative hypothermia can contribute to perioperative ischaemic events,[32] especially in the premorbid elderly. However, a figure of around 38 per cent represents a modest increase in demand and shivering may not be the actual mechanism contributing to myocardial ischaemic events in the elderly.

Effects on the cardiovascular system

Frank et al.[32] showed that a reduction in core temperature to less than 35°C increases the risk of postoperative myocardial ischaemic events in premorbid patients undergoing vascular surgery. Rewarming a premorbid and hypothermic patient during and after surgery reduced myocardial ischaemic events by 55 per cent.[32] Shivering does not contribute to myocardial ischaemia and the

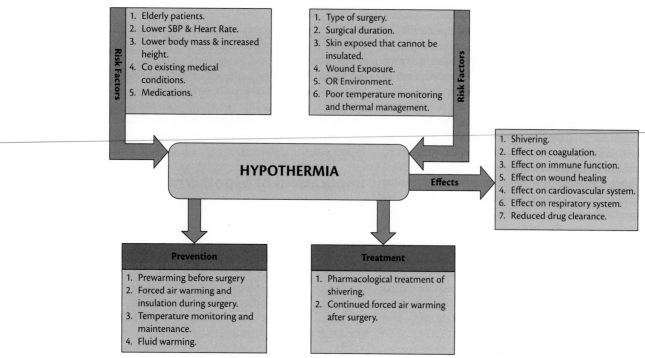

Fig. 34.1 Causes, treatment, and prevention of hypothermia.

cause of these effects likely to be due to the adrenergic response and a catecholamine surge. Frank et al.[33] found that there was a significantly higher concentration (pcg/ml) of noradrenaline in patients who did not received forced air warming therapy intraoperatively compared to those who did (480 ±70 vs 330 ±30, P = 0.02) and at 60 min (530 ±50 vs 340 ±30, P = 0.002), and 180 min (500 ± 80 vs 320 ±30, P = 0.004). This also resulted in higher systolic, mean, and diastolic blood pressures, along with increased risk of arrhythmias.

Effect on the respiratory system

Hypothermia blunts the ventilator response to CO_2. Hypothermia also causes a leftward shift of the oxygen dissociation curve. There is an increase of the affinity of oxygen to haemoglobin thereby affecting the unloading of oxygen at the tissue level.

Effect on coagulation

The contribution of hypothermia to coagulopathies is often overlooked as most coagulation testing is done in the lab at 37°C. Several studies have indicated that elderly patients have differences in coagulation function as compared to their younger counterparts.[34,35] Rohrer[36] studied the effect of hypothermia on prothrombin time and partial thromboplastin time. Mean prothrombin time results increased from 11.8 ± 0.3 (SD) seconds at 37°C to 12.9 ± 0.5, 14.2 ± 0.5, and 16.6 ± 0.2 seconds at 34°C, 31°C, and 28°C, respectively (p ≤0.001 for each). Partial thromboplastin time determinations increased from 36.0 ± 0.7 (SD) seconds at 37°C to 39.4 ± 1.0, 46.1 ± 1.1, and 57.2 ± 0.6 seconds at 34°C, 31°C, and 28°C, respectively (p ≤0.001 for each).

Hypothermia influences coagulation in three ways:

◆ Reduction of thromboxane B2 levels: this directly influences platelet function at the surgical site. This phenomenon reverses on warming. Interestingly, the use of aspirin does not significantly augment this activity and bleeding in hypothermic patients on aspirin is similar to those not on it.[37]

◆ Fibrinogen: hypothermia causes a potential deficit in fibrinogen availability and a delay in thrombin generation, consequently inhibiting coagulation function.

◆ Effect on the coagulation cascade: hypothermia influences the enzyme systems of the coagulation cascade which are sensitive to temperature changes.

Some studies have shown that hypothermia does not significantly influence blood loss during surgery.[38] However, a meta-analysis on this subject confirmed that mild hypothermia significantly increases blood loss by an estimated 16 per cent.[39]

Effect on immune function

Thermoregulatory vasoconstriction brings about a reduction in the partial pressure of oxygen in tissues. This in turn influences oxidative killing of organisms by neutrophils. Immune functions, such as the chemotaxis and phagocytosis of granulocytes, macrophage motility, and antibody production are also affected. Collagen formation in hypothermic patients is also limited as the formation of scar tissue requires adequate oxygen to be present to complete the hydroxylation reaction. Kurz et al.[40] investigated the effect of hypothermia on patients undergoing elective colon surgery and found that intraoperative core temperatures 2°C below normal triples the incidence of wound infection. They also showed delay in healing of the scar wounds in patients belonging to the hypothermic group.

Effect on drug metabolism

Hypothermia may bring about as much as a 5 per cent reduction in minimum alveolar concentration (MAC) per 1°C reduction in temperature with halothane and isoflurane anaesthesia.[41] These effects may be due to the increased lipid solubility of gases with reduced temperature. Further reduction in temperatures may directly depress CNS function causing further reduction in MAC. Nitrous oxide lipid solubility is only marginally affected since its lipid solubility is largely unaffected by hypothermia.[42] The duration of action of vecuronium is nearly doubled at 34°C.[43] The duration of atracurium is also increased by hypothermia.[44] Hypothermia also increases steady state plasma concentrations of fentanyl by approximately 5%/°C.[45] Plasma concentrations of propofol are increased by 30 per cent with a 3°C drop in temperature.

These findings are of particular importance in the elderly where MAC requirements are already reduced. Slower clearance of anaesthetic agents may further delay recover from general anaesthesia in the hypothermic patient.

Clinical monitoring

Temperature monitoring is mandatory in many countries around the world. In general, patients having surgery exceeding 30 minutes under general anaesthesia should have continuous temperature monitoring. This may also be followed in elderly patients undergoing surgeries under regional anaesthesia where hypothermia may be expected. Core temperature is usually measured at the tympanic membrane, nasopharynx, or the oesophagus. When measured, skin temperatures vary from that of the core, but when corrected, are reasonably accurate.

Pharmacological management of shivering

After the ingestion or infusion of certain nutrients, there is an increase in energy expenditure. Proteins or amino acids have been postulated to stimulate heat production. Preoperative amino acid infusions have been used to prevent hypothermia and postoperative shivering with both general and regional anaesthesia. Amino acids increase the threshold core temperature for thermoregulatory vasoconstriction as well as increase energy expenditure. Fructose also exhibits similar action.[46]

Certain drugs influence the thermoregulatory control causing reduction in symptoms (most notably shivering) and thereby greatly increasing thermal comfort. When hypothermia has already set in, these drugs may be used to rapidly comfort a symptomatic patient while other measures to correct core hypothermia are initiated.

Of the available medications to treat shivering, opioids appear to be the most effective. Intravenous meperidine (pethidine) has been extensively studied and used for this purpose. Meperidine decreases the shivering threshold almost twice as much as the vasoconstriction threshold.[47] The antishivering action of meperidine may be partially mediated by κ-opioid receptors and also its effects on biogenic monoamine reuptake inhibition, N-methyl-D-aspartate receptor antagonism, or stimulation of α2 adrenoceptors. Meperidine is usually given as a dose of 0.5 mg/kg for the treatment of shivering[48] or as a 25 mg bolus in adult patients.

Tramadol is an antishivering drug which inhibits reuptake of serotonin (5-hydroxytryptamine: 5-HT), noradrenaline, and dopamine, and, facilitates 5-HT release. Cerebral α2-adrenoceptors are also thought to play a role in the attenuation of postoperative shivering by tramadol. The dose of intravenous tramadol for the treatment of shivering is 1 mg/kg.[49]

Clonidine in the dose of 1.5–3 mcg/kg has also been used to prevent postoperative shivering.[50]

The other drugs that have been studied to manage shivering with significant results include ketanserin, doxapram, alfentanil, nefopam, ketamine and magnesium.

Pharmacological interventions may have inadvertent adverse outcomes in the elderly as most of the discussed drugs have other effects. There is insufficient evidence regarding their safety profile in the elderly. In this regard, gradual dosing, titrated to response and effect, may be prudent in the elderly.

Warming strategies and equipment

Numerous warming devices are available and various techniques for warming have been employed with varied results. The efficacy of these devices and methods often depend upon the amount of body surface area available to warm and this is dependent on the type of surgery. Efforts must be made to keep the core temperature above 36°C.

It may be beneficial to know if there are predictors of intraoperative hypothermia so as to identify which patient is at risk and intraoperative warming could be employed as soon as possible. Kasai et al.[51] in a retrospective analysis studied preoperative risk factors in patients who became hypothermic. They concluded that patients with increased age, lower weight, increased height, lower systolic blood pressure and heart rate developed hypothermia more easily. They developed a probability equation with a specificity of 83 per cent to predict which patients may become hypothermic, thus suggesting that more aggressive warming methods may be needed in these patients. Operating room environmental standards vary between countries and on average seem to be between 19–23°C, with humidity levels under 50 per cent. Temperatures in the lower range and laminar airflow patterns are recommended for orthopaedic, transplant, and cardiac surgeries to prevent airborne infections. Lower temperatures also enhance comfort for operating room staff working for long periods under operating room lights wearing surgical gowns and radiation shields. Ambient temperature may not be responsible for the initial drop in core temperature which is due to redistribution of heat, but will eventually contribute through convective heat losses in a poorly insulated patient during longer surgeries. Large air changes seen in laminar flow theatres further compound this problem. Convective and radiant heat losses may be managed by insulating the patient and providing active warming.

Thermal insulators

The simplest example of a thermal insulator is a blanket. Thermal insulators reduce heat loss by convection and radiation. This occurs by trapping air (still air). Still air is an effective insulator and can reduce heat loss by 28–45 per cent depending on the type of insulator used. Thermal mass insulators (cotton surgical drapes, commercially available disposable drapes, hospital duvets) all provide a similar quality of insulation.[52] Another type of commercially available insulator is the radiant insulator which is a metalized plastic reflective sheet. This insulator reflects back radiant heat to trap it in the layer of still air under it. Radiant insulators offer better heat trapping effects as compared to mass insulators.[53] Additional layers over the first layer of insulation do not significantly improve heat trapping. Prewarmed blankets do not provide any additional benefits as compared to unwarmed ones.[54]

Another method that has been used to provide more effective heat entrapment is the 'Hibler's method', which involves a vapour trapping layer (plastic based wrap) and an additional dry insulating layer (blanket) on top. This may be useful in settings where forced air warmers are not available.

Active warming devices

Circulating water mattresses and under body warmers placed under the patient have been marketed for prevention of hypothermia in paediatric and adult patients. There are reports that circulating water mattresses warmers may be largely ineffective when used alone because heat loss occurs from the anterior exposed surface of the body, and the posterior surface which lies on the mattress is not exposed to convective and radiant heat loss systems. Burns have also been reported on its usage.

Forced air warmers are among the most popular and effective heat management systems available today. They are effective in limiting heat loss via convection and radiation. Forced air warmers can bring about an increase in core temperature.[55] They ensure that the air surrounding the patient stays warm. Unlike normal blankets which require body heat to warm the air surrounding the patient, forced air warming blankets provide an external heat source. With a continuous supply of heat over the patient's skin, heat loss is reduced. Additionally, heat can be gained through convection into the patient.

Resistive warmers are similar to electric heating blankets which are as effective as forced air warmers.[56] Forced air warmers may potentially interfere with the pattern of airflow systems inside the operating theatre, thereby increasing the chance of infections[57] but other studies report that this is unlikely to be true.[58] Resistive warmers offer the additional benefit of not contributing to operating room noise.

Negative pressure warmers apply low vacuum and heat to the patient's extremity (hand and forearm), to conductively warm blood in the extremity which is then delivered directly to the body's core by the patient's own circulation. However, the efficacy of these warmers has been questioned.[59]

Prewarming

Prewarming a patient is a simple and effective method to preserve intrinsic heat and delay heat loss when the patient is eventually subject to anaesthesia and surgery. Prewarming a patient decreases the core–peripheral temperature gradient and reduces heat loss caused by redistribution. Prewarming also causes centrally activated vasodilation which is not affected after the induction of anaesthesia. These effects help in maintaining normothermia during surgery. Prewarming must be done for 30–60 minutes prior to surgery to be effective. Warming a patient for longer may provoke thermal discomfort and elicit sweating, which may abolish the beneficial effects of prewarming.[60]

Warmed fluids

Warmed intravenous fluids do not actively warm patients, but may slow down heat loss in patients who are being warmed by other alternative methods. Intravenous fluids that are at ambient temperature may contribute to hypothermia by reducing body temperature by 0.25°C for every 1 L.[61] The warming of fluids may be helpful in prolonged surgery where large amounts of fluids are given.

Humidification of airway gases

The respiratory tract accounts for less than 10 per cent of the total heat loss. This small amount is lost in warming and humidification of the inspired gases. There seems to be no apparent benefit in thermal management by active heating of the inspired gas flow even in longer operations as the losses are miniscule.

Conclusion

Thermal disturbances and their management are often neglected in the elderly as the clinician is often drawn to other existing problems. While the influences of hypothermia are not dissimilar when compared to younger adults, its effects may be more pronounced in the elderly who may have impaired thermoregulatory mechanisms. It is imperative that we monitor and treat hypothermia as is done for pain or any other clinical parameter.

References

1. Sund-Levander M, Forsberg C, Wahren LK. Normal oral, rectal, tympanic and axillary body temperature in adult men and women: a systematic literature review. *Scand J Caring Sci.* 2002;16(2):122–128.
2. Howell TH. Oral temperature range in old age. *Gerontol Clin.* 1975;17(3):133–136.
3. Waalen J, Buxbaum JN. Is older colder or colder older? The association of age with body temperature in 18,630 individuals. *J Gerontol A Biol Sci Med Sci.* 2011;66:487–492.
4. Kenney WL, Munce TA. Invited review: aging and human temperature regulation. J Appl Physiol. 2003;95(6):2598–2603.
5. Sessler DI. Perioperative thermoregulation. In Silverstein J, Rooke A, Reves JG, McLeskey CH (eds) *Geriatric anesthesiology* 2nd edn (pp. 107–122). Baltimore, MD: Springer, 2008.
6. Lamke LO, Nilsson GE, Reithner HL. Water loss by evaporation from the abdominal cavity during surgery. *Acta Chir Scand.* 1977;143(5):279–284.
7. Severens NM. Temperature and surgical wound heat loss during orthopedic surgery: computer simulations and measurements. *Can J Anaesth.* 2010;57(4):381–382.
8. Poulos DA. Central processing of cutaneous temperature information. *Fed Proc.* 1981;40(14):2825–2829.
9. Simon E. Temperature regulation: The spinal cord as a site of extrahypothalamic thermoregulatory functions. *Rev Physiol Biochem Pharmacol.* 1974;71:1–76.
10. De Witte J, Sessler DI. Perioperative shivering: physiology and pharmacology. *Anesthesiology.* 2002;96(2):467–484.
11. Wenger CB. The regulation of body temperature. In Rhoade RA, Tanner GA (eds) *Medical physiology*, 2nd edn (pp. 527–550). Philadelphia, PA: Lippincott Williams & Wilkins, 2003.
12. Hynson JM, Sessler DI, Moayeri A, McGuire J. Absence of nonshivering thermogenesis in anesthetized humans. *Anesthesiology.* 1993;79(4):695–703.
13. Kramer MR, Vandijk J, Rosin AJ (1989) Mortality in elderly patients with thermoregulatory failure. *Arch Intern Med.* 1989;149:1521–1523.
14. Sessler DI. Temperature regulation and monitoring. In Miller RD (ed) *Miller's anesthesia*, 7th edn (pp. 1533–1536). London: Churchill Livingstone, 2009.
15. Buggy DJ, Crossley AWA. Thermoregulation, mild perioperative hypothermia and post-anaesthetic shivering. *Br J Anaesth.* 2000;84(5):615–628.
16. Kurz A, Plattner O, Sessler DI, Huemer G, Redl G, Lackner F. The threshold for thermoregulatory vasoconstriction during nitrous oxide/isoflurane anesthesia is lower in elderly than in young patients. *Anesthesiology.* 1993;79(3):465–469.
17. Plattner O, Xiong J, Sessler DI, *et al.* Rapid core-to-peripheral tissue heat transfer during cutaneous cooling. *Anesth Analg.* 1996;82(5):925–930.

18. Ikeda T, Sessler DI, Kazama T, Ikeda K, Sato S. Less core hypothermia when anesthesia is induced with inhaled sevoflurane than with intravenous propofol. *Anesth Analg.* 1999;88(4):921–924.

19. Spencer RL, Burks TF. Alteration of thermoregulatory set point with opioid agonists. *J Pharmacol Exp Ther.* 1990;252(2):696–705.

20. Kurz A, Sessler DI, Annadata R, Dechert M, Christensen R. Midazolam minimally impairs thermoregulatory control. *Anesth Analg.* 1995;81(2):393–398.

21. Doufas AG, Sessler DI. Physiology and clinical relevance of induced hypothermia. *Neurocrit Care.* 2004;1(4):489–498.

22. Frank SM, Beattie C, Christopherson R, Norris EJ, Rock P, Parker S, Kimball AW Jr. Epidural versus general anesthesia, ambient operating room temperature, and patient age as predictors of inadvertent hypothermia. *Anesthesiology.* 1992;77(2):252–257.

23. Emerick TH, Ozaki M, Sessler DI, Walters K, Schroeder M. Epidural anesthesia increases apparent leg temperature and decreases the shivering threshold. *Anesthesiology.* 1994;81(2):289–298.

24. Leslie K, Sessler DI. Reduction in the shivering threshold is proportional to spinal block height. *Anesthesiology.* 1996;84(6):1327–1331.

25. Sessler DI. Mild perioperative hypothermia. *N Engl J Med.* 1997;336:1730–1737.

26. Minamisawa H, Nordstrom CH, Smith ML, Siesjo BK. The influence of mild body and brain hypothermia on ischemic brain damage. *J Cereb Blood Flow Metab.* 1990;10:365–374.

27. Erecinska M, Thoresen M, Silver IA. Effects of hypothermia on energy metabolism in mammalian central nervous system. *J Cereb Blood Flow Metab.* 2003;23:513–530.

28. Colbourne F, Sutherland G, Corbett D. Postischemic hypothermia. A critical appraisal with implications for clinical treatment. *Mol Neurobiol.* 1997;14:171–201.

29. Todd MM, Hindman BJ, Clarke WR, Torner JC. Mild intraoperative hypothermia during surgery for intracranial aneurysm; Intraoperative Hypothermia for Aneurysm Surgery Trial (IHAST) Investigators. *N Engl J Med.* 2005;352(2):135–145.

30. Tuma MA, Stansbury LG, Stein DM, McQuillan KA, Scalea TM. Induced hypothermia after cardiac arrest in trauma patients: a case series. *J Trauma.* 2011;71(6):1524–1527.

31. Frank SM, Fleisher LA, Olson KF, et al. Multivariate determinates of early postoperative oxygen consumption: The effects of shivering, core temperature, and gender. *Anesthesiology.* 1995;83:241–249.

32. Frank SM, Beattie C, Christopherson R, et al. Unintentional hypothermia is associated with postoperative myocardial ischemia. *Anesthesiology.* 1993;7: 468–476.

33. Frank SM, Higgins MS, Breslow MJ, et al. The catecholamine, cortisol, and hemodynamic responses to mild perioperative hypothermia. A randomized clinical trial. *Anesthesiology.* 1995;82(1):83–93.

34. Pleym H, Wahba A, Bjella L, Stenseth R. Sonoclot analysis in elderly compared with younger patients undergoing coronary surgery. *Acta Anaesthesiol Scand.* 2008;52(1):28–35.

35. Boldt J, Haisch G, Kumle B, et al. Does coagulation differ between elderly and younger patients undergoing cardiac surgery? *Intensive Care Med.* 2002;23(4):466–471.

36. Rohrer MJ, Natale AM. Effect of hypothermia on the coagulation cascade. *Crit Care Med.* 1992;20(10):1402–1405.

37. Michelson AD, Barnard MR, Khuri SF, Rohrer MJ, MacGregor H, Valeri CR. The effects of aspirin and hypothermia on platelet function in vivo. *Br J Haematol.* 1999;104(1):64–68.

38. Johansson T, Lisander B, Ivarsson I. Mild hypothermia does not increase blood loss during total hip arthroplasty. *Acta Anaesthesiol Scand.* 1999;43(10):1005–1010.

39. Rajagopalan S, Mascha E, Jie Na MS, Sessler DI. The effects of mild perioperative hypothermia on blood loss and transfusion requirement. *Anesthesiology.* 2008;108(1):71–77.

40. Kurz A, Sessler DI, Lenhardt R. Perioperative normothermia to reduce the incidence of surgical-wound infection and shorten hospitalization.

Study of Wound Infection and Temperature Group. *N Engl J Med.* 1996;334:1209–1215.

41. Vitez TS, White PF, Eger EI 2nd. Effects of hypothermia on halothane MAC and isoflurane MAC in the rat. *Anesthesiology.* 1974;41(1):80–81.

42. Antognini JF, Lewis BK, Reitan JA. Hypothermia minimally decreases nitrous oxide anesthetic requirements. *Anesth Analg.* 1994;79(5):980–982.

43. Heier T, Caldwell JE, Sessler DI, Miller RD. Mild intraoperative hypothermia increases duration of action and spontaneous recovery of vecuronium blockade during nitrous oxide-isoflurane anesthesia in humans. *Anesthesiology.* 1991;74(5):815–819.

44. Leslie K, Sessler DI, Bjorksten AR, Moayeri A. Mild hypothermia alters propofol pharmacokinetics and increases the duration of action of atracurium. *Anesth Analg.* 1995;80(5):1007–1014.

45. Fritz HG, Bauer R, Walter B, Moeritz K-U, Reinhart K. Effects of hypothermia (32°C) on plasma concentration of fentanyl in piglets (abstract). *Anesthesiology.* 1999;91:A444.

46. Mizobe T, Nakajima Y. Dietary-induced thermogenesis and perioperative thermoregulation. *Masui.* 2007;56(3):305–316.

47. Kurz A, Ikeda T, Sessler DI, et al. Meperidine decreases the shivering threshold twice as much as the vasoconstriction threshold. *Anesthesiology.* 1997;86(5):1046–1054.

48. Bhatnagar S, Saxena A, Kannan TR, Punj J, Panigrahi M, Mishra S. Tramadol for postoperative shivering: a double-blind comparison with pethidine. *Anaesth Intensive Care.* 2001;29(2):149–154.

49. de Witte J, Deloof T, Veylder JD, Housmans PR. Tramadol in the treatment of postanesthetic shivering. *Acta Anaesthesiol Scand.* 1997;41(4):506–510.

50. Horn EP, Standl T, Sessler DI, et al. Physostigmine prevents postanesthetic shivering as does meperidine or clonidine. *Anesthesiology.* 1998;88(1):108–113.

51. Kasai T, Hirose M, Yaegashi K, Matsukawa T, Takamata A, Tanaka Y. Preoperative risk factors of intraoperative hypothermia in major surgery under general anesthesia. *Anesth Analg.* 2002;95(5):1381–1383.

52. Brauer A, Perl T, Uyanik Z, English MJ, Weyland W, Braun U. Perioperative thermal insulation: minimal clinically important differences? *Br J Anaesth.* 2004;92(6):836–840.

53. Henriksson O, Lundgren JP, Kuklane K, Holmer I, Bjornstig U. Protection against cold in prehospital care-thermal insulation properties of blankets and rescue bags in different wind conditions. *Prehosp Disaster Med.* 2009;24:408–415.

54. Sessler DI, Schroeder M. Heat loss in humans covered with cotton hospital blankets. *Anesth Analg.* 1993;77(1):73–77.

55. Kurz A, Kurz M, Poeschl G, et al. Forced-air warming maintains intraoperative normothermia better than circulating-water mattresses. *Anesth Analg.* 1993;77(1):89–95.

56. Ng V, Lai A, Ho V. Comparison of forced-air warming and electric heating pad for maintenance of body temperature during total knee replacement. *Anaesthesia.* 2006;61(11):1100–1104.

57. McGovern PD Albrecht M, Belani KG, et al. Forced-air warming and ultra-clean ventilation do not mix: an investigation of theatre ventilation, patient warming and joint replacement infection in orthopaedics. *J Bone Joint Surg Br.* 2011;93(11):1537–1544.

58. Sharp RJ, Chesworth T, Fern ED. Do warming blankets increase bacterial counts in the operating field in a laminar-flow theatre? *J Bone Joint Surg Br.* 2002;84(4):486–488.

59. Taguchi A, Arkilic CF, Ahluwalia A, Sessler DI, Kurz A. Negative pressure rewarming vs. forced air warming in hypothermic postanesthetic volunteers. *Anesth Analg.* 2001;92(1):261–266.

60. Sessler DI, Schroeder M, Merrifi eld B, et al. Optimal duration and temperature of pre-warming. *Anesthesiology.* 1995;82(3):674–681.

61. Sessler DI. Complications and treatment of mild hypothermia. *Anesthesiology.* 2001;95(2):531–543.

CHAPTER 35

Infections in the elderly

Diane Monkhouse

Introduction

Providing quality healthcare for the elderly is a major challenge to all clinicians. Despite advances in clinical practice and antibiotic therapy, infectious diseases continue to be a major cause of mortality in the aged.[1] In comparison with the general population, infections tend to be more frequent and severe in the elderly. Pneumonia, influenza, and complications of bacteraemia are among the ten major causes of death in the elderly.[2] Reasons for increased susceptibility include epidemiological factors, immunosenescence, and malnutrition coupled with an abundance of age-related anatomical and physiological changes. Atypical presentation often delays diagnosis and the presence of age-related comorbid conditions with dysfunction of host defence makes management complex and challenging.[3]

Factors which predispose to infections in the elderly

Altered immunity

Studies suggest that although changes in immunity with healthy aging (termed immunosenescence) occur rapidly, it is the confounding effects of age-related diseases and environmental factors which produce a state of immune dysfunction. This combination accounts for the increased risk of infection in older adults.[4] Immunosenescence is a predisposing condition which contributes only a small risk. However, this risk increases as the immune system is further impaired as a result of chronic illness, malnutrition, long-term residential nursing care, or immunosuppressant drug therapy.[5]

Age-related decline in immunity is seen at a functional level by increased susceptibility to specific infections and poor vaccination responses. Atrophy of the thymus (the source of new T cells) and concomitant expansion of the memory T-cell population are key factors in the reduction seen in adaptive immunity and vaccination responses. There are also dramatic changes to the innate immune system with age, including reduced neutrophil bactericidal function and an increase in the constitutive circulating level of pro-inflammatory cytokines such as tumour necrosis factor alpha (TNFα), interleukin (IL)-6 and IL1β (inflamm-aging). The latter contributes to the development of several diseases including cardiovascular disease.[6] Immunoglobulins (Igs) also change with age. The IgM memory cells which are responsible for protection against encapsulated bacteria, such as *Streptococcus pneumoniae*, diminish with age. In addition, there is a decline in splenic function which increases risk of infection by encapsulated organisms.[7]

The major immunological changes associated with aging are summarized in Table 35.1.

Anatomical and physiological factors

Although the immune system has a central role in defence against infection, many other elements have an important role (Table 35.2). Epithelia from the skin, bronchi, and digestive tract form a physical barrier to prevent invasion of micro-organisms.[8] The efficiency of the mucociliary escalator, maintenance of gastric acidity, and the ability to produce rapid urine flow are all protective mechanisms designed to prevent bacterial invasion.[2] The efficiency of each diminishes with age.

The risk of pneumonia is increased by a blunting of airway protective reflexes, a decrease in mucociliary clearance, a reduction in T cells and immunoglobulin in respiratory secretions, and a reduction in gastric acid production.

Urinary tract infection is more common in the elderly because of urothelial changes which promote bacterial adherence, reduced bladder capacity, uninhibited contractions, decreased urinary flow, and significant residual volumes of urine post-voiding.

Gastroenteritis and colitis are more common in the elderly. Age-dependent factors contributing to this include reduced gastric acidity, decreased intestinal motility, alterations in intestinal mucus, and bacterial flora. The latter is exacerbated by frequent antibiotic use.[9]

Chronic diseases

The impact of chronic disease states upon susceptibility to infection in the elderly cannot be underestimated. Factors contributing to increased risk are summarized in Table 35.3.

Table 35.1 Age-related changes in the immune system

Element of the immune system	Change
Innate immunity	Normal neutrophilia during acute phase with some decrease in phagocytosis and killing
	Increase in pro-inflammatory cytokine production
	Reduced natural killer cell function
Specific immunity	Involution of thymus
T lymphocytes	Impaired T-cell proliferation
B lymphocytes	Decreased Th1 response with increased Th2 response
	Decreased production of specific antibodies
	Increased generation of autoantibodies

Table 35.2 Age-related anatomical and physiological changes which predispose to infections

Organ system	Changes
Respiratory tract	Loss of elastic tissue and tone
	Increased risk of lower airway collapse
	Weakened cough
	Reduced effectiveness of mucociliary escalator
	Colonization with multi-resistant bacteria
Gastrointestinal tract	Reduced saliva production
	Reduced oesophageal motility increasing the risk of aspiration
	Achlorhydria—linked with increased risk of *E. coli* infections
Urinary tract	Any condition resulting in urinary retention can cause chronic bacteriuria
	For example, neurogenic bladder, long-term catheterization, and prostatic hypertrophy
	Decline in renal function impairs the ability to acidify and concentrate the urine which are protective against urinary infection
Skin	Loss of elasticity and hydration with age
	More susceptible to shearing forces and tearing
	Reduced barrier to infection

Table 35.3 Chronic disease states which increase infection risk in the elderly

Chronic diseases which increase infection risk in elderly	Mechanism
Diabetes mellitus	Neutrophils, monocytes, and lymphocytes demonstrate decrease in adherence, chemotaxis, and intracellular killing
	Reduced cell-mediated immunity
Chronic obstructive pulmonary disease	Colonization with multi-drug resistant pathogens
	Immunosuppressive effect of steroid therapy
Chronic kidney disease	Defects in neutrophil function, chronically decreased proliferation of immune system
Stroke	Loss of airway protective reflexes
	Increased risk of aspiration of gastric contents
	Diminished cough
	Bulbar insufficiency
Malignancies	Lack of immunoglobulin G, defects in cell-mediated immunity
Autoimmune diseases	Lack of complement components, immunosuppressive therapy
Chronic infections	Chronic immune activation
	High levels of circulating cytokines such as TNFα which induces muscle weakness

Malnutrition

Infection and malnutrition have always been intricately linked.[10] Ten to twenty-five per cent of nursing home residents have significant nutritional deficits.[11] This figure may increase to almost 50 per cent in those admitted to hospital for treatment.[12]

Malnutrition may present as a global calorific deficit or as protein and/or micronutrient deficiency. It can create a vicious cycle of problems in that malnutrition increases the risk of infection and subsequent infection exacerbates the nutritional deficit. The severity and chronicity of infection are important as there is a huge metabolic demand placed upon an elderly individual with limited nutritional reserve. Poor nutritional status can be exacerbated by diarrhoea, malabsorption, anorexia, and diversion of nutrients to mount an immune response. In addition, fever increases both calorie and micronutrition requirements. An inadequate dietary intake leads to weight loss, decreased immunity, mucosal damage, and increased risk of invasion by pathogens.[10]

Global malnutrition, reduced intake or increased requirement for calories and protein, is the most common nutritional deficit in the elderly population. However, micronutrient deficiencies (vitamins and minerals) can occur in up to 40 per cent of elderly hospitalized patients.[13]

Clinical manifestations of malnutrition in older adults include low body weight, muscle wasting, dermatitis, angular stomatitis, poor wound healing, and peripheral oedema. Assessment of body mass index (BMI) is a simple screening test. Thorough assessment of nutritional status in the elderly is required if BMI is less than 22, if there is weight loss in excess of 5 per cent of body weight in a month or if body weight is more than 20 per cent below ideal body weight.[14] Early nutritional assessment accompanied by measurement of lean muscle mass and biochemical markers should be encouraged with early intervention from a dedicated dietetic service.[15]

Environmental factors

The vast majority of people institutionalized in long-term care facilities such as nursing homes are frail, elderly, physically dependent, and often have a degree of cognitive impairment. Nursing home residents have increased vulnerability to infection because of their frailty, significant physical comorbidities, and altered host resistance.[3] In addition, the closed institutionalized environment allows regular exposure to pathogens because of contact with other residents, staff, and visitors. Healthcare-associated infections, emergence of resistant organisms, and outbreaks (particularly respiratory and gastrointestinal infections) are all major causes for concern in long-term care facilities. Poor oral hygiene is very common in nursing homes, increasing the risk of colonization of the oral cavity. An aggressive approach to oral hygiene has been shown to decrease bacterial load.[16]

Clinical presentation and investigation

Fever and the cardinal manifestations of infection may be absent or blunted in elderly patients with serious or life-threatening infections.[17] The diagnosis of infections in elderly patients may be delayed because of an atypical presentation. A sudden onset of confusion, behavioural disturbance, lethargy, loss of appetite, dizziness, and falls may be the only clinical features even in severe life-threatening infections.[18] It should also be emphasized that vague clinical presentations are characteristic of many non-infectious diseases which further increases the diagnostic difficulty.

Studies of pyrexia of unknown origin in the elderly demonstrate that, unlike in the young, a precise diagnosis can be made in around 90 per cent of cases.[19] Most frequently, it is the result of an atypical presentation of a relatively common disease. Tuberculosis, temporal arteritis, polymyalgia rheumatica, and malignancy should be considered in the differential diagnosis.[20]

The triad of leucocytosis, neutrophilia, and left shift lacks sensitivity in the elderly.[2] Serum C-reactive protein (CRP) is a sensitive marker of infection but unfortunately lacks specificity in the elderly patients. As a diagnostic biomarker, procalcitonin (PCT) has several advantages over other inflammatory markers such as CRP. PCT shows a prompt increase in response to initial infection within 6–12 hours. Circulating PCT levels halve daily when the infection is controlled by host immune response and antimicrobial therapy.[21] Its role in the elderly still lacks a substantial evidence base.[22]

Important infections in the elderly

Pneumonia

For centuries pneumonia has often been seen as the terminal infectious disease of the elderly. In 1888 William Osler noted that 'Pneumonia remains now, as then, the most serious acute disease with which physicians have to deal; serious because it attacks the old, the feeble…persons who are not able to withstand the sudden sharp onset of the malady'.[23]

Pneumonia in elderly patients is associated with significant morbidity and mortality compared with younger adults. It is the fifth most common cause of death in the United Kingdom. Elderly hospitalized patients have a mortality of 12 per cent. Mortality rates exceed 30 per cent in those requiring ventilatory support in critical care.[24]

In general, there are three types of pneumonia: community-acquired, nursing home-acquired, and nosocomial pneumonia.[25] Kaplan and co-workers reported an incidence of 18.3 per 1000 population older than 65years with a mortality rate of 10.6 per cent. The incidence rose fivefold and mortality doubled as age increased from 65–69 to over 90years.[26] The predictors of fatal outcome in the community-acquired pneumonia are included in Table 35.4.

Patient outcome is dependent upon early recognition of the severity of pneumonia with prompt treatment in an appropriate

Table 35.4 Predictors of fatal outcome in community-acquired pneumonia in the elderly

Predictors of fatal outcome
Bedridden before the onset of pneumonia
Temperature <37°C
Swallowing disorder
Respiratory rate ≥30 breaths/minute
Acute kidney injury
Multilobar involvement
Immunosuppression
Acute Physiology and Chronic Health Evaluation (APACHE) score ≥22

Table 35.5 CURB-65 scoring system

Modified British Thoracic Society Guidelines (CURB-65)
Confusion (defined as a Mental Test Score of 8 or less, or new disorientation in person, place or time)
Urea >7mmol/L
Respiratory rate ≥30/min
Blood pressure (systolic <90mmHg or diastolic ≤60mmHg)
Age ≥65 years

Reproduced from *Thorax*, Lim WS, et al., 'British Thoracic Society guidelines for the management of community acquired pneumonia in adults: update 2009', 64, sIII, pp. iii1–iii55, copyright 2009, with permission from BMJ Publishing Group Ltd.

environment. A number of prognostic scoring systems have been developed to predict mortality risk. The CURB-65 is a modification of the British Thoracic Society guidelines and incorporates age greater than 65 as a risk factor.[27] The CURB-65 score (Table 35.5) can be used to stratify patients into three different management groups. Group 1 (score 0 or 1) have a low mortality and can be safely managed in the community. Group 2 (score of 2) have an intermediate mortality risk and should receive inpatient treatment while group 3 (score of 3 or more) have a high mortality and should be considered for critical care management. Subsequent work performed by Myint and co-workers suggested that oxygenation was the most sensitive predictor of outcome in the elderly while confusion and high urea are both relatively common and insensitive, and add little to the predictive model.[28] The SOAR (systolic blood pressure, oxygenation, age, and respiratory rate) prediction tool was developed as an alternative to CURB-65 (Table 35.6).

The classic features of pneumonia including fevers, rigors, productive cough, and shortness of breath may be absent in the elderly population. Atypical manifestations such as delirium, worsening chronic confusion, lethargy, and falls may be apparent. The non-specific symptoms may contribute to delayed diagnosis and treatment and subsequent increase in mortality.

The diagnostic workup for pneumonia remains the same for all patients. However, it is important to emphasize that the initial chest radiograph taken in a dehydrated elderly patient may show no evidence of infiltrate or consolidation. Findings may be apparent only after fluid repletion.[7] Patients should have oxygen saturations, arterial blood gases, urea and electrolytes, CRP, full blood count, and liver function tests measured on admission.[29] Blood and sputum cultures should be sent on all hospitalized patients. Acquisition of a suitable sputum sample from an elderly, dehydrated, confused patient may

Table 35.6 SOAR prediction rule for elderly patients

SOAR prediction tool—1 point for each of the following
Systolic blood pressure <90mmHg
Oxygenation (PaO$_2$:FiO$_2$ <250)
Age >65years
Respiratory rate ≥30 breaths/min

Reproduced from Myint PK, et al., 'Severity assessment criteria recommended by the British Thoracic Society (BTS) for community-acquired pneumonia (CAP) and older patients. Should SOAR (systolic blood pressure, oxygenation, age and respiratory rate) criteria be used in older people? A compilation study of two prospective cohorts', *Age and Ageing*, 2006, 35, 3, pp. 286–291, by permission of Oxford University Press and The British Geriatrics Society.

be difficult. Pneumococcal urine antigen test should be performed for all patients with moderate or high severity pneumonia.

Although *Streptococcus pneumoniae* remains the most important cause of pneumonia in the elderly, pneumonia due to *Staphylococcus* and Gram-negative organisms is increasingly common in older adults especially amongst the hospitalized or residents of long-term care facilities with complex comorbidities. *Legionella* and atypical infections such as *Mycoplasma* are less commonly seen in the elderly. Although viral pneumonia is less common, the risk of morbidity and mortality from secondary complications of influenza is increased.

Initial empirical antimicrobial therapy for pneumonia in the elderly should be guided by the severity of illness, host factors such as comorbidities, residential status, length of hospital stay, and drug allergies in conjunction with local antimicrobial prescribing guidelines. The route of administration needs careful attention. The parenteral route is recommended in severe pneumonia, in those with swallowing difficulties or reduced conscious level, and where gastric absorption is unreliable.[29] The choice of antibiotic is beyond the scope of this review but the general principle is to tailor treatment according to the microbiology results aiming for a narrow-spectrum antibiotic to decrease the risk of antibiotic resistance.

Vaccination of the elderly is an important consideration. All patients aged over 65 years or at risk of invasive pneumococcal disease who are admitted to hospital with pneumonia and who have not been vaccinated should receive 23-valent pneumococcal polysaccharide vaccine during the convalescent period in line with the UK Department of Health guidelines.[30] Annual influenza vaccine should be offered to all over 65 years.

Urinary tract infections

Urinary tract infections (UTIs) are the most common infection amongst the elderly population both in the community and institutional settings.[31] Most infections are asymptomatic with the prevalence of 15–30 per cent in men and 25–50 per cent in women, depending upon underlying disease and residential status.[32] This age-dependent increase in asymptomatic bacteriuria is paralleled by an increase in symptomatic UTI. Factors contributing to increased risk of bacterial colonization and infection of the urinary tract in the elderly include chronic comorbid conditions particularly cognitive dysfunction, incontinence, and chronic degenerative neurological conditions associated with neurogenic bladder (such as Parkinson's and cerebrovascular disease) Instrumentation of the bladder, urethral catheterization, prostatic hypertrophy in men, and hormonal changes in postmenopausal women may also contribute.[22]

For elderly patients, routine screening and treatment of asymptomatic bacteriuria are not recommended.[33] It is only recommended in older persons before transurethral resection of the prostate and before urological procedures in which mucosal bleeding is anticipated.[34]

The diagnosis of UTI requires significant bacteriuria associated with genitourinary symptoms. Among institutionalized elderly individuals, many of whom are cognitively impaired, distinguishing asymptomatic bacteriuria from UTI can be very difficult. The only clinical manifestations may be nausea, vomiting, confusion or offensive urine. Eighty per cent of UTIs in the community are caused by Gram-negative organisms (predominantly *Escherichia coli*) and 20 per cent Gram-positive organisms such as *Enterococcus*. Amongst elderly hospitalized patients, *E. coli* is still the most common pathogen isolated from the urinary tract but nosocomial pathogens such as *Pseudomonas aeruginosa*, vancomycin-resistant *Enterococcus, Candida* species, and non-*E. coli* Enterobacteriaceae are often identified.[35]

Asymptomatic bacteriuria requires no treatment. Inappropriate initiation of antimicrobial therapy tends to increase the risk of super-infection with resistant organisms and adverse side effects of antibiotics.

Treatment of UTIs should be directed at the organism identified by Gram stain and culture. Parenteral therapy is advised for elderly, hospitalized patients who are systemically unwell. If Gram-negative organisms are seen on staining, a broad-spectrum β-lactam agent or a fluoroquinolone should be prescribed. If Gram-positive organisms are identified, vancomycin would be an appropriate choice of treatment. For patients at risk of infection from multiply resistant Gram-negative organisms, a carbapenem plus aminoglycoside combination should provide effective cover. Unfortunately, polymicrobial infections occur in approximately 30 per cent of patients and more frequently in patients with long-term indwelling catheters. Catheters contain stagnant urine promoting development of a biofilm on the interior surface which can harbour a large number of micro-organisms. In these patients, broad-spectrum antimicrobial therapy may be necessary. De-escalation of antibiotics to narrow-spectrum agents should be performed as soon as culture results are available. There is also evidence that simply changing the catheter may improve clinical symptoms.[36]

Relapse of infection arises from inadequate eradication of infection with recurrence of infection with the same organism after discontinuation of antimicrobial therapy. This should prompt a thorough investigation of the entire urinary tract. Reinfection refers to the development of another infection with a different organism and is usually due to chronic conditions preventing free flow of urine or poor hygiene.[37]

Surgical site infections

Surgical site infections (SSIs) are one of the most important healthcare-associated infections seen in clinical practice (Fig. 35.1). A prevalence study reported that up to 8 per cent of patients in UK hospitals have healthcare-associated infections, of which 14 per cent could be attributed to SSIs.[38] Not only does this contribute to significant morbidity and mortality, SSI can double the length of inpatient stay and increase hospital costs. Depending upon the type of surgery and the severity of infection, additional attributable costs may be between £814 and £6626.[39]

The US Centers for Disease Control and Prevention (CDC) definition describes three levels of SSI:[40]

- *Superficial incisional* affecting the skin and subcutaneous tissue and characterized by localized signs of infection such as redness, pain, or swelling at the site of infection or by drainage of pus.

- *Deep incisional* affecting the fascial and muscle layers and characterized by the presence of pus or an abscess, fever with wound tenderness, or separation of the wound edges exposing deeper tissue layers.

- *Organ and space infection* involves any part which is opened or manipulated during the course of the surgical procedure (e.g. the

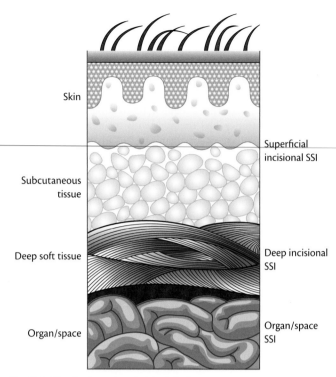

Skin

Superficial
incisional SSI

Subcutaneous
tissue

Deep soft tissue

Deep incisional
SSI

Organ/space

Organ/space
SSI

Fig. 35.1 Classifications of surgical site infections.

peritoneum or joint), and are characterized by abscess formation detected by radiological examination or during re-operation.

Advances in surgical and anaesthetic techniques have resulted in patients who are at high risk of SSIs being considered for surgery (Table 35.7). Surgical wounds are likely to become contaminated by resident skin or visceral bacterial flora. Progression from wound contamination to clinical infection is determined by the adequacy of host defence.[41] Advanced age, obesity, blood transfusion, and use of steroids or other immunosuppressive agents have all been reported to increase the risk of SSI.[42] Frequently these factors cannot be modified in the preoperative period. However, appropriate use of antibiotic prophylaxis, proper choice of operation, and meticulous surgical technique can reduce the incidence of SSI. From the anaesthetist's perspective, maintenance of blood volume, haemostasis, normothermia and oxygen carrying capacity with adequate analgesia improves tissue perfusion and helps reduce the risk of SSI.

Prophylactic antibiotics should be considered for clean procedures involving placement of prosthesis or implant, clean-contaminated or contaminated surgery.[39] The timing of delivery of antimicrobial prophylaxis should take into account the drug half-life, drug infusion time, and the need for a repeated dose depending on duration of surgery. There is evidence that administration of antibiotic prophylaxis up to 2 hours preoperatively is associated with the lowest rates of infection in clean and clean-contaminated surgery.[43] Consideration should always be given to the adverse effects of antibiotics and use of local antibiotic prescribing guidelines based on potential pathogens, patterns of infection, and antibiotic resistance.

Perioperative inadvertent hypothermia can directly impair immune function. Mild hypothermia has been shown to increase the incidence of SSIs, delay wound healing, and lengthen hospital stay.[44] The National Institute for Health and Clinical Excellence recommends that patients undergoing surgical procedures lasting longer than 30 minutes should receive active warming and monitoring of core temperature.[45]

Enhanced recovery after surgery (ERAS) is an increasingly utilized approach to perioperative management emphasizing patient pre-optimization, minimal access surgical techniques, multi-modal opioid-sparing analgesia, early nutrition, and mobilization. The aim is to achieve earlier hospital discharge and return to normal functional status with the potential benefit of reducing postoperative infection rates.[46]

Clostridium difficile-associated diarrhoea

Clostridium difficile is an anaerobic, Gram-positive, spore-forming bacterium and is the most common cause of nosocomial diarrhoea in hospital and long-term elderly care facilities. More than 80 per cent of reported *C. difficile* infections occur in hospitalized or institutionalized adults aged 65 years or over. It can cause a spectrum of disease ranging from mild diarrhoea to potentially fatal complications such as pseudomembranous colitis, toxic megacolon, bleeding, and colonic perforation.[47] The clinical manifestations are due to the production of two exotoxins, toxins A and B, which have enterotoxic and cytotoxic properties.[48] The main risk factor is exposure to broad-spectrum antibiotics, particularly cephalosporins, fluoroquinolones, and clindamycin.[7] However, the age-related reduction in gastric acid, reduced immune function, malnutrition, and the presence of chronic underlying pathology also contribute.[47]

Table 35.7 Factors influencing risk of surgical site infections

Patient factors	Anaesthetic factors	Surgical factors
Advanced age	Adequate tissue oxygenation	Preoperative preparation
Severity of underlying disease	Normovolaemia	Hand hygiene
Multiple comorbid conditions	Normothermia	Site and timing of surgery
Malnutrition	Normoglycaemia	Surgical technique
Immunosuppressive agents	Adequate pain control	Duration and extent of surgery
Obesity	Blood transfusion	Blood loss
Smoking		

Clinical features include crampy abdominal pain, offensively smelling loose stools, fever, leucocytosis, and hypoalbuminaemia. Laboratory confirmatory tests include enzyme immunoassays to detect toxins A and B. An alternative is the cell cytotoxicity assay which is more sensitive and specific but it is more expensive, more technically demanding, and has a slower turn-around time.[49] The first step in treatment is to withdraw antibiotics wherever possible. The second step is the administration of either oral metronidazole or vancomycin for 10–14 days.

A patient who is affected excretes large numbers of spores in liquid faeces. The spores can contaminate the general environment including mattresses, toilet areas, and commodes. Spores can survive simple disinfection procedures and use of chlorine-based compounds is advocated.[50] There are five key measures that hospitals need to employ to minimize risks posed by *C. difficile*:

♦ Rapid isolation of the patient with new-onset diarrhoea.

♦ Scrupulous hand hygiene to prevent person-to-person transmission of spores. Handwashing with soap and water is recommended.

♦ Personal protective equipment.

♦ Enhanced environmental cleanliness to reduce the level of spore contamination and the likelihood of further transmission to other patients.

♦ Prudent antimicrobial prescribing with rapid de-escalation where appropriate

Methicillin-resistant *Staphylococcus aureus*

Methicillin-resistant *Staphylococcus aureus* (MRSA) presents a major problem to elderly patients, particularly those who are long-stay inpatients or nursing home residents. Elderly patients who are colonized with MRSA are at increased risk of systemic infection and tend to have a poor functional status.[1] The most common reservoirs for MRSA are the nasal mucosa and oropharynx. Routine preoperative screening for MRSA is common in surgical units. Mupirocin topical nasal eradication therapy and chlorhexidine skin wash are recommended for MRSA carriers to reduce the shedding of MRSA.[51]

Prevention of MRSA transmission is vital. Thorough hand washing and isolation of infected patients with appropriate handling of bodily secretions are essential to minimize spread. While colonization by MRSA does not require systemic treatment, active infection requires intravenous antibiotic therapy. Vancomycin or teicoplanin are suitable, effective antimicrobial agents. Elderly patients require dose adjustment depending on renal function and therapeutic drug monitoring may be required.

Antibiotic therapy

Antibiotic administration in elderly patients is not without risk. The age-related physiological decline in renal and hepatic function decreases the rate of excretion of numerous antibiotics. This predisposes elderly patients to a risk of antibiotic-induced toxicity highlighting the need for careful drug selection and clinical and laboratory monitoring. In addition, elderly patients often have multiple comorbid conditions and receive polypharmacy. Concurrent use of antibiotics may increase the risk of drug interaction. Specific examples of adverse antibiotic-related events which occur more frequently in the elderly include:

♦ Aminoglycoside-induced nephrotoxicity and ototoxicity.

♦ Antibiotic-associated pseudomembranous colitis.

♦ Trimethoprim and sulfamethoxazole-induced blood dyscrasias and hyperkalaemia.

♦ Quinolone-related seizures.

There are a number of ways to prevent the development of antibiotic-related adverse reactions. The most effective method is judicious use of antimicrobials with meticulous surveillance. It must be emphasized that not all clinical or functional changes in the elderly should be attributed to infection. Antibiotics should only be administered where there is evidence to indicate potential benefit. Treatment duration should be confined to accepted practice guidelines. When a specific pathogen is isolated and sensitivities are available, de-escalation from broad-spectrum to narrow-spectrum agents is recommended.[52]

Conclusion

Infection in elderly patients may be asymptomatic and of little significance to their normal daily life or they may be life-threatening and life-changing events. The diagnosis of infection may be difficult because of atypical presentations and signs with advancing age and routine investigations such as a chest X-ray may be misleading. Some infections become more common with prolonged stay in hospital and pose serious risks to the frail elderly patient. Treatment with appropriate antibiotics, based on culture and sensitivity remains the most appropriate therapy for bacterial infections although vaccinations against influenza and pneumococcus have proved to be effective.

It is important to remember that an overwhelming infection may be an end-of-life event and in the very frail, ill elderly it is prudent to have ascertained their wishes with regard to major medical interventions, such as controlled ventilation, before escalating treatment.

References

1. Mouton CP, Bazaldua OV, Pierce B, Espino DV. Common infections in older adults. *Am Fam Physician*. 2001;63(2):257–269.
2. Gavazzi G, Krause KH. Ageing and infection. *Lancet Infect Dis*. 2002;2:659–666.
3. Yoshikawa TT. Epidemiology and unique aspects of aging and infectious diseases. *Clin Infect Dis*. 2000;30:931–933.
4. Castle SC, Uyemura K, Fulop T, Makinodan T. Host resistance and immune response in advanced age. *Clin Geriatr Med*. 2007;23:463–479.
5. Ginaldi L, Loreto MF, Corsi MP, Modesti M, De Martinis M. Immunosenescence and infectious diseases. *Microbes Infect*. 2001:3:851–857.
6. Aw D, Silva AB, Palmer DB. Immunosenescence: emerging challenges for an ageing population. *Immunology*. 2007;120:435–446.
7. Htwe TH, Mushtaq A, Robinson SB, Rosher RB, Khardori N. Infections in the elderly. *Infect Dis Clin N Am*. 2007;21:711–743.
8. Ben-Yehuda A, Weksler ME. Host resistance and the immune system. *Clin Geriatr Med*. 1992:8;701–711.
9. Pilotto A, Malfertheimer P. An approach to Helicobacter pylori infection in the elderly. *Aliment Pharmacol The.r* 2002;16:683–691.

10. Katona P, Katona-Apte J. Interaction between nutrition and infection. *Clin Infect Dis.* 2008; 46: 1582–1588.

11. Lesourd BM, MazariL, Ferry M. The role of nutrition in immunity in the aged. *Nutr Rev.* 1998;56:S113–S125.

12. Sullivan DH, Sun S, Walls RC. Protein energy undernutrition among elderly hospitalized patients. A prospective study. *JAMA.* 1999;281;2013–2019.

13. High K. Nutritional strategies to boost immunity and prevention of infection in elderly individuals. *Clin Infect Dis.* 2001;33:1892–1900.

14. Barrocas A, Belcher D, Champagne C. Nutritional assessment practical approaches. *Clin Geriatr Med.* 1995;11:675–713

15. Omran ML, Morley JE. Assessment of protein energy malnutrition in older persons, part 1: history, examination, body composition and screening tools. *Nutrition.* 2000;16:50–63.

16. Yoneyama T, YoshidaM, Ohrui T, *et al.* Oral care reduces pneumonia in older patients in nursing homes. *J Am Geriatr Soc.* 2002;50:430–433.

17. Norman DC. Fever and aging. *Infect Dis Clin Pract.* 1998:7;387–390.

18. Bellmann-Weiler R, Weiss G. Pitfalls in the diagnosis and therapy of infections in elderly patients- a mini-review. *Gerontology.* 2009;55:241–249.

19. Knockaert DC, Vanneste LJ, Bobbaers HJ. Fever of unknown origin in elderly patients. *J Am Geriatr Soc.* 1993;41:1187–1892.

20. Tal S, Guller V, Gurevich A. Fever of unknown origin in older adults. *Clin Geriatr Med.* 2007;23:649–668.

21. Scheutz P, Christ-Crain M, Muller B. Procalcitonin and other biomarkers to improve assessment and antibiotic stewardship in infections—hope for hype? *Swiss Med Wkly.* 2009;139:318–326.

22. Heppner HJ, Bertsch T, Alber B, *et al.* Prcalcitonin: inflammatory biomarker for assessing the severity of community acquired pneumonia. *Gerontology.* 2010;56:385–389.

23. Silvermann ME, Murray TJ, Bryan CS (eds). *The Quotable Osler* (p. 139). Philadelphia, PA: American College of Physicians, 1998.

24. Brito V, Niederman MS. Predicting mortality in the elderly with community acquired pneumonia: should we design a new car or set a new 'speed limit'? *Thorax.* 2010;65:944–945.

25. Chong CP, Street PR. Pneumonia in the elderly: a review of severity assessment, prognosis, mortality, prevention and treatment. *South Med J.* 2008;101:1134–1140.

26. Kaplan V, Angus DC, Griffin MF, *et al.* Hospitalized community acquired pneumonia in the elderly. *Am J Respir Crit Care Med.* 2002;165:766–772.

27. Lim WS, van der Eerden MM, Laing R, *et al.* Defining community acquired pneumonia severity on presentation to hospital: an international derivation and validation study. *Thorax.* 2003;58:377–382.

28. Myint PK, Kamath AV, Vowler SL, *et al.* Severity assessment criteria recommended by the British Thoracic Society (BTS) for community acquired pneumonia (CAP) and older patients. Should SOAR (systolic blood pressure, oxygenation, age and respiratory rate be used in older people? A compilation study of two prospective cohorts. *Age Ageing.* 2006;35:286–291.

29. Lim WS. Baudouin SV, George RC, *et al.* Guidelines for the management of community acquired pneumonia: update 2009. *Thorax.* 2009;64(Suppl III):iii1–iii55.

30. Department of Health. *JCVI statement on routine pneumococcal vaccination programme for adults aged 65 years and older.* <http://webarchive.nationalarchives.gov.uk/+/www.dh.gov.uk/ab/jcvi/dh_094744>.

31. Foxman B. Epidemiology of urinary tract infections: incidence, morbidity and economic costs. *Am J Med.* 2002;113:5–13S

32. Nicolle LE. Urinary tract infections in long-term care facilities residents. *Clin Infect Dis.* 2000;31:757–761.

33. Juthani-Mehta M. Asymptomatic bacteriuria and urinary tract infection in older adults. *Clin Geriatr Med.* 2007;23:585–594.

34. Nicolle LE, Bradley S, Colgan R, *et al.* Infectious Diseases Society of America guidelines for the diagnosis and treatment of asymptomatic bacteriuria in adults. *Clin Infect Dis.* 2005;40:643–654.

35. Nicolle LE. Resistant pathogens in urinary tract infections. *J Am Geriatr Soc.* 2002;50:S230–S235.

36. Nicolle LE. Urinary tract infection in geriatric and institutionalized patients. *Curr Opin Urol.* 2002;12(1):51–55.

37. Yoshikawa TT, Nicolle LE, Norman DC. Management of complicated urinary tract infection in older patients. *J Am Geriatr Soc.* 1996;44(10):1235–1241.

38. Smyth ET, McIlvenny G, McIlvenny GE, *et al.* Four Country Healthcare Associated Infection Prevalence Survey 2006: overview of results. *J Hosp Infect.* 2008;69:230–248.

39. National Institute for Health and Clinical Excellence. *Surgical site infection—prevention and treatment of surgical site infection.* <http://www.guidance.nice.org.uk/CG74> (accessed 28 August 2011).

40. Horan TC, Gaynes RP, Martone WJ, Jarvis WR, Emori TG. CDC definitions of nosocomial surgical site infections, 1992: a modification of CDC definitions of surgical wound infections. *Infect Control Hosp Epidemiol.* 1992;13:606–608.

41. Gifford C, Christelis N, Cheng A. Preventing postoperative infections: the anaesthetist's role. *CEACCP.* 2011;11:151–156.

42. Meakins JL. Prevention of postoperative infection. *ACS surgery.* <http://www.acssurgery.com/acs/Chapters/CH0101.mtm> (accessed 2 September 2011).

43. Classen DC, Evans RS, Pestonik SL, Horn SD, Menlove RL, Burke JP. The timing of prophylactic administration of antibiotics and the risk of surgical wound infection. *N Engl J Med.* 1992;326:281–286.

44. KurzA, Sessler DI, Lenhardt R. Perioperative normothermia to reduce the incidence of surgical-wound infection and shorten hospitalization. Study of Wound Infection and Temperature Group. *N Engl J Med.* 1996;334:1209–1215.

45. National Institute for Health and Clinical Excellence. *Perioperative hypothermia (inadvertent).* <http://www.guidance.nice.org.uk/CG65> (accessed 2 September 2011).

46. Kehlet H and Wilmore DW. Evidence based surgical care and the evolution of fast track surgery. *Ann Surg.* 2008;248:189–198.

47. Mathei C, Niclaes L, Suetens C, Jans B, Buntinx F. Infections in nursing home residents. *Infect Dis Clin N Am.* 2007;21:761–772.

48. Calfee DP. Clostridium difficile: a reemerging pathogen. *Geriatrics.* 2008;63:10–14.

49. Bartlett JG, Gerding DN. Clinical recognition and diagnosis of Clostridium difficile infection. *Clin Infect Dis.* 2008;46:S12–S18.

50. Mayfield JL, Leet T, Miller J, Mundy LM. Environmental control to reduce the transmission of Clostridium difficile. *Clin Infect Dis.* 2000;31(4):995–1000.

51. Michel M, Guttman L. Methicillin-resistant Staphylococcus aureus and vancomycin- resistant enterococci: therapeutic realities and possibilities. *Lancet.* 1997;349:1901–1906.

52. Yoshikawa TT. VRE, MRSA, PRP and DRGNB in LTCF: lessons to be learned from this alphabet. *J Am Geriatr Soc.* 1998;46:241–243.

CHAPTER 36

Medico-legal aspects

Barry N. Speker

Introduction

Life expectancy is lengthening at a rate previously unanticipated. Society needs to provide for and protect the elderly. By 2031 the British population over 75 years of age will increase to 8.2 million.[1] By 2035 the number of people aged over 85 is projected to be 2.5 times larger than in 2010, numbering 3.6 million and amounting to 5 per cent of the population. Dementia affects one person in 20 above the age of 65 and one person in five over 80.

The Mental Capacity Act 2007 which came into force in the UK on 1 October 2007, was designed to consolidate the law on capacity, consent, and best interests as well as bringing changes to protect vulnerable persons and enable medical practitioners to deal with many sensitive legal and ethical issues involved in treating the elderly.

The Human Rights Act has also emphasized the concentration of our laws on the basic human rights of individuals. The culture of complaints and the increasingly compensation-centred focus of society require that anaesthetists ensure full compliance with legal obligations and guard against situations where complaints and claims may arise. Anaesthetizing the elderly requires constant awareness of questions of capacity and consent.

Ethical issues

Law should be consistent with the ethics of the society in which it operates. In the practice of anaesthesia as with many activities, there are wide discretions within which judgement is exercised. This will involve ethical, moral, and religious factors. Medical ethics principles in relation to treatment include:

Beneficence and non-malfeasance

The aim must be to do good and not to cause harm. The cost/benefit analysis of medical treatment for older patients is much more difficult than for younger patients. The risk of harm is often greater and the likelihood of benefit is less certain. Hospitalization and treatment can result in other risks for the elderly including confusion, disruption to daily life, risks of falls, risk of pulmonary embolism, and bronchopneumonia. There will be greater problems in coping postoperatively with a higher risk of cognitive impairment after major surgery.

Autonomy

All patients should be assisted to exercise their autonomy. This is enshrined in the Mental Capacity Act. There is a greater tendency for the elderly to acquiesce in decisions and to place an over-reliance on the judgement of doctors. The elderly may also be at risk of undue influence from relatives, carers, and religious groups. In considering the autonomy of the patient it is essential that sufficient time is spent assessing the patient's level of understanding and ability to make appropriate decisions. This is guided by the tests under the Mental Capacity Act.

Justice

Various approaches may be adopted to reach a conclusion as to what is just for the patient.

Utilitarian approach

Healthcare resources should be allocated to do the most good for the largest number of people. This is difficult to judge and involves considerations such as how many quality years would be provided by the delivery of treatment to one patient rather than another. A younger patient will have more quality years. Treatment may assist him or her in getting back to work.

Idealistic approach

Resources being allocated to help the people whose need for healthcare is greatest. The elderly will require disproportionately more healthcare and can argue that they have paid more into the UK National Health Service (NHS) by way of tax over many years. Society may not tolerate an over-emphasis on such an approach.

Compromise

Expectation that allocation of health resources will be undertaken to benefit the most needy as well as the largest number of persons in a proportionate manner and with an evidence base. The law will rarely interfere with the NHS allocation of resources provided that a proper process has been followed and the allocation is not bizarre.[2]

Treatment of the elderly may be more expensive, with the need for provision of intraoperative equipment such as warming devices and antipressure sore apparatus. Anaesthesia is more risky. Recovery time as an inpatient may be longer and a higher nursing ratio required.

Sanctity of human life

The Human Rights Act 1998 incorporated the European Convention on Human Rights into English law. Article 2 (Right to Life), Article 3 (A Prohibition against inhuman and degrading treatment), and Article 8 (Respect for Private and Family Life) are often argued in support of a claim for medical treatment. However there is *no* basic human right to demand medical treatment, even where there is a known and available treatment and a patient will die without it. Health resources are finite. Every patient in need cannot receive every available treatment. A reasonable compromised allocation is necessary, and is central to the role of the National Institute for Health and Clinical Excellence.

Ethical clinical decision-making

For decisions to be made in an ethical manner, they should not be left to one individual who will be affected by personal views, ethics, and standpoints. It is implicit that decisions should be made on a multidisciplinary team basis. This involves following guidelines from the General Medical Council (GMC), British Medical Association, The Royal College of Anaesthetists, and the Association of Anaesthetists of GB and Ireland, lessons learned from audit, peer review, and, where necessary, legal advice.

Whether decisions have been made on an ethical basis is relevant in relation to medico-legal claims, to ensure that the standard of care applied is in accordance with the legal standard. In complex cases applications should be made to the Court to determine whether treatment should proceed.

Preoperative assessment for surgery

This involves an ethical approach. Age itself is not a good predictor of surgical risk. Physiological age-related changes increase the risk of surgery and anaesthesia. Comorbidities also increase with age. The purpose of the assessment is to identify within the patient the integrated responses which are clinically reduced and to review individual organ systems for functional reserve. This involves a consideration of issues such as ischaemic heart disease and valve dysfunction, the likelihood of chest infections and pulmonary complications and the steps which will be required to reduce the risk of bronchopneumonia and deep vein thrombosis (DVT). The increase of delirium and confusion with high risk of postoperative cognitive impairment argues against general anaesthesia.

The role of anaesthetists is crucial in undertaking preoperative assessments of the elderly. Can the patient withstand anaesthesia or the length of the surgery? Is the proposed operation heroic but futile? Should the emphasis be on palliation and achieving what may be an acceptable quality of life?

An adverse outcome or death may result in a complaint, claim or coroner's inquest, as to whether the preoperative assessment was appropriate, adequate, realistic, and competent and whether it justified the decision to proceed. The need for full records is essential.[3]

Consent to treatment

It is fundamental to the doctor/patient relationship that consent is obtained from the patient for all treatment. Where consent cannot be obtained, law and practice provide safeguards and identify enquiries to be made prior to determining that treatment should proceed without consent in the patient's best interests.

Respect for a patient's autonomy and the right to self-determination have been long established and are set out in the words of Cardozo J in *Schloendorff* v *Society of New York Hospital*:

Every human being of adult years and sound mind has a right to determine what shall be done with his own body: and a surgeon who performs an operation without his patient's consent commits an assault.[4]

The Mental Capacity Act 2005

The Mental Capacity Act 2005 (MCA) was enacted after many years of consultation. The purposes of the Act included clarifying the test of capacity and how it is to be assessed as well as elucidating the meaning of 'best interests' and the factors to be taken into account in assessing it. The Act also introduced empowerment for patients to make decisions for the future and to appoint individuals to exercise decision-making on their behalf, as well as requiring an advocate to be involved in decisions. The Act is the guide as to whether it is acceptable, lawful or appropriate to proceed to anaesthetize an elderly patient.

Any interference with a patient without appropriate consent amounts to an assault or battery. If the patient comes to serious harm or dies, there is the spectre of serious criminal action, professional disciplinary action and compensation claims.

Five key principles underpin the MCA

◆ A person must be assumed to have capacity unless it is established that they lack capacity to make a specific decision (i.e. lack of capacity may not apply to all decisions).

◆ A person is not to be treated as unable to make a decision unless all practicable steps to help him to do so have been taken without success.

◆ A person is not to be treated as unable to make a decision merely because he makes an unwise decision.

◆ An act done, or decision made, under the Act for or on behalf of a person who lacks capacity must be done, or made, in his best interests (as defined in the MCA) including taking into account what the person might have wanted if capable of making a decision.

◆ Before an act is done or the decision is made, regard must be had as to whether the purpose for which it is needed can be as effectively achieved in a way that is less restrictive of the person's rights and freedom of action.[5]

The legal and clinical framework provided by the MCA is to be used by professionals when assisting individuals to make treatment decisions in advance if they have capacity to do so, or to make decisions which respect the individual's known beliefs, values, and opinions if professionals are acting according to best interest principles.

Assessment of capacity

Under Section 2 of the MCA:

A person lacks capacity in relation to a matter if at the material time he is unable to make a decision for himself in relation to the matter because of an impairment of, or a disturbance in the functioning of, the mind or brain.

The disturbance may be permanent or temporary. Lack of capacity is not established merely by reference to a person's age or appearance or their medical condition; nor is it established because of behaviour which may lead others to make unjustified assumptions about capacity. Accordingly a doctor must not assume lack of capacity based upon the assessment of another. An anaesthetist prior to proceeding, must form a clear view by carrying out the assessment under the MCA.

A person does not have capacity to make a decision if he cannot:

◆ Understand information relevant to the decision.

◆ Retain that information

◆ Use or weigh that information as part of the decision-making process, or

◆ Communicate the decision (by speech, sign language or other means).[6]

The patient does not have capacity unless he can comply with *all* of points listed. In particular it must not be presumed that a patient is incapable because of advanced age or because of a diagnosed condition such as dementia. A patient may have capacity if able to retain information relevant to a decision for a short period of time even if it may then be forgotten. The ability to communicate may be by talking, using sign language, or simple movements such as blinking an eye or squeezing a hand. Interpreters must be used where necessary.

Patients may have capacity to consent to some interventions but not others. Capacity may fluctuate. The assessment by the healthcare professional should be in relation to the decision in question. Details of the assessment and the conclusions made must be recorded in the patient's notes.

The issue of capacity should not be confused with a healthcare professional's assessment of the reasonableness of a person's decision. One of the principles of the Act is that a patient is entitled to make an unwise decision which is considered by others to be irrational. If on the other hand the decision is irrational because it is based on a lack of ability to perceive the true situation then it may be the patient does not have the capacity to comprehend or make use of the information.

Voluntariness of consent

Consent is only valid if it is given voluntarily and freely and not as the result of pressure or undue influence being exerted on the patient to accept or refuse treatment. Pressure of this kind may come from partners or family members and this is a particular risk in the case of elderly patients. It may also be exerted by members of a religious sect. Doctors should be alert to this possibility where there is pressure on the patient to proceed or not to proceed with treatment. It is always advisable for practitioners to see the patient alone in order to ensure that the decision which they make is their own decision. Anaesthesia should be considered separately from the surgery itself.

Communication of information

For consent to be valid the patient needs to understand the nature and purpose of the procedure. Important information must not be withheld. Full details of the anaesthesia to be given including the nature and route of it, the drugs to be used, and the risks and possible side effects must be communicated.

Informing a patient of the nature and purpose of a procedure may secure valid consent but may not be sufficient to fulfil the legal duty of care. Failure to provide full information may expose a practitioner to a claim for negligence if the patient suffers harm as a result of the treatment.

In the Sidaway case the House of Lords held that the legal standard to be used when deciding whether adequate information had been given to a patient is the same as that used when judging whether a doctor had been negligent in the treatment.[7] This is the Bolam test.[8] A doctor is not negligent if his practice conforms to that of a responsible body of medical opinion held by practitioners skilled in the field in question. The information which should be given to a patient regarding anaesthesia is that information which a responsible body of anaesthetists would regard as appropriate in the circumstances of the individual patient. It is important to stay within acceptable peer standards.

There are some cases where a Court may be critical of a practice even if a 'responsible body' of medical practitioners holds it. In *Chester* v *Afshar*[9] the House of Lords held that a neurosurgeon who failed to warn a patient of a small risk of injury inherent in surgery was liable to the patient when that risk materialized, even though the risk was not increased by the failure to warn and even though the patient would have had the operation if she had known of the risk. The patient was entitled to make an informed choice, whether and if so when and by whom, to be operated on.

In the light of *Chester* v *Afshar* health professionals should give details of all significant possible adverse outcomes and record the information given.

Consent forms—Department of Health reference guide for examination or treatment 2009

The standard Department of Health form of consent to treatment should always be fully completed although the validity of consent does not in fact depend upon such a form. The advantage of it is as evidence of the discussion with the patient, the communication of the nature and purpose of the treatment, and the identification of the risks inherent in it. It should also be evidence that the patient has understood what has been communicated. The presence of the signature on the form does not in itself prove that the assessment of the patient's capacity has been properly undertaken or that the patient fully appreciates and understands all of the information which should have been conveyed. This should be recorded separately in the notes.

Elderly patients may have poor recollection of what they are told about anaesthesia. Relatives may complain that the patient could not or would not have understood or consented.

The taking of consent should be undertaken at a senior level, by the anaesthetist who will undertake the procedure and is able to answer questions about risks.

Refusal of consent

Where a patient has capacity and makes an informed decision to refuse treatment, whether at the time or in advance, then that decision must be respected. Similarly a patient with capacity is entitled to withdraw consent at any time even during the performance of a procedure. A judgement must be made as to whether stopping the procedure at a particular point may put the life of a person at risk, in which case the practitioner may continue until that risk no longer applies.

Advance decisions to refuse treatment

Prior to the Mental Capacity Act persons could make advance decisions known as 'living wills', indicating that they wished to refuse certain treatments which might be given to them at a future time when they may lack capacity. These previously had no formal legal standing under English law although in the Tony Bland[10] case the House of Lords indicated that such a living will would be given some weight if it existed.

The MCA gives legal enforceability to advance decisions to refuse life-sustaining treatment. In order to be valid, they must be signed and witnessed and must expressly state that the refusal of treatment is applicable even if it places life at risk.[11]

Healthcare professionals must follow an advance decision if it is valid and applicable, even if this may result in the patient's death. Legal advice should be taken as to the validity.

The MCA protects health professionals from liability where they continue to treat a patient in that person's best interests[12] until such time as they have clarified the validity of the advance directive. In rare cases the matter is referred for determination to the Court of Protection.

It is important to check that an advance decision by an elderly patient has not been the result of coercion or undue influence. Conflicts of interest may raise suspicions as to the validity.

The advance decision will not be valid if the patient has previously withdrawn it or taken any action inconsistent with it or where the circumstances which applied at the time the document was signed have changed. There may also be a change in circumstances which the patient could not have anticipated.

Increasingly elderly patients may have made advance decisions which indicate the treatment they will not accept. Doctors must check in every case whether the patient has made an advance decision and record in the notes why they consider that it is applicable and what steps they have taken to follow it. If they decide that the advance decision is not binding it can still be taken into account as a statement of the patient's wishes. Documents which merely set out treatment preferences as in the previous type of 'living will' are not legally binding.

Lasting powers of attorney

Since the implementation of the MCA a person can complete a personal welfare lasting power of attorney (PWLPA)[13] under which a donor with capacity may appoint a person (the donee) to make personal welfare and medical decisions on the donor's behalf when the donor loses capacity.

An increasing number of such documents will now be in existence and they must be carefully checked by health professionals as to their validity. A donee under a PWLPA cannot refuse life-sustaining treatment unless the PWLPA expressly authorizes this. The PWLPA can give consent for DNAR designation.

Adult patients without capacity

The Mental Capacity Act 2005 clarifies the arrangements for dealing with the situation where adult patients do not have the capacity to consent to medical treatment.[14] The Act is augmented by the detailed guidance set out in the Code of Practice.[15]

Under English law no person can give consent to the examination or treatment of any adult who lacks capacity to give consent for himself, unless they have been authorized to do so under a lasting power of attorney or have authority as a deputy appointed by the Court. Accordingly parents, relatives and members of the healthcare team have no right to consent on behalf of such a patient. Family members of elderly patients often believe they have a right to consent to treatment or to refuse it. This is not so even if they are identified in the notes as 'next of kin' or if they are named as executors in a will.

The traditional position has always been that where consent cannot be given, the doctor can proceed in what he considers to be the 'best interests' of the patient. The Act sets out clear criteria which must be applied in order to determine whether the intended treatment is in the best interests of the patient:

- Whether it is likely the patient will regain capacity to make the relevant decision and if so when that is likely to be and whether the decision could be postponed until then.

- So far as reasonably practicable the patient must be allowed and encouraged to participate in the decision as fully as possible.

- Where the determination relates to life-sustaining treatment, a decision must not be motivated by desire to bring about the patient's death.

- The professionals must so far as reasonably practicable consider the patient's past and present wishes and feelings including in particular:

  - any written statements made by him when he had capacity

  - the beliefs and values (e.g. cultural and religious) that would be likely to influence a decision if he had capacity

  - the other factors which he would be likely to consider if he were able to do so.

If it is practicable and appropriate professionals must consult with persons named by the patient, carers, including paid carers, a donee under a lasting power of attorney or a deputy appointed by the Court of Protection.[16]

These principles emphasize the need to concentrate on the interests, needs, and wishes of the individual patient whose autonomy must be respected. An appropriate entry must be made in the medical notes to indicate that the best interests test and the test of capacity under the Act have been properly applied. Health professionals are protected under the MCA from liability for giving or withholding treatment where they have a reasonable belief that the patient lacks capacity and the treatment or its omission is in the patient's best interests.

Independent medical capacity advocates

The Mental Capacity Act imposes a duty on NHS bodies to instruct an independent medical capacity advocate (IMCA) before *serious medical treatment* is given, if the health professionals are satisfied that there is no one appropriate to consult in determining the patient's best interests.[17] This would also arise where relatives have abused an elderly patient or where family members themselves are in such conflict with the patient or each other that it is not felt appropriate to consult with them.

IMCAs are appropriately trained. The duties of an IMCA are not to make decisions but to support the person who lacks capacity and to try to represent their views and interests to the decision-maker. They should also obtain and evaluate information through interviewing the patient, look at relevant records and documents and obtain the views of professionals providing treatment. They should identify alternative courses of action and if required obtain further medical evidence and prepare a report for consideration by the decision-maker.

For these purposes *serious medical treatment* includes the withdrawal or withholding of treatment. It is not only treatment which has serious consequences for the patient but also where the benefits, risks and burdens are finely balanced.

The list of treatments which come within the definition of '*serious medical treatment*' is set out Chapter 10.44–50 of the Code of Practice and is extensive. Examples are treatments causing protracted pain or side-effects, heart surgery or treatment impacting on life choices. With particular relevance to elderly patients are amputations and the withholding or withdrawal of artificial nutrition and hydration.[18]

Where a serious medical treatment is required '*urgently*' there is no need to request an IMCA but the reasons for not doing so should be documented.

Court of Protection

The Court of Protection is a specialist part of the High Court which can make decisions in individual cases on issues regarding capacity or the treatment of an individual. Such decisions can be made at very short notice.[19]

The significance of decisions made by the Court as to lawfulness of treatment is not to order a doctor to carry out any particular treatment but to declare that if the doctor decides to proceed then such treatment will be considered to be in the patient's best interests and will be lawful.

Circumstances where it is appropriate for referral to the Court for a ruling on lawfulness before the procedure is undertaken:

- Withholding or withdrawal of artificial nutrition and hydration (ANH) from patients in a persistent vegetative state.
- Organ, bone marrow, or peripheral blood stem cell donation by an adult who lacks the capacity to consent.
- Proposed non-therapeutic sterilization of a person who lacks capacity to consent.
- Other cases where there is a doubt or dispute about whether a particular treatment will be in a patient's best interests.

The Court of Protection has power to appoint deputies to make ongoing decisions for health matters.

'Do not attempt cardiopulmonary resuscitation' decisions

Cardiopulmonary resuscitation (CPR) has a low success rate (particularly where a patient has a serious condition and is in poor general health). Chest compressions, clinically assisted respiration and defibrillation carry risks of complications and harmful side effects. CPR may prolong the dying process and suffering of a seriously ill patient and may be regarded as degrading and undignified. Cardiac or respiratory arrest may be the terminal event at a time when attempts to resuscitate may be futile and of no overall benefit to the patient.

The question of whether CPR should be attempted in the event of an arrest should be considered as early as is reasonable and after careful consideration of all of the relevant factors. These include the likely clinical outcome, the patient's known or ascertainable wishes, the patient's human rights, the likelihood of the patient suffering severe unmanageable pain, or other distressing side effects and the patient's level of awareness.

Where the patients lack capacity, the views of the healthcare team should be taken as well as family members and carers.

A judgement must be made as to what to say to the patient about the do not attempt CPR (DNACPR) decision. Communicating that CPR would not be clinically successful may be burdensome to the patient. Such matters must be dealt with compassionately but still with respect to all of the issues with regard to consent and the involvement of others as set out in the MCA. Regard must also be had to any advance decision made by the patient.

The decision to record DNACPR in the notes must be taken by a senior clinician and should be reviewed regularly and the reviews recorded in the notes.

Deprivation of liberty safeguards

The Mental Capacity Act deprivation of liberty safeguards came into force on 1 April 2009.[20] These safeguards provide a legal framework for hospitals and care homes to obtain authorization to lawfully deprive people who are using their services of their liberty. Such issues will often arise where elderly patients are being treated.

In 2008 the Government published a Code of Practice to supplement the Mental Capacity Act 2005. This identifies the difference between deprivation of liberty (for which authority must be obtained from a supervisory body—the Primary Care Trust or Local Authority) and restriction of liberty (which does not require such authority). Deprivation may apply where physical restraint is used, complete control is being exercised over a patient's care or movements or medication is given forcibly against a patient's will. It may also arise where a hospital is taking responsibility for deciding if a patient can be released into the care of others. It is necessary to have in mind whether a deprivation situation arises and to ensure that the hospital policy is scrupulously followed.

The situation must be contrasted with the position where a patient is sectioned under the Mental Health Act 1983. Such sectioning is to enable patients to be restrained for treatment for their mental health; but this does not enable doctors to treat physical complaints.

End of life care

Section 4(5) of the Mental Capacity Act 2005 provides that where the determination of a patient's best interests relates to life-sustaining treatment, the decision-maker must not, in considering whether the treatment is in the best interests of the person concerned, be motivated by a desire to bring about the patient's death. Steps taken by a doctor to bring life to an end are absolutely unlawful.[21] Whether English law will change to permit euthanasia remains highly contentious. Clinicians may rely on the double-effect principle where giving therapeutic treatment is justified even if it is known that it may also have a secondary adverse effect.

The GMC guidelines on end of life treatment and care[22] were challenged in the case of *Burke* v *The General Medical Council*.[23] The Court of Appeal held that the GMC guidance was lawful in establishing that a patient cannot demand a particular treatment. Health professionals must take account of a patient's wishes when making treatment decisions. If a patient with capacity indicates his wish to be kept alive by the provision of ANH the doctor's duty of care will require him to provide ANH for so long as the treatment continues to prolong life. If the patient lacks capacity then all reasonable steps which are in the patient's best interests should be taken to prolong their life. Although there is a strong presumption in favour of providing life-sustaining treatment, there are circumstances where such treatment is no longer clinically indicated.

Mr Burke failed to obtain an injunction to prevent doctors from withdrawing ANH at some future time, when he lost capacity as a result of his terminal condition. The Court of Appeal reinforced the view that doctors, having taken into account the views of the patient, family members, and others close to the patient, were in the best position to make the judgement as to whether continuing treatment was in the best interests of the patient. This position is incorporated into the Mental Capacity Act.

Intensivists, who are regularly faced with the issue of withholding treatment or moving to palliation must take into account the need for patients to be allowed to die with dignity.

Withdrawal of artificial nutrition and hydration, where it is known that death will result, is a responsible decision if ANH is no longer in the patient's best interests. This amounts to an omission and is therefore not an intentional deprivation of life by the state contrary to Article 2 of the European Convention on Human Rights. The death of a patient in those circumstances is a result of the illness or injury from which the patient suffered and is not a breach of the right to life.

The withdrawal of treatment considered futile, does not amount to torture, inhuman or degrading treatment or punishment contrary to Article 3 of the European Convention. Anything considered necessary on a therapeutic basis, cannot be said to be either inhuman or degrading.

Clinical negligence

Medical or clinical negligence claims depend upon a Claimant (or those acting on his behalf) establishing the legal tort of negligence. This involves:

* A legal duty to take reasonable care.
* Breach of that duty by the Defendant.
* Damage caused to the Claimant as a result.

All healthcare professionals treating a patient owe him a duty of care. Breach of the duty is proved by a failure to treat the patient in accordance with the standard of care which is considered necessary. The standard test is that set out in the well-known case of *Bolam* v *Friern Hospital Management Committee*[24] in which McNair J said:

> A doctor is not guilty of negligence if he has acted in accordance with a practice accepted as proper by a responsible body of medical men skilled in that particular art…putting it the other way round, a doctor was not negligent, it he is acting in accordance with such a practice merely because there is a body of opinion that takes a contrary view.

The relevant standard of care is accordingly set by doctors. This can change as time goes on.

In *Bolitho* v *City and Hackney Health Authority*[25] the Court held that it was entitled to find in a rare case that professional opinion was not capable of '*withstanding logical analysis*'. In such cases a Judge is entitled to hold that the body of opinion supporting the medical treatment in the case was '*not reasonable or responsible*'. This enables a Court to reject what would otherwise be regarded as acceptable and therefore non-negligent practice. As a general rule, doctors should hesitate long before departing from established

professional practice or guidelines or codes of professional conduct. Anaesthetists must recognize and work within the limits of their competence.

Anaesthetizing the elderly is covered by the same test of clinical negligence as other types of medical treatment. The following are areas to which attention is particularly drawn:

* Whether an adequate preoperative assessment has been undertaken?
* Should the operation or procedure have gone ahead?
* Was the patient likely to tolerate the anaesthetic?
* Was the type and dose of anaesthetic drug given reasonable?
* Was due account taken of comorbidities?
* Was anaesthesia appropriately maintained?
* Were appropriate reversal agents used?
* Was the patient protected from harm during anaesthesia?
* Were foreseeable risks including infection, DVT, paralysis suitably considered and protected against?
* Was the patient maintained in the appropriate regimen postoperatively?

The likelihood of claims is always reduced by full and effective communication with the patient and where appropriate with the patient's family. Taking time to explain treatment at all stages in a patient and compassionate manner may well remove queries and uncertainties which can be the basis of a claim.

Family involvement in decision-making

Whilst it is a fundamental principle enshrined in common law and the MCA that patients have autonomy and that it is the patient who must be allowed to make decisions and assisted in doing so, the input of relatives is also recognized. Clinicians must inform elderly patients that they are free to involve their relatives in consultations if they wish.

Clinicians must be alert to the possibility that family pressure may amount to undue influence. There can be situations where relatives can manipulate patients indirectly to make decisions which serve interests other than those of the patient. This is a particular risk with elderly patients.

Relatives may themselves be directly affected by the treatment decision which is to be made and need to understand the options and the consequences of the decision the patient may take. Relatives may need to specify their ability to provide aftercare and support which may be required. They can assist in decision-making at a time when a patient may be distressed or making a decision from a wish not to be a burden on family members.

In most cases relatives' motives are genuine and directed by a desire for the best outcome for their loved ones. It is good practice to involve relatives in decisions made about medical treatment as well as end of life decisions. It is for clinicians to be alert to the positive advantages of relatives playing a full part in the decision-making process but to guard against the risk of conflicts of interest and undue influence.

Lord Donaldson in *Re: T*[26] stated that the test is whether 'the patient really means what he says or is merely saying it…to satisfy someone else'. Clinicians need information about the patient's relationship with the family to assess whether the patient's decision is his own.

Research

Particular care must be taken where involving elderly patients in research which may not be therapeutic. Research projects involve clear requirements to ensure that patients participating in any research project have given valid consent. Patients must not be pressurized or made to feel that they will receive inferior care if they decline to be involved.

A detailed legal framework is set out in the Mental Capacity Act for involving people who lack the capacity in research,[27] by ensuring that their wishes and feelings are respected. Full particulars are set out in Chapter 11 of the Mental Capacity Act (2005) Code of Practice. However this does not include clinical trials which are governed by the Medicines for Human Use (Clinical Trial Regulations) 2004.

The MCA requires that a family member or unpaid carer must be consulted on any proposal that a person lacking capacity takes part in research. If such a person is not identifiable then it would be appropriate to involve an IMCA. Past and present wishes, feelings and values are important to decide whether the patient should take part in the research or not.

Coroners and inquests

Coroners have a duty to enquire into deaths if the body of the deceased lies within their jurisdiction, and if the death was violent, unnatural, or sudden with cause unknown.

Doctors must comply with the requirements to report deaths to the Coroner. This includes deaths during or as an apparent consequence of an operation, or related to the effects of an anaesthetic. They are also reportable if the death was unexpected or related to treatment or drug therapy. All deaths within 24 hours of admission to hospital or after any procedure, operation, treatment or anaesthetic or discharge from hospital should be reported. This will include deaths due to or contributed to by fractures or falls or deaths related to a defect or failure of a system or procedure or where dementia is involved. Cases where there have been medical mishaps or inappropriate treatment or a critical incident must be reported, as well as late diagnosis or treatment, cases where there has been neglect, self-neglect, malnutrition, hyperthermia, or apparent suicide. Furthermore deaths caused or contributed to by unusual diseases, occupational injury, or disease must be reported.

The Coroner will usually order a postmortem if there is any uncertainty over the medical cause of death.

Where it is unclear whether a death should be reported, contact should be made with the Coroner's Office for advice. Where there are concerns in relation to end of life care and the withdrawal of treatment it is prudent to discuss with the Coroner. The same applies where there is any doubt with regard to the use of organs following death.

In the leading case of *Tony Bland*,[10] a Hillsborough survivor, who had been in a persistent vegetative state for some years, doctors were intending to withdraw artificial nutrition and hydration with the agreement of the patient's family. This was reported to the Coroner in Sheffield who indicated that if this was done he would refer the matter to the Police with a view to the doctors being prosecuted for murder. The High Court decision established guidelines whereby ANH can be withdrawn following a suitable referral to the Court.

A Coroner must hold an inquest where he has concerns as to the medical cause of death or the circumstances arising or where the family of the deceased raise concerns. He will require reports from clinicians and nursing staff. The procedure is inquisitorial and not adversarial. It is up to the Coroner to decide which witnesses must attend. He will expect hospital clinicians to provide detailed reports promptly, covering issues which he feels require explanation. The Coroner's Inquest is often used by relatives of a deceased to obtain answers to questions which have not been satisfactorily resolved and may be used as an opportunity to gather evidence for use in a subsequent claim.

Good communications with the patient during lifetime, accurate and full reporting in the notes and good communication and explanation in a compassionate way with relatives both before and after death are crucial to avoid an acrimonious Inquest and reducing the risk of a claim.

Where a death has occurred in relation to medical treatment Coroners are increasingly entering narrative verdicts rather than a verdict of '*misadventure*'. A typical narrative verdict is that 'Death was the unexpected outcome of a necessary operation'. Such a verdict is not a finding of fault. Coroners are specifically precluded from entering a verdict which holds any individual or organization responsible for the death. He does have the right to suggest that death was aggravated by lack of care. A verdict of unlawful killing may be entered in an extreme case.

The Coroner will wish to know why particular treatments were undertaken, whether they were justified and whether valid consent was given. He will explore how decisions were taken with regard to treatments or the withdrawal or withholding of treatment.

It is part of the Coroner's role to identify acts or omissions which caused or contributed to the death and to make recommendations in order to prevent similar deaths occurring in the future. Formal recommendations of this kind may be sent in a letter under Rule 43 of the Coroners' Rules requiring a Hospital Trust, for example, to reply to say what steps they have taken or will take in relation to the concerns expressed. It is prudent to anticipate the Coroner's concerns by showing action has been taken in advance of the Inquest hearing. This may discourage a Rule 43 letter.

Coroners tend to be sympathetic towards health professionals provided there has been openness and no attempt to withhold information or disguise what has occurred.

Death certification

A medical practitioner should not sign a death certificate unless he has attended the patient for the last illness, seen the patient within 14 days before death and seen the body after death. He must be satisfied as to the cause of death and that it is wholly from natural causes and not otherwise reportable to the Coroner.

In certifying death it is important not to confuse modes of dying (cardiac arrest, renal failure, shock, etc.) with the pathological cause of death. The words '*possible*' or '*probable*' should not be used.

Under the Coroners' and Justice Act 2009 brought into force in 2012 changes have been made in relation to death certification.

References

1. Office of National Statistics. *Population projections.* <http://http://www.statistics.gov.uk/hub/population/population-change/population-projections>.

2. *R v Cambridge HA ex p B* [1995] 2 All ER 129.

3. National Institute for Health and Clinical Excellence. *Preoperative tests: the use of routine preoperative tests for elective surgery.* CG3. London: NICE, 2003.

4. [1914] 211 NY125.

5. Section 1 MCA.

6. Section 3 MCA.

7. *Sidaway v Board of Governors of Bethlem Royal Hospital* [1985] 1 All ER 643.

8. [1957] 2 All ER 118.

9. [2004] UKHL 41.

10. *Airedale NHS Trust v Bland* [1993] 1 All ER 821.

11. Sections 24–26 MCA.

12. Section 25 MCA.

13. Section 9 MCA.

14. Section 3 MCA.

15. Department for Constitutional Affairs. *Mental Capacity Act 2005 Code of Practice.* London: TSO, 2007. <http://www.dca.gov.uk/legal-policy/mental-capacity/mca-cp.pdf>.

16. Section 4 MCA.

17. Section 35 MCA.

18. Section 37 MCA.

19. Section 45 MCA.

20. S4A and S4B MCA.

21. *R v Cox.*

22. GMC End of Life Treatment and Care: Good Practice and Decision-Making (New Guidelines 1.7.10).

23. *Burke v GMC.*

24. [1957] 1 WLR 583.

25. [1997] 4 All ER 771.

26. Re: T (Adult: Refusal of Medical Treatment) [1992] 4 All ER 649.

27. Section 30 MCA.

CHAPTER 37

The future: a commentary

Bernadette Th. Veering and Chris Dodds

Introduction

It is clear that anaesthetists will be providing anaesthesia care for increasing numbers of elderly patients for generations ahead. The majority of techniques we currently use were not scientifically proven or at least the science behind them was not developed, researched, or taught in this age group but in much younger patients. The data available for those patients over 90 years of age does not even include normative values. There has been a change in attitude towards caring for the elderly over the 25 years since the first anaesthetic specialist society was formed in the United Kingdom (Age Anaesthesia Association, 1988) but there is still a very long way to go before we can claim to be able to tailor anaesthesia care to their specific needs.

What is very reassuring is that there are international experts in all fields of anaesthesia caring for the elderly patient and researching into the complex problems faced by this cohort of patients. However, if there is any unifying theme throughout the preceding chapters it is the lack of a large body of evidence on which to base considered and safe anaesthetic care for the most vulnerable group of patients we will encounter. Their complexity combined with their often invisible lack of functional reserve is daunting yet all too frequently poorly explored before surgery which is then followed by unacceptable outcomes.

There are major questions that must be answered before we can develop our own practice and then develop appropriate training schemes to teach others the best anaesthetic practice for the elderly patient. Firstly we need to actually know what an average response is of patients in their 8th, 9th, and 10th decades undergoing anaesthesia and surgery. There are simply no normative data against which to judge outcomes. Very few of the anaesthetic agents in use today have been evaluated in the very elderly, and usually not in large enough studies to give confidence in their conclusions. We have minimal information on the regional or national variations of response to these drugs and rather unthinkingly extrapolate the reported conclusions into the population we are caring for.

Preoperative preparation

The reduction in reserve across many organ systems and the greater incidence of chronic diseases means that preoperative assessment has to be far more searching than for fitter younger patients. Protocol-based assessments do provide a starting point but cannot probe the degree of behavioural adaption present that allows the elderly patient to function in society. A review of prescribed and 'over-the-counter' medication is imperative as is an estimate of compliance. Teaching of these skills and the evaluation and assessment of the trainee is yet to be embedded into many national anaesthetic training schemes.

Choice of anaesthetic technique

Despite over 60 years of study we still lack a clear answer on whether a general or regional anaesthetic technique is safest. Separating expertise at the techniques is difficult as is trying to achieve consistent drug usage. Detailed *in vitro* testing and animal modelling of the effects of various anaesthetic agents has often produced conflicting results, and clinical studies are almost impossible to recruit enough patients to effectively power them appropriately. This does not mean that we should not try but that until the underlying causes of the major complications are untangled we are unlikely to be able to identify which is the better option and in which circumstances.

Outcome measures

All known major complications of surgery and anaesthesia occur more frequently in the elderly. Indeed some of most damaging complications still occur with the same incidence as when they were first described over 60 years ago. They are so common that they risk becoming 'normal for their age' and no further consideration given to trying to understand the causes of these awful complications. Beyond the impact of these frequent and disabling problems lie the true benefits to the elderly patient of, often heroic, surgery that may transform their lives proportionately more than younger patients. With the exceptions of most cardiac and some orthopaedic and vascular surgery we are handicapped by a lack of detailed audit of outcomes and of clinical practices. This is improving slowly.

Specific complications

Postoperative cognitive dysfunction

If any complication occurred in younger patients with the frequency that postoperative cognitive dysfunction does in patients over 70 years of age there would be a national outcry and public enquiries demanded to resolve the issue. It is a damming indictment of our populations that this has not happened. No other condition that affects one in four over 70s undergoing major abdominal surgery exists with so little press and public interest. Until recently the same was true for major research funding bodies and it is only in the last few years that appropriately funded research is staring to unravel the potential causes for postoperative cognitive dysfunction. Hopefully this will allow strategies to be developed that will minimize the risk and incidence of the dreadful complication.

Delirium

This is the commonest acute complication in the elderly, more importantly reaching to nearly 75 per cent of elderly cardiac surgical patients. Even non-surgical patients have an incidence that reaches up to 35 per cent. There are markers that can be used to indicate which patients are at an increased risk of developing delirium and treatment provided though multidisciplinary teams does help reduce the impact on their recovery. Even the most useful sedative medication (haloperidol) is not licensed for use in delirium in most countries!

However, this reactive approach highlights our limited understanding of the causes and possible preventative strategies that may reduce or even eliminate this complication.

Pain: assessment and management

We understand that the elderly patient handling of opioid analgesics differs from younger patients but instead of enabling practitioners to tailor effective analgesia for the elderly all too often the elderly are denied analgesia despite recognition of the pain they are suffering. This inhumane management is unacceptable.

Part of the problem is that we have relatively few reliable and easily used pain measurement scales and they are not in common usage across the globe. Even where pain is effectively scored the use of such tools as the pain escalator, which may be valuable in younger patients, is too rigid for the management of this cohort whose only consistent feature is their interindividual variability.

Fluid balance

The original NCEPOD audit of causes of death in those over the age of 80 (National Confidential Enquiry into Patient Outcome and Death. *Extremes of Age, The 1999 report of the National Confidential Enquiry into Peri-operative Death*. London: NCEPOD, 1999) identified that one of the most common avoidable culprits was poor fluid management. Both extremes were present with some postoperative patients being completely dehydrated and others overloaded, usually following central neuraxial blockade. Over 10 years later the repeat audit in 2010 (*Elective & Emergency Surgery in the Elderly: An Age Old Problem*: <http://www.ncepod.org.uk/2010eese.htm>) found no change in this situation. As this problem lies before all doctors and nurses caring for the elderly, surgeons, physicians, geriatricians, as well as anaesthetists there is clearly a need for a much broader intervention, perhaps during the early medical school or pre-registration years.

Training priorities

In common with training in geriatric medicine at large there has been very little focus on the specific problems, diseases, and management of the elderly patient in anaesthesia and critical care. This has gradually been improving with specific sections in training curricula and national assessments, but local training is still limited. In the United Kingdom one recommendation of an identified consultant with a specific interest in caring for the elderly has not yet achieved complete implementation.

Conclusion

Is all doom and gloom? Certainly not! The whole field is far more dynamic and productive than could have been imagined even 10 years ago. However, there is still so much to learn and then teach that we have little scope for self-congratulation. We hope this textbook will provide as much useful information as is possible on the fundamental changes with ageing that impact on organ systems and specific diseases that are more common in the elderly. Developments in surgical fields and critical care will continue to challenge us to expand our practice, and advances in anaesthesia will fuel even more innovation from our surgical colleagues.

Index

Page numbers in **bold** refer to figures/tables/diagrams